CW00927601

HANDBOOK OF PSYCHODYNAMIC APPROACHES TO PSYCHOPATHOLOGY

Also Available

What Works for Whom?: A Critical Review
of Psychotherapy Research, Second Edition
Anthony Roth and Peter Fonagy

What Works for Whom?: A Critical Review
of Treatments for Children and Adolescents, Second Edition
*Peter Fonagy, David Cottrell, Jeannette Phillips,
Dickon Bevington, Danya Glaser, and Elizabeth Allison*

Handbook of

Psychodynamic Approaches to Psychopathology

EDITED BY

Patrick Luyten
Linda C. Mayes
Peter Fonagy
Mary Target
Sidney J. Blatt

THE GUILFORD PRESS
New York   London

© 2015 The Guilford Press
A Division of Guilford Publications, Inc.
370 Seventh Avenue, Suite 1200, New York, NY 10001
www.guilford.com

All rights reserved

No part of this book may be reproduced, translated, stored in a retrieval system,
or transmitted, in any form or by any means, electronic, mechanical, photocopying,
microfilming, recording, or otherwise, without written permission from the publisher.

Printed in the United States of America

This book is printed on acid-free paper.

Last digit is print number: 9 8 7 6 5 4 3 2 1

The authors have checked with sources believed to be reliable in their efforts to provide
information that is complete and generally in accord with the standards of practice
that are accepted at the time of publication. However, in view of the possibility of
human error or changes in behavioral, mental health, or medical sciences, neither the
authors, nor the editors and publisher, nor any other party who has been involved in
the preparation or publication of this work warrants that the information contained
herein is in every respect accurate or complete, and they are not responsible for any
errors or omissions or the results obtained from the use of such information. Readers are
encouraged to confirm the information contained in this book with other sources.

Library of Congress Cataloging-in-Publication Data

Handbook of psychodynamic approaches to psychopathology / edited by Patrick Luyten,
Linda C. Mayes, Peter Fonagy, Mary Target, Sidney J. Blatt.
    p. ; cm.
  Includes bibliographical references and index.
  ISBN 978-1-4625-2202-6 (hardcover : alk. paper)
  I. Luyten, Patrick, editor. II. Mayes, Linda C., editor. III. Fonagy, Peter, 1952–,
editor. IV. Target, Mary, editor. V. Blatt, Sidney J. (Sidney Jules), 1928–2014, editor.
  [DNLM: 1. Mental Disorders—therapy. 2. Psychotherapy, Psychodynamic—
methods. 3. Psychopathology—methods. WM 420.5.P75]
  RC480.5
  616.89′14—dc23
                                                                        2015001484

About the Editors

Patrick Luyten, PhD, is Associate Professor in the Faculty of Psychology and Educational Sciences, University of Leuven; Reader in the Research Department of Clinical, Educational, and Health Psychology, University College London; and Visiting Professor at the Yale Child Study Center. His research focuses on the role of personality, stress, and interpersonal processes in depression, chronic fatigue syndrome, and fibromyalgia. Dr. Luyten is also currently involved in studies on mentalization-based treatment of patients with borderline personality disorder. He serves on the editorial boards of several scientific journals and is a recipient of the Psychoanalytic Research Exceptional Contribution Award from the International Psychoanalytical Association. He also maintains a private practice.

Linda C. Mayes, MD, is the Arnold Gesell Professor of Child Psychiatry, Pediatrics, and Psychology in the Yale Child Study Center and Special Advisor to the Dean, Yale School of Medicine. Her research integrates perspectives from child development, behavioral neuroscience, psychophysiology and neurobiology, developmental psychopathology, and neurobehavioral teratology. Dr. Mayes's work focuses on stress-response and regulatory mechanisms in young children at both biological and psychosocial risk. She also focuses on how adults transition to parenthood and the basic neural circuitry of early parent–infant attachment. Dr. Mayes and her colleagues have developed a series of interventions for parents, including Minding the Baby, an intensive home-based program, and Discover Together, a program to enhance community and family resilience.

Peter Fonagy, OBE, FMedSci, FBA, PhD, is Freud Memorial Professor of Psychoanalysis and Head of the Research Department of Clinical, Educational and Health Psychology, University College London; Chief Executive of the Anna Freud Centre; Consultant to the Child and Family Program at the Menninger Department of Psychiatry and Behavioral Sciences, Baylor College of Medicine; and Visiting Professor at Yale, Harvard, and Emory Medical Schools. Dr. Fonagy's clinical interests center on early attachment relationships, social cognition, borderline personality disorder, and violence. With collaborators in the United Kingdom and the United States, he co-developed an innovative research-based dynamic therapeutic approach, mentalization-based treatment. Dr. Fonagy has published more than 400 scientific papers, 250 chapters, and 17 books.

Mary Target, MSc, PhD, is Professor of Psychoanalysis in the Research Department of Clinical, Educational and Health Psychology, University College London; Clinical Professor at Yale Medical School; and Visiting Professor at the University of Vienna. She has held several leadership positions in psychology and psychoanalytic organizations. Dr. Target has a half-time psychoanalytic practice, with clinical interests in early attachment relationships, personality disorders, and disturbances of adult attachment and social cognition. Her research interests include child and adult attachment and mentalization, treatment outcomes in children and adolescents, and the development and evaluation of models of psychotherapy. Dr. Target has published more than 100 scientific papers and 11 books in collaboration, many with Peter Fonagy.

Sidney J. Blatt, PhD, until his death in 2014, was Professor Emeritus in the Departments of Psychiatry and Psychology at Yale University. He was a Life Member of the Western New England Institute for Psychoanalysis. Dr. Blatt published extensively in a wide range of journals in psychology, psychiatry, and psychoanalysis, and authored several books. He was a recipient of the Mary S. Sigourney Foundation Award for distinguished contributions to psychoanalysis, among other honors.

Contributors

Jon G. Allen, PhD, The Menninger Clinic, Houston, Texas

Anthony Bateman, MA, FRCPsych, Halliwick Psychological Therapies Service, St. Ann's Hospital, London, United Kingdom

Manfred Beutel, MD, DiplPsych, Department of Psychosomatic Medicine and Psychotherapy, University Medical Center Mainz, Johannes Gutenberg University, Mainz, Germany

Sidney J. Blatt, PhD (deceased), Departments of Psychiatry and Psychology, Yale University, New Haven, Connecticut

Robert F. Bornstein, PhD, Derner Institute of Advanced Psychological Studies, Department of Psychology, Adelphi University, Garden City, New York

Fredric N. Busch, MD, Department of Psychiatry, Weill Cornell Medical College, New York, New York; Center for Psychoanalytic Training and Research, Columbia University, New York, New York

John F. Clarkin, PhD, Department of Psychiatry, New York Presbyterian Hospital—Westchester Division, Weill Cornell Medical College, White Plains, New York

Jared A. DeFife, PhD, private practice, Atlanta, Georgia

Wendy Denham, PhD, Center for Reflective Communities, Los Angeles, California

Guy Doron, PhD, Baruch Ivcher School of Psychology, Interdisciplinary Center, Herzlyia, Israel

Peter Fonagy, OBE, FMedSci, FBA, PhD, Psychoanalysis Unit, Research Department of Clinical, Educational and Health Psychology, University College London, London, United Kingdom

Andrew J. Gerber, MD, PhD, New York State Psychiatric Institute, Columbia University, New York, New York

William H. Gottdiener, PhD, Department of Psychology, John Jay College of Criminal Justice, City University of New York, New York, New York

John Grienenberger, PhD, Center for Reflective Communities, Los Angeles, California

Susanne Harder, PhD, Department of Psychology, University of Copenhagen, Copenhagen, Denmark

Jonathan Hill, MB, BChir, MRCPsych, School of Psychology and Clinical Language Sciences, University of Reading, Reading, United Kingdom

Mark J. Hilsenroth, PhD, Derner Institute of Advanced Psychological Studies, Department of Psychology, Adelphi University, Garden City, New York

Johannes Kruse, MD, Department of Psychosomatics and Psychotherapy, University of Giessen, Giessen, Germany

Klara Kuutmann, MS, Department of Psychology, Uppsala University, Uppsala, Sweden

Michael Kyrios, PhD, School of Psychology, College of Medicine, Biology and Environment, Australian National University, Canberra, Australia

Falk Leichsenring, DSc, Department of Psychosomatics and Psychotherapy, University of Giessen, Giessen, Germany

Kenneth N. Levy, PhD, Department of Psychology, The Pennsylvania State University, University Park, Pennsylvania

Alicia F. Lieberman, PhD, Department of Psychiatry, University of California, San Francisco, San Francisco, California

Patrick Luyten, PhD, Faculty of Psychology and Educational Sciences, University of Leuven, Leuven, Belgium; Research Department of Clinical, Educational and Health Psychology, University College London, London, United Kingdom

Norka Malberg, PsyD, Yale Child Study Center, Yale University School of Medicine, New Haven, Connecticut

Linda C. Mayes, MD, Yale Child Study Center and Departments of Child Psychiatry, Pediatrics, and Psychology, Yale University School of Medicine, New Haven, Connecticut

Kevin B. Meehan, PhD, Department of Psychology, Long Island University, Brooklyn, New York

Mario Mikulincer, PhD, Baruch Ivcher School of Psychology, Interdisciplinary Center, Herzlyia, Israel

Barbara L. Milrod, MD, Department of Psychiatry, Weill Cornell Medical College, New York, New York; New York Psychoanalytic Society & Institute, New York, New York

Sven Rabung, PhD, Department of Psychology, Alpen-Adria-Universität Klagenfurt, Klagenfurt, Austria; Department of Medical Psychology, University Medical Center Hamburg–Eppendorf, Hamburg, Germany

Diane Reynolds, MFT, Center for Reflective Communities, Los Angeles, California

Lauren K. Richards, PhD, Red Sox Foundation/Massachusetts General Hospital Home Base Program and Department of Psychiatry, Harvard Medical School, Boston, Massachusetts

Joshua Roffman, MD, Martinos Center for Biomedical Imaging, Charlestown, Massachusetts

Bent Rosenbaum, MD, Department of Psychology, University of Copenhagen, Copenhagen, Denmark

Trudie Rossouw, MD, North East London NHS Foundation Trust, London, United Kingdom

Dar Sar-El, PhD, Baruch Ivcher School of Psychology, Interdisciplinary Center, Herzlyia, Israel

Marc S. Schulz, PhD, Department of Psychology, Bryn Mawr College, Bryn Mawr, Pennsylvania

Golan Shahar, PhD, Department of Psychology, Ben-Gurion University of the Negev, Beer-Sheva, Israel

Helen Sharp, PhD, Institute of Psychology, Health and Society, University of Liverpool, Liverpool, United Kingdom

Phillip R. Shaver, PhD, DClinPsy, Department of Psychology, University of California, Davis, Davis, California

Maria S. St. John, PhD, MFT, Department of Psychiatry, University of California, San Francisco, San Francisco, California

Howard Steele, PhD, Department of Psychology, New School for Social Research, New York, New York

Miriam Steele, PhD, Department of Psychology, New School for Social Research, New York, New York

Jesse J. Suh, PsyD, Department of Psychiatry, University of Pennsylvania, Philadelphia, Pennsylvania

Mary Target, MSc, PhD, Psychoanalysis Unit, Research Department of Clinical, Educational and Health Psychology, University College London, London, United Kingdom

Heather Thompson-Brenner, PhD, Center for Anxiety and Related Disorders, Department of Psychology, Boston University, Boston, Massachusetts

Jane Viner, MD, Department of Psychiatry, Massachusetts General Hospital, Boston, Massachusetts

Robert J. Waldinger, MD, Center for Psychodynamic Therapy and Research, Department of Psychiatry, Massachusetts General Hospital, Boston, Massachusetts

Acknowledgments

We are in the first place indebted to the many authors who have contributed to this volume. Their vision and dedication to have this volume reflect the latest views and findings have been truly exemplary.

Special thanks go out to the team at University College London, in particular Clare Farrar, Chloe Campbell, Elizabeth Allison, and Rose Palmer, for their editorial assistance, optimism, and warm disposition.

We also wish to thank Jim Nageotte and Jane Keislar at The Guilford Press for their support throughout the process of writing this book and, above all, their never-ending patience and determination in seeing this project to completion.

During the course of producing this volume, Sidney J. Blatt, one of our coeditors, passed away unexpectedly. He was a true pioneer in the field of psychoanalytic research whose ideas and approach have had an enormous impact on the field and will continue to do so in the future. His death is a great loss to the field, but we also miss him dearly as our mentor, colleague, and friend. It is our hope and conviction that this volume will help to keep his ideas alive. We dedicate this book to him and to all those who wish to follow in his footsteps by integrating creative empirical research with a willingness to contemplate the most complex aspects of the human psyche.

Contents

PART III. PSYCHOPATHOLOGY IN CHILDHOOD AND ADOLESCENCE

PART I

THEORETICAL BACKGROUND

CHAPTER 1

Theoretical and Empirical Foundations of Contemporary Psychodynamic Approaches

Patrick Luyten, Linda C. Mayes, Sidney J. Blatt, Mary Target, and Peter Fonagy

This volume was kindled by the need for a critical but balanced overview of contemporary psychodynamic approaches to psychopathology. The past decades have witnessed a dramatic increase in empirical research in this area, making it difficult for both researchers and clinicians to keep abreast of all the findings; it is the constructive chaos of these many findings that makes such a handbook a necessity.

Despite its ambitious-sounding title, this book's real aspirations are relatively modest: We aim to provide a sampling of the relevant literature, and it is neither our ambition nor our goal to be comprehensive. Instead, we aim to provide a representative overview of empirically supported psychodynamic approaches to understanding and treating psychopathology. We have focused this overview on the presenting problems that are most likely to appear in clinicians' offices and about which the field has generated significant empirical research, at both a basic and a clinical level. This volume is empirical in orientation, as we are strongly committed to the view that psychoanalytic ideas, just as any other approach within science, should be put to the test. This commitment has inevitably led us to exclude certain ideas and approaches that belong to the rich psychoanalytic tradition and that we believe are among the most imaginative in clinical psychology and psychiatry, but have not so far been addressed in empirical studies. It is our sincere hope that future editions of this handbook will include most of these ideas, as empirical research on them emerges.

The book is divided into four sections. The first introduces basic psychodynamic theories and approaches to psychopathology. The second reviews empirically supported psychodynamic approaches to conceptualizing and treating major psychiatric disorders in adults, and the third section focuses on psychodynamic theories about the origins and treatment of emotional and behavioral problems in childhood and adolescence. The final section discusses the empirical base of psychodynamic treatment and reviews outcome and process–outcome research.

In this introductory chapter, we first discuss the revival of psychoanalytic approaches to psychopathology over the past decades. This is followed by a summary of basic psychoanalytic assumptions concerning the nature of psychopathology and its treatment.

THE REVIVAL OF PSYCHOANALYTIC APPROACHES TO PSYCHOPATHOLOGY

Although psychoanalysis is now a less dominant force in psychiatry and clinical psychology than it was in the 1950s and 1960s, a considerable body of empirical research has emerged on psychoanalytic theory, concepts, and practice (Bornstein & Masling, 1998a, 1998b; Fisher & Greenberg, 1996; Levy, Ablon, & Kächele, 2011; Luyten, Mayes, Target, & Fonagy, 2012; Shapiro & Emde, 1993; Shedler, 2010; Westen, 1998, 1999). These studies demonstrate not only that psychoanalytic concepts can be tested empirically, but also that solid evidence supports many psychoanalytic assumptions. Furthermore, psychoanalytic research is increasingly published in major, high-ranking, mainstream psychology and psychiatry journals. There is now also considerable evidence documenting both the efficacy and effectiveness of various forms of psychodynamic psychotherapy (Abbass, Hancock, Henderson, & Kisely, 2006; Fonagy, Roth, & Higgitt, 2005; Leichsenring & Rabung, 2011; Midgley & Kennedy, 2011). Thus, although the empirical basis for psychoanalysis is still less extensive than that for some other forms of psychotherapy, such as cognitive-behavioral therapy (CBT), assertions that psychoanalysis has not produced empirical data to support its theories and therapies fail to recognize this growing empirical portfolio. In addition, as the chapters in this volume illustrate, there is growing convergence between psychoanalysis and other theoretical approaches in psychology, such as cognitive psychology (Bucci, 1997; Erdelyi, 1985; Luyten, Blatt, & Fonagy, 2013; Ryle, 1990); developmental psychology and developmental psychopathology, including attachment research (Beebe, Rustin, Sorter, & Knoblauch, 2003; Diamond & Blatt, 1999; Emde, 1988a, 1988b; Fonagy & Target, 2003; Levy & Blatt, 1999; Lyons-Ruth & Jacobvitz, 2008; Main, 2000; Stern, 1985); social psychology (Mikulincer & Shaver, 2007; Westen, 1991); and the neurosciences (Fotopoulou, Pfaff, & Conway, 2012; Kandel, 1999; Mayes, 2000; Solms & Turnbull, 2002). This convergence attests to the continued value of psychoanalysis as a theory and to the notion that psychoanalytic concepts are amenable to rigorous hypothesis testing and empirical research.

These efforts have been paralleled by a growing awareness within the psychoanalytic community of the need for systematic, empirical evidence to support psychoanalytic assumptions and therapies (Blatt, Auerbach, & Levy, 1997; Bornstein, 2001; Fonagy, 2003; Luyten, Blatt, & Corveleyn, 2006; Shedler, 2002). Within the movement to develop an evidence base for psychoanalysis, there are two different "cultures" (Luyten et al., 2006). The first, which is chiefly interpretive in orientation, emphasizes meaning and purposefulness in human behavior, and relies primarily on the traditional case study method, as introduced by Freud, for theory-building, and/or on more qualitative methods in general (Green, 2000; Hoffman, 2009). The second culture primarily relies on methods from the physical, natural, and social sciences that search for sequences of cause and effect, and on the use of probabilistic rather than individualistic models of data analysis and explanation.

We believe these two cultures within psychoanalysis are complementary: Each provides a basis for bridging the gap between psychoanalysis and other disciplines. The interpretive culture is the bridge to the humanities, whereas the neopositivistic, empirical culture is the bridge to the natural and social sciences. Methodological pluralism is needed, which implies an openness to research and theories from other theoretical and methodological perspectives including, but not limited to, linguistics, philosophy, developmental psychopathology, cognitive-behavioral research, and the neurosciences. As Fonagy (2003, p. 220) has noted, "The mind remains the mind whether it is on the couch or in the laboratory."

Psychoanalysis is one of the most comprehensive theories of human nature. In our haste to achieve scientific respectability, we should not relinquish the full richness of its approach, but neither should we retreat into an orthodox position, closing ourselves off from the world. The danger is that methodology "conceived originally as a means to the end of scientific knowledge, may come to be an end in itself" (Mishler, 1979, p. 6).

Such a tendency toward orthodoxy also brings us to the reasons behind the resistance to change that undeniably characterizes some quarters within the psychodynamic community. First, psychoanalytic researchers and clinicians need to be aware of their own preferences and dislikes that may maintain the divide between two cultures of evidence gathering in psychoanalysis. The interpretive and neopositivistic cultures are relatively isolated from one another, and, as in all human interactions, processes of both idealization and denigration can be observed in how the two cultures depict themselves and each other. Moreover, current changes in evidence-based medicine and managed care may feel threatening to clinicians, as these changes may challenge their well-practiced interpretive ways of working and their years of training in interpretive approaches. Researchers, in turn, may want to stick to "hard" methods and theories in order to maintain scientific respectability and academic recognition.

More work is needed to get these two cultures on "speaking terms" again. This work should entail the inclusion of psychoanalytic research findings in psychoanalytic training programs, the presence of clinicians in funding agencies, and the establishment of practice research networks consisting of both clinicians and researchers. These are, in our opinion, necessary steps toward creating a unified culture for evidence gathering in psychoanalysis (Luyten et al., 2006; Luyten, Mayes, et al., 2012).

THE PSYCHODYNAMIC APPROACH TO PSYCHOPATHOLOGY

The Four Psychologies of Psychoanalysis and Beyond

Psychoanalysis encompasses a broad field with a rich historical tradition, and it has commonly been said that psychoanalysis provides the most comprehensive approach to human development. However, psychoanalysis is not one unified approach: Just as in other strands of science, there are different theoretical and conceptual threads within the larger rubric of "psychoanalysis." Furthermore, just as cognitive-behavioral approaches are characterized by several "waves" of theorizing and research, there have been major shifts over time in psychodynamic approaches. In this context, Pine (1988) and others have referred to the "four psychologies of psychoanalysis," encompassing (1) the traditional Freudian approach, (2) ego psychology, (3) object relations/attachment theory, and (4) self psychology (McWilliams, 2011; Pine, 1988) (see Table 1.1).

Each of these approaches is rooted in the application of psychoanalytic ideas to different patients and problems. Historically, the different models have evolved through attempts to explain why and how individuals develop vulnerabilities for psychopathology in the course of their psychological development. The earliest models largely derived from clinical experience, with each model focusing on particular clinical problems, developmental issues, or phases, and often determined by individual analysts' own interests, their setting, and the nature of their patient group or even specific patients.

The *Freudian drive approach* essentially emerged out of the study of patients perceived to be struggling with sexual and aggressive drives. It proposed that psychopathology is related to failures of the child's mental apparatus to deal satisfactorily with the pressures inherent in a maturationally predetermined sequence of drive states, leading to fixation, and subsequent regression to these fixation points later in life when the individual is confronted with environmental adversity, intrapsychic conflicts, or a combination of both (Freud, 1905/1953).

In an effort to redress the balance of drive theory's emphasis on sexual and aggressive drives, *ego psychology* emerged, with its focus on the child's adaptive capacities, and particularly the capacity of the ego to adapt to changing external and internal demands (Hartmann, 1939; Hartmann, Kris, & Loewenstein, 1946). Anna Freud (1974/1981) developed a more comprehensive developmental theory, emphasizing the notion of different *developmental lines*, which continues to be a central tenet of developmental psychopathology (Cicchetti & Cohen, 1995). Additionally, within this focus on adaptive ego capacities, Erik Erikson (1950) formulated the still influential *epigenetic theory* of human development, which places emphasis on different developmental tasks throughout the life cycle. A rich body of developmental research continues to be based on Erikson's formulations (Cox, Wilt, Olson, & McAdams, 2010; Kroger, Martinussen, & Marcia, 2010).

Object relations and attachment theory developed out of dissatisfaction with the largely "intrapsychic" focus of both the drive approach and ego psychology and these theories' inability to explain the distortions in self and interpersonal relationships that are typically observed in individuals with psychotic and borderline features. Object relations theory is based on the central assumptions that (1) relationships are primary to drive satisfaction, rather than secondary, as is assumed in traditional drive and ego psychology, and (2) development fundamentally takes place within an interpersonal matrix, with attachment/interpersonal processes playing a key role in determining development, rather than a preprogrammed maturational process as is assumed in drive and ego psychology (Bion, 1962; Fairbairn, 1952/1954; Greenberg & Mitchell, 1983; Kernberg, 1976; Klein, 1937; Winnicott, 1960).

TABLE 1.1. Central Features of the Four Psychologies of Psychoanalysis

	Drive psychology	Ego psychology	Object relations/attachment theory	Self psychology
Central focus	Biological drives or in experiential terms: wishes, desires (sexuality, aggression)	Adaptive capacities of the ego	Development of relationships and underlying self and object representations	Development of self
Influence of past versus present	Strong emphasis on how the past influences drives, wishes, desires	More emphasis on present adaptation/coping strategies	Emphasis on how past influences present relationships and perception of self-in-relationships	Emphasis on how past influences present self-experience
Focus on unconscious factors versus consciousness	Unconscious influences central	More attention to role of consciousness	Emphasis on both conscious and unconscious factors	Emphasis on both conscious and unconscious factors
Focus on conflict versus deficit	Strong emphasis on conflict and defense	Acknowledgment of role of (developmental) deficit	Emphasis on conflict with attention to deficit	Emphasis on developmental deficit and conflict
Importance of transference	Strong emphasis on transference of past relationships from drive perspective	Less emphasis on transference	Emphasis on transference of "ways-of-being" with attachment figures that have been generalized in current relationships	Emphasis on transference of past self-experiences in relationships

Integrative approaches

Self psychology, finally, aimed to replace the abstract theoretical language typical of many psychoanalytic approaches with a more phenomenological, experience-driven language to describe the development of the self and its disruptions (Kohut, 1971). The central tenet of self psychology is that the infant needs an understanding caregiver—a need that persists throughout life in order for the individual to develop and to promote the experience of selfhood (Wolf, 1988). Empathic responses from caregivers are needed to support the infant's wishes, ambitions, and ideals. Disruptions in this process are thought to lead to vulnerability to disorders of the self, such as depression and personality disorders characterized by problems with self-esteem and hypersensitivity to criticism and/or rejection (typically, narcissistic and borderline personality disorders). The influence of self psychology extends far beyond psychoanalysis, as, for instance, is demonstrated by burgeoning theorizing and research concerning the self, self-discrepancies, self-aggrandizement, and overt and covert narcissism in social and personality psychology (Baumeister, 1987; Besser & Zeigler-Hill, 2010; Higgins, 1987; Pincus & Lukowitsky, 2011; Zeigler-Hill & Abraham, 2006).

But even these four broad psychologies do not fully embody the tradition of psychoanalytic approaches, particularly given the growing tendency toward integration among these approaches, which has led to a wide spectrum of psychodynamic approaches with varying emphases and styles (Luyten, Mayes, et al., 2012). Given this increasing integration, we use the terms *psychoanalytic* and *psychodynamic* interchangeably in this volume, as it has become impossible to distinguish neatly between psychoanalysis and psychodynamic either theoretically or with regard to treatment (Kächele, 2010), as we will discuss below. Similarly, whereas the psychoanalytic approach historically provided a unique and very specific approach toward human development, increasingly, basic psychoanalytic assumptions and viewpoints have been incorporated (although not necessarily acknowledged) in other branches of (clinical) psychology, psychiatry, social sciences, and humanities and, more recently, the neurosciences.

In the following sections we discuss the basic assumptions shared by all psychodynamic approaches. These include (1) an inherently developmental model; (2) an understanding of unconscious motivation and intentionality; (3) the ubiquity of transference, that is, the repetition of feelings from past relationships in present ones; (4) a person-centered perspective; (5) an appreciation of complexity; (6) a focus on the internal psychic world and psychological causality; and (7) the assumption of continuity between normality and psychopathology (Table 1.2). For the purpose of highlighting their core importance to psychoanalytic theories as well as technique, we will discuss each of these assumptions separately. Evidently, however, these assumptions are intrinsically related, and together they comprise the specificity of the psychodynamic approach.

Basic Assumptions of Psychodynamic Approaches

The Developmental Approach within Psychoanalysis

Psychoanalytic theories are fundamentally developmental. They share a distinct emphasis on *the formative role of early life experiences and later psychic structures*

TABLE 1.2. Basic Assumptions of Psychodynamic Approaches to Psychopathology

Developmental perspective	A developmental understanding of psychopathology is central.
Unconscious motivation and intentionality	Factors outside of the individual's awareness play an important role in explaining the development and maintenance of psychopathology.
Transference	Templates of past relationships and ways of thinking influence current relationships and perceptions.
Person-oriented perspective	Focus is on understanding the whole person, including strengths and vulnerabilities.
Recognition of complexity	Emphasis is on regression and progression on interrelated developmental lines, and on the role of deferred action (events achieving new meaning based on later experiences).
Focus on the inner world and psychological causality	Focus is on how psychological factors may mediate the influence of social and biological factors.
Continuity between normal and disrupted personality development	There is no categorical distinction between normality and psychopathology: psychopathology is dimensionally distributed.

and behavior. Psychoanalytic theories are also inherently developmental in their emphasis on a gradual unfolding of the mind and mental capacities, with there being different ways of understanding and knowing the world at different stages of development. Indeed, psychoanalysts were among the first to offer clearly explicated stage theories of development (Tyson & Tyson, 1990). From the beginnings of psychoanalysis, psychoanalytic clinicians, starting with Sigmund Freud, Karl Abraham, and Melanie Klein, to name just a few, were struck by the critical importance of early developmental disruptions to understanding their patients' complaints. They conceptualized different forms of psychopathology as dynamic conflict–defense constellations, rooted in early adverse experiences and disruptions and/or impairments of early capacities and stages of development. Unsurprisingly, the theories these early clinicians built up were thus fundamentally developmental in nature. Their clinical intuitions were further elaborated by those who have since become known as the pioneers of developmental psychology, such as René Spitz (1945), John Bowlby (1951), Anna Freud (1973), Joseph Sandler (Sandler & Rosenblatt, 1987), and Margaret Mahler (1975). Many intuitions of these highly talented clinicians have subsequently been confirmed, for example, via the findings of contemporary neurobiology on the role of early experiences and the significance of critical time windows in development, in which biological/psychological systems are especially sensitive to environmental experiences (Lupien, McEwen, Gunnar, & Heim, 2009). Broad-ranging research findings have further confirmed and extended the early psychoanalytic emphasis on the formative nature of early experiences (Luyten, Vliegen, Van Houdenhove, & Blatt, 2008). Findings concerning the central importance of early attachment experiences in setting patterns and prototypes for later expectations, attitudes, and feelings with regard to the self and others (Main, Kaplan, & Cassidy, 1985), as well as expectations about one's capacity to cope with conflict, stress, and adversity (Gunnar & Quevedo, 2007), further support psychoanalytic thinking about the importance of early developmental factors.

As discussed in more detail later in this chapter, *psychoanalytic approaches aim to explain both normal and disrupted development*, with a focus on factors explaining developmental disruptions (Fonagy & Target, 2003). Psychoanalytic developmental researchers have therefore played a key role in the field of developmental psychopathology, that is, the study of the development of psychological disorders (Fonagy, Target, & Gergely, 2006; A. Freud, 1973; Lyons-Ruth & Jacobvitz, 2008; Mahler, Pine, & Bergman, 1975).

At the same time, psychoanalytic developmental theories have often overstressed the importance of specific early experiences, resulting in overspecified theories that neglect the role of genetics, epigenetics, and later experiences (Fonagy et al., 2006). Overspecification of these theories is to be expected because of their roots in the clinical encounter, as they needed to enable psychoanalytic practitioners to make sense of highly complex clinical experiences. Examples of this overdetermined style of thinking include the link that is sometimes made between borderline personality disorder and the rapprochement subphase of separation and individuation (Masterson, 1976), or between oedipal conflict and obsessional neurosis (Freud, 1909/1955). Of particular note is the neglect of the often considerable role of genetics, as well as chance events and stochastic processes, in explaining developmental trajectories (Fraley & Roberts, 2005). Furthermore, these early theories were often at odds with developmental data. The emphasis on very early, preverbal periods was particularly problematic because it placed many hypotheses beyond any realistic possibility of empirical testing (Westen, 1990; Westen, Lohr, Silk, Gold, & Kerber, 1990). These theories also often presumed the existence of capacities in children that were simply beyond developmental probability. Because many psychoanalytic developmental theories were based on work with adult patients and often rooted in reconstruction rather than direct observation (Stern, 1985), there has also been a tendency to make unwarranted extrapolations from observations of patients to normal development in children (Fonagy & Target, 2003).

Early psychoanalytic developmental theories thus overestimated the role of specific early experiences, although several psychoanalytic authors have attempted to redress this balance. These include, as mentioned earlier, Anna Freud (1974/1981), who emphasized the importance of simultaneously considering different developmental lines and their complex interactions; Erik Erikson (1959), who developed an epigenetic theory of human development across the lifespan; and George Vaillant (1977), one of the first researchers to launch longitudinal follow-up studies of adult development that focused on complex interactions among various factors impinging on psychological development. Contemporary psychoanalytic developmental theories, as the chapters in this volume attest, have become more integrative and do more justice to the complexity of developmental processes.

Unconscious Motivation and Intentionality

Psychoanalytic approaches focus on the importance of *unconscious motivation and intentionality*, consistent with contemporary theoretical models in the neurosciences (Lieberman, 2007), cognitive science (Westen & Gabbard, 2002a, 2002b), and social psychology (Mikulincer & Shaver, 2007). Whereas historically this was a unique position, there is now increasing consensus across several fields that factors influencing psychological development often exert their influence outside of conscious awareness. Moreover, there is also consensus that motivational factors may conflict with each other, and thus that both normal and pathological psychological functioning involve conflict—which is, of course, a central tenet of psychoanalytic approaches. Specifically, the coexistence of processing units from different developmental stages inevitably leads to conflict between these units, and psychological functioning thus involves the adaptive resolution of these conflicts, referred to as *compromise formations* in psychoanalysis and *constraint satisfaction* in neuroscience (Westen, Blagov, Harenski, Kilts, & Hamann, 2006). Imaging research and priming studies have, for instance, provided confirmation of the unconscious influence of attachment representations on constraint satisfaction in both normal and disrupted personality development (Mikulincer & Shaver, 2007; Westen et al., 2006) (see also Mikulincer & Shaver, Chapter 2, and Gerber, Viner, & Roffman, Chapter 4, this volume). Hence, there is now increasing consensus that both normal and disrupted psychological development reflect a series of attempts, however maladaptive, to achieve and maintain psychological balance (see also Luyten & Blatt, Chapter 5, this volume), and that psychological forces that are largely outside of the awareness of the individual play a key role in achieving such a balance.

The Ubiquity of Transference

Key to psychoanalytic thinking is the notion that *social interactions in any context, but especially in the therapeutic setting, are filtered through internalized schemas of past relationships, specifically, early caring relationships* (Andersen & Przybylinski, 2012; Westen, 1998; Westen & Gabbard, 2002b). Largely if not primarily unconsciously, these feelings, desires, and expectations regarding earlier objects are transferred to new relationships, and they are especially important in understanding both content and process in the psychoanalytic therapeutic context.

Much has been written about techniques for "working in the transference" and the ways in which both positive and negative transferences may impede (or at times, facilitate) therapeutic change (Bradley, Heim, & Westen, 2005; Høglend, 2004; Levy et al., 2006). The idea of transference is also closely related to more contemporary notions from attachment theory about internal working models. Studies in this area similarly suggest that transference is primarily unconscious, and that early attachment templates/schemas impact reactions to relationships in adulthood as well as in other key developmental periods and are key to stress modulation (Gunnar & Quevedo, 2007; Mikulincer & Shaver, 2007). "Security" implies not just the ability to sustain positive and caring relationships or to have a positive transference (for the two may not be at all synonymous), but rather the capacity when under stress to turn to and use others effectively and adaptively for emotional regulation and comfort. The Adult Attachment Interview (George, Kaplan, & Main, 1985) and other measures that more directly assess individuals' conscious appraisal of the importance of relationships (Ravitz, Maunder, Hunter, Sthankiya, & Lancee, 2010) provide empirical approaches to capturing the ways in which early experiences may shape aspects of social expectation, stress regulation, and the overall approach to the object world (Roisman, Tsai, & Chiang, 2004).

Although there are different approaches within psychoanalysis, and certainly myriad approaches outside psychoanalysis, to using patients' unconscious but enacted views and templates of persons in their contemporary lives in an effective and therapeutic way, the idea that past relationships remain active and predispose an individual to repeat the past in the present is a core psychoanalytic concept.

A Person-Oriented Perspective

Psychoanalytic approaches typically consider the whole person. Rather than focusing on the developmental pathways implicated in a particular disorder, or one symptom, behavior, or personality feature, this *person-centered perspective* emphasizes the role of *multifinality* and *equifinality* (Cicchetti & Rogosch, 1996) in explaining different pathways of individuals. Equifinality proposes that there are many possible pathways toward one specific outcome, rather than assuming that there is a single pathway for each mental disorder or developmental outcome. Multifinality, in contrast, implies that a given factor may result in a variety of outcomes, depending on the presence of other factors. This view thus involves a shift away from disease- and variable-oriented strategies toward person-oriented research and treatment strategies. This emphasis is at the core of psychoanalytic developmental theory in clinical practice, in which the focus is always on the person and his or her developmental history rather than solely on a particular symptom, disorder, or developmental outcome (Luyten et al., 2008). Indeed, psychoanalysis is strongly rooted in an individual epistemology that emphasizes the importance of specialized knowledge from the individual and individual meaning-making (Fajardo, 1998). Furthermore, multifinality characterizes the psychoanalytic approach to psychopathology in the implications for how "disorders" are defined more by an understanding of how an individual's presentation is serving adaptive and maladaptive functions, how mechanisms for these "disorders" are understood in terms of the individual's history and current circumstances, and how treatments are oriented toward understanding the role the "disorder" serves for the individual and how the maladaptive aspects of the "disorder" may be mitigated.

On the other hand, this broad focus may historically have led to overly lengthy treatments that inadequately specify the relationship between particular developmental problems and disorders and technical interventions. Furthermore, the focus on an individual epistemology and heuristic of individual meaning makes it difficult to generalize across patients and understand the relative effectiveness of specific techniques. Currently, there is a clear movement within psychoanalysis toward more specified and targeted interventions for particular problems and disorders in children and adolescents (Fonagy & Target, 2002), and toward research that combines person- and variable- or disorder-centered perspectives (Luyten, Blatt, & Mayes, 2012).

Recognition of Complexity

Psychoanalytic approaches emphasize the *complexity of psychological functioning.* Specifically, they emphasize the importance of nonlinear processes, regression, and progression on multiple interrelated developmental lines, and the role of deferred action, which refers to the reciprocal relationship between developmental events and circumstances and their later reinvestment with new meaning (e.g., a girl realizing only in adolescence that her father's behavior toward her as a child involved sexual abuse) (Mayes, 2001).

As we have discussed, many early psychoanalytic developmental theories were too linear and overspecified. In recognition of the simplicity of these earlier models, contemporary psychodynamic developmental models are both more sophisticated and more in line with current knowledge about the complexity of development (Sroufe, 2005). Interestingly, Freud (1920/1955, pp. 167–168) himself cautioned about attempts to predict later development from childhood to later adulthood:

> So long as we trace the development from its final outcome backwards, the chain of events appears continuous, and insight which is completely satisfactory or even exhaustive. But if we proceed the reverse way . . . then we no longer get the impression of an inevitable sequence of events which could not have been otherwise determined. We notice at once that there might have been another result, and that we might have been just as well able to understand and explain the latter. *The synthesis is thus not so satisfactory as the analysis; in other words, from a knowledge of the premises we could not have foretold the nature of the result* [emphasis added]. . . . We never know beforehand which of the determining factors will prove the weaker or the stronger. We only say at the end that those which succeeded must have been the stronger. Hence the chain of causation can always be recognized with certainty if we follow the line of analysis, *whereas to predict it along the line of synthesis is impossible* [emphasis added].

Focus on the Inner World and Psychological Causality

Psychoanalytic approaches are characterized by a focus on the *inner psychological world and psychological causality across the lifespan.* Psychological development can be seen as involving a move toward increasing complexity, differentiation, and integration of feelings, thoughts, and representations of self and others. These range from the most primitive undifferentiated feelings, thoughts, and fantasies of the infant to more elaborated, differentiated, and integrated representations of self and others, or internal working models, hopes, desires, fantasies, dreams, and fears (Blatt et al., 1997). Although early psychoanalytic developmental models sometimes attributed improbable cognitive abilities to infants, their intuition has been shown to be correct in that current research has amply demonstrated the essentially social nature of human infants and that the human capacity for social cognition is key to understanding the confluence of social and biological factors in determining both normal and disrupted development (Fonagy, Gergely, & Target, 2007). These views open up interesting perspectives for both research and intervention at a time when biological reductionism may again be on the rise.

Continuity between Normal and Disrupted Personality Development

The growing evidence for dimensional approaches to psychopathology (Costa & McCrae, 2010; Krueger, Skodol, Livesley, Shrout, & Huang, 2007; Lahey et al., 2008; Skodol, 2012) parallels the emphasis in psychoanalytic approaches on the *essential continuity between normality and pathology* (Blatt & Luyten, 2010; see also Luyten & Blatt, Chapter 5, this volume). As noted earlier, from the psychodynamic perspective, both normal and disrupted psychological development involve attempts to find a dynamic equilibrium between the impact (psychological and biological) of past experiences and current needs in the context of an individual's environment.

Given the ubiquity of conflict in human development and the inevitably imperfect resolution of life's important developmental tasks, human beings are fundamentally vulnerable to developing psychological problems, especially when faced with adversity that may trigger latent vulnerabilities and/or challenge coping strategies that were previously adaptive but have outlived their usefulness. These views have increasingly been adopted by other theoretical frameworks, not least by cognitive-behavioral approaches such as schema therapy (Beck, 2009; Luyten et al., 2013; Young, 1999).

PSYCHODYNAMIC TREATMENT APPROACHES

A growing evidence base for the effectiveness of psychoanalytic treatments has built up over recent years. An increasing number of controlled and naturalistic trials provide evidence for the effectiveness of psychoanalytic treatments for children and adolescents as well as adults (Abbass et al., 2006; Fonagy et al., 2015; Leichsenring, Abbass, Luyten, Hilsenroth, & Rabung, 2013; Leichsenring & Rabung, 2011; Roth & Fonagy, 2004; Shedler, 2010). However, given the lag in accumulating evidence compared to other treatments, particularly pharmacotherapy and CBT, much work remains to be done. This is further highlighted by the fact that, over the course of its history, psychoanalysis has not only developed a considerable number of theories about different aspects of human functioning, but many variations in treatment techniques have emerged in response to these different theories. As an increasingly diverse set of patients sought help with psychoanalytically trained therapists, psychoanalytic theory expanded and new treatment approaches developed accordingly. These new treatments focused on patients in different settings (e.g., inpatient, outpatient, and day-hospitalization-based treatments), different presentations (e.g., substance abuse, borderline personality disorder), and different populations (e.g., children, adolescents, adults). Psychoanalytic researchers now face the daunting task of systematically categorizing and evaluating these various treatments. Thus, there is no such thing as "psychoanalytic treatment"; rather, there are spectra of psychodynamic treatments that vary greatly in terms of their length (with some psychoanalytic treatments being as brief as eight sessions), structure, population, and setting.

As an illustration, Table 1.3 summarizes the basic features of major types of psychodynamic therapies for adults. As the table shows, these treatments vary considerably in terms of the nature of the interventions, their frequency and setting, and their goals and central focus. Briefly, psychoanalysis, historically the first treatment approach to emerge from the psychoanalytic tradition, is a high-frequency treatment of long duration that is indicated in patients with complex and chronic personality and relational problems who have the motivation and capacity for insight—as well as time and money—that is needed to achieve sustained personality changes, the ultimate aim of psychoanalysis. Such sustained changes are achieved through a long process involving the in-depth examination of the influence of the past on the present, in large part through examining the transference of patterns of feeling and thinking on to the relationship with the analyst.

Needless to say, only a minority of patients—estimates suggest fewer than 5% of all patients who are in any psychoanalytic treatment—is suitable for this intensive treatment or has the motivation and means to pursue a personal analysis, although studies suggest it can be highly effective in these patients (de Maat et al., 2013). Research indicates that these patients may derive a similar benefit from long-term individual psychodynamic psychotherapy, although studies that directly compare these two types of treatment are largely lacking (de Maat et al., 2013). Within the spectrum of long-term psychodynamic treatments, the number of sessions may vary greatly, depending on the patients' presenting problems, the specific type of long-term treatment, and the patients' wishes. Typically, in higher functioning patients there is a greater emphasis on techniques that foster insight into one's own past and present patterns of thinking and feeling and the relationship between both. For patients whose capacity for insight and affect tolerance is more compromised (e.g., those with borderline personality features), more structured and supportive treatments have been developed and empirically evaluated (see also Clarkin, Fonagy, Levy, & Bateman, Chapter 17, this volume). Brief dynamic psychotherapies can similarly be situated on a so-called expressive–supportive spectrum, with some therapies emphasizing expressive features that foster insight, while others place greater emphasis on providing structure and support. Although brief dynamic treatments aim for more modest changes in symptoms and adaptive capacities, and therefore are more suited for patients with less complex and chronic psychological problems, changes as a result of brief treatment may be considerable and long lasting (Abbass et al., 2006). Because of its more limited scope and brief nature, the examination of transference patterns plays, relatively speaking, a more limited role in brief dynamic treatments.

Recent trends have also witnessed the development of intervention and prevention strategies aimed at at-risk populations (Suchman et al., 2010), and Internet-based interventions (Andersson et al., 2012; Johansson et al., 2013; Lemma & Fonagy, 2013). The various chapters in this volume similarly attest to the broadening scope of psychodynamic treatment approaches, ranging from more traditional brief and longer-term individual treatments for adults with substance abuse (Gottdiener

TABLE 1.3. Major Types of Psychodynamic Therapy within the Spectrum of Psychodynamic Therapies for Adults

	Psychoanalyis	Longer-term psychodynamic psychotherapy	Brief psychodynamic psychotherapy
Aims	Personality change as a result of insight into the relationship between past and present	Personality change as a result of insight into the relationship between past and present, but targeted changes are typically more limited	Changes in symptoms and adaptive capacities
Role of free association	Central feature	Important role, though more limited	Limited, emphasis on dialogue between patient and therapist
Therapist stance	Technical neutrality, evenly hovering attention	Technical neutrality less strict, more active stance	More active, supportive and often directive stance
Role of repeated working through of conflicts	Repeated focus on relationship between past and present conflicts	More limited focus on relationship between past and present conflicts	More limited, focus on conflicts in here-and-now
Role of countertransference (feelings in the therapist engendered by the patient)	Major tool to inform interventions and working through	Informs interventions and working through	Informs interventions
Major interventions	• Clarification and confrontation are used to broaden the patient's perspective • Central role of interpretation of the relationship between past and present ("there-and-then" and "here-and-now") • Limited use of supportive and directive interventions	• Clarification and confrontation are used to broaden the patient's perspective • Interpretation of relationship between "here-and-now" and "there-and-then," but also more attention to current conflicts and problems • Supportive interventions and directive interventions may be used, particularly in more supportive variants	• Clarification and confrontation are used to broaden the patient's perspective • Interpretation is limited to a specific focus in the "here-and-now" • Supportive and directive interventions are used more to help the patient adapt to current problems and circumstances and to foster change
Intrapsychic–interpersonal focus	Mainly intrapsychic focus	Intrapsychic–interpersonal focus	Intrapsychic–interpersonal focus often emphasis on the interpersonal
Frequency	3–5 times a week	1–3 times a week	1–2 times a week
Setting	Couch	Face to face	Face to face

& Suh, Chapter 11) or dependent personality disorder (Bornstein, Chapter 16), to novel combined individual and group treatments for borderline personality disorder (Clarkin et al., Chapter 17), and early prevention and intervention programs (Grienenberger, Denham, & Reynolds, Chapter 21). Table 1.4 presents a summary of the typical outcomes associated with successful psychodynamic treatment, with greater effects typically associated with greater treatment length, showing that these effects potentially stretch far beyond the relief of symptoms, congruent with assumptions about the aims of psychoanalytic treatments (see also Table 1.3). Research evidence supporting the spectrum of psychodynamic treatments is discussed in greater detail by Leichsenring, Kruse, and Rabung in Chapter 23.

Common and Specific Features of Psychoanalytic Treatments

It is increasingly recognized that different types of psychotherapy in general, and psychoanalytic treatments in particular, have many elements in common. The specific techniques used in each type of psychotherapy can therefore be only partially responsible for treatment outcomes. Other factors must account for a larger portion of the variance in treatment outcome, and there are estimates of around only 15% of the variance in outcome being predicted by specific techniques, 30% by common factors (e.g., providing support), 15% by expectancy and placebo effects, and 35–40% by extratherapeutic effects (e.g., spontaneous remission, positive life events or changes) (Lambert & Barley, 2002). This does not mean that psychoanalytic treatment approaches have no unique, distinguishing features, or that there can be no specific set of predictions with regard to mutative factors. Research shows that relative to cognitive-behavioral therapists, for instance, psychodynamic therapists tend to place a stronger emphasis on (1) affect and emotional expression; (2) the exploration of patients' tendency to avoid topics (i.e., defenses); (3) the identification of recurring patterns in behavior, feelings, experiences, and relationships; (4) the past and its influence on the present; (5) interpersonal experiences; (6) the therapeutic relationship; and (7) the exploration of wishes, dreams, and fantasies (Blagys & Hilsenroth, 2000) (see Table 1.5). The Improving Access to Psychological Therapies initiative in

---

TABLE 1.4. Outcomes of Successful Psychodynamic Treatment

- Symptomatic improvement
- Improvements in relationship functioning and well-being
- Increased capacity for self-analysis
- Ability to experiment with new behaviors, particularly in interpersonal relationships
- Finding pleasure in new challenges
- Greater tolerance for negative affect
- Greater insight into how the past may determine the present
- Use of self-calming and self-supportive strategies

Note. Based on Leichsenring, Abbass, Luyten, Hilsenroth, & Rabung (2013); Shedler (2010); Falkenstrom, Grant, Broberg, and Sandell (2007); and Luyten, Blatt, and Mayes (2012).

the United Kingdom has similarly shown that although the therapist competencies required for psychodynamic treatment overlap to some extent with those required for other treatments (such as the ability to engage the client and establish a positive therapeutic alliance), a number of specific competencies distinguish psychodynamic therapy (such as the ability to work with transference and countertransference, and to recognize and work with defenses) (Lemma, Roth, & Pilling, 2009). Continuing to develop the evidence base for psychoanalytic treatments will require research into the specifics of a given psychoanalytic therapeutic approach, as well as into the core set of competencies and therapeutic skills shared by other mental health interventions.

What Works in Psychoanalytic Treatments?

With regard to the factors responsible for therapeutic change in psychoanalysis, several different theories have been formulated. These include changes in ego, id, and superego in traditional psychoanalytic formations (Freud, 1923/1961); changes in ego capacities (and defenses and coping strategies in particular) from the perspective of ego psychology (Hartmann, 1939); changes in the differentiation, articulation, and integration in object representations, according to object relations approaches (Blatt & Behrends, 1987; Levy et al., 2006); changes in self-structures from the self psychology perspective, leading to a so-called restoration of the self (Kohut, 1977); changes in the individual's position with regard to the desire of the Other, as conceptualized in Lacanian approaches (Lacan, 2006); and, more recently, changes in states of mind with regard to attachment experiences (Levy et al., 2006), and reflective

TABLE 1.5. Common and Distinguishing Features of Psychoanalytic Treatment Approaches

Common features
- Ability to engage the client
- Ability to develop and maintain a good therapeutic alliance, and to understand the client's perspective and general "worldview"
- Ability to deal with emotional content
- Ability to manage endings in therapy
- Ability to assess client's relevant history and suitability for intervention
- Ability to engage with and derive benefit from supervision

Distinguishing features involve greater focus on . . .
- Affect and emotional expression
- Exploration of patients' tendency to avoid topics (i.e., defenses)
- Identification of recurring patterns in behavior, feelings, experiences, and relationships
- Focus on the past and its influence on the present
- Focus on interpersonal relationships
- Exploration of the therapeutic relationship
- Exploration of wishes, dreams, and fantasies

Note. Based on Blagys and Hilsenroth (2000); Lemma, Roth, and Pilling (2009); and Shedler (2010).

functioning or mentalizing, that is, the capacity to understand the self and others in terms of mental states (Fonagy & Luyten, 2009).

A common denominator among these (and other) theories of therapeutic action is that psychoanalytic treatment results in what has been called the *internalization of the analytic function*—that is, the capacity to continue self-analysis after the end of treatment, leading to greater inner freedom, creativity, and self-reflectiveness and the ability to proceed with analysis after the end of treatment, leading to sustained efficacy underpinned by increased adaptive capacities to deal with stressors (Blatt, Zuroff, Hawley, & Auerbach, 2010) (see also Table 1.4). In this context, it is important to note that successful psychoanalytic treatment is associated with sustained and continuing improvement after the end of treatment (so-called sleeper effects) (de Maat et al., 2013; Leichsenring & Rabung, 2008). These findings support the view that psychodynamic treatments are associated with increased security of internal mental exploration (Fonagy & Luyten, 2009), leading to greater resilience in the face of adversity (Luyten, Fonagy, Lemma, & Target, 2012).

More research, however, is needed to determine whether a causal relation indeed exists between specific psychoanalytic techniques and these outcomes, and whether these outcomes are unique to psychoanalytic treatments. As noted, research findings suggest that these outcomes are probably not unique (Luyten, Blatt, & Mayes, 2012). An important question is whether the effects of (long-term) psychoanalytic treatments and traditional psychoanalysis are qualitatively different, as is sometimes claimed in the psychoanalytic literature. The few extant studies on this subject point primarily to quantitative differences; that is, traditional psychoanalysis may be associated with greater change, but perhaps only because of the higher frequency and longer duration, and potentially because of the interaction between duration and frequency. Importantly, studies have also failed to identify different rates of change between psychoanalysis and psychodynamic therapy (Grant & Sandell, 2004; Kächele, 2010). Hence, successful psychotherapy seems to set in motion a process of change that begins during treatment but, crucially, is thought to continue after treatment. Different treatments may be able to activate such a process via different routes. For instance, challenging dysfunctional assumptions about the self and others in CBT may activate this process just as effectively as the repeated exploration and interpretation of relationship patterns in psychoanalytic treatments and, at least for some patients, may result not only in changes in patients' representations of self and others, but also in an increased ability to reflect on one's own self and others, leading to "broaden and build" cycles (Fredrickson, 2001). One implication of these views is that psychoanalytic treatment—and most other treatments for that matter—may have relatively neglected the transferring of insight and knowledge gained in treatment to situations and relationships outside the treatment setting (Fonagy, Luyten, & Allison, in press).

At the same time, the extent to which such a process of change is set in motion may differ considerably between different treatments. Furthermore, treatments may also contain interventions that reflect "superstitious behavior," that is, practices inherited through tradition and training that are unrelated to outcome but repeated simply because they are believed to be associated with outcome (Fonagy, 2010).

Moreover, psychoanalytic treatments (or indeed any mental health treatment) may also contain elements that hamper such a process and thus may be iatrogenic. These factors point to the need for careful research to understand which elements of a treatment are essential to change, which are a part of core competencies across treatments, and which may be either inert or, at worst, damaging.

CONCLUSIONS

This book seeks to draw attention to the benefits that can be reaped from an intellectually creative interaction among psychoanalysts, psychoanalytic researchers, and workers in other fields. We also aim to demonstrate the considerable gains to be made if we can achieve a considered balance among clinical work, engagement with psychoanalytic theory, and empirical research focused on a critical evaluation of psychodynamic approaches.

In 1994, Henry, Strupp, Schacht, and Gaston (1994, p. 498) concluded their review of the evidence supporting psychodynamic therapies as follows:

> By their very nature, psychodynamic concepts have been the most intractable to scientific scrutiny. Perhaps then, the most important observation that can be made about the current research is that it exists at all. Psychodynamic researchers have made a promising start to a most challenging endeavor—that of operationalizing complex constructs and developing replicable measurement procedures.

We hope and are convinced that this volume not only demonstrates that psychoanalytic researchers have heeded this call, but also that they will continue to do so in the future.

REFERENCES

Abbass, A. A., Hancock, J. T., Henderson, J., & Kisely, S. R. (2006). Short-term psychodynamic psychotherapies for common mental disorders. *Cochrane Database of Systematic Reviews*, Issue 7 (Article No. CD004687), DOI: 10.1002/14651858.CD004687.pub4.

Andersen, S. M., & Przybylinski, E. (2012). Experiments on transference in interpersonal relations: Implications for treatment. *Psychotherapy, 49*, 370–383.

Andersson, G., Paxling, B., Roch-Norlund, P., Östman, G., Norgren, A., Almlöv, J., et al. (2012). Internet-based psychodynamic versus cognitive behavioral guided self-help for generalized anxiety disorder: A randomized controlled trial. *Psychotherapy and Psychosomatics, 81*, 344–355.

Baumeister, R. F. (1987). How the self became a problem: A psychological review of historical research. *Journal of Personality and Social Psychology, 52*, 163–176.

Beck, A. T. (2009). Cognitive aspects of personality disorders and their relation to syndromal disorders: A psychoevolutionary approach. In C. R. Cloninger (Ed.), *Personality and psychopathology* (pp. 411–429). Washington, DC: American Psychiatric Press.

Beebe, B., Rustin, J., Sorter, D., & Knoblauch, S. (2003). An expanded view of intersubjectivity in infancy and its application to psychoanalysis. *Psychoanalytic Dialogues, 13*, 805–841.

Besser, A., & Zeigler-Hill, V. (2010). The influence of pathological narcissism on emotional and motivational responses to negative events: The role of visibility and concern about humiliation. *Journal of Research in Personality, 44*, 520–534.

Bion, W. R. (1962). A theory of thinking. *International Journal of Psychoanalysis, 43*, 306–310.

Blagys, M., & Hilsenroth, M. (2000). Distinctive features of short-term psychodynamic-interpersonal psychotherapy: A review of the comparative psychotherapy process-literature. *Clinical Psychology: Science and Practice, 7*, 167–188.

Blatt, S. J., Auerbach, J. S., & Levy, K. N. (1997). Mental representations in personality development, psychopathology, and the therapeutic process. *Review of General Psychology, 1*, 351–374.

Blatt, S. J., & Behrends, R. S. (1987). Internalization, separation–individuation, and the nature of therapeutic action. *International Journal of Psychoanalysis, 68*, 279–297.

Blatt, S. J., & Luyten, P. (2010). Reactivating the psychodynamic approach to the classification of psychopathology. In T. Millon, R. F. Krueger, & E. Simonsen (Eds.), *Contemporary directions in psychopathology: Scientific foundations of the DSM-V and ICD-11* (pp. 483–514). New York: Guilford Press.

Blatt, S. J., Zuroff, D. C., Hawley, L. L., & Auerbach, J. S. (2010). Predictors of sustained therapeutic change. *Psychotherapy Research, 20*, 37–54.

Bornstein, R. F. (2001). The impending death of psychoanalysis. *Psychoanalytic Psychology, 18*, 3–20.

Bornstein, R. F., & Masling, J. M. (1998a). *Empirical perspectives on the psychoanalytic unconscious.* Washington, DC: American Psychological Association.

Bornstein, R. F., & Masling, J. M. (1998b). *Empirical studies of the therapeutic hour.* Washington, DC: American Psychological Association.

Bowlby, J. (1951). *Maternal care and mental health. WHO Monograph Series, No. 2.* Geneva, Switzerland: World Health Organization.

Bradley, R., Heim, A. K., & Westen, D. (2005). Transference patterns in the psychotherapy of personality disorders: empirical investigation. *British Journal of Psychiatry, 186*, 342–349.

Bucci, W. (1997). *Psychoanalysis and cognitive science: A multiple code theory.* New York: Guilford Press.

Cicchetti, D., & Cohen, D. J. (1995). Perspectives on developmental psychopathology. In D. Cicchetti & D. J. Cohen (Eds.), *Developmental psychopathology: Vol. 1: Theory and methods* (pp. 3–23). New York: Wiley.

Cicchetti, D., & Rogosch, F. A. (1996). Equifinality and multifinality in developmental psychopathology. *Development and Psychopathology, 8*, 597–600.

Costa, P. T., & McCrae, R. R. (2010). Bridging the gap with the five-factor model. *Personality Disorders, 1*, 127–130.

Cox, K. S., Wilt, J., Olson, B., & McAdams, D. P. (2010). Generativity, the big five, and psychosocial adaptation in midlife adults. *Journal of Personality, 78*, 1185–1208.

de Maat, S., de Jonghe, F., de Kraker, R., Leichsenring, F., Abbass, A., Luyten, P., et al. (2013). The current state of the empirical evidence for psychoanalysis: A meta-analytic approach. *Harvard Review of Psychiatry, 21*, 107–137.

Diamond, D., & Blatt, S. (Eds.) (1999). Attachment research and psychoanalysis: 2. Clinical implications [Special issue]. *Psychoanalytic Inquiry, 19*, 669–941.

Emde, R. N. (1988a). Development terminable and interminable: I. Innate and motivational factors from infancy. *International Journal of Psycho-Analysis, 69*, 23–42.

Emde, R. N. (1988b). Development terminable and interminable: II. Recent psychoanalytic theory and therapeutic considerations. *International Journal of Psycho-Analysis, 69*, 283–286.

Erdelyi, M. H. (1985). *Psychoanalysis: Freud's cognitive psychology.* New York: Freeman.

Erikson, E. H. (1950). *Childhood and society.* New York: Norton.

Erikson, E. H. (1959). *Identity and the life cycle.* New York: International Universities Press.

Fairbairn, W. R. D. (1954). *An object-relations theory of the personality.* New York: Basic Books. (Original work published 1952)

Fajardo, B. (1998). A new view of developmental research for psychoanalysts. *Journal of the American Psychoanalytic Association, 46,* 185–207.

Falkenstrom, F., Grant, J., Broberg, J., & Sandell, R. (2007). Self-analysis and post-termination improvement after psychoanalysis and long-term psychotherapy. *Journal of the American Psychoanalytic Association, 55,* 629–674.

Fisher, S., & Greenberg, R. (1996). *Freud scientifically reappraised: Testing the theories and therapy.* New York: Wiley.

Fonagy, P. (2003). Genetics, developmental psychopathology and psychoanalytic theory: The case for ending our (not so) splendid isolation. *Psychoanalytic Inquiry, 23,* 218–247.

Fonagy, P. (2010). The changing shape of clinical practice: Driven by science or by pragmatics? *Psychoanalytic Psychotherapy, 24,* 22–43.

Fonagy, P., Cottrell, D., Phillips, J., Bevington, D., Glaser, D., & Allison, E. (2015). *What works for whom?: A critical review of treatments for children and adolescents* (2nd ed.). New York: Guilford Press.

Fonagy, P., Gergely, G., & Target, M. (2007). The parent–infant dyad and the construction of the subjective self. *Journal of Child Psychology and Psychiatry, 48,* 288–328.

Fonagy, P., & Luyten, P. (2009). A developmental, mentalization-based approach to the understanding and treatment of borderline personality disorder. *Development and Psychopathology, 21,* 1355–1381.

Fonagy, P., Luyten, P., & Allison, E. (in press). Epistemic petrification and the restoration of epistemic trust: A new conceptualization of borderline personality disorder and its psychosocial treatment. *Journal of Personality Disorders.*

Fonagy, P., Roth, A., & Higgitt, A. (2005). Psychodynamic psychotherapies: Evidence-based practice and clinical wisdom. *Bulletin of the Menninger Clinic, 69,* 1–58.

Fonagy, P., & Target, M. (2002). Psychodynamic approaches to child therapy. In F. W. Kaslow & J. Magnavita (Eds.), *Comprehensive handbook of psychotherapy: Vol. I. Psychodynamic/object relations* (pp. 105–129). New York: Wiley.

Fonagy, P., & Target, M. (2003). *Psychoanalytic theories: Perspectives from developmental psychopathology.* London: Whurr.

Fonagy, P., Target, M., & Gergely, G. (2006). Psychoanalytic perspectives on developmental psychopathology. In D. Cicchetti & D. J. Cohen (Eds.), *Developmental psychopathology: Vol. 1. Theory and method* (2nd ed., pp. 701–749). Hoboken, NJ: Wiley.

Fotopoulou, A., Pfaff, D., & Conway, M. A. (2012). *From the couch to the lab: Trends in psychodynamic neuroscience.* Oxford, UK: Oxford University Press.

Fraley, R. C., & Roberts, B. W. (2005). Patterns of continuity: A dynamic model for conceptualizing the stability of individual differences in psychological constructs across the life course. *Psychological Review, 112,* 60–74.

Fredrickson, B. L. (2001). The role of positive emotions in positive psychology. The broaden-and-build theory of positive emotions. *American Psychologist, 56,* 218–226.

Freud, A. (1973). *The writings of Anna Freud, Vol. III: Infants without families. Reports on the Hampstead Nurseries (1939–1945).* New York: International Universities Press.

Freud, A. (1981). A psychoanalytic view of developmental psychopathology. In *The writings of Anna Freud* (Vol. 8, pp. 119–136). New York: International Universities Press. (Original work published 1974)

Freud, S. (1953). Three essays on the theory of sexuality. In J. Strachey (Ed. & Trans.), *The standard edition of the complete psychological works of Sigmund Freud* (Vol. 7, pp. 123–230). London: Hogarth Press. (Original work published 1905)

Freud, S. (1955). Notes upon a case of obsessional neurosis. In J. Strachey (Ed. & Trans.), *The standard edition of the complete psychological works of Sigmund Freud* (Vol. 10, pp. 153–320). London: Hogarth Press. (Original work published 1909)

Freud, S. (1955). The psychogenesis of a case of homosexuality in a woman. In J. Strachey (Ed. & Trans.), *The standard edition of the complete psychological works of Sigmund Freud* (Vol. 18, pp. 145–172). London: Hogarth Press. (Original work published 1920)

Freud, S. (1961). The ego and the id. In J. Strachey (Ed. & Trans.), *The standard edition of the complete psychological works of Sigmund Freud* (Vol. 19, pp. 1–59). London: Hogarth Press. (Original work published 1923)

George, C., Kaplan, N., & Main, M. (1985). *The Adult Attachment Interview.* Unpublished manuscript, Department of Psychology, University of California, Berkeley.

Grant, J., & Sandell, R. (2004). Close family or mere neighbors?: Some empirical data on the differences between psychoanalysis and psychotherapy. In P. Richardson, H. Kächele, & C. Renlund (Eds.), *Research on psychoanalytic psychotherapy with adults* (pp. 81–108). London: Karnac Books.

Green, A. (2000). What kind of research for psychoanalysis? In J. Sandler, A.-M. Sandler, & R. Davies (Eds.), *Clinical and observational psychoanalytic research: Roots of a controversy* (pp. 21–27). London: Karnac Books.

Greenberg, J. R., & Mitchell, S. A. (1983). *Object relations in psychoanalytic theory.* Cambridge, MA: Harvard University Press.

Gunnar, M., & Quevedo, K. (2007). The neurobiology of stress and development. *Annual Review of Psychology, 58,* 145–173.

Hartmann, H. (1939). *Ego psychology and the problem of adaptation.* New York: International Universities Press, 1958.

Hartmann, H., Kris, E., & Loewenstein, R. (1946). Comments on the formation of psychic structure. *Psychoanalytic Study of the Child, 2,* 11–38.

Henry, W. P., Strupp, H. H., Schacht, T. E., & Gaston, L. (1994). Psychodynamic approaches. In A. E. Bergin & S. L. Garfield (Eds.), *Handbook of psychotherapy and behavior change* (4th ed., pp. 467–508). New York: Wiley.

Higgins, E. T. (1987). Self-discrepancy: A theory relating self and affect. *Psychological Review, 94,* 319.

Hoffman, I. Z. (2009). Doublethinking our way to "scientific" legitimacy: The desiccation of human experience. *Journal of the American Psychoanalytic Association, 57,* 1043–1069.

Høglend, P. (2004). Analysis of transference in dynamic psychotherapy: A review of empirical research. *Canadian Journal of Psychoanalysis, 12,* 279–300.

Johansson, R., Björklund, M., Hornborg, C., Karlsson, S., Hesser, H., Ljótsson, B., et al. (2013). Affect-focused psychodynamic psychotherapy for depression and anxiety through the Internet: A randomized controlled trial. *PeerJ, 1,* e102.

Kächele, H. (2010). Distinguishing psychoanalysis from psychotherapy. *International Journal of Psychoanalysis, 91,* 35–43.

Kandel, E. R. (1999). Biology and the future of psychoanalysis: A new intellectual framework for psychiatry revisited. *American Journal of Psychiatry, 156,* 505–524.

Kernberg, O. F. (1976). *Object relations theory and clinical psychoanalysis.* New York: Jason Aronson.

Klein, M. (1937). Love, guilt and reparation. In *Love, guilt and reparation: The writings of Melanie Klein, Vol. I* (pp. 306–343). New York: Macmillan, 1984.

Kohut, H. (1971). *The analysis of the self.* New York: International Universities Press.

Kohut, H. (1977). *The restoration of the self.* New York: International Universities Press.

Kroger, J., Martinussen, M., & Marcia, J. E. (2010). Identity status change during adolescence and young adulthood: A meta-analysis. *Journal of Adolescence, 33,* 683–698.

Krueger, R. F., Skodol, A. E., Livesley, W. J., Shrout, P. E., & Huang, Y. (2007). Synthesizing dimensional and categorical approaches to personality disorders: Refining the research agenda for DSM-V Axis II. *International Journal of Methods in Psychiatric Research, 16* (Suppl. 1), S65–S73.

Lacan, J. (2006). *Écrits: The first complete edition in English* (B. Fink, Trans.) New York: Norton.

Lahey, B. B., Rathouz, P. J., Van Hulle, C., Urbano, R. C., Krueger, R. F., Applegate, B., et al. (2008). Testing structural models of DSM-IV symptoms of common forms of child and adolescent psychopathology. *Journal of Abnormal Child Psychology, 36,* 187–206.

Lambert, M. J., & Barley, D. E. (2002). Research summary on the therapeutic relationship and psychotherapy outcome. In J. C. Norcross (Ed.), *Psychotherapy relationships that work* (pp. 17–32). Oxford, UK: Oxford University Press.

Leichsenring, F., Abbass, A., Luyten, P., Hilsenroth, M., & Rabung, S. (2013). The emerging evidence for long-term psychodynamic therapy. *Psychodynamic Psychiatry, 41*, 361–384.

Leichsenring, F., & Rabung, S. (2008). Effectiveness of long-term psychodynamic psychotherapy: A meta-analysis. *Journal of the American Medical Association, 300*, 1551–1565.

Leichsenring, F., & Rabung, S. (2011). Long-term psychodynamic psychotherapy in complex mental disorders: Update of a meta-analysis. *British Journal of Psychiatry, 199*, 15–22.

Lemma, A., & Fonagy, P. (2013). Feasibility study of a psychodynamic online group intervention for depression. *Psychoanalytic Psychology, 30*, 367–380.

Lemma, A., Roth, A. D., & Pilling, S. (2009). *The competences required to deliver effective psychoanalytic/psychodynamic therapy.* London: Research Department of Clinical, Educational and Health Psychology, University College London. Retrieved from *www.ucl.ac.uk/clinical-psychology/CORE/Psychodynamic_Competences/Background_Paper.pdf.*

Levy, K. N., & Blatt, S. J. (1999). Attachment theory and psychoanalysis: Further differentiation within insecure attachment patterns. *Psychoanalytic Inquiry, 19*, 541–575.

Levy, K. N., Clarkin, J. F., Yeomans, F. E., Scott, L. N., Wasserman, R. H., & Kernberg, O. F. (2006). The mechanisms of change in the treatment of borderline personality disorder with transference focused psychotherapy. *Journal of Clinical Psychology, 62*, 481–501.

Levy, R. A., Ablon, J. S., & Kächele, H. (2011). *Psychodynamic psychotherapy research: Evidence-based practice and practice-based evidence.* New York: Springer.

Lieberman, M. D. (2007). Social cognitive neuroscience: A review of core processes. *Annual Review of Psychology, 58*, 259–289.

Lupien, S. J., McEwen, B. S., Gunnar, M. R., & Heim, C. (2009). Effects of stress throughout the lifespan on the brain, behaviour and cognition. *Nature Reviews. Neuroscience, 10*, 434–445.

Luyten, P., Blatt, S. J., & Corveleyn, J. (2006). Minding the gap between positivism and hermeneutics in psychoanalytic research. *Journal of the American Psychoanalytic Association, 54*, 571–610.

Luyten, P., Blatt, S. J., & Fonagy, P. (2013). Impairments in self structures in depression and suicide in psychodynamic and cognitive behavioral approaches: Implications for clinical practice and research. *International Journal of Cognitive Therapy, 6*, 265–279.

Luyten, P., Blatt, S. J., & Mayes, L. C. (2012). Process and outcome in psychoanalytic psychotherapy research: The need for a (relatively) new paradigm. In R. A. Levy, J. S. Ablon, & H. Kächele (Eds.), *Handbook of evidence-based psychodynamic psychotherapy. Bridging the gap between science and practice* (2nd ed.). New York: Humana Press/Springer.

Luyten, P., Fonagy, P., Lemma, A., & Target, M. (2012). Depression. In A. Bateman & P. Fonagy (Eds.), *Handbook of mentalizing in mental health practice* (pp. 385–417). Washington, DC: American Psychiatric Association.

Luyten, P., Mayes, L. C., Target, M., & Fonagy, P. (2012). Developmental research. In G. O. Gabbard, B. Litowitz, & P. Williams (Eds.), *Textbook of psychoanalysis* (2nd ed., pp. 423–442). Washington, DC: American Psychiatric Press.

Luyten, P., Vliegen, N., Van Houdenhove, B., & Blatt, S. J. (2008). Equifinality, multifinality, and the rediscovery of the importance of early experiences: Pathways from early adversity to psychiatric and (functional) somatic disorders. *Psychoanalytic Study of the Child, 63*, 27–60.

Lyons-Ruth, K., & Jacobvitz, D. (2008). Attachment disorganization: Genetic factors, parenting contexts, and developmental transformation from infancy to adulthood. In J. Cassidy & P. R. Shaver (Eds.), *Handbook of attachment: Theory, research, and clinical applications* (2nd ed., pp. 666–697). New York: Guilford Press.

Mahler, M. S. (1975). On human symbiosis and the vicissitudes of individuation. *Journal of the American Psychoanalytic Association, 23*, 740–763.

Mahler, M. S., Pine, F., & Bergman, A. (1975). *The psychological birth of the human infant: symbiosis and individuation.* New York: Basic Books.

Main, M. (2000). The organized categories of infant, child and adult attachment: Flexible vs. inflexible attention under attachment-related stress. *Journal of the American Psychoanalytic Association, 48,* 1055–1096.

Main, M., Kaplan, N., & Cassidy, J. (1985). Security in infancy, childhood and adulthood: A move to the level of representation. In I. Bretherton & E. Waters (Eds.), Growing points of attachment theory and research. *Monographs of the Society for Research in Child Development, 50,* 66–104.

Masterson, J. F. (1976). *Psychotherapy of the borderline adult: A developmental approach.* New York: Brunner/Mazel.

Mayes, L. C. (2000). A developmental perspective on the regulation of arousal states. *Seminars in Perinatology, 24,* 267–279.

Mayes, L. C. (2001). The twin poles of order and chaos: Development as a dynamic, self-ordering system. *Psychoanalytic Study of the Child, 56,* 137–170.

McWilliams, N. (2011). *Psychoanalytic diagnosis: Understanding personality structure in the clinical process* (2nd ed.). New York: Guilford Press.

Midgley, N., & Kennedy, E. (2011). Psychodynamic psychotherapy for children and adolescents: A critical review of the evidence base. *Journal of Child Psychotherapy, 37,* 1–29.

Mikulincer, M., & Shaver, P. R. (2007). *Attachment in adulthood: Structure, dynamics and change.* New York: Guilford Press.

Mishler, E. G. (1979). Meaning in context: Is there any other kind? *Harvard Educational Review, 49,* 1–19.

Pincus, A. L., & Lukowitsky, M. R. (2011). Pathological narcissism and narcissistic personality disorder. *Annual Review of Clinical Psychology, 6,* 421–446.

Pine, F. (1988). The four psychologies of psychoanalysis and their place in clinical work. *Journal of the American Psychoanalytic Association, 36,* 571–596.

Ravitz, P., Maunder, R., Hunter, J., Sthankiya, B., & Lancee, W. (2010). Adult attachment measures: A 25-year review. *Journal of Psychosomatic Research, 69,* 419–432.

Roisman, G. I., Tsai, J. L., & Chiang, K.-H. S. (2004). The emotional integration of childhood experience: Physiological, facial expressive, and self-reported emotional response during the Adult Attachment Interview. *Developmental Psychology, 40,* 776–789.

Roth, A., & Fonagy, P. (2004). *What works for whom?: A critical review of psychotherapy research* (2nd ed.). New York: Guilford Press.

Ryle, A. (1990). *Cognitive analytic therapy: Active participation in change.* Chichester, UK: Wiley.

Sandler, J., & Rosenblatt, B. (1987). The representational world. In J. Sandler (Ed.), *From safety to superego: Selected papers of Joseph Sandler* (pp. 58–72). London: Karnac Books.

Shapiro, T., & Emde, R. N. (1993). *Research in psychoanalysis: Process, development, outcome.* Madison, CT: International Universities Press.

Shedler, J. (2002). A new language for psychoanalytic diagnosis. *Journal of the American Psychoanalytic Association, 50,* 429–456.

Shedler, J. (2010). The efficacy of psychodynamic psychotherapy. *American Psychologist, 65,* 98–109.

Skodol, A. E. (2012). Personality disorders in DSM-5. *Annual Review of Clinical Psychology, 8,* 317–344.

Solms, M., & Turnbull, O. (2002). *The brain and the inner world: An introduction to the neuroscience of subjective experience.* New York: Other Press.

Spitz, R. (1945). Hospitalism: An inquiry into the genesis of psychiatric conditions in early childhood. *Psychoanalytic Study of the Child, 1,* 53–73.

Sroufe, L. A. (2005). Attachment and development: A prospective, longitudinal study from birth to adulthood. *Attachment and Human Development, 7,* 349–367.

Stern, D. N. (1985). *The interpersonal world of the infant: A view from psychoanalysis and developmental psychology.* New York: Basic Books.

Suchman, N. E., DeCoste, C., Castiglioni, N., McMahon, T. J., Rounsaville, B., & Mayes, L. (2010). The Mothers and Toddlers Program, an attachment-based parenting intervention for substance using women: Post-treatment results from a randomized clinical pilot. *Attachment and Human Development, 12,* 483–504.

Tyson, P., & Tyson, R. L. (1990). *Psychoanalytic theories of development: An integration.* New Haven, CT: University Press.

Vaillant, G. E. (1977). *Adaptation to life.* Toronto: Little, Brown.

Westen, D. (1990). Towards a revised theory of borderline object relations: Contributions of empirical research. *International Journal of Psycho-Analysis, 71,* 661–694.

Westen, D. (1991). Social cognition and object relations. *Psychological Bulletin, 109,* 429–455.

Westen, D. (1998). The scientific legacy of Sigmund Freud: Toward a psychodynamically informed psychological science. *Psychological Bulletin, 124,* 333–371.

Westen, D. (1999). The scientific status of unconscious processes: Is Freud really dead? *Journal of the American Psychoanalytic Association, 47,* 1061–1106.

Westen, D., Blagov, P. S., Harenski, K., Kilts, C., & Hamann, S. (2006). Neural bases of motivated reasoning: An FMRI study of emotional constraints on partisan political judgment in the 2004 U.S. Presidential election. *Journal of Cognitive Neuroscience, 18,* 1947–1958.

Westen, D., & Gabbard, G. O. (2002a). Developments in cognitive neuroscience: I. Conflict, compromise, and connectionism. *Journal of the American Psychoanalytic Association, 50,* 53–98.

Westen, D., & Gabbard, G. O. (2002b). Developments in cognitive neuroscience: II. Implications for theories of transference. *Journal of the American Psychoanalytic Association, 50,* 99–134.

Westen, D., Lohr, N., Silk, K., Gold, L., & Kerber, K. (1990). Object relations and social cognition in borderlines, major depressives, and normals: A TAT analysis. *Psychological Assessment: A Journal of Consulting and Clinical Psychology, 2,* 355–364.

Winnicott, D. W. (1960). The theory of the parent-infant relationship. In *The maturational process and the facilitating environment* (pp. 37–55). New York: International Universities Press.

Wolf, E. S. (1988). Case discussion and position statement. *Psychoanalytic Inquiry, 8,* 546–551.

Young, J. E. (1999). *Cognitive therapy for personality disorder: A schema-focused approach* (3rd ed.). Sarasota, FL: Professional Resource Press/Professional Resource Exchange.

Zeigler-Hill, V., & Abraham, J. (2006). Borderline personality features: Instability of self-esteem and affect. *Journal of Social and Clinical Psychology, 25,* 668–687.

CHAPTER 2

Attachment-Related Contributions to the Study of Psychopathology

Mario Mikulincer and Phillip R. Shaver

The originator of attachment theory, John Bowlby, was, as most readers of this volume know, a British psychoanalyst who maintained a practice at the Tavistock Clinic in London throughout the years he was writing his influential trilogy on attachment (Bowlby, 1973, 1980, 1982) and his book about applying the theory in psychotherapy (e.g., Bowlby, 1988). His major intellectual collaborator, Mary Ainsworth, was an expert on developmental psychopathology and clinical assessment, and had coauthored a book about the Rorschach Inkblot Test (Klopfer, Ainsworth, Klopfer, & Holt, 1954) before meeting Bowlby. From the beginning, therefore, attachment theory was intended to contribute to the study, assessment, understanding, and treatment of psychopathology. In recent years, the theory has influenced the conceptualization and treatment of childhood, adolescent, and adult psychological disorders, as indicated by numerous chapters in the 2008 edition of the *Handbook of Attachment* (Cassidy & Shaver, 2008), especially the chapters in Part V, "Psychopathology and Clinical Applications of Attachment Theory and Research."

In the present chapter we focus mainly on our own line of research on adolescent and adult attachment processes—work based on a wide variety of self-report, social-cognitive, and behavioral measures.[1] We consider how this research relates to the study and amelioration of psychopathology. Beginning with a brief overview of attachment theory and our elaboration of it, we go on to explain how the study of individual differences in adult attachment intersects with the study of psychopathology,

---

[1] We generally use continuous dimensional measures rather than categorical ones because Fraley and Waller (1998), using taxometric analyses, showed that there are no distinct categories in the self-report domain. Some researchers (e.g., Bartholomew & Horowitz, 1991; Hazan & Shaver, 1987) have used categorical self-report methods, but the three or four categories they assessed are more accurately viewed as regions in a two-dimensional (anxiety-by-avoidance) space.

as illuminated by members of our research groups as well as many other investigators. Attachment insecurity is a major contributor to psychological problems and disorders, and the enhancement of attachment security is an important part of successful treatment of these problems and disorders.

ATTACHMENT THEORY: BASIC CONCEPTS

According to attachment theory (Bowlby, 1982), human beings are born with an innate psychobiological system (the *attachment behavioral system*) that motivates them to seek proximity to and support from significant others (*attachment figures*), especially in times of need. Bowlby (1973) also described important individual differences in attachment-system functioning, which he attributed mainly to experiences in close relationships. Interactions with attachment figures who are available and responsive in times of need facilitate the normal development and operation of the attachment system, promote a stable sense of attachment security, and heighten confidence in support seeking as a distress-regulation strategy. When a person's attachment figures are not reliably available and supportive, however, proximity seeking fails to relieve distress, a sense of attachment security is not attained, and strategies of affect regulation other than proximity seeking are developed. These secondary attachment strategies are conceptualized in terms of two major dimensions of insecurity, which we call *anxiety* and *avoidance.*

In studies of adolescents and adults by personality and social psychologists, tests of attachment theory have focused on a person's *attachment style*—the pattern of relational expectations, emotions, and behaviors that results from internalizing a particular history of attachment experiences (Shaver & Mikulincer, 2002). Research beginning with Ainsworth, Blehar, Waters, and Wall (1978) and continuing through recent studies by social and personality psychologists (reviewed by Mikulincer & Shaver, 2007a) indicates that attachment styles can be located in a two-dimensional space defined by the two roughly orthogonal dimensions of attachment-related anxiety and avoidance (Brennan, Clark, & Shaver, 1998). The avoidance dimension reflects the extent to which a person distrusts the goodwill of relationship partners and defensively strives to maintain behavioral independence and emotional distance. The anxiety dimension reflects the degree to which a person worries that a partner will not be available in times of need, partly because of the person's own self-doubt and self-deprecation. People who score low on both dimensions are said, in our research field, to be secure with respect to attachment. A person's location in the two-dimensional space can be measured with reliable and valid self-report scales (e.g., Brennan et al., 1998) and is associated in theoretically predictable ways with a wide variety of measures of relationship quality and psychological adjustment (see Mikulincer & Shaver, 2007a, for a review).

Attachment styles begin in interactions with primary caregivers during early childhood, as a large body of research has shown (see Cassidy & Shaver, 2008, for an anthology of reviews). Bowlby (1988), however, claimed that memorable interactions with other relationship partners throughout life can alter a person's working models of self and others, moving a person (in our terms) from one region to another of the anxiety-by-avoidance space. Moreover, although attachment style is often conceptualized as a single global orientation toward close relationships, and can definitely be measured as such, a person's orientation to attachment is rooted in a complex cognitive and affective associative neural network that includes many different episodic, context-specific, and relationship-specific, as well as fairly general, attachment representations (Mikulincer & Shaver, 2003). A growing body of research shows that attachment style can change, subtly or dramatically, depending on current context, recent experiences, and recent relationships (e.g., Baldwin, Keelan, Fehr, Enns, & Koh Rangarajoo, 1996; Mikulincer & Shaver, 2001).

We (Mikulincer & Shaver, 2003) have proposed a three-phase model of attachment-system activation and functioning in adulthood (see Figure 2.1). Following Bowlby (1982), we assume that the routine monitoring of internal and external events and experiences results in activation of the attachment system when a potential or an actual threat is perceived. When the attachment system is activated, an affirmative answer to the question "Is an attachment figure available and likely to be responsive to my needs?" results in a sense of attachment security and increases general faith in other people's goodwill; a related sense of being loved, esteemed, and accepted by relationship partners; and optimistic beliefs about one's ability to handle frustration and distress. According to Bowlby (1988), attachment security also fosters optimal functioning of other behavioral systems (such as exploration, sexuality, and caregiving) and is therefore an important and pervasive mainstay of mental health, personality development, and social adaptation.

Perceived unavailability of an attachment figure results in attachment insecurity, which compounds the distress aroused by the appraisal of a particular situation as threatening. This state of insecurity forces a decision about the viability (or nonviability) of further (more active) proximity seeking as a protective strategy. The appraisal of proximity as essential—because of attachment history, temperamental factors, or contextual cues—results in energetic, insistent attempts to attain proximity, support, and care. These attempts are called *hyperactivating strategies* in attachment theory (Cassidy & Kobak, 1988) because they involve the upregulation of the attachment system, including perpetual vigilance and intense concern until an attachment figure is perceived to be adequately available and supportive. Hyperactivating strategies include attempts to elicit a partner's involvement, care, and support through crying, begging, clinging, and controlling responses (Davis, Shaver, & Vernon, 2003); overdependence on relationship partners as sources of protection (Shaver & Hazan, 1993); and perception of oneself as relatively helpless in emotion regulation (Mikulincer & Shaver, 2003). These aspects of attachment-system hyperactivation account for many of the empirically documented correlates of measurable attachment-related anxiety (Mikulincer & Shaver, 2007a).

Appraising proximity seeking as unlikely to alleviate distress encourages deactivation of the attachment system, inhibition of support seeking, and a decision to handle distress alone, especially distress that arises from the failure of attachment figures to be available and responsive. This set of affect-regulation strategies has been labeled *deactivating* (Cassidy & Kobak, 1988) because their aim is to keep the

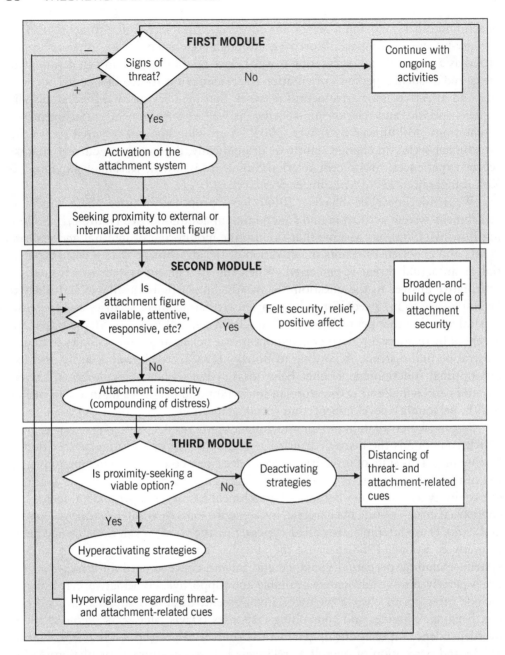

FIGURE 2.1. A model of attachment-system activation and functioning in adulthood.

attachment system downregulated to avoid the frustration and pain of attachment-figure unavailability. Deactivating strategies include avoidance of intimacy, avoidance of dependence on close relationship partners, and maintenance of emotional distance from others. These tendencies are supplemented by a self-reliant stance that decreases dependence on others. Deactivating strategies account for the empirically documented correlates of measurable attachment-related avoidance (Mikulincer & Shaver, 2007a).

Hyperactivating and deactivating strategies shape the quality of a person's relationships and emotional experiences. Because this volume deals with psychopathology, we focus here mainly on the implications of attachment insecurities for mental health and psychopathology.

ATTACHMENT, MENTAL HEALTH, AND PSYCHOPATHOLOGY

According to attachment theory (Main, 1990; Mikulincer & Shaver, 2003, 2007a; Shaver & Mikulincer, 2002), secondary attachment strategies (anxious hyperactivation and avoidant deactivation) are defenses against the psychological pain induced by unavailability, unreliability, or unresponsiveness of attachment figures. Although these secondary strategies are initially adaptive, in the sense that they conform a child's behavior to the requirements of an inconsistently available, or consistently distant or unavailable, attachment figure, they prove maladaptive when used in later relationships where proximity-seeking and collaborative interdependence could be productive and rewarding. They also foster the continued use of nonoptimal working models of self, others, and relationships (mental representations or schemas) and affect-regulation strategies that interfere with social adjustment and mental health. Hundreds of studies, summarized in our 2007 book (Mikulincer & Shaver, 2007a), confirm that attachment insecurities place a person at risk for emotional difficulties and psychopathology.

In this section of the chapter, we review research on connections between attachment insecurity and psychopathology in relation to four important questions:

1. Are particular forms of attachment insecurity associated with particular forms of psychological dysfunction?
2. Can attachment insecurities by themselves produce psychopathology?
3. Is the association between attachment insecurity and psychopathology unidirectional?
4. Can increased attachment security contribute to mental health and decrease the likelihood or severity of psychopathology?

Are Particular Forms of Attachment Insecurity Associated with Particular Disorders?

According to attachment theory, interactions with inconsistent, unreliable, or insensitive attachment figures interfere with the development of a secure, stable psychological foundation, reduce resilience in coping with stressful life events, and predispose a person to break down psychologically in times of crisis (Bowlby, 1988). Attachment insecurity can therefore be viewed as a *general* vulnerability to psychological disorders (as explained in greater detail by DeKlyen & Greenberg, 2008), with the particular symptomatology depending on genetic, developmental, and environmental factors.

In our book (Mikulincer & Shaver, 2007a), we reviewed hundreds of crosssectional, longitudinal, and prospective studies of both clinical and nonclinical samples and found that attachment insecurity was common among people with a wide variety of psychological disorders, ranging from mild distress to severe personality disorders and even schizophrenia. Consistently compatible results have also been reported in recent articles. For example, attachment insecurities (of both anxious and avoidant varieties) are associated with the likelihood and severity of depression (e.g., Catanzaro & Wei, 2010), clinically significant anxiety (e.g., Bosmans, Braet, & Van Vlierberghe, 2010), obsessive–compulsive disorder (OCD) (e.g., Doron, Moulding, Kyrios, Nedeljkovic, & Mikulincer, 2009), posttraumatic stress disorder (PTSD) (e.g., Ein-Dor, Doron, Solomon, Mikulincer, & Shaver, 2010), suicidal tendencies (e.g., Gormley & McNiel, 2010), eating disorders (e.g., Illing, Tasca, Balfour, & Bissada, 2010), behavioral problems (e.g., McWilliams & Bailey, 2010), and personality disorders (e.g., Crawford et al., 2007). Separation anxiety, complicated grief following the loss of a loved one, and posttraumatic reactions to physical, sexual, or psychological abuse are especially closely related to what Bowlby (1982) called the attachment behavioral system (the biological basis of attachment), so it is easy to understand why they are related to insecurities that can be traced back to the unavailability or insensitivity of attachment figures (e.g., Boelen, 2009; Prigerson & Jacobs, 2001).

However, research showing that particular forms of attachment insecurity contribute to particular forms of psychological disorder has caused us to alter our 2007 conclusion slightly. For example, attachment anxiety and avoidance are related to different types of depression (e.g., Catanzaro & Wei, 2010; Davila, 2001): attachment anxiety is related to interpersonal aspects of depression, such as overdependence, lack of autonomy, and neediness, whereas avoidance is related to achievement-related aspects of depression, such as perfectionism, self-punishment, and self-criticism (see also Luyten & Blatt, 2011).

Differences related to particular forms of attachment insecurity have also been found in studies of PTSD (e.g., Mikulincer, Florian, & Weller, 1993; Solomon, Dekel, & Mikulincer, 2008). Anxious attachment is associated with what Horowitz (1982) called intrusion symptoms: unwanted and uncontrollable reactivation of thoughts, images, emotions, and nightmares related to a traumatic event. Avoidant attachment predisposes a traumatized person to deny or downplay the trauma and avoid direct or symbolic exposure to trauma reminders, thereby encouraging what Horowitz (1982) called posttraumatic avoidance responses, including psychic numbing, denial of the significance and consequences of the traumatic event, and behavioral inhibition.

Although attachment insecurity is a key feature of many personality disorders, the specific kind of attachment insecurity differs among disorders (e.g., Brennan & Shaver, 1998; Meyer & Pilkonis, 2005). Anxious attachment is associated with dependent, histrionic, and borderline disorders, whereas avoidant attachment is associated with schizoid and avoidant disorders. Crawford and colleagues (2007) found that attachment anxiety is associated with what Livesley (1991) called the "emotional dysregulation" component of personality disorders, which includes identity confusion, anxiety, emotional lability, cognitive distortions, submissiveness, oppositionality, self-harm, narcissism, and suspiciousness. Crawford and colleagues also found that avoidant attachment is associated with what Livesley called the "inhibitedness" component of personality problems, including restricted expression of emotions, problems with intimacy, and social avoidance.

In an earlier study, Crawford and colleagues (2006) assessed personality disorders (via parental reports, self-reports, and psychiatric interviews) and self-reported attachment orientations at ages 16, 22, and 33 in a nonclinical community sample. In this study, avoidant attachment was associated with Cluster A symptoms (paranoid, schizoid, and schizotypal), whereas attachment anxiety was associated with Cluster B symptoms (antisocial, borderline, histrionic, and narcissistic) and Cluster C symptoms (avoidant, dependent, and obsessive–compulsive).

In summary, attachment insecurities contribute nonspecifically to many kinds of psychopathology, but in addition, particular forms of attachment insecurity seem to predispose individuals to particular kinds and configurations of psychological disorders. That is, it seems that attachment insecurities have a "pathoplastic" relationship (Enns & Cox, 1997) with psychological disorders, by which they can modify the expression and course of a disorder without necessarily having a direct etiological role.

Can Attachment Insecurities by Themselves Produce Psychopathology?

We suspect that the eventual answer to this question will be no. Beyond disorders such as separation anxiety and pathological grief, in which attachment injuries are the main causes and themes, attachment insecurities per se are unlikely to be sufficient causes of adolescent and adult psychological disorders (see DeKlyen & Greenberg, 2008, for a similar perspective on child psychopathology). Other factors (e.g., genetically determined temperament, intelligence, and life history, including abuse) are likely to converge with or amplify the effects of attachment experiences on the causal path to psychopathology. For example, extensive evidence shows that early relational traumas (e.g., abuse, neglect) have dramatic negative effects on brain development (e.g., Glaser, 2001; Teicher et al., 2004).

Consider, for example, the relationship between attachment-related avoidance and psychological distress. Many studies of large community samples have found no association between avoidant attachment and self-report measures of global distress (see Mikulincer & Shaver, 2007a, for a review). However, studies focusing on highly stressful events, such as exposure to missile attacks, living in a dangerous neighborhood, or giving birth to an infant with a congenital heart defect, found that avoidance was related to greater distress and poorer long-term adjustment (e.g., Berant, Mikulincer, & Shaver, 2008; Mikulincer et al., 1993; Mikulincer, Horesh, Eilati, & Kotler, 1999).

Some studies have identified moderators of the link between attachment and psychopathology. For example, Wautier and Blume (2004) found that attachment insecurity was associated with depression and anxiety disorders during adolescence mainly among adolescents whose sense of personal identity was unstable. Other researchers found that marital dissatisfaction amplified the detrimental effects of attachment insecurity on the severity of depression (Scott & Cordova, 2002) and that unsupportive husbands were more likely to increase the probability of their wives having postpartum depression if the wives had previously scored high on a measure of attachment anxiety (Simpson, Rholes, Campbell, Tran, & Wilson, 2003).

Life-history factors are also important. For example, the association between attachment insecurity and depression is higher among adults with a childhood history of physical, psychological, or sexual abuse (e.g., Whiffen, Judd, & Aube, 1999). Stressful life events, poverty, physical health problems, and involvement in turbulent romantic relationships during adolescence also strengthen the link between attachment insecurity and psychopathology (e.g., Besser, Priel, & Wiznitzer, 2002; Davila, Steinberg, Kachadourian, Cobb, & Fincham, 2004).

Is the Association between Attachment Insecurity and Psychopathology Unidirectional?

We suspect that the association is bidirectional. Although attachment insecurities can contribute to mental disorders, as we have already documented, psychological problems can also increase attachment insecurity. In such cases, a psychological disorder can be viewed as a source of stress or distress that activates the attachment system and brings to mind attachment-related worries about being unloved, rejected, or unsupported during previous crises. These worries can be amplified by the social stigma associated with psychological disorders, and the insults and ostracism that mentally ill people frequently encounter, even in interactions with their closest relationship partners (e.g., Joiner & Coyne, 1999).

Only a few studies have examined the "scarring" effects of psychopathology (e.g., Rohde, Lewinsohn, & Seeley, 1990) on attachment—the possibility that psychological disorders affect attachment insecurities (e.g., Cozzarelli, Karafa, Collins, & Tagler, 2003; Davila, Burge, & Hammen, 1997; Davila & Cobb, 2003). Davila and colleagues (1997), for example, found that late adolescent women who became less securely attached over periods of 6 to 24 months were more likely than their peers to have a history of psychopathology. Cozzarelli and colleagues (2003) found that women who moved in the direction of insecure attachment over a 2-year period following abortion were more likely than other women who underwent the procedure to have a history of depression or abuse. Solomon and colleagues (2008) assessed attachment insecurities and PTSD symptoms among Israeli ex-prisoners of war (POWs), along with a matched control group of veterans, 18 and 30 years after their release from captivity. Attachment anxiety and avoidance increased over time among the ex-POWs, and the increases were predicted by the severity of PTSD symptoms at the first wave of measurement.

Can Increased Attachment Security Contribute to Mental Health and Decrease the Likelihood or Severity of Psychopathology?

If attachment insecurities are risk factors for psychopathology, then the initiation, maintenance, or restoration of a sense of attachment security should increase resilience and improve mental health. According to attachment theory, interactions with available and supportive attachment figures impart a sense of safety, arouse positive emotions (e.g., relief, satisfaction, gratitude, love), and provide psychological resources for dealing with problems and adversities. Secure individuals remain relatively unperturbed during times of stress, recover faster from episodes of distress, and experience longer periods of positive affectivity, which contribute to overall emotional well-being and mental health.

In some of our studies, we have examined the effects of increased security on various indicators of mental health by experimentally activating mental representations of supportive attachment figures (e.g., Mikulincer, Hirschberger, Nachmias, & Gillath, 2001; Mikulincer & Shaver, 2001). These research techniques, which we (Mikulincer & Shaver, 2007b) refer to as "security priming," include subliminal pictures suggesting attachment-figure availability, subliminal names of people designated by participants as security-enhancing attachment figures, guided imagery highlighting the availability and supportiveness of an attachment figure, and visualization of the faces of security-enhancing attachment figures. In each study, we have compared the effects of security priming with those of emotionally positive but attachment-unrelated stimuli (e.g., pictures of a large amount of money, names or faces of acquaintances who are not attachment figures) or emotionally neutral stimuli (e.g., neutral words, pictures of furniture).

Security priming improves participants' mood even in threatening contexts and eliminates the detrimental effects of threats on positive moods (e.g., Mikulincer et al., 2001). Mikulincer, Shaver, and Horesh (2006) found that subliminal priming with security-related words mitigated cognitive symptoms of PTSD (heightened accessibility of trauma-related words in a Stroop color-naming task) in a nonclinical sample. Admoni (2006) found that priming with the names of each participant's security providers mitigated two cognitive symptoms of eating disorders (distorted body perception and heightened accessibility of food-related words in a Stroop task) in a sample of women hospitalized for eating disorders.

There is preliminary evidence that a sense of security provided by a psychotherapist improves a client's mental health. In a study based on data from the multisite National Institute of Mental Health Treatment of Depression Collaborative Research Program, Zuroff and Blatt (2006) found that a client's positive appraisals of his or her therapist's sensitivity and supportiveness predicted relief from depression and self-criticism and maintenance of therapeutic benefits over an 18-month period. The results were not attributable to patient characteristics or severity of depression. In a one-year prospective study of the effectiveness of residential treatment of high-risk adolescents, Gur (2006) found that staff members' provision of a sense of attachment security resulted in lower rates of anger, depression, and behavioral problems in the adolescents. Although these preliminary findings are encouraging, there is still a great need for additional well-controlled research examining the long-term effects of security-enhancing therapeutic figures on adult clients' mental health. There is already encouraging evidence for early-childhood interventions (reviewed by Berlin, Zeanah, & Lieberman, 2008). We particularly like the Circle of Security intervention program designed by Powell, Cooper, Hoffman, and Marvin (2007), which contains hints about a combination of education and emotional support that might also work with adults.

MEDIATING PROCESSES

According to attachment theory (e.g., Bowlby, 1988), the linkage between attachment insecurities (whether in the form of anxiety, avoidance, or both) and psychopathology is mediated by several pathways: negative mental representations of self and others; inadequate methods of regulating distress; ineffective strategies for coping with problems; difficulties in interpersonal relationships; and interference with goal pursuit and regulation of impulses, thoughts, and actions. Although each of these mediating pathways may be sufficient to predispose an insecurely attached person to develop psychopathology of a particular kind, they form such a densely interwoven web of cognitions, emotions, motives, behaviors, and patterns of relating to others that they may constitute instead a general vulnerability to breakdown rather a route to a particular dysfunctional outcome. Thus, searching for a single mediating mechanism may be fruitless because the different difficulties typically reinforce each other in self-expanding cycles of maladjustment. Instead of focusing on mediators of particular kinds of psychopathology, we will review studies documenting associations between attachment insecurities and each of the *mediators* of psychopathology.

Mental Representations of Self and Others

According to attachment theory, and as confirmed by research, lack of parental sensitivity and responsiveness contributes to disorders of the self, characterized by lack of self-cohesion, doubts about one's internal coherence and continuity over time, unstable self-esteem, and overdependence on other people's approval (Bartholomew & Horowitz, 1991; Kohut & Wolf, 1978; Mikulincer, 1998; Park, Crocker, & Mickelson, 2004). Insecure people are likely to be overly self-critical, plagued by self-doubts, or prone to using defenses such as destructive perfectionism to counter feelings of worthlessness and hopelessness (e.g., Wei, Heppner, Russell, & Young, 2006; Zuroff & Fitzpatrick, 1995). These dysfunctional beliefs about the self leave insecure people vulnerable to forms of distress that are diatheses (vulnerabilities) for psychopathology, as often claimed by cognitive therapists (e.g., Wright, Thase, & Beck, 2011).

Although both anxious and avoidant people have difficulty constructing a cohesive self and a stable sense of self-worth, their reliance on different secondary attachment strategies results in different disorders of the self. Anxious people's desire to gain a partner's love and protection keeps them from "owning" their anger toward a partner and causes them to take responsibility for their frustration and pain, thereby reinforcing their sense of worthlessness and contributing to hopeless, helpless patterns of causal explanation and continual self-derogation (e.g., Mikulincer, 1995; Williams & Riskind, 2004). Avoidant people's commitment to self-reliance causes them to push negative self-representations out of awareness and to defensively inflate their self-image (e.g., Mikulincer, 1998) (see also Waldinger & Schulz, Chapter 6, this volume). As a result, they often report high levels of explicit self-esteem and describe themselves in positive terms. Nevertheless, their efforts to self-enhance are accompanied by unrealistically high self-standards—to be as strong and as perfect as possible—which leads them to rely on external sources of validation combined with self-criticism, perfectionism, and renewed self-doubts. These dynamic processes create a self-exacerbating cycle in which self-criticism and defensive self-inflation reinforce each other. However, when defensive self-inflation is interfered with by a high cognitive or emotional load, the suppressed negative self-conceptions erupt into avoidant people's consciousness, as we have demonstrated experimentally (Mikulincer, Dolev, & Shaver, 2004) in strong support of a psychodynamic model of the mind.

Adult attachment research has shown that both major forms of insecurity, anxiety and avoidance, are associated with pathological narcissism (e.g., Dickinson & Pincus, 2003). But avoidant attachment predisposes a person to *overt* narcissism or grandiosity, which includes both self-praise and denial of weaknesses (Wink, 1991). Attachment anxiety, in contrast, predisposes a person to *covert* narcissism, characterized by self-focused attention, hypersensitivity to other people's evaluations, and appraisal of oneself in terms of unrealistic, exaggerated expectations and a sense of entitlement (Wink, 1991) (see also Meehan & Levy, Chapter 15, this volume).

Distress Regulation and Coping

The attachment system plays an important role in emotion regulation, which is deficient in most forms of psychopathology. According to attachment theory, interactions with available attachment figures and the resulting sense of attachment security provide actual and symbolic supports for learning constructive emotion-regulation strategies. For example, interactions with emotionally accessible and responsive others provide a context in which a child can learn that acknowledgment and display of emotions is an important step toward restoring emotional balance, and that it is useful and socially acceptable to express, explore, and try to understand one's feelings (Cassidy, 1994). Adult attachment researchers have found that secure individuals, as compared with their less secure peers, tend to score higher on self-report and behavioral measures of emotional expressiveness (e.g., Feeney, 1995) and self-disclosure (e.g., Keelan, Dion, & Dion, 1998), and have readier access to early memories of painful emotions (Mikulincer & Orbach, 1995).

Interactions with available and supportive attachment figures promote and reaffirm optimistic and hopeful appraisals of life's challenges. During these interactions, children learn that distress is manageable, external obstacles can be overcome, and restoration of emotional equanimity is only a matter of time. As a result, secure people can make self-soothing reappraisals of distress-eliciting events, a process that reduces distress and fosters resilience. Indeed, as compared with anxious and avoidant people, secure individuals make more optimistic appraisals of stressful events (e.g., Mikulincer & Florian, 1998). For example, Berant, Mikulincer, and Florian (2001) found that securely attached mothers of infants who were diagnosed with congenital heart defects reported more positive appraisals of maternal tasks, both immediately after the diagnosis and one year later, than anxious or avoidant mothers. Six years later, the effects of insecure mothers on their children were evident in both objective and projective measures administered to the then 7-year-old children (Berant et al., 2008).

Experiences of attachment-figure availability also offer opportunities to learn that one's own efforts and actions are often able to reduce distress. For example, a child learns that his or her bids for proximity alter a partner's behavior and result in the restoration of emotional balance. Gradually, these experiences strengthen the child's confidence in his or her ability to self-soothe in ways similar to their soothing by helpful attachment figures (Mikulincer & Shaver, 2004). As a result, although they might seem to foster dependency, security-enhancing interactions with attachment figures encourage a person's acquisition of and reliance on active, instrumental approaches to problem solving. In support of this view, secure individuals tend to rely on active problem-focused strategies, not just self-focused emotion-regulation strategies, when coping with stressful events (e.g., Mikulincer & Florian, 1998).

Unlike relatively secure people, avoidant individuals often prefer to cordon off emotions from their thoughts and actions, using what Lazarus and Folkman (1984) called "distancing coping." As a result, they tend to present a façade of security and composure, but leave suppressed distress unresolved in ways that impair their ability to deal with life's inevitable adversities. This impairment is particularly likely during prolonged, demanding stressful experiences that require active coping with a problem and mobilization of external sources of support (e.g., Berant et al., 2001).

People with high attachment anxiety, in contrast, often find negative emotions to be congruent with their attachment-system hyperactivation. For them, "emotion regulation" can mean emotion amplification and exaggeration of attachment-related and -unrelated worries, depressive reactions to actual or potential losses and failures, and intrusion of PTSD symptoms following traumas. Attachment anxiety is also associated with socially destructive outbursts of anger and impulsive, demanding behavior toward relationship partners, sometimes including violence (Mikulincer & Shaver, 2007a).

Difficulties in Interpersonal Relationships

According to attachment theory, recurrent failure to obtain support from attachment figures and to sustain a sense of security, and the resulting reliance on secondary attachment strategies, interfere with the acquisition of social skills. For example, hyperactivating strategies involve anxious people focusing on their unsatisfied needs, weaknesses, and vulnerabilities. As a result, they are relatively unskilled at expressing positive mental states, such as satisfaction, happiness, and gratitude, and their negative attentional focus draws cognitive and empathic resources away from accurately interpreting others' emotional signals and needs (e.g., Fraley, Niedenthal, Marks, Brumbaugh, & Vicary, 2006). Deactivating strategies, in contrast, involve avoidant people inhibiting the expression of thoughts and feelings to others and makes them less likely than their peers to attend to relationship partners' verbal and nonverbal messages and signals (Collins, Cooper, Albino, & Allard, 2002; Schachner, Shaver, & Mikulincer, 2005).

The difficulties insecurely attached people encounter in social relations are especially evident when it comes to conflict management. Conflicts threaten the wish of anxious individuals to gain approval and support, and they heighten fears of rejection and abandonment. These individuals are therefore likely to appraise conflicts in catastrophic terms, display intense negative emotions as a result, fail to attend to and understand what their partner is saying, have difficulty maintaining open communication and engaging in constructive negotiation, or accede too quickly to a partner's demands as a way of avoiding rejection. Avoidant people are likely to view conflicts as unpleasant primarily because they interfere with autonomy and call for expressions of love, care, forgiveness, need, or vulnerability, all of which are perceived as entangling and unpleasant. When circumstances do not allow escape from a conflict, avoidant people are likely to attempt to dominate their partner, which obviously interferes with calm discussion and compromise (e.g., Creasey & Hesson-McInnis, 2001; Pistole & Arricale, 2003).

These skill deficits, combined with the difficulty of insecure individuals in maintaining a flexible balance between dependency and autonomy, and between self-concern and concern for others, create serious problems in relationships. Bartholomew and Horowitz (1991), using the Inventory of Interpersonal Problems (IIP; Horowitz, Rosenberg, Baer, Ureno, & Villasenor, 1988), which arrays different kinds of problems in a circular pattern, found that attachment anxiety was associated with more interpersonal problems in general. Secure individuals did not show notable elevations in any sections of the problem circle, but avoidant people generally had problems with nurturance (being cold, introverted, or competitive), and anxious people had problems with emotionality (e.g., being overly expressive). Interestingly, fearfully avoidant individuals (those who scored high on both anxious and avoidant attachment) had problems in the low-dominance portion of the circle (i.e., they were overly submissive and exploitable).

Problems in interpersonal relations are associated, subjectively, with the self-reported loneliness and social isolation of insecure individuals (e.g., Hazan & Shaver, 1987; Larose & Bernier, 2001) and their relatively low relationship satisfaction, more frequent relationship dissolution, and more frequent coercion and violence (see Mikulincer & Shaver, 2007a, for a review). The inability or unwillingness of insecure individuals to care sensitively for a relationship partner in need (e.g., Collins & Feeney, 2000) and their sexual inhibitions and difficulties (e.g., Tracy, Shaver, Albino, & Cooper, 2003) can alienate relationship partners, arouse feelings of rejection, anger, and isolation, and contribute to relationship failure. According to interpersonal theories of psychopathology (e.g., Joiner & Coyne, 1999), these negative relationship experiences, attributable in part to the ways in which insecure people often relate to their partners, can contribute to psychopathology.

Problems in Self-Regulation

Insecure individuals' problems in the area of behavioral self-regulation also increase their vulnerability to psychopathology. Their difficulty in creating effective plans, organizing effective problem-solving efforts, selecting among alternative actions, and abandoning unobtainable goals cause frustration, failure, and distress in couple relationships, at school, and at work (see Mikulincer & Shaver, 2007a, for a review of studies of insecurity and problems with self-regulation).

One example of difficulties outside the domain of romantic and marital relationships is in the area of choosing and developing a career. O'Brien, Friedman, Tipton, and Linn (2000) reported a longitudinal study showing that insecure attachment to parents during adolescence predicted problems in career decision making and possession of less ambitious career aspirations five years later. Roisman, Bahadur, and Oster (2000) found that attachment insecurities in infancy and adolescence (measured with the Adult Attachment Interview [AAI]; see Hesse, 2008, for a discussion of that measure) uniquely predicted poorer career planning.

Attachment-related difficulties in self-regulation also occur in the areas of academic performance and school adjustment (e.g., Aspelmeier & Kerns, 2003). For example, Larose, Bernier, and Tarabulsy (2005) conducted a longitudinal study of the transition from high school to college and found that both anxious and avoidant students (assessed with the AAI) reported poorer preparation for examinations and poorer attention to academic tasks at the end of high school and again at the end of the first semester of college. Moreover, anxiously attached students reported an increase in fear of academic failure and a decrease in the priority they placed on studies during the transition to college. Attachment-related avoidance was associated with a decrease in the quality of attention and exam preparation during the college transition and lower grades after each of the first three semesters of college (even when controlling for high school grades).

Researchers have found effects of attachment orientation in work settings (e.g., Hardy & Barkham, 1994; Hazan & Shaver, 1990). More anxious or avoidant adults report lower levels of work satisfaction. Moreover, those who score higher on attachment anxiety are more worried about their job performance, and those who score higher on avoidance have more conflicts with coworkers. These associations were also evidenced in two longitudinal studies. Burge and colleagues (1997) found that attachment insecurities in parent–child or romantic relationships predicted decreases in the work performance of female adolescents 2 years later, and Vasquez, Durik, and Hyde (2002) observed that insecure attachment in a sample of parents assessed one year after the birth of a child predicted greater self-reported work overload 3.5 years later. These associations persisted even when other psychological problems (e.g., depression) were statistically controlled.

DISCUSSION AND CONCLUSIONS

Attachment theory emerged in the context of Bowlby's experiences in the field of child and family psychotherapy. His original interest was the influence of attachment relationships in early childhood on later psychological functioning. The concepts he proposed for this purpose turned out to apply across the lifespan, and attachment theory has become a major influence on the study of close relationships of all kinds and on the study of resilience and psychopathology. Here we have provided an overview of research on the connections between, on the one hand, social-personality psychologists' measures of individual differences in attachment orientations, and, on the other hand, psychological problems and forms of psychopathology. Attachment insecurities clearly play a role in psychopathology, and in some cases the different forms of insecurity are related to different forms of psychopathology.

The concepts of attachment, anxious and avoidant attachment, and attachment-related defenses arose in the context of psychoanalytic theories and therapies. Our research, which borrows methods from the increasingly psychodynamic study of social cognition and emotion, offers solid support for a psychodynamic approach to psychopathology, including the milder forms of psychological problems found in the "normal" population. Further research is needed before the relationships between attachment insecurities and forms of psychopathology, both mild and severe, are fully understood. In particular, we need more longitudinal studies tracing the developmental trajectory of attachment insecurities and psychopathology, while taking into account the joint contribution of genetic and life-history factors.

REFERENCES

Admoni, S. (2006). *Attachment security and eating disorders.* Unpublished doctoral dissertation, Bar-Ilan University, Ramat Gan, Israel.

Ainsworth, M. D. S., Blehar, M. C., Waters, E., & Wall, S. (1978). *Patterns of attachment: Assessed in the Strange Situation and at home.* Hillsdale, NJ: Erlbaum.

Aspelmeier, J. E., & Kerns, K. A. (2003). Love and school: Attachment/exploration dynamics in college. *Journal of Social and Personal Relationships, 20,* 5–30.

Baldwin, M. W., Keelan, J. P. R., Fehr, B., Enns, V., & Koh Rangarajoo, E. (1996). Social-cognitive conceptualization of attachment working models: Availability and accessibility effects. *Journal of Personality and Social Psychology, 71,* 94–109.

Bartholomew, K., & Horowitz, L. M. (1991). Attachment styles among young adults: A test of a four-category model. *Journal of Personality and Social Psychology, 61,* 226–244.

Berant, E., Mikulincer, M., & Florian, V. (2001). The association of mothers' attachment style and their psychological reactions to the diagnosis of infant's congenital heart disease. *Journal of Social and Clinical Psychology, 20,* 208–232.

Berant, E., Mikulincer, M., & Shaver, P. R. (2008). Mothers' attachment style, their mental health, and their children's emotional vulnerabilities: A seven-year study of children with congenital heart disease. *Journal of Personality, 76,* 31–66.

Berlin, L. J., Zeanah, C. H., & Lieberman, A. F. (2008). Prevention and intervention programs for supporting early attachment security. In J. Cassidy & P. R. Shaver (Eds.), *Handbook of attachment: Theory, research, and clinical applications* (pp. 745–761). New York: Guilford Press.

Besser, A., Priel, B., & Wiznitzer, A. (2002). Childbearing depressive symptomatology in high-risk pregnancies: The roles of working models and social support. *Personal Relationships, 9,* 395–413.

Boelen, P. A. (2009). The centrality of a loss and its role in emotional problems among bereaved people. *Behaviour Research and Therapy, 47,* 616–622.

Bosmans, G., Braet, C., & Van Vlierberghe, L. (2010). Attachment and symptoms of psychopathology: Early maladaptive schemas as a cognitive link? *Clinical Psychology and Psychotherapy, 17,* 374–385.

Bowlby, J. (1973). *Attachment and loss: Vol. 2. Separation: Anxiety and anger.* New York: Basic Books.

Bowlby, J. (1980). *Attachment and loss: Vol. 3. Loss: Sadness and depression.* New York: Basic Books.

Bowlby, J. (1982). *Attachment and loss: Vol. 1. Attachment* (2nd ed.). New York: Basic Books. (Original work published 1969)

Bowlby, J. (1988). *A secure base: Clinical applications of attachment theory.* London: Routledge.

Brennan, K. A., Clark, C. L., & Shaver, P. R. (1998). Self-report measurement of adult romantic attachment: An integrative overview. In J. A. Simpson & W. S. Rholes (Eds.), *Attachment theory and close relationships* (pp. 46–76). New York: Guilford Press.

Brennan, K. A., & Shaver, P. R. (1998). Attachment styles and personality disorders: Their connections to each other and to parental divorce, parental death, and perceptions of parental caregiving. *Journal of Personality, 66,* 835–878.

Burge, D., Hammen, C., Davila, J., Daley, S. E., Paley, B., Herzberg, D., et al. (1997). Attachment cognitions and college and work functioning two years later in late adolescent women. *Journal of Youth and Adolescence, 26,* 285–301.

Cassidy, J. (1994). Emotion regulation: Influences of attachment relationships. *Monographs of the Society for Research in Child Development, 59,* 228–283.

Cassidy, J., & Kobak, R. R. (1988). Avoidance and its relationship with other defensive processes. In J. Belsky & T. Nezworski (Eds.), *Clinical implications of attachment* (pp. 300–323). Hillsdale, NJ: Erlbaum.

Cassidy, J., & Shaver, P. R. (Eds.). (2008). *Handbook of attachment: Theory, research, and clinical applications* (2nd ed.). New York: Guilford Press.

Catanzaro, A., & Wei, M. (2010). Adult attachment, dependence, self-criticism, and depressive symptoms: A test of a mediational model. *Journal of Personality, 78,* 1135–1162.

Collins, N. L., Cooper, M., Albino, A., & Allard, L. (2002). Psychosocial vulnerability from adolescence to adulthood: A prospective study of attachment style differences in relationship functioning and partner choice. *Journal of Personality, 70,* 965–1008.

Collins, N. L., & Feeney, B. C. (2000). A safe haven: An attachment theory perspective on support seeking and caregiving in intimate relationships. *Journal of Personality and Social Psychology, 78,* 1053–1073.

Cozzarelli, C., Karafa, J. A., Collins, N. L., & Tagler, M. J. (2003). Stability and change in adult attachment styles: Associations with personal vulnerabilities, life events, and global construals of self and others. *Journal of Social and Clinical Psychology, 22,* 315–346.

Crawford, T. N., Livesley, W. J., Jang, K. L., Shaver, P. R., Cohen, P., & Ganiban, J. (2007). Insecure attachment and personality disorder: A twin study of adults. *European Journal of Personality, 21,* 191–208.

Crawford, T. N., Shaver, P. R., Cohen, P., Pilkonis, P. A., Gillath, O., & Kasen, S. (2006). Self-reported attachment, interpersonal aggression, and personality disorder in a prospective community sample of adolescents and adults. *Journal of Personality Disorders, 20,* 331–351.

Creasey, G., & Hesson-McInnis, M. (2001). Affective responses, cognitive appraisals, and conflict tactics in late adolescent romantic relationships: Associations with attachment orientations. *Journal of Counseling Psychology, 48,* 85–96.

Davila, J. (2001). Refining the association between excessive reassurance seeking and depressive symptoms: The role of related interpersonal constructs. *Journal of Social and Clinical Psychology, 20,* 538–559.

Davila, J., Burge, D., & Hammen, C. (1997). Why does attachment style change? *Journal of Personality and Social Psychology, 73,* 826–838.

Davila, J., & Cobb, R. J. (2003). Predicting change in self-reported and interviewer-assessed adult attachment: Tests of the individual difference and life stress models of attachment change. *Personality and Social Psychology Bulletin, 29,* 859–870.

Davila, J., Steinberg, S. J., Kachadourian, L., Cobb, R., & Fincham, F. (2004). Romantic involvement and depressive symptoms in early and late adolescence: The role of a preoccupied relational style. *Personal Relationships, 11,* 161–178.

Davis, D., Shaver, P. R., & Vernon, M. L. (2003). Physical, emotional, and behavioral reactions to breaking up: The roles of gender, age, emotional involvement, and attachment style. *Personality and Social Psychology Bulletin, 29,* 871–884.

DeKlyen, M., & Greenberg, M. T. (2008). Attachment and psychopathology in childhood. In J. Cassidy & P. R. Shaver (Eds.), *Handbook of attachment: Theory, research, and clinical applications* (2nd ed., pp. 637–665). New York: Guilford Press.

Dickinson, K. A., & Pincus, A. L. (2003). Interpersonal analysis of grandiose and vulnerable narcissism. *Journal of Personality Disorders, 17,* 188–207.

Doron, G., Moulding, R., Kyrios, M., Nedeljkovic, M., & Mikulincer, M. (2009). Adult attachment insecurities are related to obsessive compulsive phenomena. *Journal of Social and Clinical Psychology, 28,* 1022–1049.

Ein-Dor, T., Doron, G., Solomon, Z., Mikulincer, M., & Shaver, P. R. (2010). Together in pain: Attachment-related dyadic processes and posttraumatic stress disorder. *Journal of Counseling Psychology, 57,* 317–327.

Enns, M. W., & Cox, B. J. (1997). Personality dimensions and depression: Review and commentary. *Canadian Journal of Psychiatry, 42,* 274–284.

Feeney, J. A. (1995). Adult attachment and emotional control. *Personal Relationships, 2,* 143–159.

Fraley, R. C., Niedenthal, P. M., Marks, M., Brumbaugh, C., & Vicary, A. (2006). Adult attachment and the perception of emotional expressions: Probing the hyperactivating strategies underlying anxious attachment. *Journal of Personality, 74,* 1163–1190.

Fraley, R. C., & Waller, N. G. (1998). Adult attachment patterns: A test of the typological model. In J. A. Simpson & W. S. Rholes (Eds.), *Attachment theory and close relationships* (pp. 77–114). New York: Guilford Press.

Glaser, D. (2001). Child abuse and neglect and the brain: A review. *Journal of Child Psychology and Psychiatry and Allied Disciplines, 41,* 97–116.

Gormley, B., & McNiel, D. E. (2010). Adult attachment orientations, depressive symptoms, anger, and self-directed aggression by psychiatric patients. *Cognitive Therapy and Research, 34,* 272–281.

Gur, O. (2006). *Changes in adjustment and attachment-related representations among high-risk adolescents during residential treatment: The transformational impact of the functioning of caregiving figures as a secure base.* Unpublished doctoral dissertation, Bar-Ilan University, Ramat Gan, Israel.

Hardy, G. E., & Barkham, M. (1994). The relationship between interpersonal attachment styles and work difficulties. *Human Relations, 47,* 263–281.

Hazan, C., & Shaver, P. R. (1987). Romantic love conceptualized as an attachment process. *Journal of Personality and Social Psychology, 52,* 511–524.

Hazan, C., & Shaver, P. R. (1990). Love and work: An attachment-theoretical perspective. *Journal of Personality and Social Psychology, 59,* 270–280.

Hesse, E. (2008). The Adult Attachment Interview: Protocol, method of analysis, and empirical studies. In J. Cassidy & P. R. Shaver (Eds.), *Handbook of attachment: Theory, research, and clinical applications* (2nd ed., pp. 552–598). New York: Guilford Press.

Horowitz, L. M., Rosenberg, S. E., Baer, B. A., Ureno, G., & Villasenor, L. (1988). Inventory of

Interpersonal Problems: Psychometric properties and clinical applications. *Journal of Consulting and Clinical Psychology, 56,* 885–892.

Horowitz, M. J. (1982). Psychological processes induced by illness, injury, and loss. In T. Millon, C. Green, & R. Meagher (Eds.), *Handbook of clinical health psychology* (pp. 53–68). New York: Plenum Press.

Illing, V., Tasca, G. A., Balfour, L., & Bissada, H. (2010). Attachment insecurity predicts eating disorder symptoms and treatment outcomes in a clinical sample of women. *Journal of Nervous and Mental Disease, 198,* 653–659.

Joiner, T. E., & Coyne, J. C. (Eds.). (1999). *The interactional nature of depression: Advances in interpersonal approaches.* Washington, DC: American Psychological Association.

Keelan, J. R., Dion, K. K., & Dion, K. L. (1998). Attachment style and relationship satisfaction: Test of a self-disclosure explanation. *Canadian Journal of Behavioral Science, 30,* 24–35.

Klopfer, B., Ainsworth, M. D. S., Klopfer, W. F., & Holt, R. R. (1954). *Developments in the Rorschach technique* (Vol. 1). Yonkers-on-Hudson, NY: World Book.

Kohut, H., & Wolf, E. (1978). The disorders of the self and their treatment: An outline. *International Journal of Psychoanalysis, 59,* 413–425.

Larose, S., & Bernier, A. (2001). Social support processes: Mediators of attachment state of mind and adjustment in late adolescence. *Attachment and Human Development, 3,* 96–120.

Larose, S., Bernier, A., & Tarabulsy, G. M. (2005). Attachment state of mind, learning dispositions, and academic performance during the college transition. *Developmental Psychology, 41,* 281–289.

Lazarus, R. S., & Folkman, S. (1984). *Stress, appraisal, and coping.* New York: Springer.

Livesley, W. J. (1991). Classifying personality disorders: Ideal types, prototypes, or dimensions? *Journal of Personality Disorders, 5,* 52–59.

Luyten, P., & Blatt, S. (2011). Integrating theory-driven and empirically-derived models of personality development and psychopathology: A proposal for DSM V. *Clinical Psychology Review, 31,* 52–68.

Main, M. (1990). Cross-cultural studies of attachment organization: Recent studies, changing methodologies, and the concept of conditional strategies. *Human Development, 33,* 48–61.

McWilliams, L., & Bailey, J. (2010). Associations between adult attachment ratings and health conditions: Evidence from the National Comorbidity Survey Replication. *Health Psychology, 29,* 446–453.

Meyer, B., & Pilkonis, P. A. (2005). An attachment model of personality disorders. In M. F. Lenzenweger & J. F. Clarkin (Eds.), *Major theories of personality disorder* (2nd ed., pp. 231–281). New York: Guilford Press.

Mikulincer, M. (1995). Attachment style and the mental representation of the self. *Journal of Personality and Social Psychology, 69,* 1203–1215.

Mikulincer, M. (1998). Adult attachment style and affect regulation: Strategic variations in self-appraisals. *Journal of Personality and Social Psychology, 75,* 420–435.

Mikulincer, M., Dolev, T., & Shaver, P. R. (2004). Attachment-related strategies during thought suppression: Ironic rebounds and vulnerable self-representations. *Journal of Personality and Social Psychology, 87,* 940–956.

Mikulincer, M., & Florian, V. (1998). The relationship between adult attachment styles and emotional and cognitive reactions to stressful events. In J. A. Simpson & W. S. Rholes (Eds.,) *Attachment theory and close relationships* (pp. 143–165). New York: Guilford Press.

Mikulincer, M., Florian, V., & Weller, A. (1993). Attachment styles, coping strategies, and post-traumatic psychological distress: The impact of the Gulf War in Israel. *Journal of Personality and Social Psychology, 64,* 817–826.

Mikulincer, M., Hirschberger, G., Nachmias, O., & Gillath, O. (2001). The affective component of the secure base schema: Affective priming with representations of attachment security. *Journal of Personality and Social Psychology, 81,* 305–321.

Mikulincer, M., Horesh, N., Eilati, I., & Kotler, M. (1999). The association between adult attachment style and mental health in extreme life-endangering conditions. *Personality and Individual Differences, 27*, 831–842.

Mikulincer, M., & Orbach, I. (1995). Attachment styles and repressive defensiveness: The accessibility and architecture of affective memories. *Journal of Personality and Social Psychology, 68*, 917–925.

Mikulincer, M., & Shaver, P. R. (2001). Attachment theory and intergroup bias: Evidence that priming the secure base schema attenuates negative reactions to out-groups. *Journal of Personality and Social Psychology, 81*, 97–115.

Mikulincer, M., & Shaver, P. R. (2003). The attachment behavioral system in adulthood: Activation, psychodynamics, and interpersonal processes. In M. P. Zanna (Ed.), *Advances in experimental social psychology* (Vol. 35, pp. 53–152). New York: Academic Press.

Mikulincer, M., & Shaver, P. R. (2004). Security-based self-representations in adulthood: Contents and processes. In W. S. Rholes & J. A. Simpson (Eds.), *Adult attachment: Theory, research, and clinical implications* (pp. 159–195). New York: Guilford Press.

Mikulincer, M., & Shaver, P. R. (2007a). *Attachment in adulthood: Structure, dynamics, and change.* New York: Guilford Press.

Mikulincer, M., & Shaver, P. R. (2007b). Boosting attachment security to promote mental health, prosocial values, and inter-group tolerance. *Psychological Inquiry, 18*, 139–156.

Mikulincer, M., Shaver, P. R., & Horesh, N. (2006). Attachment bases of emotion regulation and posttraumatic adjustment. In D. K. Snyder, J. A. Simpson, & J. N. Hughes (Eds.), *Emotion regulation in families: Pathways to dysfunction and health* (pp. 77–99). Washington, DC: American Psychological Association.

O'Brien, K. M., Friedman, S. M., Tipton, L. C., & Linn, S. G. (2000). Attachment, separation, and women's vocational development: A longitudinal analysis. *Journal of Counseling Psychology, 47*, 301–315.

Park, L. E., Crocker, J., & Mickelson, K. D. (2004). Attachment styles and contingencies of self-worth. *Personality and Social Psychology Bulletin, 30*, 1243–1254.

Pistole, M., & Arricale, F. (2003). Understanding attachment: Beliefs about conflict. *Journal of Counseling and Development, 81*, 318–328.

Powell, B., Cooper, G., Hoffman, K. & Marvin, R. (2007). The Circle of Security project: A case study—"It hurts to give that which you did not receive." In D. Oppenheim & D. Goldsmith (Eds.), *Attachment theory in clinical work with children: Bridging the gap between research and practice* (pp. 172–202). New York: Guilford Press.

Prigerson, H. G., & Jacobs, S. C. (2001). Traumatic grief as a distinct disorder: A rationale, consensus criteria, and a preliminary empirical test. In M. S. Stroebe, R. O. Hansson, W. Stroebe, & H. A. W. Schut (Eds.), *Handbook of bereavement research: Consequences, coping, and care* (pp. 613–647). Washington, DC: American Psychological Association.

Rohde, P., Lewinsohn, P. M., & Seeley, J. R. (1990). Are people changed by the experience of having an episode of depression?: A further test of the scar hypothesis. *Journal of Abnormal Psychology, 99*, 264–271.

Roisman, G. I., Bahadur, M. A., & Oster, H. (2000). Infant attachment security as a discriminant predictor of career development in late adolescence. *Journal of Adolescent Research, 15*, 531–545.

Schachner, D. A., Shaver, P. R., & Mikulincer, M. (2005). Patterns of nonverbal behavior and sensitivity in the context of attachment relationships. *Journal of Nonverbal Behavior, 29*, 141–169.

Scott, R. L., & Cordova, J. V. (2002). The influence of adult attachment styles on the association between marital adjustment and depressive symptoms. *Journal of Family Psychology, 16*, 199–208.

Shaver, P. R., & Hazan, C. (1993). Adult romantic attachment: Theory and evidence. In D. Perlman & W. Jones (Eds.), *Advances in personal relationships* (Vol. 4, pp. 29–70). London: Jessica Kingsley.

Shaver, P. R., & Mikulincer, M. (2002). Attachment-related psychodynamics. *Attachment and Human Development, 4,* 133–161.

Simpson, J. A., Rholes, W. S., Campbell, L., Tran, S., & Wilson, C. L. (2003). Adult attachment, the transition to parenthood, and depressive symptoms. *Journal of Personality and Social Psychology, 84,* 1172–1187.

Solomon, Z., Dekel, R., & Mikulincer, M. (2008). Complex trauma of war captivity: A prospective study of attachment and post-traumatic stress disorder. *Psychological Medicine, 38,* 1427–1434.

Teicher, M. H., Dumont, N. L., Ito, Y., Vaituzis, C., Giedd, J. N., & Andersen, S. L. (2004). Childhood neglect is associated with reduced corpus callosum area. *Biological Psychiatry, 56,* 80–85.

Tracy, J. L., Shaver, P. R., Albino, A. W., & Cooper, M. L. (2003). Attachment styles and adolescent sexuality. In P. Florsheim (Ed.), *Adolescent romance and sexual behavior: Theory, research, and practical implications* (pp. 137–159). Mahwah, NJ: Erlbaum.

Vasquez, K., Durik, A. M., & Hyde, J. S. (2002). Family and work: Implications of adult attachment styles. *Personality and Social Psychology Bulletin, 28,* 874–886.

Wautier, G., & Blume, L. B. (2004). The effects of ego identity, gender role, and attachment on depression and anxiety in young adults. *Identity, 4,* 59–76.

Wei, M., Heppner, P. P., Russell, D. W., & Young, S. K. (2006). Maladaptive perfectionism and ineffective coping as mediators between attachment and future depression: A prospective analysis. *Journal of Counseling Psychology, 53,* 67–79.

Whiffen, V. E., Judd, M. E., & Aube, J. A. (1999). Intimate relationships moderate the association between childhood sexual abuse and depression. *Journal of Interpersonal Violence, 14,* 940–954.

Williams, N. L., & Riskind, J. H. (2004). Adult romantic attachment and cognitive vulnerabilities to anxiety and depression: Examining the interpersonal basis of vulnerability models. *Journal of Cognitive Psychotherapy, 18,* 7–24.

Wink, P. (1991). Two faces of narcissism. *Journal of Personality and Social Psychology, 61,* 590–597.

Wright, J. H., Thase, M. E., & Beck, A. T. (2011). Cognitive therapy. In R. E. Hales, S. C. Yudofsky, & G. Gabbard (Eds.), *Essentials of psychiatry* (3rd ed., pp. 559–587). Arlington, VA: American Psychiatric Publishing.

Zuroff, D. C., & Blatt, S. J. (2006). The therapeutic relationship in the brief treatment of depression: Contributions to clinical improvement and enhanced adaptive capacities. *Journal of Consulting and Clinical Psychology, 74,* 199–206.

Zuroff, D. C., & Fitzpatrick, D. K. (1995). Depressive personality styles: Implications for adult attachment. *Personality and Individual Differences, 18,* 253–365.

CHAPTER 3

The Developmental Perspective

Norka Malberg and Linda C. Mayes

From its very roots, psychoanalysis is inherently a developmental theory in that it focuses on the relationship between early experiences and ongoing mental development and especially adult character. At the same time, the psychoanalytic developmental theory originally emerged not from longitudinal studies of children, but rather from retrospective construction from analyses with adults. Not until psychoanalysts began working with children and pulling in observations from nurseries and preschool programs did the psychoanalytic developmental model become more multidimensional and focus on normative as well as nonnormative change.

Psychoanalytic theories of development have now evolved from their original stage-based developmental map to incorporate models of developmental psychopathology and of nonlinear systems and change (Fonagy & Target, 2003). As a result, contemporary psychoanalytic developmental theory has been increasingly able to capture the complexity and interactive nature of the developing mind across the lifespan. This shift has been facilitated by:

- The influence of attachment theory as a perspective on how early relationships and caring shape social and emotional development (Eagle, 2013).
- The increasing influence of social neuroscience in understanding the impact of early relationships on neural development and on key domains such as emotion and stress regulation (Mayes, Fonagy & Target, 2007).
- The emergence of developmental psychopathology in the early 1990s as a field dedicated to uncovering the developmental course of psychological disorders of childhood and adulthood as a means of highlighting the role of intergenerational transmission of psychopathology and the importance of early intervention (Lyden & Suchman, 2013).

Furthermore, as highlighted by Fonagy, Target, and Gergely (2006), the contemporary expansion of developmental psychoanalysis in the context of developmental psychopathology is evidenced by:

- Increased awareness of the importance of the cultural and social contexts of development.
- The focus on and understanding of the significance of early-childhood experiences.
- Understanding of the role of dependency, attachment, and safety in development alongside the role of instinctual drives.

Today's developmental psychoanalysis creates a narrative that emphasizes the impact of early relational experience on a range of emerging capacities in children (e.g., affect regulation, reward sensitivity, social engagement) and the longitudinal pathways to psychopathology. This approach influences not only theoretical conceptualizations, but also the nature of clinical practice. It places significant emphasis on the intersubjective aspects of the psychoanalytic therapeutic relationship, both on the nonverbal or implicit and on the verbal or explicit dimensions of therapeutic action, as well as their potentially mutative effects.

In this chapter, we explore how the understanding of psychopathology from a developmental psychoanalytic perspective has evolved and been transformed by findings in neuroscience, developmental psychopathology, attachment, and developmental research. We seek to illustrate how this evolution integrates and builds on the work of early theorists and to highlight the contributions of contemporary psychoanalysts to both the theory and the practice of developmental psychoanalysis.

DEFINING THE DEVELOPMENTAL PERSPECTIVE

A developmental perspective has been part of psychoanalytic theory and clinical thinking since its inception. Freud's (1905/1953) *Three Essays on the Theory of Sexuality*, in which he outlined his theory of psychosexual phases, introduced the idea of a staged developmental ontogeny for libidinal change and orientation, setting the scene for what was to be a continuous reworking and evolution of these ideas. This theory of development offered broadly conceived phases of psychosexual maturation based largely on the psychic experience of bodily change and defined through clinical work with adults. The result was what Kennedy (1971) described as the "genetic–reconstructive" approach, in which the focus was placed on the adult's analytic material and how it informs our reconstruction of the childhood experience. Freud (1905/1953, p. 201) himself recognized that reconstructions inevitably contained distortions and recommended that psychoanalytic investigations be supplemented by direct observations of children. Out of this awareness emerged a "developmental approach" concerned with both internal and external influences on children's development. This approach to a psychoanalytic theory of development relied on direct child observation and external sources for evidence of influences on mental development, such as the quality of the child–parent relationship. Thus, from these early roots grew a framework for integration and the emergence of a developmentally informed psychoanalysis with both children and adults.

Anna Freud's work in Vienna and later in London as a clinical observer in the context of the Hampstead War Nurseries exemplifies this approach. As described by Mayes and Cohen (1996), Anna Freud was

> at her natural bent an observer of children, and her observational skills, colored by a psychoanalytic environment, were honed pragmatically. . . . On the one hand, she argued for meticulous, carefully recorded observations of children's moment-to-moment activities and behaviors; on the other, she felt that one of the dangers of academic psychology ran the risk of deriving meaning solely from conscious behaviors with little to no understanding that one behavior might have multiple unconscious determinants. (pp. 119–120)

MAPPING DEVELOPMENT

Psychoanalysis and developmental psychology use different investigative tools to gather their observations. Psychoanalysis draws on principles that originated in clinical research with adults and were then elaborated by work with children, whereas developmental psychology draws on naturalistic observational as well as experimental studies of children. Different research and observational approaches do not always integrate easily. Confusion and controversy have also obstructed discourse. Such confusion can usually be reduced to definitional differences, although controversy often erupts over more substantive matters (Abrams & Solnit, 1998). By the early 20th century, a number of scholars in Europe and the United States were beginning to map various domains of developmental change, from motor to cognitive skills (Gesell, 1937; Piaget, 1937/1954). These domains were typically observable and measurable, and were only loosely related in maturational progression to the psychosexual developmental phases. The challenge for psychoanalysts working with children was to create a more detailed map of development that incorporated changes in the child's internal as well as external landscape.

The psychoanalytic developmental approach therefore had the challenge of integrating the work of theorists from the field of developmental psychology and the emerging field of child psychoanalysis. The strong tendency toward stagelike theories of development bears witness to the influence of existing developmental psychology theories of the time. Furthermore, the motivation of these early theorists came from their wish to extend the understanding of psychopathology from the observation of children in both clinical and naturalistic settings. Spitz (1945), for example, based his thinking about development on his observations of institutionalized infants who had limited access to consistent caregiving and stimulation. He saw new affective expressions such as the social smile as psychic organizers and indicators of a new level in psychic structural organization. For him, development was both cumulative and epigenetic, meaning that each stage was built on the previous one whether the developmental path was normal or pathological, and individual variation in each stage was shaped by environmental and caring experiences. Each stage brought new psychic formations as well as new observable cognitive, motor, and socioemotional capacities.

Another influence on the developing field of developmental psychoanalysis was the work of Jean Piaget (1937/1954), who thought of behavior as an adaptation to the demands of the external world. Indeed, Anne-Marie Sandler (1975), in her review of Piaget's contribution to psychoanalysis, points out that psychoanalysis, rich though it is in many ways, is relatively impoverished in its conceptualization of cognitive processes. In that context, Piaget's detailed study of cognition showed how this field might be relevant to psychoanalysis, both theoretically and clinically, through deepening our understanding of conscious and unconscious processes. Piaget thought of the child's adaptation to the environment as coming to an equilibrium between assimilating new information within already available categories and accommodating new information by forming new categories. Piaget saw this process as altering the development of internal cognitive schemas, while emphasizing the role of external influences in both cognitive and emotional development.

Anna Freud (1965) was a significant contributor to the emergence of a cohesive and integrative developmental psychoanalysis. Her interest in learning about the developmental process beyond the understanding of children's neurotic psychopathology, together with her departure from a rigid and stagelike conceptualization of psychopathology, contributed to the emergence of a more integrated and fluid developmental view of normality and pathology. One of her principal legacies is the blending of innovative perspectives into established facts and theories of psychoanalysis (Abrams & Solnit, 1998). Her concept of lines of development represents perhaps the best-known psychoanalytic developmental map. The lines stand as "historical realities which, when assembled, convey a convincing picture of an individual child's personal achievements or, on the other hand, of his failures in personality development" (Freud, 1965, p. 64).

This contribution was a major step forward in the application of an approach that viewed personality and pathology as being the interaction between major mental agencies (ego, superego, and id) and external reality. From this perspective, psychopathology was understood as the result of disharmonies between the different lines of development—an interactive process involving both internal and external realities. This was reflected in the emphasis on understanding the ego in all its aspects: developmental, integrative, adaptive and economic. Anna Freud stressed the fact that psychological development does not end with childhood but continues throughout the lifespan. A picture of development emerged as an active, dynamic process, always interactive with experience and environment, and always purposeful in providing the child with the optimal available adaptation, given external and internal needs and demands. This view of development invited the inclusion of both the influence and interaction of the individual's biology and his or her relational environment.

In accordance with this view, the contemporary field of developmental psychopathology further promotes a move away from the stage-based developmental map, to incorporate new ideas involving models of nonlinear systems and change. Work in this new field focuses on understanding the interplay and genesis between normality and pathology. The goal is to comprehend the processes of adaptation and maladaptation across the lifespan by pursuing multiple levels of analysis and a multidomain approach to mapping development (Cicchetti & Cohen, 2006). In many ways, the field of developmental psychopathology has come to provide, in psychoanalytic terms, a "container" for the integration of both developmental psychology and psychoanalytic methods of studying and understanding development and psychopathology. As a result, a contemporary developmental psychoanalytic perspective is characterized by a focus on an increasing level of integration and adaptation, and the capacity, in both theoretical and clinical settings, to capture the complexity and interactive nature of the developing mind across the lifespan in its theory and its clinical applications (Matthew, 1998).

CLASSICAL PSYCHOANALYTIC DEVELOPMENTAL THEORY: EMERGENCE AND EVOLUTION

The developmental perspective is acknowledged by all genuinely psychoanalytic theories to some degree (Fonagy, Target, & Gergely, 2006), transcending the different versions of development of the various classical psychoanalytic schools. This point of view is now expanding in the light of current scientific evidence and ongoing clinical exploration in the contemporary developmental psychodynamic landscape. The shift away from a "genetic–reconstructive" understanding of psychopathology began early on in the history of psychoanalysis with Freud's development of the structural model of the mind (Sandler, Holder, Dare, & Dreher, 1997), and with it came the understanding of anxiety as a response to both internal and external stimuli. In this way, Freud restored adaptation to the external world as an essential part of the psychoanalytic account and set the scene for the emergence of several models of development that still influence the work of contemporary developmental psychoanalysis. These models ranged from those that conceive of development as relying on "an average expectable environment" that affirms the importance of the actual parent (Hartmann, 1950/1964) to later modified versions describing all mental activity—both interactional and intersubjective—as relational, and defining internalization as the basic psychological process that propels development (Loewald, 1978). Increasingly, a shift occurred from a one-person psychology toward an interactional approach (a two-person system) that informed the field's understanding of development: That is, psychological development requires the care (and mind) of the parent and affirms that it is the infant's place in the mind of the parent that gives rise to the quality of the infant's own mental life.

Within the evolution of developmental psychoanalysis there have been several different narratives regarding progression along the developmental path across the lifespan, all of which have come to coexist and influence both psychoanalytic theory and clinical technique. Initially, the psychoanalytic developmental model emphasized the centrality of the drives, in which the primary motivation was the reduction of internal tension in a quest for homeostasis. Viewed through this lens, the interest in object relations emerges in the course of development and comes secondary to the primitive motives. As a result, psychopathology was equated with very early development. For example, early conceptualizations in child psychoanalysis depicted the infant going through subjective phases that paralleled adult psychotic states (Klein, 1946/1952). However, as this model evolved, informed by observational studies of children, interest grew in motives and processes separate from the drives and a reconceptualization of psychopathology in terms of developmental deficits instead of solely as a result of drive–defense conflict. This view slowly moved away from the centrality of the Oedipus complex and focused on the impact of early dyadic processes as the foundation of ego development. In other words, the quality of the early relationship (object relation) and its influence in the development of the internal organization was seen as central. Informed by this shift away from the primacy of the drives, other models of development attempted to portray the physically dependent infant while depicting his or her social nature from the beginning and its importance in terms of personality development. Descriptions of the early gradual process of separation and differentiation depicted an infant ready to engage in the drama of finding him- or herself in the eyes of his or her primary caregiver (Winnicott, 1965). A focus on the importance of the quality and psychological availability of early care and interpersonal organization became increasingly central in the conceptualizations of child psychoanalysis and developmental theory. In the words of Clarke and Scharff (2014), "A fundamental contribution of object relations theory comes from the principle inherent in the formulation of the complex relationship between the infant and the mother. It is the notion that one must understand the subjective experience of the child to understand the meaning of the object relationships involved" (p. 19).

An early example of this lens is found in the work of Margaret Mahler (Mahler, Pine, & Bergman, 1975), who studied the mother–child relationship and the longitudinal correlation between object relations and psychic structure formation. Mahler's work is a good example of how the primacy of object relations is assumed and the basically "object-seeking" character of instincts is emphasized. This description of object relations contributed significantly to the clinical understanding of borderline personality disorder patients—specifically Mahler's view of patients as fixated in a rapprochement, wishing to cling but fearing the loss of their fragile sense of self, wishing to be separate but also fearing to move away from the parental figure (Fonagy & Target, 2003).

However, Mahler's description of the infant in a state of primary narcissism, that is, a state in which there is no differentiation and complete dependency, is disputed by contemporary evidence on infant development that depicts a newborn infant actively perceiving and learning, with specific expectations about the structure of the physical and social world (Gergely, 1992). The infant is seen as an active agent in the relationship, with an emerging sense of intentionality and an innate capacity to seek, encourage, and (when necessary) avoid relating (Tronick, 2007).

The integration of these findings on newborn and infant learning within an object relations frame seeks to explore the epigenetic evolution of fundamental constructs such as cognition and affect in the context of the relational sphere (Dodge & Rutter, 2011). For example, early formulations initiated by Sandler and Rosenblatt (1962) and expanded by Fonagy, Gergely, Jurist, and Target (2002) place feeling states and the notion of a feeling of safety at the center of the psychoanalytic theory of motivation. In this model, the affect state is seen as the key organizer of interpersonal relationships as well as cognition in infancy throughout the developmental continuum. Psychopathology is no longer equated solely with disruptive experiences in infancy and a fixation at an earlier developmental stage, but instead it is understood as a more complex interaction of early caring, biology, and endowment/genetic factors.

Contemporary developmental psychoanalytic models are systemic in nature. Development is viewed as a consequence of the continuous interaction between the person (psychology and endowment) and the environment (the relationship between the person and the social systems). In order to predict development under this transactional model (Sameroff, 2009), one must examine a system of interactional exchanges and continual restructuring. In many ways, this idea is similar to Anna Freud's invitation to child analysts always to keep in mind the question "What moves development along?" and to gather conceptual approaches from multiple disciplines while maintaining a respect for the analytic observational tool (Freud, 1958). Out of the contemporary push toward the integration of multiple investigative tools, and with new knowledge coming from multiple fields (neuroscience, attachment theory, clinical case studies, developmental psychology and psychopathology, and genetics, among others), a new brand of contemporary developmental psychoanalysis has emerged, which enhances its capacity to influence other fields as well as its ability to develop interventions that translate psychoanalytic theory and practice in the context of multidisciplinary systems.

TOWARD AN INTEGRATIVE CONTEMPORARY PSYCHOANALYTIC MODEL

Developmental psychoanalysis has become more explicitly integrative in its quest for new ways to understand the development of psychopathology. It seeks the integration of earlier psychoanalytic theories with contemporary ideas, and it promotes a more active dialogue and process of cross-fertilization with other fields that study development, such as cognitive and affective neuroscience, psychology, and education. In addition, its focus is not solely on an individual, but also on the many systems in which that individual develops and functions. Furthermore, specific conceptual constructs that are developed from clinical data facilitate and inform this integration.

The Concept of Intersubjectivity and its Centrality in Contemporary Developmental Psychoanalysis

Contemporary psychoanalytic developmental theory emerges from an object relations tradition in which psychological development is viewed as occurring in an interpersonal matrix (Blatt & Levy, 2003). In recent years, different psychoanalytic schools of thought have converged in an effort to formulate psychoanalysis as a relational theory. In this context, intersubjectivity has been defined in the context of the analytic situation as the field of intersection between two subjectivities, the interplay between two different subjective worlds (Benjamin, 1990). A common thread is found in the belief that the human mind is interactive, that is, inherently social, rather than monadic, and that the psychoanalytic process should be understood as occurring between subjects rather than within the individual. From this perspective, mental life is seen though an intersubjective lens (Benjamin, 1990; Fonagy et al., 2002). This shift, in combination with the groundbreaking work of infant researchers (Beebe, 2005; Stern, 1985) that documented intersubjectivity at the outset of human development, has allowed developmental psychoanalysis in the past 25 years to tap into the rich vein of research on attachment. As described by Fonagy and Target (2007),

> Infant research teaches us that human external reality is inherently shared because it is constructed out of shared feelings, shared intentions and shared plans. . . . This shared reality, which is largely built within attachment relationships, may well give knowledge of the external world a lasting sense of significance and pleasure (or more negative qualities such as danger, depending on the quality of the early relationship). (p. 921)

From this point of view, relationships are the organizers of psychic life. The focus is thus on the dynamic interchange between people instead of within the individual mind. As a result, the dyad, rather than the individual, becomes the fundamental unit of development, and dyadic structures organize mental life from the start. This opens up new ways of conceptualizing the developmental pathways of specific psychopathologies that guide our clinical formulations and practice (Fonagy et al., 2002). The field of trauma is an example of how this evolution has benefited our understanding and clinical practice with this population. There has been much progress, for example, in understanding the link between an early history of abusive or neglectful environments and the development of psychopathology (Cicchetti & Lynch, 1993; Raineki, Cortés, Belnoue, & Sullivan, 2012). The relevance of this research extends to changes in social policy and effective clinical interventions with high-risk populations (Midgley & Vouvra, 2012; Solomon & George, 2011), allowing the psychoanalytic developmental tradition to reclaim its legacy of informing social change.

Attachment Theory and Its Impact on Contemporary Developmental Psychoanalysis

Although psychoanalysis and attachment theory were originally seen as incompatible perspectives, it is now evident that there are important synergies between them (Blatt & Levy, 2003; Eagle, 2013). In the past 25 years, attachment theory, rooted in the premise that a continuous exchange between theory, practice, and research is essential, has become an integrative force that has facilitated interdisciplinary dialogue and exchange. Today, the language of attachment has become probably one of the most common of the developmental perspectives familiar to psychologists, social workers, counselors, and other allied professionals such as pediatricians and teachers (Tyson, 2000).

Bowlby (1979), a psychoanalyst himself, felt that actual events such as loss and separation affected the development of the child and the later functioning of the individual in adulthood. He emphasized the importance of understanding infant–mother attachment as being based on a primary and autonomous instinctual system instead of a derivative of the drives. Because it emerged through observations of real-life separations and losses in childhood, attachment theory reflects the emphasis on an integrative view of human development that brings together internal and external experience, relationships among children and adults, and a broader systemic view of a child's environment.

Contemporary clinical researchers working using the attachment lens, such as Steele and Steele (2008), have built on the efforts of Ainsworth (1970), who operationalized the study of the effect the quality of maternal care has on the development of the child's behavioral patterns of attachment. Ainsworth's work using the Strange Situation and Mary Main's work on the Adult Attachment Interview (AAI; Main, 1991) was pivotal in facilitating a bridge between contemporary attachment research and its clinical applications and developmental psychoanalysis. For example, Main's research using the AAI first suggested that a parent's metacognitive capacity, that is, the ability to reflect on one's experiences, serves as a significant protective factor. In follow-up studies, Carlson and Sroufe (1995) and van IJzendoorn (1995) focused on the importance of a mother's capacity to regulate and organize her thoughts and feelings about her own childhood history of receiving care. They found that this capacity linked to her ability to regulate, organize, and respond sensitively to her child's own attachment needs (comfort, safety, and closeness). This was a significant shift toward an emphasis on the impact of the quality of the relationship on the child's emotional and social development and on defining a "developmental environment."

Working from an interactional model, developmental psychoanalysis has further explored and expanded on this notion, while retaining its focus on the investigation of mental processes as experienced and constructed from a subjective perspective. A clear link exists between adult psychopathology and having a "good enough" experience of a parental mind that can "keep the child in mind" in a way that allows the child to experience and develop his or her own separate and unique sense of self within a safe and predictable intersubjective space. Fonagy and colleagues (2002) addressed this link by integrating developmental psychoanalytic constructs with emerging findings from the fields of social cognition, neuroscience, and genetics under the umbrella of attachment theory and research, and redefined the already existing construct of *mentalization*. Mentalization, which was developed as an empirically testable construct, was first operationalized as *reflective functioning*, an overt manifestation in narrative of an individual's mentalizing capacity (Fonagy, Target, Steele, & Steele, 1998; Slade, 2005). This core psychological capacity is defined as the ability to understand the behaviors of the self and others in terms of underlying mental states and intentions. More specifically, through the capacity to mentalize, individuals are able to explain the behaviors of the self and others by reference to the present state and intentions of the agent (such as beliefs, hopes, and wishes). From this perspective, mentalizing can be described as the key to social communication and information gathering (Fonagy, Luyten & Strathearn, 2011).

Follow-up studies have extended Main's original findings (Main, 1991; Main & Goldwyn, 1984), suggesting that a primary caregiver who is able to hold on to complex mental states (that is, one who is able to mentalize effectively) is able to hold her child's internal affective experience in mind, thereby facilitating her understanding of her child's behavior with respect to the child's own feelings and intentions. The caregiver, functioning from this *reflective stance*, imparts meaning to the child's affective experiences in a way that promotes the child's affect regulation and emerging sense of self. In this way, the caregiver fosters the child's emotional security (Fonagy, Steele, & Steele, 1991; Steele, Steele, Croft, & Fonagy, 1999). Especially in circumstances of adversity, mentalizing capacity on the part of the caregiver is vital to maintain and facilitate a range of progressive developmental processes in the child. Conversely, the absence of this experience of effective parental mentalizing is seen as underlying the development of various forms of psychopathology in the child. By operationalizing reflective functioning as a measure of mentalizing capacity and studying the impact of parental reflective functioning on a child's development, psychoanalytic researchers have demonstrated the importance of the caregiver's mentalizing capacity to the normative developmental outcome of the child. The findings of this research have highlighted—for child psychotherapists and for other allied professionals working with children—the importance of working with parents in exploring the meaning of the parenting experience and how it impacts their reflective capacities (Toth, Rogosch, & Cicchetti, 2008). This issue is particularly relevant in the context of intergenerational transmission of relational trauma (Suchman, Decoste, Ordsay, & Beers, 2013).

INTEGRATION AND CROSS-FERTILIZATION FROM A DEVELOPMENTAL PERSPECTIVE

Social Neuroscience and the Developing Social Brain

An example of cross-fertilization from other fields is found in the strong evidence provided by social neuroscience for the role of early attunement in relationships on the longitudinal development of affect regulation and capacity to engage in relationships (Schore, 2003). For instance, there is now strong evidence demonstrating the negative impact of neglectful and/or abusive early relationships on development and an association with a diverse range of adverse neurodevelopmental outcomes, including long-term cognitive and academic delays. Similarly, there is now good evidence about adverse effects on the overall development of a child's brain architecture (National Scientific Council on the Developing Child, 2008). This evidence has resulted in the development of innovative dyadic modalities of treatment (Lieberman & Van Horn, 2008; Suchman et al., 2013) that integrate psychoanalytic thinking based on clinical data (Fraiberg, Adelson, & Shapiro, 1975) and research findings from the fields of neuroscience and attachment.

The empirical findings from these clinical applications facilitate the conceptualization of psychopathology as more than the results of maladaptive internal working models resulting from experiences of relational and environmental trauma. Rather, the integration of the social-cognitive lens into the conceptualizations of developmental psychoanalysis allows for movement away from a disorder-centered approach and introduces a conceptualization of the patient's pathology as the result of difficulties in social adaptation and stress regulation. An example of this integration is found in the work of Csibra and Gergely (2011), who have coined the term *the pedagogic stance* to describe a human-specific, cue-driven social-cognitive adaptation of mutual design, dedicated to ensuring efficient transfer of relevant cultural knowledge. From this point of view, humans are predisposed to "teach" and "learn" new and relevant cultural knowledge. This adaptation is part of a developmental progression throughout life, but it is particularly relevant at certain key stages in development such as adolescence, when the capacity to learn from others is most required. Gergely, Egyed, and Kiraly (2007) speak of "ostensive communicative cues" as a means by which "teachers" (caregivers) indicate to a child that information that is about to be transmitted is trustworthy and generalizable beyond the current situation ("epistemic trust") (see also Luyten, Beutel, & Shahar, Chapter 14, and Mayes, Luyten, Blatt, Fonagy, & Target, Chapter 25, this volume). In infancy, these cues include eye contact, turn-taking contingent reactivity, and the use of special vocal tone by the caregiver, and they establish the adult as having the infant's subjective experience in mind. This empirical developmental research has direct relevance to therapeutic work. By mentalizing the other in the context of a developmentally informed clinical intervention, the therapist is providing the patient with the experience of feeling as if someone sees the world from his or her perspective, having established a situation of epistemic trust. In this way, the therapy offers a new developmental experience and an environment of "safety" in which the patient is able to feel understood and to open up to learning about both his or her internal world and external world (Fonagy & Bateman, 2012).

Gene × Environment Interactions and the Impact of Care on Gene Regulation

Most mental disorders are multifactorial, meaning that their etiology involves multiple genetic and multiple environmental factors. In the past decade, researchers have moved away from the study of purely genetic effects and toward the research of gene × environment interactions in the field of psychiatric genetics (Bakermans-Kranenburg & van IJzendoorn, 2007). Rutter and Silberg (2002) described three reasons justifying the exploration of this interaction. First, a genetically influenced differential response to the environment constitutes the mechanism thought to give rise to evolutionary change. Second, to suppose that there are no gene × environment interactions would seem to require the assumption that environmental responsivity is the one biological feature that is uniquely outside genetic influence. Third, a wide range of naturalistic and experimental studies in humans and animals have shown great heterogeneity in response to all manner of environmental features, both physical and psychosocial, confirming in this way the inevitable involvement of genetic influence.

Initial support for this field came from animal studies such as those conducted with rhesus macaque monkeys by Suomi (2011) and colleagues, which showed that an environmental feature, namely, whether monkeys were peer-reared or mother-reared, altered the impact of genes. More recent human studies, such as those conducted by Gunnar and Vazquez (2006), support the importance of exploring gene

× environment interactions in the context of the impact of care on gene regulation. Gunnar and Vazquez found that secure attachment plays a crucial role in buffering the effects of stress in early development, leading to what is called "adaptive hypo-activity" of the hypothalamic–pituitary–adrenal axis in early development, which in turn results in resilience in the face of adversity. This work has great potential to significantly influence interventions with children involved with the child welfare system, just as Bowlby's work and the naturalistic observations of Spitz (1945) changed policies regarding the hospitalization of children and the understanding of the meaning of loss and separation to children. Furthermore, research on gene × environment interactions supports a shift away from a deterministic view of developmental psychopathology, as well as supporting the value of relationally based psychoanalytic interventions. In the context of early-childhood maltreatment and neglect, for instance, the identification of susceptibility genes and how environmental factors interact with these genes facilitates our ability to identify risk and targets for developing interventions to preempt the onset of illness, and guides efforts to tailor and personalize treatments for individuals with stress-related mental health problems (Perepletchikova et al., 2011).

HOW DEVELOPMENTAL PSYCHOANALYSIS INFORMS CONTEMPORARY MODALITIES OF TREATMENT

Perhaps the greatest challenge to the classical conceptualization of adult psychopathology as being directly linked with infantile experiences comes from the ever-growing understanding in developmental psychoanalysis of the complexity and fluidity of the developmental continuum. This understanding is in turn informed by contemporary findings in neuroscience, genetics, and developmental psychopathology. This shift is evident in the clinical accounts of contemporary child psychoanalysts, who often reflect on the need for clinical modification when working with specific pathologies and the importance of a research-informed systemic approach to intervention (Boston Charge Process Study Group, 2007).

The work of infant researchers within the attachment tradition supports the need to revisit not only our theoretical understanding of psychopathology but also the components of our clinical practice. This evolution represents a challenge to the classical view of the psychoanalyst as a neutral and somewhat passive agent of change. Infant research in combination with the ever-growing literature on parent–infant psychotherapy (Baradon, 2010) has resulted in new ways of conceptualizing adult clinical material from a developmental perspective. This has influenced the way we think about important technical concepts such as countertransference in both adult and child treatment. For instance, viewed from a "dyadic systemic perspective" (Beebe & Lachmann, 2002), the relationship between the patient and the psychotherapist is thought of in the context of "interactive tilts" in which the patient's unconscious goals—for instance, his or her need to obtain the love and approval of the therapist—affect the patient's self-regulatory range and interactive patterns in the room. Faced with these "tilts," the therapist, in the same way as a sensitive parent, attempts to respond to them by exploring his or her own need for the patient and remains aware of a state of "interactive vigilance in the room" as the interactive system is tilted toward regulating the patient's state. As the psychotherapist allows the reinstatement of a flexible movement back and forth in the room, the process of psychotherapy is understood from this systems perspective as a continual co-construction of experience.

This explanatory process is similar to that described by Fonagy and Bateman (2012) in their work with borderline patients using mentalization-based treatment (MBT). In this approach, the psychotherapist assesses the current stress-regulation capacities and interpersonal functioning of the patient, framed by a developmental understanding of the patient's relational history and how it has impacted his or her current functioning. Much of this formulation of the patient's functioning is informed by both the therapist's experience of the patient in the "here-and-now," and the emerging knowledge and understanding of the patient's internal representations of the self in the context of relationships. In this way, the contemporary developmental psychoanalytic perspective is one that explores the intersubjective processes that informed psychic development from the beginning of life through to adulthood, and attempts to translate this evolving body of clinical and research findings to the development of cohesive and integrative interventions. Here we briefly describe two such interventions.

Mentalization-Based Treatment for Adolescents: A Clinical Intervention Informed by the Contemporary Developmental Perspective

An example of a psychoanalytically informed developmental intervention is the work of Trudie Rossouw with self-harming adolescents. Mentalization-based treatment for adolescents (MBT-A) has produced valuable clinical insights regarding the importance of integrating modalities when working with such adolescents. One of the landmarks of Rossouw's intervention is the exploration of what Fonagy and Bateman (2012) have termed "the alien self." The alien self is an internal representation of the self that emerges in the context of a relational exchange filled with parental projection, characterized by the absence of curiosity and inquisitiveness regarding the child's intentions, wishes, and feelings. Like other MBT interventions, Rossouw's (2012) work seeks to help young persons and their families to improve their awareness of their own mental states and the mental states of others by enhancing their capacity to mentalize. MBT-A integrates explicit and implicit ways of encouraging the reflective capacities of the young person and family. Family interventions consist of focused and experiential approaches to psychoeducation, insight, and modeling of a reflective and inquisitive stance by the psychotherapist. By working with the young person and the family in the here-and-now, the intervention seeks to provide a new relational experience for both the young person and the family. In this experience, internal representations can be revisited with the aim of producing more coherent narratives of the self in the context of relationships and, most importantly, increasing a sense of agency and with it an improved capacity for "mentalized affectivity" (thinking while experiencing strong and activating feelings; Fonagy et al., 2002; Jurist, 2005).

Outcome research from this intervention provides support for the clinical hypothesis, with young people's self-harming behaviors showing significant reduction, coupled with improvements in their parents' reflective capacities (Midgley & Vrouva, 2012).

Mothering from the Inside Out: A Dyadic Clinical Intervention

Mothering from the Inside Out (Suchman et al., 2013) is a 20-week individual attachment-based therapy intervention that aims to help mothers with substance abuse problems develop more balanced representations of their children and improve their capacity to mentalize (operationalized for research as reflective functioning). The program seeks to intervene individually with mothers in order to improve their capacity to respond sensitively to their young children's cues, to respond and soothe their children when distressed, and to foster progressive social and emotional development in their children (all characteristics of reflective functioning). The program assesses the mothers' attachment patterns and the quality of their attributions regarding their children's behaviors. The intervention seeks to identify and prevent potential intergenerational transmission of maladaptive patterns of attachment behavior, which had potentially already influenced the psychological trajectory of the parent. By tackling intergenerational transmission of representations, this intervention offers the mother the opportunity of a new developmental experience, one that allows her to consider new ways of responding and interacting with her child. The aim of this approach is to improve the mother's representational balance and reflective functioning capacities.

As evidenced in these examples of work with adolescents and mother–toddler dyads, contemporary developmental psychoanalysis seeks to integrate disciplines and clinical modalities in the same fashion as it did more than 50 years ago. However, the ever-growing link between research and practice, and the technological advances in fields such as neurology and genetics, allow a wider scope of ideas to influence our clinical practice and confirm some of the basic tenets of the field. However, at its core the developmental psychoanalytic intervention continues to seek the same goals— namely, to foster progressive development by facilitating the emergence of a coherent sense of self, the capacity to handle emotions (affect regulation), and the general capacity for self-observation in the context of relationships.

CONCLUSIONS AND FUTURE DIRECTIONS

Developmental psychoanalysis has both expanded and evolved in the context of developmental psychopathology, as evidenced by increased awareness of the importance of the cultural and social contexts of development; the focus on and understanding of the significance of early-childhood experiences; and the expansion of a conceptualization that considers understanding the role of dependency, attachment, and safety in development alongside the role of instinctual drives and also the awareness regarding the synthesizing function of the self (Fonagy et al., 2006). Developmental psychoanalysis has evolved and taken on a developmental psychopathology perspective that acknowledges the constant interplay between biology/endowment and experience/ environment. Child psychoanalysts and developmentally oriented psychodynamic clinicians are taking their work to outreach settings (hospitals, schools, prisons) and are translating the rich language of contemporary developmental psychoanalysis into models that are accessible and innovative (Zanetti, Powell, Cooper, & Hoffman, 2011).

In general, advances in the fields of cognitive neuroscience and genetics have informed a progression toward a more flexible, integrative, and systemic developmental psychodynamic approach. The psychoanalytic focus on the representation of subjectivity and how it emerges from early development has much to contribute to the understanding of individual differences in the quality of functioning of basic mental mechanisms and how they are affected by early adversity. Most important, developmental psychoanalysis and its conceptualization of the mind as an immediate experience, a sensation, a motivation, an action, and perceptions rooted in the body and its developmental experiences (Klin & Jones, 2007), bring further depth to the analysis. Furthermore, psychoanalytic developmental conceptualizations add to the understanding of processes such as resilience and the long-term sequelae of chronic stress. The examples of clinical conceptualization and practice in this chapter illustrate how contemporary developmental psychoanalysis tells a story of a developing mind in the context of the interpersonal matrix as it is influenced by both internal and external variables. A psychoanalytic perspective on development and psychopathology identifies and operationalizes central constructs and agents of change responsible for the continuities and discontinuities along a developmental continuum.

REFERENCES

Abrams, S., & Solnit, A. J. (1998). Coordinating developmental and psychoanalytic processes: Conceptualizing technique. *Journal of the American Psychoanalytic Association, 46*, 85–103.

Ainsworth, M. D. S. (1970). Attachment, exploration and separation: Illustrated by the behaviour of one-year olds in a strange situation. *Child Development, 41*, 49–67.

Bakermans-Kranenburg, M. J., & van IJzendoorn, M. H. (2007). Genetic vulnerability or differential susceptibility in child development: The case of attachment. *Journal of Child Psychology and Psychiatry, 48*, 1160–1173.

Baradon, T. (2010). *Relational trauma in infancy: Psychoanalytic, attachment and neuropsychological contributions to parent–infant psychotherapy*. London: Routledge.

Beebe, B. (2005). Mother–infant research informs mother–infant treatment. *Psychoanalytic Study of the Child, 60*, 7–46.

Beebe, B., & Lachmann, F. M. (2002). *Infant research and adult treatment: Co-constructing interactions*. New York: Analytic Press.

Benjamin, J. (1990). An outline of inter-subjectivity: The development of recognition. *Psychoanalytic Psychology, 7*, 33–46.

Blatt, S. J., & Levy, K. N. (2003). Attachment theory, psychoanalysis, personality development, and psychopathology. *Psychoanalytic Inquiry, 23*, 102–150.

Boston Change Process Study Group. (2007). The foundation level of psychodynamic meaning: Implicit process in relation to conflict, defense and the dynamic unconscious. *International Journal of Psychoanalysis, 88*, 843–860.

Bowlby, J. (1979). *The making and breaking of affectional bonds*. London: Tavistock.

Carlson, E., & Sroufe, L. A. (1995). The contribution of attachment theory to developmental psychopathology. In D. Cicchetti & D. Cohen (Eds.), *Developmental processes and psychopathology: Vol. 1. Theoretical perspectives and methodological approaches* (pp. 581–617). New York: Cambridge University Press.

Cicchetti, D., & Cohen, D. J. (Eds.). (2006). *Developmental psychopathology: Vol. I. Theory and method* (2nd ed.). Hoboken, NJ: Wiley.

Cicchetti, D., & Lynch, M. (1993). Toward an ecological/transactional model of community violence and child maltreatment: Consequences for children's development. *Psychiatry, 56,* 96–118.

Clarke, G. S., & Scharff, D. E. (2014). *Fairbairn and the object relations tradition.* London: Karnac Books.

Csibra, G., & Gergely, G. (2011). Natural pedagogy as evolutionary adaptation. *Philosophical Transaction of the Royal Society of London. Series B, Biological Sciences, 36,* 1149–1157.

Dodge, K. A., & Rutter, M. (2011). *Gene–environment interactions in developmental psychopathology.* New York: Guilford Press.

Eagle, M. N. (2013). *Attachment and psychoanalysis: Theory, research, and clinical implications.* New York: Guilford Press.

Fonagy, P., & Bateman, A. (2012). *Handbook of mentalizing in mental health practice.* Washington, DC: American Psychiatric Publishing.

Fonagy, P., Gergely, G., Jurist, E., & Target, M. (2002). *Affect regulation, mentalization, and the development of the self.* New York: Other Press.

Fonagy, P., Luyten, P., & Strathearn, L. (2011). Borderline personality disorder, mentalization, and the neurobiology of attachment. *Infant Mental Health Journal, 32,* 47–69.

Fonagy, P., Steele, H., & Steele, M. (1991). Maternal representations of attachment during pregnancy predict the organization of infant–mother attachment at one year. *Child Development. 62,* 891–905.

Fonagy, P., & Target, M. (2003). Psychoanalytic theories: Perspectives from developmental psychopathology. London: Whurr.

Fonagy, P., & Target, M. (2007). Playing with reality: IV. A theory of external reality rooted in intersubjectivity. *International Journal of Psychoanalysis, 88,* 917–937.

Fonagy, P., Target, M., & Gergely, G. (2006). Psychoanalytic perspectives on developmental psychopathology. In D. Cicchetti & D. J. Cohen (Eds.), *Developmental psychopathology. Vol. 1: Theory and method* (2nd ed., pp. 701–749). Hoboken, NJ: Wiley.

Fonagy, P., Target, M., Steele, H., & Steele, M. (1998). Reflective-functioning manual (Version 5) for application to Adult Attachment Interviews. Unpublished manual. Psychoanalysis Unit, University College London.

Fraiberg, S., Adelson, E., & Shapiro, V. (1975). Ghosts in the nursery: A psychoanalytic approach to the problems of impaired infant–mother relationships. *Journal of the American Academy of Child Psychiatry, 14,* 387–421.

Freud, A. (1958). Child observation and prediction of development. *Psychoanalytic Study of the Child, 13,* 117–124.

Freud, A. (1965). *Normality and pathology in childhood: Assessments of development.* New York: International Universities Press.

Freud, S. (1953). Three essays on the theory of sexuality. In J. Strachey (Ed. & Trans.), *The standard edition of the complete psychological works of Sigmund Freud* (Vol. 7, pp. 123–230). London: Hogarth Press. (Original work published 1905)

Gergely, G. (1992). Developmental reconstructions: Infancy from the point of view of psychoanalysis and developmental psychology. *Psychoanalysis and Contemporary Thought, 15,* 3–55.

Gergely, G., Egyed, K., & Kiraly, I. (2007). On pedagogy. *Developmental Science, 10,* 139–146.

Gesell, A. (1937). Infants are individuals. *Vital Speeches of the Day, 4,* 132.

Gunnar, M., & Vazquez, D. (2006). Stress neurobiology and developmental psychopathology. In D. Cicchetti & D. J. Cohen (Eds.), *Developmental psychopathology: Vol. II. Developmental neuroscience* (pp. 533–577). Hoboken, NJ: Wiley.

Hartmann, H. (1964). *Comments on the psychoanalytic theory of the ego*. New York: International Universities Press, 1964. (Original work published 1950)

Jurist, E. L. (2005). Mentalized affectivity. *Psychoanalytic Psychology, 22*, 426–444.

Kennedy, H. (1971). Problems in reconstruction in child analysis. *Psychoanalytic Study of the Child, 26*, 386–402.

Klein, M. (1952). Notes on some schizoid mechanisms. In M. Klein, P. Heimann, S. Isaacs, & J. Riviere (Eds.), *Developments in psychoanalysis* (pp. 292–320). London: Hogarth Press. (Original work published 1946)

Klin, A., & Jones, W. (2007). Embodied psychoanalysis? Or, on the confluence of psychodynamic theory and developmental science. In L. Mayes, P. Fonagy, & M. Target (Eds.), *Developmental science and psychoanalysis: Integration and innovation* (pp. 5–38). London: Karnac Books.

Lieberman, A. F., & Van Horn, P. (2008). *Psychotherapy with infants and young children: Repairing the effects of stress and trauma on early attachment*. New York: Guilford Press.

Loewald, H. W. (1978). Instinct theory, object relations and psychic structure formation. In *Papers on Psychoanalysis* (pp. 207–218). New Haven, CT: Yale University Press.

Lyden, H. M., & Suchman, N. E. (2013). Transmission of parenting models at the level of representation: Implications for mother-child dyads affected by maternal substance abuse. In N. E. Suchman, M. Pajulo, & L. C. Mayes (Eds.), *Parenting and substance abuse: Developmental approaches to intervention* (pp. 100–120). New York: Oxford University Press.

Mahler, M., Pine, F., & Bergman, A. (1975). *The psychological birth of the human infant: Symbiosis and individuation*. New York: Basic Books.

Main, M. (1991). Metacognitive knowledge, metacognitive monitoring, and singular (coherent) vs. multiple (incoherent) models of attachment: Some findings and some directions for future research. In P. Marris, J. Stevenson-Hinde, & C. Parkes (Eds.), *Attachment across the life cycle* (pp. 127–159). New York: Routledge.

Main, M., & Goldwyn, R. (1984). Predicting rejection of her infant from mother's representation of her experiences: Implications for the abused-abusing intergenerational cycle. *Child Abuse and Neglect, 8*, 203–217.

Matthew, J. (1998). Psychological differential diagnosis: Alternatives to the DSM system. *Journal of Contemporary Psychotherapy, 28*, 91–95.

Mayes, L. C., & Cohen, D. J. (1996). Anna Freud and developmental psychoanalytic psychology. *Psychoanalytic Study of the Child, 51*, 117–141.

Mayes, L. C., Fonagy, P., & Target, M. (2007). *Developmental science and psychoanalysis: Integration and innovation*. London: Karnac Books.

Midgley, N., & Vrouva, I. (2012). *Minding the child: Mentalization-based interventions with children, young people and their families*. London: Routledge.

National Scientific Council on the Developing Child. (2008). Mental problems in early childhood can impair learning and behavior for life (Working Paper No. 6). Retrieved from *www.cpeip.fsu.edu/resourceFiles/Mental_Health%20Problems_Early%20Childhood.pdf*.

Perepletchikova, F., Axelrod, S. R., Kaufman, J., Rounsaville, B. J., Douglas-Palumberi, H., & Miller, A. L. (2011). Adapting dialectical behaviour therapy for children: Towards a new research agenda for paediatric suicidal and non-suicidal self-injurious behaviours. *Child and Adolescent Mental Health, 16*, 116–121.

Piaget, J. (1954). *The construction of reality in the child*. New York: Basic Books. (Original work published 1937)

Raineki, C., Cortés, M. R., Belnoue, L., & Sullivan, R. M. (2012) Effects of early-life abuse differ across development: Infant social behavior deficits are followed by adolescent depressive-like behaviors mediated by the amygdala. *Journal of Neuroscience, 32*, 7758–7765.

Rossouw, T. (2012). Self-harm in young people: Is MBT the answer? In N. Midgley & I. Vrouva (Eds.), *Minding the child: Mentalization-based interventions with children, young people and their families* (pp. 131–144). London: Routledge.

Rutter, M., & Silberg, J. (2002). Gene–environment interplay in relation to emotional and behavioral disturbance. *Annual Review of Psychology, 53*, 463–490.

Sameroff, A. (Ed.). (2009). *The transactional model of development: How children and contexts shape each other*. Washington, DC: American Psychological Association.

Sandler, A-M. (1975). Comments on the significance of Piaget's work for psychoanalysis. *International Review of Psychoanalysis, 2*, 365–377.

Sandler, J., Holder, A., Dare, C., & Dreher, A. (1997). *Freud's models of the mind*. London: Karnac Books.

Sandler, J., & Rosenblatt, B. (1962). The concept of the representational world. *Psychoanalytic Study of the Child, 17*, 128–145.

Schore, A. N. (2003). *Affect regulation and the repair of the self*. New York: Norton.

Slade, A. (2005). Parental reflective functioning: An introduction. *Attachment and Human Development, 7*, 269–281.

Solomon, J., & George, C. (Eds.). (2011). *Disorganized attachment and caregiving*. New York: Guilford Press.

Spitz, R. (1945). Hospitalism: An inquiry into the genesis of psychiatric conditions in early childhood. *Psychoanalytic Study of the Child, 1*, 53–73.

Steele, H., Steele, M., Croft, C., & Fonagy, P. (1999). Infant–mother attachment at one year predicts children's understanding of mixed emotions at six years. *Social Development, 8*, 161–178.

Steele, H., & Steele, M. (2008). *Clinical applications of the Adult Attachment Interview*. New York: Guilford Press.

Stern, D. (1985). *The interpersonal world of the infant: A view of psychoanalysis and developmental psychology*. New York: Basic Books.

Suchman, N. E., Decoste, C., Ordway, M. R., & Bers, S. (2013). Mothering from the Inside Out: A mentalization-based individual therapy for mothers with substance-use disorders. In N. E. Suchman, M. Pajulo, & L. C. Mayes (Eds.), *Parenting and substance abuse: Developmental approaches to intervention*. New York: Oxford University Press.

Suomi, S. J. (2011). Risk, resilience, and gene-environment interplay in primates. *Journal of the Canadian Academy of Child and Adolescent Psychiatry, 20*, 289–297.

Toth, S. L., Rogosch, F. A., & Cicchetti, D. (2008). Attachment-theory-informed intervention and reflective functioning in depressed mothers. In H. Steele & M. Steele (Eds.), *Clinical applications of the Adult Attachment Interview* (pp. 154–174). New York: Guilford Press.

Tronick, E. (2007). *The neurobehavioral and social emotional development of infants and children*. New York: Norton.

Tyson, P. (2000). Psychoanalysis, development and the life cycle. *Journal of the American Psychoanalytic Association, 48*, 1045–1049.

van IJzendoorn, M. H. (1995). Adult attachment representations, parental responsiveness, and infant attachment. A meta-analysis on the predictive validity of the Adult Attachment Interview. *Psychological Bulletin, 117*, 387–403.

Winnicott, D. W. (1965). *The maturational processes and the facilitating environment: Studies in the theory of emotional development*. London: Hogarth Press.

Zanetti, C. A., Powell, B., Cooper, G., & Hoffman, K. (2011). The Circle of Security intervention: Using the therapeutic relationship to ameliorate attachment security in disorganized dyads. In J. Solomon & C. George (Eds.), *Disorganized attachment and caregiving* (pp. 318–342). New York: Guilford Press.

CHAPTER 4

Neuroscience and Psychoanalysis

Andrew J. Gerber, Jane Viner, and Joshua Roffman

Psychoanalysis and neuroscience have a fraught and complicated relationship. On the one hand, they can be seen as fierce allies—even "saviors" of one another. Some individuals with backgrounds in neuroscience or psychoanalysis have at times proclaimed that the merger of these two fields—sometimes even using a single term, *neuropsychoanalysis*—is the natural culmination of progress on both sides and will soon lead to a synthesis of the two perspectives. Meanwhile, others have claimed that this relationship is premature or even completely wrongheaded. From the psychoanalytic side, an emphasis on neuroscience is sometimes seen as a threat to the very core of a psychoanalytic worldview, that is, an emphasis on subjectivity and meaning. From the neuroscience side, an alliance of an up-and-coming, empirically based science with an old-fashioned, unfalsifiable, and "cultish" (or even "disproven") historical branch of psychology may appear to be pure folly.

In this chapter we hope to demonstrate that, as is so often the case, a middle position is much more reasonable. The rapid growth of the neuroscience literature over the past few decades, with particular emphasis on human cognition, offers an unprecedented opportunity to examine the constructs of a psychoanalytic metapsychology and gather empirical data where once patient and therapist report or theory were the only viable strategies. Psychoanalysis as a metapsychological theory and a clinical intervention has developed significantly over the past few decades as well and now offers new, agreed-upon constructs that are more amenable to empirical testing.

Meanwhile, despite the strength of its methods and its meticulous exploration of neuron-level behavior, neuroscience is still a long way from developing more general theories of cognition, affect, and motivated behavior. To investigate those paths, it looks to other fields—cognitive psychology, neuroeconomics, and even philosophy of mind—to suggest potential models for behavior. It only stands to reason that one of the most long-standing and meticulously written about theories of cognition, affect, and behavior—psychoanalysis—should be a part of that conversation.

We have divided this chapter into two major areas of theoretical focus and empirical research: (1) affect and (2) memory and learning. The work of many important contributors to the discussion of neuroscience and psychoanalysis, including Mark Solms, Jaak Panksepp, Aikaterini Fotopoulou, Douglas Watt, and Oliver Turnbull, is not discussed in this chapter and has been well summarized recently elsewhere (Fotopoulou, Pfaff, & Conway, 2012). Other areas could easily have been included as well, particularly social cognition (Roffman, Gerber, & Glick, 2012), attachment (Buchheim, George, Kächele, Erk, & Walter, 2006), and the neurobiology of stress-response systems (Luyten, Blatt, & Mayes, 2012). Finally, the recent major initiative led by Thomas Insel and Bruce Cuthbert at the National Institute of Mental Health (Morris & Cuthbert, 2012) to use continuous measures or Research Domain Criteria (RDoC) to improve upon the use of psychiatric diagnoses in research, though a natural complement to the psychoanalytic approach to neuroscience, is not discussed here (see, however, Chapters 1, 5, and 8). However, we feel that our two chosen areas represent a natural beginning to this exploration and offer a demonstration of how reasonable links can be built between psychoanalysis and neuroscience.

AFFECT

Psychodynamic thinkers have long recognized the importance of affect and considered its impact on individuals' lives and its role in psychotherapy. Cognitive neuroscientists were initially reticent to delve into the study of affect, since it seemed too vague and amorphous to measure. However, as theories of emotion and research methods have progressed, affect has become a major topic of research in relation to both psychopathology and normal functioning (Barrett, Ochsner, & Gross, 2007). For our purposes, we use "affect" synonymously with "emotion"—that is, a mental state with psychological and physiologic components. We review the ways investigators have defined and measured the elements of affect in typically developing individuals, and discuss interpretations of the neural correlates of affect. Our focus is on the following themes: (1) the circumplex model of affect, (2) emotion–cognition interactions, (3) levels of awareness, (4) typology of affect, (5) emotion schemas, (6) memes, (7) imitation, and (8) the mirror neuron system (MNS). Finally, we propose ways in which a more comprehensive, neurobiologically based understanding of affect may ultimately shape clinical practice.

Circumplex Model

The circumplex model of emotion (see Figure 4.1) captures the continuous nature of affective states and describes emotion along two axes, *valence* (unpleasant vs. pleasant) and *arousal* (activation vs. deactivation) (Peterson, 2005; Posner, Russell, & Peterson, 2005). Studies using functional magnetic resonance imaging (fMRI) have looked at subjects' blood oxygen level–dependent (BOLD) signal in their brains while

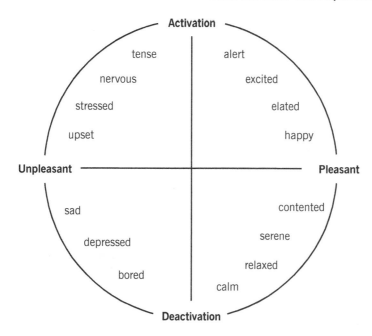

FIGURE 4.1. The affective circumplex model shows how different affective states may be represented on two continuous, unrelated scales: activation–deactivation (vertical axis) and unpleasant–pleasant (horizontal axis).

they were viewing emotional faces (Gerber et al., 2008) and emotion-denoting words (Posner et al., 2009), and have found evidence for two neural networks subserving the affective dimensions of valence and arousal. Moreover, there seems to be a "dose–response" relationship between neural activity and affective ratings that is predicted by dimensional models of emotion.

Another fMRI study sought to remove semantic and facial processing that may have confounded the results of the aforementioned studies; this study explicitly asked participants to rate the arousal and valence of their emotions as they imagined themselves in various emotion-evoking situations (e.g., "Imagine that you just won the lottery and you will have all the money you could ever want") while measuring the BOLD signal in subjects' brains (Vogt, 2005). Findings demonstrated that distinct networks are recruited for processing the valence and arousal dimensions of emotions: specifically, more negative emotions caused increased neural activity in the dorsolateral prefrontal cortex (DLPFC), frontal pole, the anterior midcingulate cortex (aMCC)/rostrodorsal anterior cingulate cortex (ACC), supplementary motor area, occipitotemporal junction, and cerebellar hemisphere. Furthermore, the intensity of signal change in these regions increased in a linear fashion with greater degrees of unpleasantness. The authors interpreted their findings to mean that negatively valenced (i.e., unpleasant) emotions engage executive-motor and attentional systems through the aMCC/rostral dorsal ACC (dACC). This network is thought to coordinate the exchange of emotional information between the supplementary motor area, DLPFC, frontal pole, and cerebellar hemispheres, enabling emotional appraisal and preparation for withdrawal from an inciting unpleasant stimulus (Vogt, 2005). The researchers also speculated that negatively valenced emotions engage a particular attentional circuit that is biased toward detecting and responding to unpleasant stimuli. Conversely, positively valenced emotions may preferentially engage the delayed activation of classic reward circuits, specifically, midline and medial temporal lobe (MTL) structures mediating arousal and dorsal cortical areas and mesolimbic pathways mediating valence (Colibazzi et al., 2010).

The circumplex model measures affect along two continuous distinct scales, captures the dimensionality of emotional experience in healthy control subjects, and can be correlated with neural activity in specific brain circuits. Application of the circumplex model to a patient population may be useful as a tool to assess suicidality in depressed individuals. One study found, in 104 participants, that reports of positive and negative affect predicted suicidal thoughts and behaviors over and above the cognitive factor of hopelessness. Thus, assessment of suicidal risk can be improved by assessing for negatively valenced affect (Yamokoski, Scheel, & Rogers, 2011).

Emotion–Cognition Interactions

Psychodynamic models are not concerned solely with how affects are generated, but also with how they are regulated and expressed. The interplay of cognition and emotion is a rich topic of study and debate. Some theorists contend that emotion and cognition are constantly interacting and intermingling, precluding pure emotional and cognitive states (Izard, 2009). Other emotion theorists have described the experience of emotion as a result of the integration of concurrent activity in brain structures and circuits, including the brainstem, amygdala, insula, ACC, and orbitofrontal cortex (Damasio, 2003; Lane, Ahern, Schwartz, & Kaszniak, 1997). Izard (2009) describes seven principles of emotion that relate emotional experience to cognitive processes. First, he describes emotion feeling as a stage of neurobiological activity that is experienced as motivational and informational, which subsequently influences thought and action (e.g., a felt cognition or an action tendency). He contends that "emotion feelings" can be activated and influenced by perceptual, appraisal, and subjective processes, but cannot be created by them. Izard contrasts phenomenal (primary) and access (reflective) consciousness, phenomenal being described as a low-level of awareness without being perceived, but not "unconscious" as it registers at a reportable level of consciousness (Chalmers, 1996), and access being described as a higher level of consciousness (Izard, 2009). Izard proposes the following:

> Level of awareness of an emotion feeling depends in part on its intensity and expression, and after language acquisition, on labeling, articulating, and acknowledging the emotion experience. These capacities, critical to personality and social development, depend on the neural activity and resultant processes involved in symbolization and language. (p. 6)

In summary, Izard suggests that conceptualizing levels of awareness may provide a better way of understanding human mentality and mind–brain functions.

Levels of Awareness

Many aspects of social interactions occur without conscious awareness, and interested researchers have hypothesized about how relationships between individuals' neural activity and levels of consciousness relate to their emotional experiences.

Etkin and colleagues (2004) studied conscious and unconscious awareness of affect by focusing on activation in the basolateral amygdala in response to fearful faces. This study found that when the stimuli are presented subliminally (i.e., so that they are not consciously seen), activity in the basolateral amygdala is related to a subject's own baseline trait level of anxiety. However, when stimuli are presented with the subject's conscious awareness, activity in this region is not related to baseline anxiety. The authors hypothesize that conscious compensatory or regulatory responses account for the apparent lack of association between conscious fearful stimuli and amygdalar activity. Thus, any theory of the neural underpinnings of affect must take into account the level of consciousness at which the stimuli are observed.

Lane's typology of affect (Figure 4.2) cites behavioral and neurobiological evidence for four overlapping categories of affective processes, as follows: (1) background feeling, (2) implicit affect, (3) focal attention, and (4) reflective awareness (Lane & Garfield, 2005). Background feelings do not require consciousness; rather, they are states that impact experience and give information about one's state of well-being, which likely involve the ventromedial prefrontal cortex, ventral and pregenual ACC, anterior insula, somatosensory cortex, and right parietal cortex (for a review, see

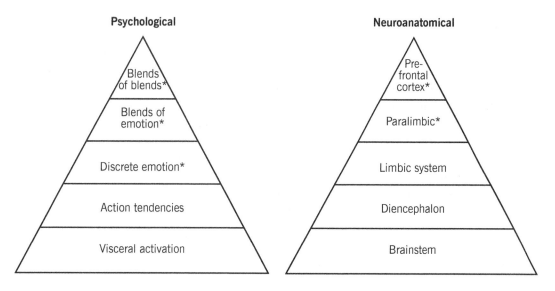

FIGURE 4.2. Parallels between the hierarchical organization of psychological/emotional experience and its neuroanatomical substrates. Each succeeding level adds to and modulates lower levels but does not replace them. Although each model contains five levels, there is not a one-to-one correspondence between each level in the two models. Lower levels correspond to implicit processes. Higher levels (indicated with *) correspond to explicit processes.

Lane, 2008). Implicit affect is unconscious, while focal attention shines a conscious light on affect and can invoke reappraisal of affect.

Ochsner, Bunge, Gross, and Gabrieli (2002) showed that people could manipulate their affect by reappraising a visual image in a way contrary to an initial impression. These authors further showed that particular brain regions are involved, namely, increased activation of the lateral and medial prefrontal regions and decreased activation of the amygdala and medial orbitofrontal cortex.

Reflective awareness requires an understanding of affect in relation to self and other representations, and therefore is probably essential to psychodynamic theories. All of the above-described levels of emotion have the potential to contribute to psychopathology as well as mechanisms of change; however, across most psychotherapeutic approaches, reflective awareness directs specific attention to problematic thoughts and maladaptive negative feelings to enable individuals to harness control over and improve the effects of these mental contents.

The hierarchical organization of psychological aspects of emotional experience, and the correlation of these aspects with associated neural substrates, can be used to guide therapeutic approaches. For example, body-based therapies (e.g., massage, yoga, acupuncture) may be appropriate for targeting implicit affect and making it available for explicit processing. In contrast, mind-based approaches, such as emotion-focused therapies, in conjunction with psychoeducational methods, might enhance explicit processing. This integrated model provides a principled approach to individualizing psychotherapy (Lane, 2008).

Emotion Schemas

Neural systems and mental processes involved in emotion feeling, perception, and cognition interact continually and dynamically into direct levels of awareness, vary from low to high, and generate and monitor thought and action (Izard, 2009). For all basic emotions, motivational and action processes occur in a similar fashion across situations. In contrast, there are wide differences in motivational and cognitive processes and behavior across individuals related to emotion schemas. Emotion schemas are defined as the most frequently occurring emotion experiences; they are dynamic emotion–cognition interactions that may consist of momentary/situational responding or enduring traits of personality that emerge over developmental time (Izard, 1993). Izard (1993) describes emotion-specific experiences (e.g., anger schemas) that have a consistent core feeling state but different perceptual tendencies (biases), thoughts, and action plans. Emotion schemas are influenced by characterological differences such as personality traits and temperament. Izard argues that emotion schemas should enhance the regulatory, motivational, and functional capacities of an individual's emotional capacities; however, gene–environment interactions can make schemas become maladaptive, and when individuals establish connections between emotion feelings and negative actions, psychopathology can develop (Izard, 2009).

Development and application of emotion schemas has been studied in, for instance, borderline personality disorder (BPD) (Unoka, Fogd, Fuzy, & Csukly,

2011). Study participants with BPD made more errors on a facial emotion recognition task than did control participants, and individuals with BPD demonstrated a pattern of misreading cues, specifically overidentifying disgust (a rejection cue) and underidentifying fear and sadness (empathy-provoking cues). These distortions may be part of interpersonal affective schemas for individuals with BPD—a finding consistent with BPD patients' clinical symptoms of fear of abandonment, a core DSM-5 diagnostic feature of BPD. Furthermore, insecure attachment styles (Agrawal, Gunderson, Holmes, & Lyons-Ruth, 2004), high levels of rejection sensitivity (Ayduk et al., 2008), and the prevalence of early maladaptive schemas (Specht, Chapman, & Cellucci, 2009) experienced by individuals with BPD may relate to aberrant interpersonal emotional schemas.

Memes

Although memes, or "replicant units," were originally described as cognition and behavior patterns that can be transmitted through imitative learning, can be readily copied, and become subject to natural selection (Dawkins, 1989), some argue that memes involving emotion, specifically emotion-schema memes (ESMs), emerged to serve unique adaptive functions in social interactions (Izard, 2009). Some authors propose that the brain evolved with human evolution to enable learning via imitation, which eventually became an important mechanism by which children acquire memes and subsequently learn to interact within their social environment. Imitating the expressive behavior of another person may activate neural and sensory motor processes that increase the likelihood of experiencing the emotion (and action tendencies) of the other person (Izard, 1990; Niedenthal, 2007). Children's imitation of their parents' positive emotion expressions and interactions may be an epigenetic phenomenon of evolutionary processes that contributes to the formation of ESMs (Izard, 2009).

Reciprocal Imitation

Children are not the only players in the development of ESMs; the parents or caregivers whom the children imitate are also involved. Researchers interested in studying the effect of reciprocal imitation used fMRI to evaluate neurobiology while people were being imitated (Guionnet et al., 2011). These authors observed that the dorsal part of the left anterior insular cortex (dAIC) and dACC were activated to a greater extent when the subject was being imitated than while they were engaged in imitation. The dAIC is thought to have a function of integrating one's own perceptions, feelings, thoughts, and planning (Kurth, Zilles, Fox, Laird, & Eickhoff, 2010). The dACC has been shown to be involved in conflict monitoring and adjustments in control (Kerns, Cohen, & MacDonald, 2004) and salience processing (Seeley et al., 2007). It has been suggested that the joint activation of the left dAIC and dACC observed while individuals were being imitated could reflect the feeling of "visceral connectedness" to other people (Hari & Kujala, 2009). The transfer of emotion, cognition, and action patterns between family members, across and within generations, raises questions about the transfer of healthy (adaptive) or pathological (maladaptive) ESMs.

Mirror Neuron System

Mirror neurons were first described in the F5 sector of the ventral premotor cortex in the macaque (Gallese, Fadiga, Fogassi, & Rizzolatti, 1996; Rizzolatti, Fadiga, Gallese, & Fogassi, 1996). These neurons, like most neurons in F5, discharge in association with movements that have a specific goal (motor acts). Neuroimaging demonstrated the existence of two main networks with mirror properties: one residing in the parietal lobe and the premotor cortex plus the caudal part of the inferior frontal gyrus (parietofrontal mirror system), and the other formed by the insula and the anterior mesial frontal cortex (limbic mirror system) (Cattaneo & Rizzolatti, 2009). The parietofrontal mirror system is involved in recognition of voluntary behavior, while the limbic mirror system is devoted to the recognition of affective behavior (Cattaneo & Rizzolatti, 2009). Mirror neuron system (MNS) involvement in empathy has been suggested by four functional neuroimaging studies that each reported a positive correlation between MNS activation and empathy scores (Gazzola, Aziz-Zadeh, & Keysers, 2006; Jabbi, Swart, & Keysers, 2007; Kaplan & Iacoboni, 2006; Pfeifer, Iacoboni, Mazziotta, & Dapretto, 2008).

Taken together, these studies suggest a positive correlation between self-reported empathy and MNS activation (see Table 4.1). Findings are generally considered to support MNS involvement in emotional empathy, most commonly seen as increased activation of the inferior frontal gyrus either unilaterally or bilaterally. Methodological differences between these studies also question the strength of the conclusions (Baird, Scheffer, & Wilson, 2011); however, this is an area of active research, and future evidence may clarify the relationship between empathy and MNS neural networks.

Mirror Neuron System and Autism Spectrum Disorders

Clinically, some functional deficits typical of autism spectrum disorder (ASD), such as deficits in imitation, emotional empathy, and ability to attribute intentions to others, have a clear counterpart in the functions of the mirror system (Cattaneo & Rizzolatti, 2009). This "broken mirror" hypothesis has been controversial since its inception, with some arguing that theory as it relates to ASD is premature and undersupported (Southgate & Hamilton, 2008). In a transcranial magnetic stimulation study in which corticospinal excitability was measured in individuals with ASD and typically developing controls as they observed hand gestures, the ASD participants failed to show activation of the MNS relative to controls. Furthermore, ASD subjects' scores on a self-reported social impairment scale were negatively associated with the presence of MNS activity, a relationship that did not exist for control subjects (Enticott et al., 2012). The authors interpreted this to mean that a deficit within mirror neurons, or dysfunction of the broader MNS, limits one's ability to understand the behavior of others. Implicated dysfunction of the MNS may account for the deficits

TABLE 4.1. Summary of Neuroimaging Studies Showing a Positive Correlation between Self-Reported Empathy and Mirror Neuron System Activation

Author (year)	N (mean age) of participants	Imaging task and stimuli	Empathy measure	Main findings
Gazzola et al. (2006)	16 (31 years)	Listening to or performing mouth or hand action sounds (e.g., kissing, ripping paper)	IRI	Positive correlation between left premotor cortex and inferior parietal lobule activation (during hand and environmental sounds) and perspective-taking scale scores. *Note:* Subjects were categorized into high-empathy and low-empathy groups.
Jabbi et al. (2007)	18 (24 years)	Observing film clips of actors drinking liquids and displaying different facial expressions (pleased, disgusted, neutral), and also ingesting pleasant, unpleasant, and neutral-tasting liquids	IRI	Positive correlation between bilateral anterior insula and frontal operculum activation and total IRI score (most evident for the personal distress and fantasy scale scores). No correlation between IRI score and brain activation during ingesting liquids.
Kaplan & Iacobini (2006)	26 (26 years)	Observing film clips of drinking cups in different contexts (being cleaned, drunk from, no context) and with different hand grips (precision or whole hand)	IRI	Positive correlation between right inferior frontal gyrus activation and empathic concern scale (averaged across all film clips), and fantasy scale scores (during incongruent and context-alone clips). Negative correlation with personal scale scores (during congruent actions and action in context clips).
Pfeifer et al. (2008)	16 (10 years)	Imitating and observing five facial expressions (happy, fearful, sad, angry, neutral)	IRI and Interpersonal Competence Scale (parent report)	Positive correlation between inferior frontal gyrus activation (as well as right insula, left amygdala, and left fusiform gyrus) and IRI scale scores (except perspective-taking scale) during observation and imitation of expressions.

Note. IRI, Interpersonal Reactivity Index (Davis, 1983).

in socialization that are observed in ASD (Oberman & Ramachandran, 2007) and in antisocial personality disorder, and perhaps in any disorder that involves deficits or dysfunction in social skills. The issue of causation in this study remains unresolved, with mirror neuron impairment either a cause or a consequence of social impairments in ASD.

Summary

In this section, we described theoretical models and scientific methods used to investigate affect, beginning with the circumplex model of affect, which measures affect along two variables of valence and arousal. We reviewed theories about the interface between affect and cognition neurophysiologically and psychologically, specifically the levels of awareness and typology of affect. We discussed the development of affect processing and associated neural activity in interpersonal contexts with emotion schemas, memes, imitation, and the MNS. Finally, we considered evidence for MNS dysfunction in individuals with ASDs. Clinically, an individual's ability to recognize, understand, and compensate in response to emotional cues impacts his or her ability to cope with stressors and function productively in the world. Although specific approaches vary, an aim of psychotherapy is to enable individuals to become more psychologically minded; researchers have investigated how the process of psychotherapy translates to bringing about changes in individuals' lives. Greater understanding of typical functioning and the differences that result from psychopathology will enable clinicians to appropriately tailor therapeutic interventions.

MEMORY AND LEARNING

Throughout history, writers, philosophers, and scientists have contemplated how knowledge is acquired, stored, and recalled. Many of these great thinkers accepted that what we know and remember is not in our conscious awareness; some information is not even accessible to awareness. Over time, advances in our understanding of the human brain and its means of learning and organizing information have illuminated the mechanisms of memory. However, the study of memory and learning remains limited by investigators' reliance on people's subjective reports of their experiences. Studies in experimental animals provide evidence about the event-like memory processing capabilities of these species, but these experiments may not be appropriate models for capturing the essence of human episodic memory.

Freud extrapolated from his scholarly work and clinical experiences to propose that a significant portion of possible thought is actively excluded from awareness (Ellenberger, 1970). He theorized that due to the objectionable nature of these thoughts, they were forced into the "dynamic unconscious." Also referred to as "motivated unconscious," these thoughts are purposely excluded from consciousness; however, they continue to exert a significant influence on behavior and conscious processes. Thoughts and behaviors influenced by the dynamic unconscious are most relevant to psychotherapy and psychoanalysis. In contrast, the "descriptive unconscious," a more inclusive category, encompasses not only the dynamic unconscious, but also the preconscious, which is easily accessible by consciousness if one were to focus attention on it, as well as the nonconscious, which is inherently inaccessible to consciousness because it has never been symbolized. An example of nonconscious content is procedural knowledge about how to ride a bicycle (Sandler & Fonagy, 1997). Since Freud, many alternative theories have been offered, and traditional perspectives of memory have evolved. In recent decades, cognitive neuroscientists have attempted to delineate the systems responsible for memory and learning. Controversies remain about the structure, relationship, and overlap of the systems, as well as their relationships to consciousness. Approaches to studying memory have expanded widely with the development of neuroimaging, single-neuron recordings, electrical and magnetic signals, pharmacologic manipulation of cognition, studies of patients with brain injuries, and animal models.

Explicit Memory

Explicit or *declarative* memory describes the encoding (i.e., formation) of episodic and semantic memories. Episodic memories capture knowledge about unique events, and hence require a memory system that immediately, in one attempt, encodes information automatically. This system encodes as much of what is perceived as is possible without conscious awareness (Squire, 1987).

Explicit memory is divided into *episodic* and *semantic* memory. As described by Tulving (1972), episodic memories are composed of specific details of the spatial and temporal aspects of a memory, whereas semantic knowledge is more general, "gist-type" knowledge. Early fMRI studies in neurologically intact individuals established that retrieving remote, as well as recent, episodic memories robustly activates the hippocampus (Ryan et al., 2001). Because only the hippocampus represents spatial comprehension, this provided links to all of the details to make up a fully elaborated episodic memory. Nadel and O'Keefe (1974) further elaborated the distinction between episodic and semantic knowledge to explain why patients with amnesia could or could not learn and not recall. They argued that the hippocampus was critical for episodic learning and memory due to its role in spatial processing; however, semantic memory encoding and retrieval were independent of the hippocampus.

Investigations into the neural underpinnings of the multiple memory systems established key structures essential for memory retrieval. The medial temporal lobe (MTL) system is a fundamental structure involved in binding memory systems together (Nadel & Hardt, 2011). In particular, MTL function is critical for short-term or working memory and perception. Ranganath and D'Esposito (2001) performed a neuroimaging task to investigate the role of the hippocampus in short-term memory encoding. In this study, neurologically intact subjects were presented with novel faces followed by a brief (7-second) delay and a probe face, in response to which the subjects had to state whether it was the same or different. Continuous activation was observed bilaterally in the hippocampus in this working memory task, which was interpreted to substantiate the role of the hippocampus in working memory. Another task was designed to probe long-term memory function. In this paradigm, subjects were shown novel faces and then, after a substantial delay, were asked to respond if they recognized the probe faces. During this task, no appreciable hippocampal activation was seen in study subjects (Ranganath & D'Esposito, 2001). Hannula and Ranganath (2008) performed an experiment in which subjects completed a task where they saw four objects in a specific spatial pattern within a three-dimensional grid. After a short delay, the grid was rotated by 90 degrees, and a pattern that was either the same as or different from the original was displayed. Results showed that increased activation in the hippocampus and perirhinal cortex during encoding predicted subsequent accuracy in the short-term decision task. The authors interpreted this finding as evidence that the hippocampus and perirhinal cortices are involved in visual short-term memory.

Studies of electrical activity in the hippocampus indicate that items accompanied by hippocampal activation were more likely to be remembered, whereas those accompanied by hippocampal deactivation were less likely to be remembered (Axmacher, Elger, & Fell, 2009). Cashdollar and colleagues (2009) found theta-range activity in frontal and parietal cortices in association with a working-memory task and subsequently proposed that this network may operate in conjunction with hippocampal activation during working-memory tasks.

The idea that perception proceeds without influence from previous experience is no longer accepted; hence, the MTL's role in memory naturally leads to questioning its role in *perception*. A sizeable body of evidence shows that even the simplest perceptual processes, such as figure–ground separation, are subject to top-down modifications from memory systems (e.g., Peterson & Skow, 2008). For example, studies in animals and humans suggest that damage to the MTL causes deficits in visual discrimination, which cannot be attributed to impaired long-term memory and occur independent of the perceptual nature or memory of the task (Buckley & Gaffan, 2006; Bussey & Saksida, 2007). From animal literature, we know that when monkeys have to distinguish between complex stimuli that share certain features, their perirhinal cortex plays an essential role in resolving ambiguity (Bussey, Saksida, & Murray, 2003). These results argue against the view that perception and memory are separated in the brain; rather, both appear to depend on the same representational systems.

Although the role of the MTL in memory and perception has been substantiated, the time course of its involvement is an area of ongoing research. Traditional understanding of the MTL memory system, often called the standard systems consolidation model (SCM), assumed that the hippocampus was crucial for encoding memories (i.e., short-term "cellular consolidation") but was not essential for retrieving memories. By contrast, *multiple trace theory* (MTT) (Nadel & Moscovitch, 1997) argues instead that hippocampal involvement is necessary for both encoding and retrieving episodic memory regardless of a memory's age. The MTT proposes that when remote episodic memories are recalled, the reactivated memory causes re-encoding, which modifies existing memory (Nadel & Moscovitch, 1997). This theory contends that when memory traces are recalled, they are expanded and strengthened, and new content can be added. This theory of modification of recalled memories is also called the *reconsolidation phenomenon*. For a review of neurobiological evidence related to memory reconsolidation, see Nader and Hardt (2009).

In summary, there is compelling evidence that retrieval of long-term memories can change both the content and strength of recalled memories on behavioral, physiological, and molecular levels of analysis. Neurobiological evidence of the postreactivation neural plasticity of memory systems corroborates the psychoanalytic view of revisiting memories as a dynamic process. The psychoanalytic concept *Nachträglichkeit*, which is translated as "deferred action," is relevant here. This idea—that experiences, impressions, and memory traces may be revised at a later date to fit in with fresh experiences or with the attainment of a new stage of development—asserts that recalled memories may be endowed with a new meaning. Furthermore, the plasticity of these revisited memories can be imbued with psychical effectiveness. Neurobiological evidence of the neural plasticity of recalled memories substantiates the psychoanalytic concept of deferred action whereby a subject may revise memories.

Implicit Memory

The study of *implicit* or *nondeclarative*, nonconscious memory is an area of interest to neuroscientists and psychodynamic therapists. Functional imaging experiments have demonstrated that the brain regions subserving the encoding and retrieval of explicit and implicit memory do not fully overlap (for a review, see Nadel & Hardt, 2011). Procedural memory is a type of implicit memory in which subjects learn motor or behavioral tasks without developing language to describe what they have learned, sometimes without even being aware that they have learned something. The "Weather Prediction Task" (Knowlton, Mangels, & Squire, 1996) revealed important insight into the formation of implicit memory. In this task, subjects are shown one or more of a set of four symbols and asked, with no prior information, to use them to predict whether it will rain or shine. After responding, they are told whether they are right or wrong, and the task is repeated for many trials. Subjects report feeling as if they are guessing at every answer and not learning anything during the course of the task. In fact, unbeknownst to the subject, the correct answer to each trial is calculated on the basis of combinations of fixed probabilities assigned to each symbol. Although subjects say that they are guessing, their performance improves steadily during the course of the task, demonstrating that they are learning outside of their awareness. Progressive, gradual acquisition of implicit knowledge parallels the psychoanalytic concept of schema formation.

Investigators sought to elaborate on the Weather Prediction Task to see whether strategy could be learned implicitly. To this end, Ghinescu, Schachtman, Stadler, Fabiani, and Gratton (2010) used the implicit learning procedure called the Eriksen flanker task. Subjects were divided into three groups: explicit instructions (i.e., "cues are predictive"), partially explicit instructions ("cues have *some* predictive value"), and implicit instructions ("no information about the meaning of the cues"). All groups were presented with a conscious cue, then an "imperative stimulus" (a stimulus eliciting a motor response). The conscious cues had predictive values of a "compatible" or "incompatible" stimulus (i.e., a response that was congruent or incongruent with the motor response). Results showed that instruction conditions did not produce any significant main effect or interaction. In addition, subjects in all three instruction groups performed similarly on both reaction time and accuracy. Participants in the partially explicit and implicit instruction groups were not aware of the specific predictive value of the cues. The authors concluded that explicit knowledge of contingencies is not necessary for strategy development. Furthermore, they contrasted perceptual awareness versus contingency awareness and proposed that contingency awareness can occur outside of perceptual awareness. They suggest that contingency learning does not depend on MTL structures, but rather on basal ganglia (involved in implicit learning) and lateral frontal structures involved in working memory (e.g., Braver & Cohen, 2001).

Neuroimaging studies of professional opera singers compared with untrained individuals show cortical (DLPFC and sensorimotor area) as well as subcortical and cerebellar differences in activation (Kleber, Veit, Birbaumer, Gruzelier, & Lotze, 2010). A regression analysis of functional activation with years of singing practice indicated that vocal skills training correlates with increased activity of a cortical network for enhanced motor control and sensorimotor guidance, together with increased involvement of implicit motor memory areas at the subcortical and cerebellar level—hence, different activation in self-monitoring/executive function regions in addition to motor skill regions. This study offers new and important validation for the theory that experience causes changes to the conscious regulatory system, which can impact implicit systems. Common to opera training and psychotherapy is that people are required to build and practice skills over time, which seems to elicit appreciable changes in brain activation.

Processes and consequences of reactivation of memory and schematization are complicated and controversial. Reactivation of a memory can strengthen the underlying memory; however, it strengthens only the elements that are activated at that time. The effects of reconsolidation have been described in several studies from a number of groups, corroborating this phenomenon and lending evidence that memory reactivation can indeed lead to alterations in the representations underlying memory (Chan, 2009; Forcato, Rodríguez, Pedreira, & Maldonado, 2010; Zhao, Zhang, Shi, Epstein, & Lu, 2009). Concurrently, schematization can lead to distortions that become solidified or "locked in" to the memory. Studies indicate that when repeated recalls are elicited, any distortions produced on the first recall become highly likely to be repeated on subsequent recalls (Roediger, Jacoby, & McDermott, 1996). Within the context of stress and trauma, this phenomenon has important potential clinical implications. For example, it suggests that the act of eliciting a description of a past trauma in psychotherapy may have important implications for what is "remembered" later on, and potentially for even distorting that memory. This is explored in more detail in the hotly debated "recovered memory" literature (Sandler & Fonagy, 1997).

Schematic knowledge permits quick conceptual coding, a process that can be seen in animal models. Tse and colleagues (2007) showed that if rats can acquire schematic knowledge, they are much faster to learn in subsequent food-foraging tasks. The conclusion is that schemas speed up system consolidation of new event-related knowledge, which quickly becomes independent of the hippocampus. Schemas are high-level conceptual frameworks that organize past experiences and enable rapid interpretation of new situations. They allow the individual to predict or infer unknown information in completely new situations. The schema employed while interpreting a new situation strongly influences what is encoded and remembered about a situation. Schema-inconsistent information is remembered better than schema-consistent information (Rojahn & Pettigrew, 1992). Categorizing objects using a schema-based approach can, however, lead to mistakes in the encoding process. For example, young children show better memory for items than adults because adults process according to well-established categories/schemas (Sloutsky & Fisher, 2004).

The concept of schematic augmentation describes the mind's ability to fill in the "blind spots" of memory—just as it does our blind spots in perception (Bartlett, 1932). Bartlett emphasized this concept, drawing the parallel that as nature abhors a vacuum, so the psyche abhors gaps and actively tends to fill in these gaps in a "fundamental effort after meaning" (Bartlett, 1932, p. 227). Psychologists have proposed that mental schemas, reflecting cultural habits, biases, and logical expectations, intrude upon and distort memory in an effort to fill in meaning.

Autobiographical memory describes a person's subjective perspective on specific events experienced at particular time points linked together on a personal timeline (Fivush, 2011). Autobiographical memory develops gradually across childhood and adolescence and is heavily socially and culturally variable. It is distinguished from episodic memory because of the subjective sense of self. Autobiographical memory serves three interrelated self functions: self-definition, self-in-relation, and self-regulation. However, no strong evidence separates the neural processes of encoding episodic memory from those of encoding autobiographical memory. The hippocampus is implicated in both episodic and autobiographical memory processes.

We have reviewed the acquisition and encoding of explicit and implicit memory, memory schemas, and autobiographical memory, as well as associated neural networks; we now turn our focus to remembering previously acquired memories.

Repression

The term *repression* was defined by Herbart (1816/1891) as the nondefensive inhibition of ideas by other ideas to prevent them from reaching consciousness (Erdelyi, 2006). In the two centuries since then, clinicians, philosophers, and others have debated the cause, purpose, and implications of repression. Freud's clinical experience revealed early on that exclusion from consciousness was effected not just by simple repression (i.e., inhibition) but also by a variety of distorting techniques, some utilized to degrade underlying contents (i.e., denial), all eventually subsumed under the rubric of *defense mechanisms* ("repression in the widest sense"; Freud, 1894/1966). He described his patients' conflicts that unfolded beneath their conscious awareness, and the inhibition and inaccessibility of conflicting content.

Since Freud, some clinicians contend that the "inaccessible materials" are often available and emerge indirectly (e.g., procedurally, implicitly; for a review, see Bechara et al., 1995). In recent years, psychologists and neuroscientists have focused on the "adaptive" function of inhibition of memory retrieval and consequent for-getting. These studies of "executive function" processes and associated neural cir-cuits are described below. Freud's concept of repression as a means for dealing with unpleasant, socially unacceptable desires and conflicts represents "repression in the narrow sense." However, our expanding knowledge about the adaptive features of nonconscious control of memory content enables a more complete understanding of the utility of repression.

Cognitive psychology now has several model paradigms to study memory con-trol. Anderson and Green (2001) pioneered a version of the go/no-go task called the think/no-think paradigm to demonstrate that executive control could be recruited to prevent unwanted explicit memories from coming into awareness. Furthermore, this cognitive act has enduring consequences for the rejected memories. The task involved first training subjects to remember 40 unrelated word pairs. Next, subjects engaged in a critical task in which they had to exert executive control over the retrieval pro-cess. During each trial, a cue from one of the pairs appeared on the computer screen and, depending on which cue appeared, subjects were told either to recall and say the associated response word, that is, the "think" condition, or not to think about the response, that is, the "no-think" condition. Results showed that subjects had impaired memory for "no-think" suppression items. These findings indicate that the need to prevent retrieval is an example of the need to override responses that are inap-propriate, a function associated with executive functions.

The go/no-go paradigm has been extensively used to study executive function and has been shown to recruit the DLPFC, ACC, and ventral prefrontal cortex (Casey et al., 1997; de Zubicaray, Andrew, Zelaya, Williams, & Dumanoir, 2000; Garavan, Ross, & Stein, 1999). All these authors proposed that the think/no-think paradigm activated the DLPFC and ACC, possibly with medial temporal regions, to control awareness of the memory, and suggested that this network is responsible for memory control through inhibition.

Unconscious Will

In the past, theorists assumed that many of the mental processes that make goal pur-suit possible require consciousness. Within the past decade, scientific study of goal pursuit has revealed that these processes can also operate without conscious aware-ness. In contrast to implicit learning, wherein new knowledge is gained below the level of consciousness, *subliminal* cues draw on the existence of previously acquired implicit memories. Subjects are exposed to stimuli so briefly that the stimuli do not reach the threshold of their conscious awareness, yet affect their performance on later tasks. For example, change in performance after priming of achievement-related words, enhanced fluid consumption in a taste task after priming of drinking-related words, and an increase in instrumental behavior leading to specific goals (such as helping another person by providing useful comments) after priming of names of sig-nificant others (such as a good friend) or occupations (such as nurse) associated with these goals have all been demonstrated experimentally (Aarts et al., 2005; Custers, Maas, Wildenbeest, & Aarts, 2008).

These authors took this a step further by demonstrating that subliminal exposure to reward influences the nature of the priming. They asked a group of healthy young adults to squeeze a handgrip and exposed some of them subliminally to words about physical exertion and others to words about physical exertion paired with positive rewards. Subjects primed with both sets of words squeezed the ball harder and longer than those primed with the words about physical exertion alone. Goal-directed intentional behaviors can be influenced by goal priming, which occurs outside of awareness. Subliminal priming can motivate people to deploy skills associated with the primed goal without conscious effort. Furthermore, goal pursuits that emerge unconsciously are distinct from conscious intentions and can operate independently. It has been suggested that different neural networks and processes could serve these independent processes (Dijksterhuis & Aarts, 2010).

Neuroimaging research in the past several decades has shown that reward cues are processed by limbic structures such as the nucleus accumbens and the ventral striatum (Carlson, 2011). Subcortical areas play a central role in determining the rewarding value of outcomes and are connected to frontal areas in the cortex that facilitate goal pursuit. These reward centers in the brain respond not only to evolutionarily relevant rewards such as food and sexual stimuli, but also to learned rewards (e.g., money or status), or words (e.g., "good" or "nice") associated with praise or rewards. Positive stimuli induce a reward signal that is readily picked up by the brain.

Through priming with positive stimuli, subjects could be "primed" by consciously perceived information so that later, although they did not specifically recall the information they were previously taught, their answers to questions were influenced by previous exposure (Ochsner, Chiu, & Schacter, 1994). This observable finding facilitates a way to evaluate the influence of *goals to achieve*. Bargh, Gollwitzer, Lee-Chai, Barndollar, and Trötschel (2001) primed U.S. students without their becoming aware of being influenced. Students were seated at a table to work on two seemingly unrelated language puzzles. One group of students' first puzzle included words related to achievement (such as "win" or "achieve"), and a puzzle for another group did not. Students who were exposed to achievement words were found to outperform the others on the second puzzle. Achievement priming was found to prompt behaviors characteristic of motivated states, for example, persistence in solving puzzles and increased flexibility on the Wisconsin Card Sorting Test. Extensive debriefing indicated that the students did not knowingly perceive an influence of the first task (in which they were exposed to consciously visible achievement-related words) on their responses to the second. The authors concluded that the effect of achievement priming on subsequent performance and cognitive flexibility was likely to be the result of unconscious processes.

Summary

Our understanding of memory as being composed of multiple memory systems impacts psychodynamic theory and practice. Given the functional and anatomical differences of these various memory systems, it is important to delineate to which memory system a particular learned thought or behavior belongs. Substantial evidence exists that much of learning and memory does take place outside of awareness, raising the possibility for its importance in psychopathology and mental life. Conditions such as schizophrenia, depression, and various anxiety disorders all have been shown to involve impairments in how individuals use—or misuse—previous experience (e.g., Barch, 2006; Gibbs & Rude, 2004; Jacobs & Nadel, 1985). Striving for a more comprehensive understanding of the psychological and neurobiological underpinnings of memory and learning will elucidate the impairments seen in psychopathology.

REFERENCES

Aarts, H., Chartrand, T. L., Custers, R., Danner, U., Dik, G., Jefferis, V., et al. (2005). Social stereotypes and automatic goal pursuit. *Social Cognition, 23*, 464–489.

Agrawal, H. R., Gunderson, J., Holmes, B. M., & Lyons-Ruth, K. (2004). Attachment studies with borderline patients: A review. *Harvard Review of Psychiatry, 12*, 94–104.

Anderson, M. C., & Green, C. (2001). Suppressing unwanted memories by executive control. *Nature, 410*, 366–369.

Axmacher, N., Elger, C. E., & Fell, J. (2009). Working memory-related hippocampal deactivation interferes with long-term memory formation. *Journal of Neuroscience, 29*, 1052–1060.

Ayduk, O., Zayas, V., Downey, G., Cole, A. B., Shoda, Y., & Mischel, W. (2008). Rejection sensitivity and executive control: Joint predictors of borderline personality features. *Journal of Research in Personality, 42*, 151–168.

Baird, A. D., Scheffer, I. E., & Wilson, S. J. (2011). Mirror neuron system involvement in empathy: A critical look at the evidence. *Social Neuroscience, 6*, 327–335.

Barch, D. M. (2006). What can research on schizophrenia tell us about the cognitive neuroscience of working memory? *Neuroscience, 139*, 73–84.

Bargh, J. A., Gollwitzer, P. M., Lee-Chai, A., Barndollar, K., & Trötschel, R. (2001). The automated will: Nonconscious activation and pursuit of behavioral goals. *Journal of Personal and Social Psychology, 81*, 1014–1027.

Barrett, L., Ochsner, K. N., & Gross, J. (2007). The experience of emotion. *Annual Review of Psychology, 58*, 373–403.

Bartlett, F. (1932). *Remembering: A study in experimental and social psychology*. Cambridge, UK: Cambridge University Press.

Bechara, A., Tranel, D., Damasio, H., Adolphs, R., Rockland, C., & Damasio, A. R. (1995). Double dissociation of conditioning and declarative knowledge relative to the amygdala and hippocampus in humans. *Science, 269*, 1115–1118.

Braver, T. S., & Cohen, J. D. (2001). Working memory, cognitive control, and the prefrontal cortex: Computational and empirical studies. *Cognitive Processing, 2*, 25–55.

Buchheim, A., George, C., Kächele, H., Erk, S., & Walter, H. (2006). Measuring adult attachment representation in an fMRI environment: Concepts and assessment. *Psychopathology, 39*, 136–143.

Buckley, M. J., & Gaffan, D. (2006). Perirhinal cortical contributions to object perception. *Trends in Cognitive Sciences, 10*, 100–107.

Bussey, T. J., & Saksida, L. M. (2007). Memory, perception and the ventral visual perirhinal-hippocampal stream: Thinking outside of the boxes. *Hippocampus, 17*, 898–908.

Bussey, T. J., Saksida, L. M., & Murray, E. A. (2003). Impairments in visual discrimination after perirhinal cortex lesions: Testing "declarative" vs. "perceptual–mnemonic" views of perirhinal cortex function. *European Journal of Neuroscience, 17*, 649–660.

Carlson, J. M. (2011). Ventral striatal and medial prefrontal BOLD activation is correlated with reward-related electrocortical activity: A combined ERP and fMRI study. *NeuroImage, 57*, 1608–1611.

Casey, B. J., Trainor, R. J., Orendi, J. L., Schubert, A. B., Nystrom, L. E., Giedd, J. N., et al. (1997). A developmental functional MRI study of prefrontal activation during performance of a go–no–go task. *Journal of Cognitive Neuroscience, 9*, 835–847.

Cashdollar, N., Malecki, U., Rugg-Gunn, F. J., Duncan, J. S., Lavie, N., & Duzel, E. (2009). Hippocampus-dependent and -independent theta-networks of active maintenance. *Proceedings of the National Academy of Sciences of the United States of America, 106*, 20493–20498.

Cattaneo, L., & Rizzolatti, G. (2009). The mirror neuron system. *Archives of Neurology, 66*, 557–560.

Chalmers, D. J. (1996). *The conscious mind: In search of a fundamental theory.* New York: Oxford University Press.

Chan, J. C. K. (2009). When does retrieval induce forgetting and when does it induce facilitation? Implications for retrieval inhibition, testing effect, and text processing. *Journal of Memory and Language, 61*, 153–170.

Colibazzi, T., Posner, J., Wang, Z., Gorman, D., Gerber, A., Yu, S., et al. (2010). Neural systems subserving valence and arousal during the experience of induced emotions. *Emotion, 10*, 377–389.

Custers, R., Maas, M., Wildenbeest, M., & Aarts, H. (2008). Nonconscious goal pursuit and the surmounting of physical and social obstacles. *European Journal of Social Psychology, 38*, 1013–1022.

Damasio, A. (2003). Mental self: The person within. *Nature, 423*, 227.

Davis, M. H. (1983). Measuring individual differences in empathy: Evidence for a multidimensional approach. *Journal of Personality and Social Psychology, 44*, 113–126.

Dawkins, R. (1989). *The selfish gene* (rev. ed.). Oxford, UK: Oxford University Press.

de Zubicaray, G. I., Andrew, C., Zelaya, F. O., Williams, S. C. R., & Dumanoir, C. (2000). Motor response suppression and the prepotent tendency to respond: A parametric study. *Neuropsychologia, 38*, 1280–1291.

Dijksterhuis, A., & Aarts, H. (2010). Goals, attention, and (un)consciousness. *Annual Review of Psychology, 61*, 467–490.

Ellenberger, H. (1970). *The discovery of the unconscious: The history and evolution of dynamic psychiatry.* New York: Basic Books.

Enticott, P. G., Kennedy, H. A., Rinehart, N. J., Tonge, B. J., Bradshaw, J. L., Taffe, J. R., et al. (2012). Mirror neuron activity associated with social impairments but not age in autism spectrum disorder. *Biological Psychiatry, 71*: 427–433.

Erdelyi, M. H. (2006). The unified theory of repression. *Behavioral and Brain Sciences, 29*, 499–511.

Etkin, A., Klemenhagen, K. C., Dudman, J. T., Rogan, M. T., Hen, R., Kandel, E. R., et al. (2004). Individual differences in trait anxiety predict the response of the basolateral amygdala to unconsciously processed fearful faces. *Neuron, 44*, 1043–1055.

Fivush, R. (2011). The development of autobiographical memory. *Annual Review of Psychology, 62*, 559–582.

Forcato, C., Rodríguez, M. L., Pedreira, M. E., & Maldonado, H. (2010). Reconsolidation in humans opens up declarative memory to the entrance of new information. *Neurobiology of Learning and Memory, 93*, 77–84.

Fotopoulou, A., Pfaff, D., & Conway, M. A. (2012). *From the couch to the lab: Trends in psychodynamic neuroscience.* Oxford, UK: Oxford University Press.

Freud, S. (1966). The neuro-psychoses of defence. In J. Strachey (Ed. & Trans.), *The standard edition of the complete psychological works of Sigmund Freud* (Vol. 3, pp. 43–61). London: Hogarth Press. (Original work published 1894)

Gallese, V., Fadiga, L., Fogassi, L., & Rizzolatti, G. (1996). Action recognition in the premotor cortex. *Brain, 119*, 593–609.

Garavan, H., Ross, T. J., & Stein, E. A. (1999). Right hemispheric dominance of inhibitory control:

An event-related functional MRI study. *Proceedings of the National Academy of Sciences of the United States of America, 96*, 8301–8306.

Gazzola, V., Aziz-Zadeh, L., & Keysers, C. (2006). Empathy and the somatotopic auditory mirror system in humans. *Current Biology, 16*, 1824–1829.

Gerber, A. J., Posner, J., Gorman, D., Colibazzi, T., Yu, S., Wang, Z., et al. (2008). An affective circumplex model of neural systems subserving valence, arousal, and cognitive overlay during the appraisal of emotional faces. *Neuropsychologia, 46*, 2129–2139.

Ghinescu, R., Schachtman, T. R., Stadler, M. A., Fabiani, M., & Gratton, G. (2010). Strategic behavior without awareness?: Effects of implicit learning in the Eriksen flanker paradigm. *Memory and Cognition, 38*, 197–205.

Gibbs, B. R., & Rude, S. S. (2004). Overgeneral autobiographical memory as depression vulnerability. *Cognitive Therapy and Research, 28*, 511–526.

Guionnet, S., Nadel, J., Bertasi, E., Sperduti, M., Delaveau, P., & Fossati, P. (2011). Reciprocal imitation: Toward a neural basis of social interaction. *Cerebral Cortex, 22*, 971–978.

Hannula, D. E., & Ranganath C. (2008). Medial temporal lobe activity predicts successful relational memory binding. *Journal of Neuroscience, 28*, 116–124.

Hari, R., & Kujala, M. V. (2009). Brain basis of human social interaction: From concepts to brain imaging. *Physiological Reviews, 89*, 453–479.

Herbart, J. F. (1891). (M. K. Smith, Trans). *A textbook in psychology* (2nd ed.). New York: Appleton. (Original work published 1816).

Izard, C. E. (1990). Facial expressions and the regulation of emotions. *Journal of Personality and Social Psychology, 58*, 487–498.

Izard, C. E. (1993). Four systems for emotion activation: Cognitive and noncognitive processes. *Psychological Review, 100*, 68–90.

Izard, C. E. (2009). Emotion theory and research: Highlights, unanswered questions, and emerging issues. *Annual Review of Psychology, 60*, 1–25.

Jabbi, M., Swart, M., & Keysers, C. (2007). Empathy for positive and negative emotions in the gustatory cortex. *NeuroImage, 34*, 1744–1753.

Jacobs, W. J., & Nadel, L. (1985). Stress-induced recovery of fears and phobias. *Psychological Review, 92*, 512–531.

Kaplan, J., & Iacoboni, M. (2006). Getting a grip on other minds: Mirror neurons, intention understanding, and cognitive empathy. *Social Neuroscience, 1*, 175–183.

Kerns, J. G., Cohen, J. D., & MacDonald, A. W. (2004). Anterior cingulate conflict monitoring and adjustments in control. *Science, 303*, 1023–1026.

Kleber, B., Veit, R., Birbaumer, N., Gruzelier, J., & Lotze, M. (2010). The brain of opera singers: Experience-dependent changes in functional activation. *Cerebral Cortex, 20*, 1144–1152.

Knowlton, B. J., Mangels, J. A., & Squire, L. R. (1996). A neostriatal habit learning system in humans. *Science, 273*, 1399–1402.

Kurth, F., Zilles, K., Fox, P. T., Laird, A. R., & Eickhoff, S. B. (2010). A link between the systems: Functional differentiation and integration within the human insula revealed by meta-analysis. *Brain Structure and Function, 214*, 519–534.

Lane, R. D. (2008). Neural substrates of implicit and explicit emotional processes: A unifying framework for psychosomatic medicine. *Psychosomatic Medicine, 70*, 214–231.

Lane, R. D., Ahern, G. L., Schwartz, G. E., & Kaszniak, A. W. (1997). Is alexithymia the emotional equivalent of blindsight? *Biological Psychiatry, 42*, 834–844.

Lane, R. D., & Garfield, D. A. S. (2005). Becoming aware of feelings: Integration of cognitive-developmental, neuroscientific, and psychoanalytic perspectives. *Neuropsychoanalysis, 7*, 5–30.

Luyten, P., Blatt, S. J., & Mayes, L. C. (2012). Process and outcome in psychoanalytic psychotherapy research: The need for a (relatively) new paradigm. In R. A. Levy, J. S. Ablon, & H. Kächele (Eds.), *Psychodynamic psychotherapy research: Evidence-based practice and practice-based evidence* (pp. 345–360). New York: Humana Press/Springer.

Morris, S. E., & Cuthbert, B. N. (2012). Research domain criteria: Cognitive systems, neural circuits, and dimensions of behavior. *Dialogues in Clinical Neuroscience, 14,* 29–37.

Nadel, L., & Hardt, O. (2011). Update on memory systems and processes. *Neuropsychopharmacology, 36,* 251–273.

Nadel, L., & Moscovitch, M. (1997). Memory consolidation, retrograde amnesia, and the hippocampal complex. *Current Opinion in Neurobiology, 7,* 217–227.

Nadel, L., & O'Keefe, J. (1974). The hippocampus in pieces and patches: An essay on modes of explanation in physiological psychology. In R. Bellairs & E. G. Gray (Eds.), *Essays on the nervous system: A Festschrift for Professor J. Z. Young* (pp. 367–390). Oxford, UK: Clarendon Press.

Nader, K., & Hardt, O. (2009). A single standard for memory: The case for reconsolidation. *Nature Reviews. Neuroscience, 10,* 224–234.

Niedenthal, P. M. (2007). Embodying emotion. *Science, 316,* 1002–1005.

Oberman, L. M., & Ramachandran, V. S. (2007). The simulating social mind: The role of the mirror neuron system and simulation in the social and communicative deficits of autism spectrum disorders. *Psychological Bulletin, 133,* 310–327.

Ochsner, K. N., Bunge, S. A., Gross, J. J., & Gabrieli, J. D. (2002). Rethinking feelings: An FMRI study of the cognitive regulation of emotion. *Journal of Cognitive Neuroscience, 14,* 1215–1229.

Ochsner, K. N., Chiu, C.-Y. P., & Schacter, D. (1994). Varieties of priming. *Current Opinion in Neurobiology, 4,* 189–194.

Peterson, B. S. (2005). Clinical neuroscience and imaging studies of core psychoanalytic constructs. *Clinical Neuroscience Research, 4,* 349–365.

Peterson, M. A., & Skow, E. (2008). Suppression of shape properties on the ground side of an edge: Evidence for a competitive model of figure assignment. *Journal of Experimental Psychology. Human Perception and Performance, 34,* 251–267.

Pfeifer, J. H., Iacoboni, M., Mazziotta, J. C., & Dapretto, M. (2008). Mirroring others' emotions relates to empathy and interpersonal competence in children. *NeuroImage, 39,* 2076–2085.

Posner, J., Russell, J. A., Gerber, A., Gorman, D., Colibazzi, T., Yu, S., et al. (2009). The neurophysiological bases of emotion: An fMRI study of the affective circumplex using emotion-denoting words. *Human Brain Mapping, 30,* 883–895.

Posner, J., Russell, J. A., & Peterson, B. S. (2005). The circumplex model of affect: An integrative approach to affective neuroscience, cognitive development, and psychopathology. *Development and Psychopathology, 17,* 715–734.

Ranganath, C., & D'Esposito, M. (2001). Medial temporal lobe activity associated with active maintenance of novel information. *Neuron, 31,* 865–873.

Rizzolatti, G., Fadiga, L., Gallese, V., & Fogassi, L. (1996). Premotor cortex and the recognition of motor actions. *Cognitive Brain Research, 3,* 131–141.

Roediger, H. L., Jacoby, D., & McDermott, K. B. (1996). Misinformation effects in recall: Creating false memories through repeated retrieval. *Journal of Memory and Language, 35,* 300–318.

Roffman J., Gerber, A. J., & Glick, D. M. (2012). Neural models of psychodynamic concepts and treatments: Implications for psychodynamic psychotherapy. In R. A. Levy, J. S. Ablon, & H. Kächele (Eds.), *Psychodynamic psychotherapy research: Evidence-based practice and practice-based evidence* (pp. 193–218). New York: Humana Press/Springer.

Rojahn, K., & Pettigrew, T. F. (1992). Memory for scheme-relevant information: A meta-analytic resolution. *British Journal of Social Psychology, 31,* 81–109.

Ryan, L., Nadel, L., Keil, K., Putnam, K., Schnyer, D., Trouard, T., et al. (2001). Hippocampal complex and retrieval of recent and very remote autobiographical memories: Evidence from functional magnetic resonance imaging in neurologically intact people. *Hippocampus, 11,* 707–714.

Sandler, J., & Fonagy, P. (Eds.). (1997). *Recovered memories of abuse: True or false?* London: Karnac Books.

Seeley, W. W., Menon, V., Schatzberg, A. F., Keller, J., Glover, G. H., Kenna, H., et al. (2007). Dissociable intrinsic connectivity networks for salience processing and executive control. *Journal of Neuroscience, 27*, 2349–2356.

Sloutsky, V. M., & Fisher, A. V. (2004). When learning and development decrease memory: Evidence against category-based induction. *Psychological Science, 15*, 553–558.

Southgate, V., & Hamilton, A. F. (2008). Unbroken mirrors: Challenging a theory of autism. *Trends in Cognitive Sciences, 12*, 225–229.

Specht, M. W., Chapman, A., & Cellucci, T. (2009). Schemas and borderline personality disorder symptoms in incarcerated women. *Journal of Behavior Therapy and Experimental Psychiatry, 40*, 256–264.

Squire, L. R. (1987). *Memory and brain.* New York: Oxford University Press.

Tse, D., Langston, R. F., Kakeyama, M., Bethus, I., Spooner, P. A., Wood, E. R., et al. (2007). Schemas and memory consolidation. *Science, 316*, 76–82.

Tulving, E. (1972). Episodic and semantic memory. In E. Tulving & W. Donaldson (Eds.), *Organization of memory* (pp. 381–403). New York: Academic Press.

Unoka, Z., Fogd, D., Fuzy, M., & Csukly, G. (2011). Misreading the facial signs: Specific impairments and error patterns in recognition of facial emotions with negative valence in borderline personality disorder. *Psychiatry Research, 189*, 419–425.

Vogt, B. A. (2005). Pain and emotion interactions in subregions of the cingulate gyrus. *Nature Reviews. Neuroscience, 6*, 533–544.

Yamokoski, C. A., Scheel, K. R., & Rogers, J. R. (2011). The role of affect in suicidal thoughts and behaviors. *Suicide and Life-Threatening Behavior, 41*, 160–170.

Zhao, L., Zhang, X., Shi, J., Epstein, D. H., & Lu, L. (2009). Psychosocial stress after reactivation of drug-related memory impairs later recall in abstinent heroin addicts. *Psychopharmacology, 203*, 599–608.

CHAPTER 5

The Psychodynamic Approach to Diagnosis and Classification

Patrick Luyten and Sidney J. Blatt

Issues of classification and diagnosis have been much debated over the past decades. For many years, psychiatry and clinical psychology have been dominated by a largely descriptive, atheoretical, and disorder-centered approach, exemplified by the various editions of the *Diagnostic and Statistical Manual of Mental Disorders* (DSM; American Psychiatric Association, 2013) and the *International Classification of Diseases* (ICD; World Health Organization, 1992), which has overshadowed other approaches, including psychoanalytic ones (Blatt & Luyten, 2010). Indeed, core assumptions of psychoanalytic approaches to diagnosis and classification are clearly at odds with currently prevailing models (Blatt & Luyten, 2010; Blatt & Shichman, 1983; McWilliams, 1994; PDM Task Force, 2006; Westen, Shedler, & Bradley, 2006; Westen & Weinberger, 2004). Psychodynamic approaches characteristically (1) combine a disorder-centered with a more person-centered approach, and (2) are fundamentally developmentally oriented, tracing various pathways from infancy to adulthood and identifying how complex interactions among biological and psychosocial factors are expressed across the lifetime (Luyten, Mayes, Target, & Fonagy, 2012). This contrasts with the rather static and largely nondevelopmental approach of DSM and ICD. Furthermore, rather than assuming that disorders are categorically distinct from "normality," psychoanalytic approaches assume a fundamental continuity between normality and pathology (Blatt & Shichman, 1983; Luyten, Mayes, et al., 2012; McWilliams, 2011).

Continuing criticism of the descriptive approach in psychiatry, however, has led to the beginning of major changes. First, there are clear signs that psychodynamic views and language are finding their way back into the DSM. The DSM-5 Personality Disorders Work Group, for example, proposed a classification based on impairments in representations of self and other as key in diagnosing personality disorder (Skodol et al., 2011). Although these efforts were intended to be transtheoretical, psychodynamic formulations and research played a clear role in them (Bender, Morey, & Skodol, 2011). Furthermore, even though the DSM-5 Personality Disorders Work Group proposal was not accepted, it is now included in Section III for further research, and several field trials are ongoing investigating the validity of this new approach (American Psychiatric Association, 2013) (see also Meehan & Levy, Chapter 15, this volume).

Second, the move to a more dimensional approach in classification is most evident in the Research Domain Criteria (RDoC) initiative undertaken by the National Institute of Mental Health (NIMH; Cuthbert & Insel, 2013). The RDoC initiative certainly contrasts with psychoanalysis's emphasis on psychosocial factors, as it is predominantly focused on neurobiology. However, like psychoanalytic views, the RDoC considers psychopathology as a combination of disruptions in several dimensions, or developmental lines, to use Anna Freud's concept (Freud, 1963), that are implicated across disorders, rather than assuming that each disorder has its own relatively unique etiology.

Finally, this developmental approach has started to influence views on treatment development and research. Whereas the DSM has fostered the development of treatments for specific disorders, this new approach suggests a transdiagnostic view of treatment that is congruent with the traditional psychodynamic focus on broad-spectrum rather than disorder-specific treatment (Fonagy, Target, & Gergely, 2006) (see also Parts II and III in this volume).

This chapter focuses on three major contemporary psychodynamic approaches to classification and diagnosis as examples of approaches that have received empirical support. First, we review the seminal contributions of Shedler and Westen's prototype approach. Second, we discuss formulations based on considerations concerning the developmental level or level of personality organization. Third, we summarize theoretical and empirical research relevant to the so-called two polarities models of personality and psychopathology initiated by Blatt and colleagues (Blatt, 2008; Blatt & Shichman, 1983; Luyten & Blatt, 2011). We then outline an integrative classificatory model that we have been developing over the past decade, and the implications of these views for clinical practice. Before this, however, we will outline the core assumptions of psychodynamic approaches to diagnosis and classification.

BASIC ASSUMPTIONS OF CONTEMPORARY PSYCHODYNAMIC APPROACHES TOWARD CLASSIFICATION

A major problem for the development of any classification of mental disorders is the lack of an objective standard: a set of "naturally occurring" or theoretically derived categories that can be used to validate a classification system (Westen et al., 2006). As Gödel (1933) noted in mathematics, a higher order of abstraction is needed to test the validity of an earlier or lower-level system. A conceptualization cannot be used to test its own validity; one needs an external higher order of generality to test the validity of propositions within a given system (Blatt & Blatt, 1984). One approach to this issue is empirical—that is, to delineate the criteria for a classification of psychopathology based on empirical research. Considerable consensus has now been reached concerning the following principles.

Empirically Based

Any categorization system must be based on empirical research. This may seem self-evident, but in fact, as noted earlier, DSM is fundamentally based on professional consensus rather than research findings. The NIMH launched the RDoC initiative for precisely this reason; it seeks to establish classification in an empirically based dimensional approach to psychopathology (Cuthbert & Insel, 2013).

Developmental Perspective

Although any classification system should rest on solid empirical ground, classification systems should also be firmly rooted in an encompassing developmental theory of normal and disrupted personality development. Multivariate trait models such as the Five Factor (Costa & McCrae, 2010) and the tripartite (Watson, Clark, & Chmielewski, 2008) models, for instance, though providing empirical data concerning largely genetically determined "building blocks" of normal and disrupted personality development, are too static because they lack a developmental perspective that could facilitate consideration of the distorted efforts at adaptation that occur in psychopathology (Luyten & Blatt, 2011).

It is difficult to imagine an understanding of psychopathology other than a developmental one. Hence, just as a reliance on consensus, as in the DSM, may have led to arbitrary criteria that lack empirical foundation, an overreliance on atheoretical multivariate approaches threatens to lead to a classification system that neither provides a theoretically consistent view of psychopathology nor appeals to clinicians' intuitive ways of conceptualizing psychiatric disorders (Luyten & Blatt, 2011; Shedler et al., 2010). Research increasingly demonstrates the complex pathways and the multifactorial and often recursive causality involved in both normal and abnormal development from infancy through childhood to senescence. This implies that a classification system should ideally be based in research driven by an encompassing theory concerning the nature of adaptive and maladaptive personality development.

Functionality of Psychopathology

From this perspective, forms of psychopathology should be seen as distorted modes of adaptation that derive from variations and disruptions of normal psychological development, not so much or exclusively as diseases (Blatt & Shichman, 1983). This view is increasingly being incorporated in other theories (Luyten & Blatt, 2011), often without mentioning its origin in psychoanalytic thought. This view implies that assessment should focus not only on impairments and vulnerabilities, but also on strengths and resilience as well as contextual factors.

Dimensional and Categorical

Although discrete categorical disorders may exist, a dimensional view of psychopathology appears to better fit the data for most disorders. Some disorders, however, might represent true "taxa." Furthermore, both clinicians and insurance companies will continue to prefer categorical diagnoses (e.g., this patient "has" depression). Future classification systems should thus combine the advantages of a dimensional and a categorical view (Westen et al., 2006). Although the hallmark of psychodynamic approaches to psychopathology is a developmental perspective that takes into account the function of disruptions in personality development expressed in different types of psychopathology (Luyten & Blatt, 2011), this more developmental, person-centered approach and a more descriptive, disorder-centered approach are not necessarily mutually exclusive. Psychoanalytic researchers and clinicians also use diagnostic labels and have actually been the first to delineate several types of psychopathology. Freud (1894/1962), for instance, was the first to delineate obsessive–compulsive disorder. Later, Fenichel (1945) proposed a classification of psychopathology that influenced classification and diagnosis in psychology and psychiatry for decades. Around the same time, psychoanalytic writers delineated borderline personality disorder (Knight, 1953; Stern, 1938), and Kohut and Wolf (1978) and Kernberg (1975) made substantial contributions to descriptions of the phenomenology of the personality disorders more broadly. More recently, the *Psychodynamic Diagnostic Manual* (PDM) was launched; it provides a multiaxial approach to classification and diagnosis combining a disorder-centered and a person-centered approach (PDM Task Force, 2006). All these examples clearly demonstrate that disorder-centered and person-centered approaches to psychopathology are complementary.

Both of these approaches in fact reflect the intrinsic difficulties in categorizing psychiatric disorders, and psychiatric nosology has constantly shifted between these two approaches. Earlier editions of the DSM embraced a hybrid approach, yet, from DSM-III onward, the descriptive, categorical, atheoretical approach became more prominent because there was no consensus at the time concerning the value of theory-driven approaches to psychopathology (Blatt & Luyten, 2010).

Clinical Utility

Finally, a classification system, to be clinically useful, should be "nature friendly but also user friendly" (Westen, Heim, Morrison, Patterson, & Campbell, 2002, p. 222). The DSM includes distinctions that are not only to some extent arbitrary, but also often difficult to make and cumbersome (as anyone who has ever administered a Structured Clinical Interview for DSM will endorse). The clinical utility of most DSM diagnoses is further limited because they offer little information concerning treatment and prognosis (Spitzer, First, Shedler, Westen, & Skodol, 2008).

CONTEMPORARY PSYCHODYNAMIC APPROACHES TO CLASSIFICATION AND DIAGNOSIS

The Shedler–Westen Assessment Procedure

In a creative series of studies, Shedler and Westen developed the Shedler–Westen Assessment Procedure (SWAP), a method to assess personality disorder prototypes that has had considerable influence on contemporary thinking about personality disorder diagnosis and classification (Shedler & Westen, 2010; Westen et al., 2006). The SWAP involves clinicians' Q-sort ratings of jargon-free descriptions of both descriptive phenomenology and psychological processes (including motives, defenses, and conflicts) typical of personality pathology, based on a minimum 6 hours of clinical contact or on a semistructured Clinical Diagnostic Interview.

The SWAP differs in major ways from contemporary approaches to diagnosing personality pathology, such as DSM, because these approaches typically are based on semistructured interviews that attempt to minimize clinical inference (Westen & Shedler, 1999). By contrast, the SWAP combines empirical rigor with an emphasis on clinical inference. Hence, clinicians include in their ratings not only *what* is typical of a patient but also *how* a patient tells something, the way the patient relates to others (including the clinician), and the countertransferential reactions evoked in the clinician.

Based on this procedure, Shedler, Westen, and colleagues found evidence for seven distinct "naturally occurring" personality disorder prototypes (dysphoric, antisocial, schizoid, paranoid, obsessional, histrionic, and narcissistic) (see Table 5.1 for an example). Importantly, several personality disorders included in DSM-IV-TR (American Psychiatric Association, 2000) and DSM-5 (American Psychiatric Association, 2013) did not emerge as prototypes (e.g., borderline personality disorder), whereas some prototypes emerged that are not included in DSM-IV (e.g., dysphoric personality disorder) (see also Meehan & Levy, Chapter 15, this volume).

Moreover, subsequent research showed that diagnostic comorbidity using this diagnostic system was greatly reduced; patients typically had elevated scores on only one prototype. Additionally, clinicians from various orientations can reliably categorize patients based on the SWAP, with greater clinical utility than with the DSM categorical approach and other dimensional personality models such as the Five-Factor Model (Spitzer et al., 2008). Further studies have also identified subtypes within each of these prototypes that seem to be meaningfully related to etiological factors and clinical presentation (DeFife et al., 2013; Russ, Shedler, Bradley, & Westen, 2008). Recent research also suggests that the identified prototypes are hierarchically organized within internalizing, externalizing, and borderline superordinate factors (Shedler & Westen, 2010), a finding discussed in more detail in the next section because it provides important support for psychodynamic assumptions concerning classification and diagnosis.

The SWAP not only enables clinicians to use a simple prototype-matching approach in diagnosis, rather than a cumbersome count/cutoff approach as in DSM, but it also enables them to generate hypotheses concerning the dynamics and functions

TABLE 5.1. Prototypical Description of Narcissistic Personality Disorder Using the Shedler–Westen Assessment Procedure

- Appears to feel privileged and entitled, expects preferential treatment
- Has an exaggerated sense of self-importance
- Tends to be controlling
- Tends to be critical of others
- Tends to get into power struggles
- Tends to feel misunderstood, mistreated, or victimized
- Tends to be competitive with others (whether consciously or unconsciously)
- Is articulate; can express self well in words
- Tends to react to criticism with feelings of rage and humiliation
- Tends to be angry or hostile (whether consciously or unconsciously)
- Has little empathy, seems unable to understand or respond to others' needs and feelings unless they coincide with his or her own
- Tends to blame others for own failures or shortcomings; tends to believe his or her problems are caused by external factors
- Seeks to be the center of attention
- Tends to be arrogant, haughty, or dismissive
- Seems to treat others primarily as an audience to witness of importance, brilliance, beauty, etc.

Note. Items reproduced with permission of Jonathan Shedler.

of personality features. For instance, if a patient has high scores on the SWAP items "Has an exaggerated sense of self-importance (e.g., feels special superior, grand, or envied)" and "Tends to feel s/he is inadequate, inferior or a failure," this may indicate that this patient uses grandiosity to defend against underlying feelings of inferiority and unworthiness (see Table 5.1). Hence, the combination of SWAP items leads to hypotheses concerning the dynamic conflict–defense constellations typical of personality disorders, which cannot be assessed using other dimensional models that assume that a person is high or low on a specific trait, but not both (Luyten & Blatt, 2011). Finally, the SWAP provides clinicians with a focus in the course of treatment and has been shown to be sensitive to capture therapeutic change.

In summary, the SWAP provides clinicians with an empirically supported and clinically relevant, jargon-free language to diagnose personality pathology on the basis of descriptive features and underlying psychodynamics. It is a researcher- and clinician-friendly approach to diagnosis and classification that is deeply rooted in the psychodynamic tradition of emphasizing the function of personality pathology and the importance of clinical judgment in diagnosis. This approach markedly contrasts with DSM's static view and its striving to exclude clinicians' subjective responses from psychiatric diagnosis. Remarkably, whereas the DSM approach has led to very limited reliability in psychiatric diagnosis, the Shedler–Westen approach has led to high levels of reliability across clinicians from different orientations.

Limitations of the SWAP include the absence of a developmental perspective, although a version of the SWAP for adolescents has been validated. Also, the atheoretical approach of the SWAP limits its integration with contemporary neuroscience and psychosocial approaches.

Levels of Personality Organization

Psychodynamic approaches to diagnosis and classification distinguish between *types of personality disorder* (e.g., borderline or narcissistic personality disorder), as emphasized by the Shedler–Westen approach and most other classification systems, and what has been called the *developmental* or *structural level* or the *level of personality organization* (PO). The first approach emphasizes the descriptive features of a given personality disorder (i.e., habitual patterns of behavior, cognition, emotion, motivation, and ways of relating to others), whereas the second approach refers to a set of observable features that together represent the underlying organizational level of personality, a theoretical construct used to explain the relationship between descriptive features.

This focus on the level of PO is rooted in Freudian thought, distinguishing between more "primitive" or preoedipal and more integrated "oedipal" types of psychopathology, implying different developmental levels of psychopathology. Kernberg and Caligor (2005) and McWilliams (1994, 2011) have been instrumental in introducing this distinction within the psychoanalytic literature and in delineating core features central to determining the level of PO (Caligor & Clarkin, 2010; Kernberg & Caligor, 2005; McWilliams, 1994) (see also Meehan & Levy, Chapter 15, and Clarkin, Fonagy, Levy, & Bateman, Chapter 17, this volume). These features are (see also Table 5.2):

1. The level of identity integration.
2. The predominant level of defenses (ranging from primitive defense mechanisms, such as splitting and projective identification, to more mature defense mechanisms, such as repression and rationalization) to cope with external and internal stressors and conflicts.
3. The capacity for reality testing.
4. The quality of object relations (and underlying representations of self and others).
5. The capacity for self-observation.
6. The nature of primary conflicts.
7. The transference and countertransference potential of patients (i.e., whether they evoke strong transference/countertransference feelings).

These features define a continuum of personality pathology ranging from (1) neurotic PO, hypothesized to be characterized by relatively high levels of identity integration, intact reality testing, and the predominant use of more mature (i.e., higher level) defense mechanisms; to (2) borderline PO, assumed to be characterized by identity diffusion and the use of more primitive defense mechanisms with relatively intact reality testing; and to (3) psychotic PO, hypothesized to be characterized by marked identity diffusion, impaired reality testing, and the use of primitive defense mechanisms (see Table 5.2).

TABLE 5.2. Features Distinguishing Levels of Personality Organization

	Psychotic	Borderline	Neurotic
Level of identity integration	Severely disturbed	Marked identity diffusion	Relatively integrated
Predominant level of defenses	Primary defense mechanisms (projection, splitting)	Primary defense mechanisms (splitting, projective identification)	Secondary defense mechanisms (repression, rationalization, reaction formation)
Capacity for reality testing	May be seriously disturbed (prone to delusions, hallucinations)	Relatively intact, may be temporarily disturbed, particularly in high arousal conditions	Intact
Quality of object relations and self/other representations	Serious disturbances in object relations and (threatening) disintegration of self and object representations	Troubled interpersonal relationships, often marked by chaos, idealization–denigration, instability of self and other representations	Relationships may be characterized by more subtle conflicts around autonomy/relatedness, integration of love and aggression
Capacity for self-observation	Severely disturbed	Often severely disturbed	Relatively intact
Nature of primary conflicts	Existential (life, death, identity)	Relational	Conflicts around autonomy/relatedness (e.g., guilt, shame, sexual intimacy)
Typical transference and countertransference	Very strong, often very positive, but may also be terrifying	Strong, characterized by feelings of idealization and/or denigration	More subtle

Note. Based on Kernberg and Caligor (2005) and McWilliams (2011).

The level of PO, thought to reflect the severity of personality pathology, is considered to be an important predictor of prognosis and treatment response, even more important than the "type" of personality disorder (Caligor & Clarkin, 2010). Congruent with this assumption, studies suggest that level of PO is related to treatment outcome and may be the single most important predictor of course and response to treatment, although more research is needed in this area (Koelen et al., 2012).

Another important difference between the PO-level approach and current descriptive DSM and ICD approaches is the assumption that there is no one-to-one relationship between the type of personality disorder and the level of PO, with the exception of Kernberg (e.g., see Kernberg & Caligor, 2005), who assumes that most personality disorders reflect borderline PO. Only obsessive–compulsive, depressive, and hysterical personality disorders would reflect neurotic PO, according to Kernberg. Yet, most approaches within this area assume that these axes (i.e., descriptive and level of PO) are relatively independent, and thus each type of personality pathology can manifest itself at different levels of PO (e.g., hysterical personality can manifest itself at psychotic, borderline, and neurotic levels) (McWilliams, 2011). Further research in this area is clearly needed. From this perspective, borderline PO refers to a much broader category of disorders than borderline personality disorder as defined in the DSM, which tends to focus on the more interpersonal and "spectacular" expression of borderline features that have historically been delineated (Fonagy & Luyten, in press). As noted earlier, studies by Shedler and Westen support this broader view, showing that the concept of borderline is a hierarchically higher level of functioning under which several disorders can be subsumed (e.g., histrionic–impulsive and emotionally dysregulated personality disorders). More research concerning this approach is still needed, particularly in view of the wide variety of measures used in this tradition, with little investigation of their interrelationships and the lack of large population-representative studies. Existing research, however, suggests that features referring to level of PO can be reliably assessed by both self-report and observer-report measures (Bender et al., 2011; Lowyck, Luyten, Verhaest, Vandeneede, & Vermote, 2013). Studies have shown that these measures are able to distinguish patients with various diagnoses (Huprich & Greenberg, 2003) and are associated with treatment outcome (Koelen et al., 2012). As noted, recent studies also suggest that severity of personality pathology might be the single most important predictor of course and treatment response. It is thus no surprise that psychodynamic considerations concerning levels of personality functioning have been incorporated in future DSM proposals (Skodol, 2012) (see also Meehan & Levy, Chapter 15, this volume).

Work on the Operationalized Psychodynamic Diagnostics (OPD) is also relevant in this context. The OPD resembles the PDM classification system in many respects. Whereas field trials concerning the PDM are still largely ongoing (PDM Task Force, 2006), the OPD has received considerable support over recent years (Cierpka, Grande, Rudolf, von der Tann, & Stasch, 2007; OPD Task Force, 2008). Briefly, the OPD contains five diagnostic axes: (1) illness experience and motivation for/assumptions about treatment, (2) interpersonal relationships, (3) mental conflicts, (4) level of PO, and (5) mental and psychosomatic disorders. These five axes can be reliably rated by clinicians based on a 1- to 2-hour clinical interview, and a detailed manual contains definitions, description, and examples. As with the other psychodynamic diagnostic systems discussed, the OPD is aimed primarily at informing treatment planning, although research relating the different axes to treatment outcome is still sparse. Furthermore, validity findings are still mainly limited to OPD Axis 1 and 4, with both axes being able to differentiate patients with personality disorders from those without, with large effect sizes (Doering et al., 2014). Yet, training and scoring of the various axes are relatively cumbersome processes, and the clinical utility of the OPD therefore remains a topic of some concern.

Blatt's Two-Polarities Model

Blatt's synthetic efforts offer an integration that provides a bridge among psychodynamic approaches, as well as providing a relationship to other approaches in the field of diagnosis and treatment (Blatt, 2008; Blatt & Luyten, 2010; Blatt & Shichman, 1983). Congruent with the emphasis on impairments in self and others in recent theoretical approaches to personality disorder (Livesley, 2008) and in proposals for DSM-5 (Skodol & Bender, 2009), Blatt has argued, from both a descriptive and a theoretical point of view, that personality disorders are fundamentally characterized by problems with *relatedness* (or *attachment*) on the one hand and problems with *self-definition* (or *self and identity*) on the other, and thus can be parsimoniously situated in a two-dimensional space spanned by relatedness and self-definition. More specifically, Blatt (2008) argues that relatedness and self-definition are two fundamental psychological dimensions that provide an integrated theoretical matrix for understanding processes of personality development, variations in normal PO, concepts of psychopathology, and mechanisms of therapeutic action.

According to Blatt (2008), well-functioning personality involves an integration (or balance) in the development of interpersonal relatedness and of self-definition, such that more mature levels of relatedness facilitate the development of an essentially positive and stable sense of self, identity, and autonomy, which in turn enable more differentiated and integrated interpersonal relationships (see Figure 5.1). Hence, across development, a dialectic interaction between the relatedness and self-definition developmental lines mutually reinforces the development of the other line. Disruptive experiences and biological predispositions, together with their interaction, can result in exaggerated distortions of one developmental line to the neglect of the other, reflecting compensatory or defensive maneuvers in response to developmental disruptions. Different forms of psychopathology are thus not static entities resulting from deficits in development, but can be thought of as dynamic, conflict–defense constellations that attempt to maintain a balance, however disturbed, between relatedness and self-definition.

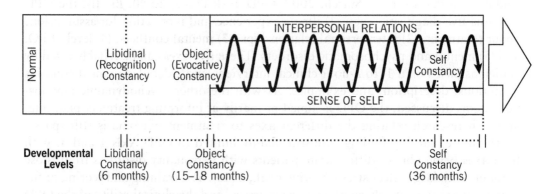

FIGURE 5.1. Blatt's dialectic model of personality development. From Blatt (1990). Copyright 1990 by the University of Chicago. Reprinted by permission.

Congruent with these assumptions, studies in both inpatients and outpatients have found that the various personality disorders, in meaningfully and theoretically expected ways, are organized into two primary configurations—one organized around issues of relatedness and the other around issues of self-definition (Blatt & Luyten, 2010). For instance, individuals with a dependent, histrionic, or borderline personality disorder typically have significantly greater concern with issues of interpersonal relatedness than with issues of self-definition. Individuals with a paranoid, schizoid, schizotypal, antisocial, narcissistic, avoidant, obsessive–compulsive, or self-defeating personality disorder usually have significantly greater preoccupation with issues of self-definition than with issues of interpersonal relatedness.

These views are further supported by both attachment research and contemporary interpersonal approaches (Luyten & Blatt, 2011) showing that personality disorders can be similarly organized in a two-dimensional space defined by *attachment anxiety* or *communion* (reflecting concerns concerning relatedness) and *attachment avoidance* or *agency* (reflecting issues with regard to identity and autonomy), respectively (Meyer & Pilkonis, 2005; Mikulincer & Shaver, 2007; Pincus, 2005) (see also Mikulincer & Shaver, Chapter 2, this volume, and Figures 5.2 and 5.3).

Studies suggest that there is not necessarily a one-to-one relationship between these two dimensions and descriptive DSM categories (Luyten & Blatt, 2011). Levy, Edell, and McGlashan (2007), for instance, found that the then-current DSM-IV criteria did not capture different underlying dynamics of patients diagnosed with DSM

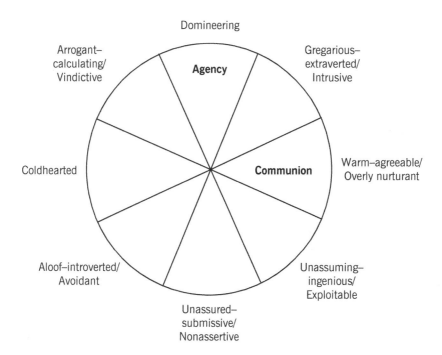

FIGURE 5.2. The interpersonal circumplex. From Pincus (2005). Copyright 2005 by The Guilford Press. Adapted by permission.

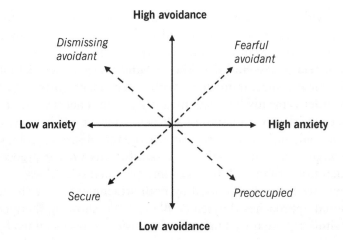

FIGURE 5.3. Two-dimensional space defined by attachment anxiety and avoidance. From Mikulincer and Shaver (2007). Copyright 2007 by The Guilford Press. Adapted by permission.

borderline personality disorder. These findings suggest that patients with DSM borderline personality disorder diagnosis are notably heterogeneous (see also Meehan & Levy, Chapter 15, and Clarkin, Fonagy, Levy, & Bateman, Chapter 17, this volume). Yet, Levy and colleagues were able to identify a hysteroid and paranoid type of borderline personality disorder that resembled a preoccupation with relatedness versus autonomy and identity, respectively, and these differences could be accounted for by the two-polarities model (Blatt & Auerbach, 1988).

The two-polarities model has also been theoretically and empirically related to current extant multivariate models of personality, which opens up many interesting perspectives for both research and clinical practice (Luyten & Blatt, 2011). The clinical utility of the model is further supported by findings that the model may explain comorbidity between "symptom disorders" and between these disorders and personality disorders (Blatt, 2008; Blatt & Luyten, 2009). Research has implicated maladaptive expressions of relatedness and self-definition in depression (Blatt, 2004; Luyten & Blatt, 2012), eating disorders (Boone, Claes, & Luyten, 2014; Thompson-Brenner et al., 2008), substance abuse (Blatt, Rounsaville, Eyre, & Wilber, 1984; Blatt & Shichman, 1983; Fonagy & Luyten, in press), posttraumatic stress disorder (Cox, MacPherson, Enns, & McWilliams, 2004; Gargurevich, Luyten, & Corveleyn, 2008), conduct disorder (Blatt & Shichman, 1983), and functional somatic disorders (Luyten et al., 2011), which may explain the high comorbidity between these disorders and their high comorbidity with personality disorders.

Although more research concerning Blatt's two-polarities model is needed, findings such as these promise to provide both researchers and clinicians with a parsimonious and theoretically encompassing model that has immediate relevance for therapeutic intervention. Studies indicate that patients with an excessive emphasis on relatedness (*anaclitic* patients) versus patients who overemphasize self-definition (*introjective* patients) respond differently to treatments and show a different process of change in psychotherapy across different treatment modalities (Blatt, Zuroff, Hawley, & Auerbach, 2010; see also Blatt, Chapter 7, this volume). Briefly, introjective features have been negatively related to outcome in brief, structured treatments, regardless of their theoretical orientation. Furthermore, congruent with their cognitive-affective style, introjective patients seem primarily responsive to more insight-oriented interventions, while anaclitic patients seem to respond better to more supportive interventions. These findings suggest that deviations of these two developmental lines can be best considered as transdiagnostic vulnerability factors that are also related to treatment outcome across treatment approaches.

AN INTEGRATIVE APPROACH TO CLASSIFICATION AND DIAGNOSIS

In recent years, we have described our attempts to reconcile various approaches and findings concerning personality pathology (Blatt & Luyten, 2009, 2010; Luyten & Blatt, 2007, 2011, 2013). Here, we summarize and update these views.

Based on the research reviewed, we have proposed that different forms of psychopathology can be situated within a hierarchical model that integrates theory-driven models that emphasize relatedness and self-definition as central coordinates in normal and disrupted personality development with empirically derived models of basic temperament and personality factors. This integration is based on four central assumptions concerning the nature of personality pathology, which we outline here.

A Circumplex View of Normal and Disrupted Personality Development

As we outline above, research indicates a growing consensus that psychopathological disorders, congruent with contemporary interpersonal approaches (Horowitz et al., 2006; Pincus, 2005), can be arranged in a two-dimensional space defined by (1) *relatedness*, ranging from high to low anxiety or warmth in relationships and (2) *self-definition*, ranging from low to high avoidance of others (see Figure 5.4). The cognitive-affective interpersonal schemas or internal working models of self and others underlying these dimensions range from relatively broad schemas to more relationship-specific working models (Blatt & Luyten, 2010; Sibley & Overall, 2010) that are part of connectionist networks that develop over the lifespan and that, at least in normal development, become increasingly complex, differentiated, and integrated.

This view implies a fundamental continuity between normal personality features and psychopathology. Thus, research should examine the developmental pathways from more basic, largely genetically determined, temperament and personality dimensions that, in interaction with environmental factors, lead to disruptions at different developmental levels of cognitive-affective schemas of self and others across the lifespan.

This view contrasts with assumptions that each disorder has a relatively unique (biological) cause, as promoted by the DSM approach. This approach rather implies

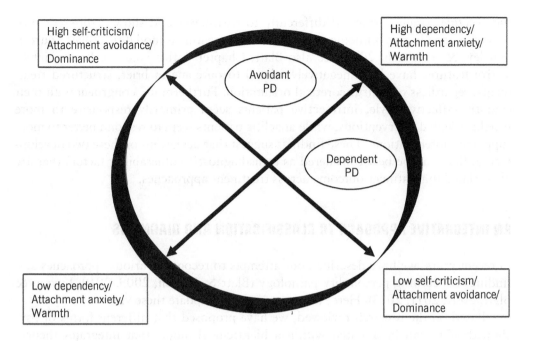

FIGURE 5.4. Dependent and avoidant personality disorder (PD) within an integrative prototype approach to psychopathology. From Luyten and Blatt (2011). Copyright 2011 by Elsevier. Adapted by permission.

that correlations between different disorders situated in the two-dimensional circumplex space are expected to decrease as one moves around the circumplex, which could lead to further understanding of the troublesome high comorbidity of disorders in DSM. Furthermore, the emphasis on cognitive-affective schemas or internal working models provides a common language across disciplines, ranging across cognitive science, cognitive-behavioral research, social and personality psychology, developmental psychopathology, psychodynamic, and neuroscience approaches. Moreover, a host of validated measures, from self-report questionnaires to interviews and observer-rated scales, are available to assess various expressions of relatedness and self-definition at different levels of abstraction (Locke, 2011; Luyten & Blatt, 2007; Sibley & Overall, 2007, 2010).

A Prototype Approach

The proposed model assumes that psychopathological disorders are best conceptualized as *prototypes* in this two-dimensional space. This contrasts markedly with the categorical approach of DSM, and with the arbitrary or empirically determined cutoff scores in multivariate dimensional models. Our approach defines different disorders in terms of *prototypical, conflict–defense constellations*, however maladaptive, that reflect attempts to establish and maintain a sense of interpersonal relatedness and self-definition at different developmental levels (Blatt & Shichman, 1983;

McWilliams, 1994). Hence, individual patients may resemble, to a greater or lesser extent, prototypical ways of dealing with issues of relatedness and self-definition, ranging from "normal" personality functioning to subclinical psychopathology to full-blown symptom and/or personality disorders. This approach also facilitates the identification of fundamental similarities among the characteristics of traditional diagnoses, such as the preoccupation with the integrity of sense of self at different developmental levels in paranoid, obsessive–compulsive, depressive, and narcissistic disorders, and the preoccupation with interpersonal relatedness at different developmental levels in dependent and histrionic personality disorders (Blatt & Shichman, 1983).

As noted earlier, the Shedler–Westen approach (Shedler & Westen, 2010; Spitzer et al., 2008) has demonstrated the advantages of prototypes as compared to the DSM categorical approach or multivariate personality models. Human beings prefer prototypes, which reflect their natural tendency when they are asked to categorize objects. Cognitive science has demonstrated that prototypes are indeed characterized by a good time:effort ratio (Spitzer et al., 2008) and enable clinicians to consider the psychodynamics underlying diagnosis, which symptom-based descriptive diagnoses and multivariate personality models do not allow (Shedler & Westen, 2010).

The hierarchical organization of different disorders in a prototype approach also offers a parsimonious way of conceptualizing comorbidity (Egan, Wade, & Shafran, 2011). Rather than being different "diseases," disorders situated close to each other in the circumplex reflect similar responses to and attempts to cope with issues of relatedness and self-definition (Luyten & Blatt, 2012). For instance, the high comorbidity among depression and functional somatic disorders such as chronic fatigue and pain disorders may not only reflect shared etiological features such as struggles with issues of self-worth and failure (self-definition issues), leading to a biopsychosocial collapse of the stress system associated with dysfunctions in immune and pain-processing systems (Luyten, Van Houdenhove, Lemma, Target, & Fonagy, 2012, 2013). Their high comorbidity may also result from the fact that depression and functional somatic complaints both involve a serious challenge to issues of self-worth and autonomy.

A Dynamic, Developmental Psychopathology Perspective

A common criticism of the DSM is its lack of developmental sensitivity because it typically uses the same criteria for disorders irrespective of the age and developmental stage of the individual. Moreover, most children and adults present with multiple problems, and therefore the DSM has resulted in an artificial distinction between disorders and problems in childhood/adolescence and in adulthood. DSM-5 has provided important steps to rectify this problem, but more work is needed.

Developmental psychopathology has abundantly shown that vulnerability to psychopathology is best conceptualized in terms of *equifinality* and *multifinality* across the lifespan (Cicchetti & Rogosch, 1996). Rather than trying to distinguish between different disorders and assuming that each disorder has a relatively unique etiology, it may be the case that different etiological factors may lead to the same developmental outcome (equifinality). In addition, depending on other factors, a given developmental factor (e.g., temperament) may lead to different developmental outcomes (multifinality). Hence, classification should be based on the consideration of complex developmental pathways that lead to a range of end states, rather than focusing on the purported unique etiology of specific disorders—an issue to which we will return in more detail later in this chapter.

As noted, these views can be integrated with extant multivariate models of personality that focus on lower-level temperament factors such as the Five-Factor Model (Costa & McCrae, 2010) and inform the study of these complex pathways in which temperament and personality factors influence these developmental trajectories. For instance, basic temperament features such as effortful control and negative affect predict whether psychological problems are expressed in terms of internalizing or externalizing problems or a combination of both (Boone et al., 2014; Casalin et al., 2014). A combination of person-centered and variable-centered research is needed in this context to unravel these influences in both normal and disrupted personality development. The identification of the neurobiological underpinnings of fundamental "building blocks of personality," consistent with the RDoC project of the NIMH (Cuthbert & Insel, 2013), will be very important in this context (see also Mayes, Luyten, Blatt, Fonagy, & Target, Chapter 25, this volume).

Let us illustrate these views by considering the relationship between two common personality disorders, dependent and avoidant personality disorder. Studies suggest that dependent personality disorder is situated in the Low-Avoidance, High-Anxiety quadrant of the circumplex (see Figure 5.4), reflecting strong desires for attachment and love in combination with strong fears of abandonment and loss of love (Luyten & Blatt, 2011; Meyer & Pilkonis, 2005). Avoidant personality disorder is situated in the High-Anxiety, High-Avoidance quadrant, suggesting that individuals with this disorder are involved in approach–avoidance conflicts. Although they wish to be accepted and admired, these individuals also fear that they will be criticized and rejected by others. As a result, they often show high levels of avoidance of others.

These two disorders thus reflect two different ways of dealing with issues of relatedness and self-definition. Basic temperament/personality factors are likely to play an important role in determining whether these issues are expressed in internalizing or externalizing symptoms. Studies suggest, for instance, that young adolescents with low levels of effortful control attempt to cope with issues of self-criticism by externalizing these issues (e.g., by blaming authority figures and society, or through antisocial behavior). Those with higher levels of effortful control (disinhibition), however, often tend to express these same issues in internalizing symptoms (e.g., self-critical depression) (Leadbeater, Kuperminc, Blatt, & Hertzog, 1999). Disorders thus are not static end states, but complex, multidetermined, dynamic conflict–defense constellations. This has also been demonstrated by priming studies. Individuals in the High-Avoidance, Low-Anxiety quadrant, for instance, often present a positive model of self on self-report questionnaires, but priming studies suggest that this positive bias toward the self is the result of a continuous defense against underlying feelings of insecurity and inferiority (Mikulincer & Shaver, 2007). Dependent individuals similarly do not simply have positive models of others; they also harbor feelings of jealousy and anger toward others, which they typically inhibit out of fear of abandonment and rejection (Mikulincer & Shaver, 2007) (see also Bornstein, Chapter 16, this volume).

Prototypes, Categories, Spectra, and Diagnoses of Disorders

The views expressed in this chapter imply that different disorders are typically part of spectra of disorders and that disorders within these spectra can be distinguished on the basis of a prototype approach. From this perspective, different spectra (e.g., based on genetic, neural, or psychosocial factors) may be distinguished. This emphasizes the importance of differentiating between prototypes, categories, spectra, and diagnoses.

Prototypes are multidimensional and hierarchically structured; they are more than simple descriptors such as anxious, frightened, depressed, or a list of such descriptors, and are more complex than conditional statements such as "He becomes depressed when confronted with failure." Prototypes involve conjunctive statements, for example, "He becomes depressed when confronted by failure and deals with the depression with defense mechanisms such as overcompensation, which then results in more experiences of failure, leading to a more extensive and lasting depression" (Blatt, Engel, & Mirmow, 1961). Prototypes are abstractions; they do not exist in reality, in contrast to *categories*, which are presumed to exist in nature. Moreover, there is a relatively limited number of prototypical ways in which human beings commonly confront conflict (e.g., issues at different developmental levels related to identity, sexuality, or aggression). The boundaries between prototypes are, by definition, fuzzy, so individuals typically can have features of different prototypes.

This brings us to the notion of *spectra* of disorders. This concept may have at least two meanings: (1) disorders can be organized in spectra because of similarities in the prototypes (e.g., narcissistic and antisocial personality disorders share prototypical ways of dealing with conflicts), and (2) they may also be organized in spectra based on similar etiological factors. The two do not need to overlap, although they may often do. Depending on the theoretical framework adopted, disorders may thus be organized along different spectra.

Finally, the notion of *diagnosis* refers to consensus statements that seek to provide meaningful labels for research and clinical practice.

Implications for the Development, Evaluation, and Dissemination of Treatments

The views expressed in this chapter emphasize the need for future investigation of the efficacy and effectiveness of broad *transdiagnostic treatments* that address basic underlying personality issues in psychopathology (Egan et al., 2011; Kazdin, 2011; Luyten & Blatt, 2007, 2011), rather than the development and evaluation of specific treatments for specific disorders. For instance, the neuropeptide oxytocin is currently being evaluated as a treatment in a spectrum of disorders marked by severe problems in relatedness, such as autism, schizophrenia, social phobia, and borderline personality disorder (Striepens, Kendrick, Maier, & Hurlemann, 2011). This makes perfect sense, rather than assuming that the effects of oxytocin would be limited to one specific disorder, as oxytocin has been implicated in attachment behavior and social cognition (Bartz, Zaki, Bolger, & Ochsner, 2011). Similarly, there is now consensus that so-called common factors (e.g., providing hope, structure, and a safe context to discuss problems) may be primarily responsible for treatment outcome in evidence-based treatments of both "symptom"-based and "personality"-based disorders (Bateman, 2012; Blatt et al., 2010; Wampold, Minami, Baskin, & Callen Tierney, 2002; Westen, Novotny, & Thompson-Brenner, 2004). Certain patient features have also been shown to explain treatment outcome across disorders and treatment approaches. As discussed earlier, patients who are preoccupied mainly with issues of relatedness or self-definition, for instance, are differentially responsive to different aspects of the treatment process, regardless of their specific diagnosis (Blatt et al., 2010).

These findings suggest that a fundamental parallel may exist between normal psychological development and the processes of therapeutic change (Blatt & Behrends, 1987; Luyten, Blatt, & Mayes, 2012). Therapeutic change may result, as in normal personality development, from a synergistic interaction of experiences of interpersonal relatedness and self-definition, of experiences of closeness and separation, of mutuality and incompatibility, and of understanding and misunderstanding, in the therapeutic relationship. Therapeutic change may thus involve a reactivation of the normal synergistic interaction between interpersonal experiences and the development of the sense of self, leading to more mature expressions of interpersonal relatedness that, in turn, further foster the development of the self (Safran, Muran, & Eubanks-Carter, 2011; Safran, Muran, Samstag, & Steven, 2002). Any effective treatment approach may provide the patient with the opportunity to examine important and intense personal issues, in a context of feeling understood and appreciated by an other, which eventually encourages and enables the patient to understand and appreciate not only his or her own feelings and thoughts, but also the thoughts and feelings of others—that is, to establish reciprocal, mutually facilitating, intersubjective interpersonal relationships (Fonagy, Luyten, & Allison, in press; Luyten & Blatt, 2013).

CONCLUSIONS AND FUTURE DIRECTIONS

This chapter has reviewed current empirically supported psychodynamic approaches to the diagnosis and classification of mental disorder. The findings reviewed show that these approaches are gaining ground, and are increasingly being incorporated into current work on classification and diagnosis. Yet, much work remains to be done; in particular, large-scale, interdisciplinary studies tracing the origins of different forms of psychopathology across the lifespan are needed. Further research is also needed on the implication of the views described in this chapter for treatment research.

With regard to diagnosis and assessment, more efforts should be devoted to developing user- and clinician-friendly classification systems and related assessment instruments. Given the increasing realization that psychopathology is essentially dimensional and results from a complex interaction among a large variety of factors, this will not be an easy task. In fact, the demand for "simple" classification systems and measures contrasts markedly with current trends in medicine, where complex, time-consuming, expensive techniques have become standard in making a diagnosis. Perhaps psychoanalysis, and clinical psychology and psychiatry more generally, should embrace these technological innovations as well and invest more in the development of innovative diagnostic methods, encompassing more person-centered and computerized assessments as well as drawing on innovations in the neurosciences.

REFERENCES

American Psychiatric Association. (2000). *Diagnostic and statistical manual of mental disorders* (4th ed., text rev.) Washington, DC: Author.

American Psychiatric Association. (2013). *Diagnostic and statistical manual of mental disorders* (5th ed.). Arlington, VA: Author.

Bartz, J. A., Zaki, J., Bolger, N., & Ochsner, K. N. (2011). Social effects of oxytocin in humans: Context and person matter. *Trends in Cognitive Sciences, 15*, 301–309.

Bateman, A. (2012). Treating borderline personality disorder in clinical practice [Editorial]. *American Journal of Psychiatry, 169*, 560–563.

Bender, D. S., Morey, L. C., & Skodol, A. E. (2011). Toward a model for assessing level of personality functioning in DSM-5, Part I: A review of theory and methods. *Journal of Personality Assessment, 93*, 332–346.

Blatt, S. J. (1990). Interpersonal relatedness and self-definition: Two personality configurations and their implications for psychopathology and psychotherapy. In J. L. Singer (Ed.), *Repression and dissociation: Implications for personality theory, psychopathology, and health* (pp. 299–335). Chicago: University of Chicago Press.

Blatt, S. J. (2004). *Experiences of depression: Theoretical, clinical and research perspectives.* Washington, DC: American Psychological Association.

Blatt, S. J. (2008). *Polarities of experience: Relatedness and self definition in personality development, psychopathology, and the therapeutic process.* Washington, DC: American Psychological Association.

Blatt, S. J., & Auerbach, J. S. (1988). Differential cognitive disturbances in three types of borderline patients. *Journal of Personality Disorders, 2*, 198–211.

Blatt, S. J., & Behrends, R. S. (1987). Internalization, separation-individuation, and the nature of therapeutic action. *International Journal of Psychoanalysis, 68*, 279–297.

Blatt, S. J., & Blatt, E. S. (1984). *Continuity and change in art: The development of modes of representation.* New York: Erlbaum.

Blatt, S. J., Engel, M., & Mirmow, E. L. (1961). When inquiry fails. *Journal of Projective Techniques, 25*, 32–37.

Blatt, S. J., & Luyten, P. (2009). A structural-developmental psychodynamic approach to psychopathology: Two polarities of experience across the life span. *Development and Psychopathology, 21*, 793–814.

Blatt, S. J., & Luyten, P. (2010). Reactivating the psychodynamic approach to the classification of psychopathology. In T. Millon, R. F. Krueger, & E. Simonsen (Eds.), *Contemporary directions in psychopathology: Scientific foundations of the DSM-V and ICD-11* (pp. 483–514). New York: Guilford Press.

Blatt, S. J., Rounsaville, B., Eyre, S. L., & Wilber, C. (1984). The psychodynamics of opiate addiction. *Journal of Nervous and Mental Disease, 172,* 342–352.

Blatt, S. J., & Shichman, S. (1983). Two primary configurations of psychopathology. *Psychoanalysis and Contemporary Thought, 6,* 187–254.

Blatt, S. J., Zuroff, D. C., Hawley, L. L., & Auerbach, J. S. (2010). Predictors of sustained therapeutic change. *Psychotherapy Research, 20,* 37–54.

Boone, L., Claes, L., & Luyten, P. (2014). Too strict or too loose? Perfectionism and impulsivity: The relation with eating disorder symptoms using a person-centered approach. *Eating Behaviors, 15,* 17–23.

Caligor, E., & Clarkin, J. F. (2010). An object relations model of personality and personality pathology. In J. F. Clarkin, P. Fonagy, & G. O. Gabbard (Eds.), *Psychodynamic psychotherapy for personality disorders. A clinical handbook* (pp. 3–35). Washington, DC: American Psychiatric Publishing.

Casalin, S., Luyten, P., Besser, A., Wouters, S., & Vliegen, N. (2014). A longitudinal cross-lagged study of the role of parental self-criticism, dependency, depression, and parenting stress in the development of child negative affectivity. *Self and Identity, 13,* 491–511.

Cicchetti, D., & Rogosch, F. A. (1996). Equifinality and multifinality in developmental psychopathology. *Development and Psychopathology, 8,* 597–600.

Cierpka, M., Grande, T., Rudolf, G., von der Tann, M., & Stasch, M. (2007). The Operationalized Psychodynamic Diagnostics System: Clinical relevance, reliability and validity. *Psychopathology, 40,* 209–220.

Costa, P. T., & McCrae, R. R. (2010). Bridging the gap with the five-factor model. *Personality Disorders, 1,* 127–130.

Cox, B. J., MacPherson, P. S. R., Enns, M. W., & McWilliams, L. A. (2004). Neuroticism and self-criticism associated with posttraumatic stress disorder in a nationally representative sample. *Behaviour Research and Therapy, 42,* 105–114.

Cuthbert, B., & Insel, T. (2013). Toward the future of psychiatric diagnosis: The seven pillars of RDoC. *BMC Medicine, 11,* 126.

DeFife, J. A., Peart, J., Bradley, B., Ressler, K., Drill, R., & Westen, D. (2013). Validity of prototype diagnosis for mood and anxiety disorders. *JAMA Psychiatry, 70,* 140–148.

Doering, S., Burgmer, M., Heuft, G., Menke, D., Baumer, B., Lubking, M., et al. (2014). Assessment of personality functioning: Validity of the Operationalized Psychodynamic Diagnosis Axis IV (Structure). *Psychopathology, 47,* 185–193.

Egan, S. J., Wade, T. D., & Shafran, R. (2011). Perfectionism as a transdiagnostic process: A clinical review. *Clinical Psychology Review, 31,* 203–212.

Fenichel, O. (1945). *The psychoanalytic theory of neurosis.* New York: Norton and Routledge.

Fonagy, P., & Luyten, P. (in press). A multilevel perspective on the development of borderline personality disorder. In D. Cicchetti (Ed.), *Developmental psychopathology* (3rd ed.). New York: Wiley.

Fonagy, P., Luyten, P., & Allison, E. (in press). Epistemic petrification and the restoration of epistemic trust: A new conceptualization of borderline personality disorder and its psychosocial treatment. *Journal of Personality Disorders.*

Fonagy, P., Target, M., & Gergely, G. (2006). Psychoanalytic perspectives on developmental psychopathology. In D. Cicchetti & D. J. Cohen (Eds.), *Developmental psychopathology: Vol. 1. Theory and method* (2nd ed., pp. 701–749). Hoboken, NJ: Wiley.

Freud, A. (1963). The concept of developmental lines. *Psychoanalytic Study of the Child, 18,* 245–265.

Freud, S. (1962). The neuro-psychoses of defence. In J. Strachey (Ed. & Trans.), *The standard edition of the complete psychological works of Sigmund Freud* (Vol. 3, pp. 43–61). London: Hogarth Press. (Original work published 1894)

Gargurevich, R., Luyten, P., & Corveleyn, J. (2008). Dependency, self-criticism, social support and posttraumatic stress disorder symptoms in Peruvian university students. *International Journal of Psychology, 43*(Special Issue 3–4), 435.

Gödel, I. (1933). On intuitionistic arithmetic and number theory. In M. Travis (Ed.), *The undecidable: Basic papers on on undecidable propositions, unsolvable problems and computable functions* (pp. 75–81). Hewlett, NJ: Raven Press.

Horowitz, L. M., Wilson, K. R., Turan, B., Zolotsev, P., Constantino, M. J., & Henderson, L. (2006). How interpersonal motives clarify the meaning of interpersonal behavior: A revised circumplex model. *Personality and Social Psychology Review, 10*, 67–86.

Huprich, S. K., & Greenberg, R. P. (2003). Advances in the assessment of object relations in the 1990s. *Clinical Psychology Review, 23*, 665–698.

Kazdin, A. E. (2011). Evidence-based treatment research: Advances, limitations, and next steps. *American Psychologist, 66*, 685–698.

Kernberg, O. F. (1975). *Borderline conditions and pathological narcissism.* New York: Jason Aronson.

Kernberg, O. F., & Caligor, E. (2005). A psychoanalytic theory of personality disorders. In M. F. Lenzenweger & J. F. Clarkin (Eds.), *Major theories of personality disorder* (2nd ed., pp. 114–156). New York: Guilford Press.

Knight, R. (1953). Borderline states. *Bulletin of the Menninger Clinic, 17*, 1–12.

Koelen, J., Luyten, P., Eurelings-Bontekoe, E. H., Diguer, L., Vermote, R., Lowyck, B., et al. (2012). The impact of level of personality organization on treatment response: A systematic review. *Psychiatry: Interpersonal and Biological Processes, 75*, 355–374.

Kohut, H., & Wolf, E. S. (1978). The disorders of the self and their treatment: An outline. *International Journal of Psycho-Analysis, 59*, 413–426.

Leadbeater, B. J., Kuperminc, G. P., Blatt, S. J., & Hertzog, C. (1999). A multivariate mode of gender differences in adolescents' internalizing and externalizing problems. *Developmental Psychology, 35*, 1268–1282.

Levy, K. N., Edell, W. S., & McGlashan, T. H. (2007). Depressive experiences in inpatients with borderline personality disorder. *Psychiatric Quarterly, 78*, 129–143.

Livesley, J. (2008). Toward a genetically-informed model of borderline personality disorder. *Journal of Personality Disorders, 22*, 42–71.

Locke, D. (2011). Circumplex measures of interpersonal constructs. In L. M. Horowitz & S. Strack (Eds.), *Handbook of interpersonal psychology: Theory, research, assessment, and therapeutic intervention* (pp. 313–324). Hoboken, NJ: Wiley.

Lowyck, B., Luyten, P., Verhaest, Y., Vandeneede, B., & Vermote, R. (2013). Levels of personality functioning and their association with clinical features and interpersonal functioning in patients with personality disorders. *Journal of Personality Disorders, 27*, 320–336.

Luyten, P., & Blatt, S. J. (2007). Looking back towards the future: Is it time to change the DSM approach to psychiatric disorders?: The case of depression. *Psychiatry: Interpersonal and Biological Processes, 70*, 85–99.

Luyten, P., & Blatt, S. J. (2011). Integrating theory-driven and empirically-derived models of personality development and psychopathology: A proposal for DSM-V. *Clinical Psychology Review, 31*, 52–68.

Luyten, P., & Blatt, S. J. (2012). Psychodynamic treatment of depression. *Psychiatric Clinics of North America, 35*, 111–129.

Luyten, P., & Blatt, S. J. (2013). Relatedness and self-definition in normal and disrupted personality development: Retrospect and prospect. *American Psychologist, 68*, 172–183.

Luyten, P., Blatt, S. J., & Mayes, L. C. (2012). Process and outcome in psychoanalytic psychotherapy research: The need for a (relatively) new paradigm. In R. A. Levy, J. S. Ablon, & H. Kächele (Eds.), *Handbook of evidence-based psychodynamic psychotherapy: Bridging the gap between science and practice* (2nd ed.). New York: Humana Press/Springer.

Luyten, P., Kempke, S., Van Wambeke, P., Claes, S. J., Blatt, S. J., & Van Houdenhove, B. (2011). Self-critical perfectionism, stress generation and stress sensitivity in patients with chronic fatigue syndrome: Relationship with severity of depression. *Psychiatry: Interpersonal and Biological Processes, 74*, 21–30.

Luyten, P., Mayes, L. C., Target, M., & Fonagy, P. (2012). Developmental research. In G. O.

Gabbard, B. Litowitz, & P. Williams (Eds.), *Textbook of psychoanalysis* (2nd ed., pp. 423–442). Washington, DC: American Psychiatric Press.

Luyten, P., Van Houdenhove, B., Lemma, A., Target, M., & Fonagy, P. (2012). An attachment and mentalization-based approach to functional somatic disorders. *Psychoanalytic Psychotherapy, 26*, 121–140.

Luyten, P., Van Houdenhove, B., Lemma, A., Target, M., & Fonagy, P. (2013). Vulnerability for functional somatic disorders: A contemporary psychodynamic approach. *Journal of Psychotherapy Integration, 23*, 14–27.

McWilliams, N. (1994). *Psychoanalytic diagnosis.* New York: Guilford Press.

McWilliams, N. (2011). *Psychoanalytic diagnosis: Understanding personality structure in the clinical process* (2nd ed.). New York: Guilford Press.

Meyer, B., & Pilkonis, P. A. (2005). An attachment model of personality disorders. In M. F. Lenzenweger & J. F. Clarkin (Eds.), *Major theories of personality disorder* (2nd ed., pp. 231–281). New York: Guilford Press.

Mikulincer, M., & Shaver, P. R. (2007). *Attachment in adulthood: Structure, dynamics and change.* New York: Guilford Press.

OPD Task Force. (Ed.) (2008). *Operationalized Psychodynamic Diagnosis (OPD-2): Manual of diagnosis and treatment planning.* Kirkland, WA: Hogrefe & Huber.

PDM Task Force. (2006). *Psychodynamic Diagnostic Manual.* Silver Spring, MD: Alliance of Psychoanalytic Organizations.

Pincus, A. L. (2005). A contemporary integrative interpersonal theory of personality disorders. In M. F. Lenzenweger & J. F. Clarkin (Eds.), *Major theories of personality disorder* (2nd ed., pp. 282–331). New York: Guilford Press.

Russ, E., Shedler, J., Bradley, R., & Westen, D. (2008). Refining the construct of narcissistic personality disorder: Diagnostic criteria and subtypes. *American Journal of Psychiatry, 165*, 1473–1481.

Safran, J. D., Muran, J. C., & Eubanks–Carter, C. (2011). Repairing alliance ruptures. *Psychotherapy, 48*, 80–87.

Safran, J. D., Muran, J. C., Samstag, L. W., & Steven, C. (2002). Repairing alliance ruptures. In J. C. Norcross (Ed.), *Psychotherapy relationships that work* (pp. 235–254). Oxford, UK: Oxford University Press.

Shedler, J., Beck, A., Fonagy, P., Gabbard, G. O., Gunderson, J., Kernberg, O., et al. (2010). Personality Disorders in DSM-5. *American Journal of Psychiatry, 167*, 1026–1028.

Shedler, J., & Westen, D. (2010). The Shedler–Westen Assessment Procedure: Making personality diagnosis clinically meaningful. In J. F. Clarkin, P. Fonagy, & G. O. Gabbard (Eds.), *Psychodynamic psychotherapy for personality disorders. A clinical handbook* (pp. 125–161). Washington, DC: American Psychiatric Publishing.

Sibley, C., & Overall, N. (2007). The boundaries between attachment and personality: Associations across three levels of the attachment network. *Journal of Research in Personality, 41*, 960–967.

Sibley, C., & Overall, N. (2010). Modeling the hierarchical structure of personality-attachment associations: Domain diffusion versus domain differentiation. *Journal of Social and Personal Relationships, 27*, 47–70.

Skodol, A. E. (2012). Personality disorders in DSM-5. *Annual Review of Clinical Psychology, 8*, 317–344.

Skodol, A. E., & Bender, D. S. (2009). The future of personality disorders in DSM-V? *American Journal of Psychiatry, 166*, 388–391.

Skodol, A. E., Bender, D. S., Morley, L. C., Clark, L. A., Oldham, J. M., Alarcon, R. D., et al. (2011). Personality disorder types proposed for DSM-5. *Journal of Personality Disorders, 25*, 136–169.

Spitzer, R. L., First, M. B., Shedler, J., Westen, D., & Skodol, A. E. (2008). Clinical utility of five dimensional systems for personality diagnosis: A "consumer preference" study. *Journal of Nervous and Mental Disease, 196*, 356–374.

Stern, A. (1938). Psychoanalytic investigation and therapy in borderline group of neuroses. *Psychoanalytic Quarterly, 7,* 467–489.

Striepens, N., Kendrick, K. M., Maier, W., & Hurlemann, R. (2011). Prosocial effects of oxytocin and clinical evidence for its therapeutic potential. *Frontiers in Neuroendocrinology, 32,* 426–450.

Thompson-Brenner, H., Eddy, K. T., Franko, D. L., Dorer, D. J., Vashchenko, M., Kass, A. E., et al. (2008). A personality classification system for eating disorders: A longitudinal study. *Comprehensive Psychiatry, 49,* 551–560.

Wampold, B. E., Minami, T., Baskin, T. W., & Callen Tierney, S. (2002). A meta-(re)analysis of the effects of cognitive therapy versus 'other therapies' for depression. *Journal of Affective Disorders, 68,* 159–165.

Watson, D., Clark, L. A., & Chmielewski, M. (2008). Structures of personality and their relevance to psychopathology II. Further articulation of a comprehensive unified trait structure. *Journal of Personality, 76,* 1485–1522.

Westen, D., Heim, A., Morrison, K., Patterson, M., & Campbell, L. (2002). Simplifying diagnosis using a prototype-matching approach: Implications for the next edition of the DSM. In L. E. Beutler & M. L. Malik (Eds.), *Rethinking the DSM: A psychological perspective* (pp. 221–250). Washington, DC: American Psychological Association.

Westen, D., Novotny, C. M., & Thompson-Brenner, H. (2004). The empirical status of empirically supported psychotherapies: Assumptions, findings, and reporting in controlled clinical trials. *Psychological Bulletin, 130,* 631–663.

Westen, D., & Shedler, J. (1999). Revising and assessing axis II, part I: Developing a clinically and empirically valid assessment method. *American Journal of Psychiatry, 156,* 258–272.

Westen, D., Shedler, J., & Bradley, R. (2006). A prototype approach to personality disorder diagnosis. *American Journal of Psychiatry, 163,* 846–856.

Westen, D., & Weinberger, J. (2004). When clinical description becomes statistical prediction. *American Psychologist, 59,* 595–613.

World Health Organization. (1992). *International statistical classification of diseases and related health problems* (10th ed.). Geneva, Switzerland: Author.

CHAPTER 6

Defenses as a Transdiagnostic Window on Psychopathology

Robert J. Waldinger and Marc S. Schulz

A recent approach to understanding and treating psychopathology highlights common psychological mechanisms that might underlie multiple diagnostic entities (Brown & Barlow, 2009; Kring, 2010). The rationale for this transdiagnostic approach is that the same fundamental psychological process can be responsible for multiple manifestations of pathology. Among the psychological mechanisms that are most important diagnostically and therapeutically are those that we employ in the service of managing discomforting emotional experiences. In this chapter we explore defenses as a framework for understanding how emotion-regulatory processes can shape adaptation and maladaptation at three different points in the life cycle.

In functional terms, defenses have been defined as habitual styles of emotion-focused coping or emotion regulation directed toward modulation of internal distress (Vaillant, 2000). Defense mechanisms can alter our perceptions of the self, others, ideas, and feelings (Vaillant, 1971). There is ample evidence that defense styles make an important contribution to individual differences in responses to stressful environments (Cramer, 2008; Schulz, Waldinger, Hauser, & Allen, 2005; Vaillant, 1992).

After a brief review of some of the relevant literature, we present three examples of ways in which defenses have been operationalized and used to inform our understanding of developmental challenges and clinical problems. These examples involve challenges that are salient at each of the three developmental periods examined—adolescents' abilities to cope with family conflicts, adult intimate partners' management of anger and aggressive impulses, and older adults' abilities to maintain subjective well-being in the face of their physical and mental decline. We have chosen this structure to underscore the importance of a developmental approach to psychopathology, which is central to psychoanalytic theories. This approach emphasizes the differing psychological needs, tasks, and capabilities that come to prominence at different points in the human life cycle. Longitudinal research that follows individuals across developmental epochs is essential to our understanding of how defenses shape and are shaped by life experience. Two of the three examples presented here use empirical data from such studies—a study following adolescents into young adulthood (Hauser, Powers, & Noam, 1991), and a study following adolescents into old age (Vaillant, 2002).

THEORETICAL BACKGROUND

Freud (1894/1997) originally conceptualized defenses as mechanisms for managing potentially threatening mental contents that were, for the most part, unconscious. These contents could take the form of thoughts, feelings, impulses, or fantasies. From a psychodynamic perspective, unacceptable or threatening contents stimulate anxiety (Brenner, 1994; Brenner & Cooper, 2006). So, for example, one person could be struggling with an impulse to physically injure a parent, another with angry feelings toward a spouse, and another with the fantasy of making love with a coworker. Whether and to what extent these generate anxiety depends on the degree to which they are unacceptable to the individual who harbors them. This emphasis on anxiety as the initiator of defensive processes is consistent with the notion that the primary purpose of such mental mechanisms is to regulate discomforting emotions. In this way, defenses can be viewed as a subset of emotion-regulatory processes. Modern conceptualizations of emotion regulation (Gross & Thompson, 2007; Schulz & Lazarus, 2012) emphasize that emotion-regulatory efforts (of which defenses are a subset) are driven by an individual's goals, and these goals may include priorities other than trying to minimize discomforting emotions.

In the past several decades, research has focused on defenses as normative mental phenomena that operate to reduce distress. In a review of recent empirical work, Cramer (2008) identified several key aspects of defense mechanisms that have been supported by research and that we explore in the studies presented in this chapter: (1) defenses develop in predictable ways across the lifespan; (2) defenses are part of normal functioning; (3) the use of defenses is related to one's affective well-being; and (4) excessive use of less mature defenses is associated with psychopathology. Other researchers have confirmed additional adaptational consequences of the use of particular types of defenses. For example, Fraley, Garner, and Shaver (2000) demonstrated that the use of avoidant defenses inhibits encoding of information in interpersonal situations, and they noted that it may contribute to dysfunction and dissatisfaction in intimate relationships. All of these aspects of defensive functioning have been described in clinical writings for over a century.

McWilliams (2004) has noted that the term *defense* is unfortunate. She argues that the implied military metaphor was fitting for a model that posited defenses as obstacles to be overcome so that unconscious aspects of mental life could come into awareness. It is less fitting, however, when we recognize that human beings need ways of coping with emotions that threaten to disrupt relationships, work life, and one's own internal well-being (Lazarus, 2000). During Freud's lifetime, ego psychologists, with their emphasis on adaptation, began to examine defenses as vital coping mechanisms that were more than merely signs of problems. Anna Freud (1936) began to point to higher-level or adaptive defenses that were essential to healthy functioning and were distinguished from more primitive defenses by their ability to alleviate distress without significant distortion of reality. Vaillant (1971) and Haan (1977) elaborated this perspective on the adaptive hierarchy of defenses into productive research programs in the 1970s.

Both Vaillant and Haan ranked defenses hierarchically according to their relative adaptiveness with respect to real-world functioning. By definition, defenses involve minimizing or keeping threatening information out of awareness to bring about short-term reduction of anxiety. Vaillant (1971) argued that the adaptiveness of a particular defense can be assessed by the degree to which this reduction in immediate discomfort comes at the cost of longer-term dysfunction. From this perspective, a defense such as repression—dealing with an uncomfortable reality by banishing it from awareness—can be relieving in the moment but quite costly over time. Take, for example, a woman who feels a mass in her breast. This event would typically arouse anxiety, and denying the experience (i.e., telling herself that she did not in fact feel the mass) may make her feel better in the moment but would result in neglect of a potentially life-threatening health problem. By contrast, a defense mechanism that allows her to manage emotion while staying engaged with reality would be considered more adaptive. For example, the defense of suppression is a conscious or semiconscious decision to postpone but not avoid paying attention to an uncomfortable feeling or situation. Using suppression in this case, the woman might make an appointment with her doctor for the following week and then put the subject out of her mind until she can get more information at her medical appointment. Suppression allows her to manage anxiety that might interfere with her daily functioning. Repression would be considered a less adaptive defense because it banishes from awareness a vital piece of reality, whereas suppression of worry until a problem can be dealt with appropriately would be considered a more adaptive defense because it is beneficial rather than costly in terms of reality testing and functioning.

To be sure, the adaptiveness of particular defenses is context-dependent (Lazarus, 1983). That is, what may be useful in one situation may be maladaptive in another. However, across a variety of challenging situations, some individuals have been found to rely on a limited repertoire of defenses. Indeed, one approach to personality typing involves delineation of one's habitual modes of dealing with emotional discomfort (Brenner, 1981; McWilliams, 2004; Shapiro, 1965). "Obsessional" individuals, for example, tend to manage anger by draining feelings from their experiences so that conscious representations of evocative events are largely devoid of affect ("I'm not angry about being fired; it was a perfectly rational business decision"). "Histrionic" individuals typically cope with stress in a strikingly different manner, emphasizing feelings while banishing disconcerting thoughts ("I'm furious, but I can't remember what it's about").

Studies have shown some maturation of defense mechanisms as people age (Costa et al., 1991; Vaillant, 2000). Nevertheless, patterns of coping with stress are thought to be relatively stable throughout adulthood. Psychodynamic conceptions of personality posit such continuity of coping styles (Shapiro, 1965), as do developmental theories such as "dynamic interactionism" views (Luyten, Blatt, & Corveleyn, 2005; Zuroff, Mongrain, & Santor, 2004) that emphasize the individual's role in constructing or selecting environmental conditions that are congruent with his or her vulnerabilities and preoccupations.

Hierarchical conceptualizations of defenses have been central to psychodynamic formulations and characterizations of levels of psychopathology. For example, at the heart of Kernberg's (1967, 2004) seminal definition of borderline personality organization lies the borderline individual's reliance on the primitive defenses of splitting, denial, projection, and projective identification—mental mechanisms that bring a reduction in anxiety at the cost of severe dysfunction in reality testing, impulse control, and personal relationships. Maladaptive defenses such as denial are the hallmarks not only of severe personality disorders but also of other serious forms of psychopathology such as bipolar disorder (e.g., Keck, McElroy, Strakowski, Bourne, & West, 1997).

Characterization of individual defense styles offers a window on basic problems in personality and interpersonal functioning that cuts across the descriptive diagnostic categories. Indeed, recent initiatives among major funding agencies (e.g., the National Institute of Mental Health) emphasize the need to move beyond simple categories of illness to investigate basic processes and mechanisms in order to be able to translate such knowledge into improved treatments (Insel et al., 2010). Delineating the maladaptive defenses that contribute to emotion-regulation difficulties can inform both diagnostic formulations and treatment strategies of all varieties, including cognitive-behavioral, psychopharmacological, and psychodynamic interventions.

The three examples described in this chapter all focus on links between defenses and adaptation at particular stages of life. Each study uses ratings of coping and defending strategies that are based on a hierarchical conception of defenses. Each examines these strategies in ways that are developmentally salient. So, for example, in the study of adolescents' abilities to cope with interparental conflict, coping and defending strategies are used to construct indices of capacities for affect tolerance and affect modulation, and these capacities are studied for developmental trends and their ability to predict responses to conflict. In examining intimate partner violence among men in adult couples, a hierarchy of adaptiveness of defenses is used to examine links between defensive style and both verbal and psychological aggression. In the study of octogenarians, we operationalize defenses according to whether they are more engaging or avoidant of reality in trying to understand how defenses are linked with the ability to maintain emotional well-being amidst the very real physical and psychological challenges of aging.

Although each study is based on a hierarchical conception of defenses, they use different systems to rate defensive functioning: the Haan (1977) Q-sort approach in adolescence, Perry's Defense Mechanism Rating Scales in early adulthood (Perry & Ianni, 1998), and Vaillant's rating of vignettes (Vaillant, 1992) in predicting late-life well-being. Each method applies a reliable coding system to rich sources of data— individual interviews and couple and family interactions. All three illustrate how the concept of defensive function sheds light on basic psychological processes that are central to emotional well-being and adaptive functioning.

ADOLESCENTS' AFFECT TOLERANCE AND AFFECT MODULATION IN THE FACE OF INTERPARENTAL CONFLICT

What factors allow some adolescents to respond more adaptively to family conflict than others? We explored this question by examining affect tolerance and regulation as capacities that adolescents bring to potentially threatening situations and that guide behavior. This study demonstrates how constructs and methods developed in the literature on defenses can be adapted to capture phenomena central to modern investigations of emotion regulation.

Researchers have found consistent links between exposure to marital conflict and problematic functioning in children (e.g., Davies, Forman, Rasi, & Stevens, 2002; Katz & Woodin, 2002). There has been considerable interest in understanding mechanisms that might account for this link, along with potential buffers that protect children from exposure to conflict. Much of the theoretical and empirical inquiry about mechanisms has focused on the idea that conflict between parents is emotionally disequilibrating for children (e.g., Crockenberg & Forgays, 1996; Crockenberg & Langrock, 2001). Research on potential buffers that attenuate the link between conflict and problematic functioning has begun to focus on person-based characteristics that may shape emotion-regulatory responses. For example, the work of Katz and Gottman (1995) has demonstrated that vagal tone may protect children from some of the negative effects of witnessing interparental conflict. Using data from a longitudinal study of adolescent and family development (Hauser, Powers, et al., 1992), we observed family interactions at three time points—when adolescents were ages 14, 15, and 16—to understand the role that stable emotion-regulatory capacities may play in shaping adolescents' responses to the challenge of witnessing interparental conflict.

We studied two emotion-regulatory capacities that differ across adolescents and that might help them weather hostile parental behavior and reduce their tendency to respond to family discord with negative behaviors. The first dimension is the capacity to tolerate, experience, and acknowledge a range of affective states, which we labeled *Affective Tolerance*. The second dimension focuses on the adolescent's ability to modulate his or her behavioral and expressive reactivity to negative emotional arousal, which we called *Modulation of Emotional Expression*. This latter dimension captures the capacity to control or modify one's expression of negative emotions to achieve personal and social goals (Schulz & Lazarus, 2012). Both of these dimensions have been cited in previous reviews of the literature as indicative of healthy emotion regulation (e.g., Cole, Michel, & Teti, 1994). Similar dimensions are discussed in the clinical literature on defenses. For example, Kernberg (1967) posits that the capacity for anxiety tolerance is one of the central features that distinguishes between levels of personality organization.

We expected that variations in adolescents' capacities to tolerate negative affect and to modulate their emotional expression would be predictive of whether adolescents were more likely to respond to interparental discord with hostility or with positive engagement. More specifically, we hypothesized that stronger emotion-regulatory capacities would be associated with less hostility and more positive engagement in the context of increased interparental hostility.

Participants in this study (for study details, see Schulz et al., 2005) were 72 two-parent families drawn from the Adolescent and Family Development Project, a longitudinal study of psychological development (see details in Hauser, Powers, et al., 1992). Adolescents were ages 14–15 (M = 14.6 years) on entering the study and were members of primarily Caucasian middle-class and upper middle-class families. Thirty-seven of these adolescents were recruited from the freshman class of a local high school, and 35 were recruited during an in-patient psychiatric hospitalization. The predominant diagnoses of the hospitalized adolescents were mood or disruptive behavior disorders. The high school sample was selected from a larger group of volunteers to match the characteristics of the psychiatric sample with respect to age, gender, birth order, number of siblings, and whether one or two parents were living in the home. Each year, when they were ages 14–16, adolescents came to the laboratory for individual interviews and completion of questionnaires in addition to the family interaction task.

The adolescents' emotion-regulatory capacities were assessed using data derived from semistructured one-hour interviews at each time point that asked the adolescents about their current lives and past experiences, including relationships with parents and siblings, friendships, school, and other activities (Hauser, 1978). In the interviews, adolescents were asked explicitly about how they managed the feelings that arose in each of these areas.

Haan's (1977) Q-sort of Defending and Coping Processes was used to code transcripts of these interviews. Coders who were blind to all other data sorted 60 descriptors of mature (coping) and immature defensive processes into forced distributions with nine piles from "most descriptive" to "least descriptive." The average interrater reliability was .68, indicating satisfactory reliability. Eighteen of the 60 descriptors in the Q-sort captured the relevant dimensions of adolescents' capacity to regulate emotion. Ten of the items described the capacity to experience and recall a range of negative feelings (e.g., unable to recall painful experiences, focuses attention on pleasant aspects of problems and ignores others, ignores aspects of situations that are potentially threatening). Eight of the items captured the ability to modulate emotional and behavioral reactions when challenged by difficulty or when experiencing distressing feelings (e.g., controls expression of affective reactions when not appropriate to express them, regulates expression of feelings proportionate to the situation, inhibits his or her reactions for the time being when appropriate). High internal consistency was obtained for both of these two scales (α = .94–.97 over the three years of the study). A principal axis factor analysis at each time period of all 60 Q-sort items yielded scales that were largely consistent with the rationally derived scales. The three-year average on each of the two scales was used in analyses to capture a reliable indicator of enduring differences in adolescents' capacities to regulate emotion.

Adolescents and their parents participated in a "revealed-differences" interaction task (Strodtbeck, 1958) designed to present families with the challenge of acknowledging and discussing differences of opinion. Family members first completed a Kohlberg Moral Judgment Interview (Colby, Kohlberg, & Candee, 1986) independently of one another. In this interview, specific moral dilemmas were presented and the participant was asked to state his or her opinion about how the dilemma should be resolved. Family members were brought together to discuss differences in their resolutions to the moral dilemmas. The Constraining and Enabling Coding System (Allen, Hauser, Eickholt, Bell, & O'Connor, 1994; Hauser, Houlihan, et al., 1991; Hauser et al., 1992) was applied to transcripts of the family interactions to measure adolescents' hostile and facilitating behaviors toward parents, hostility between parents, and parents' hostility to their adolescent.

As expected, adolescents with psychiatric backgrounds were rated as having less tolerance for negative affect and less ability to modulate their emotional expression than their high school peers. This finding is consistent with a transdiagnostic approach that posits common psychological mechanisms underlying different psychiatric diagnoses. The predominance of mood disorders and behavioral disorders among the psychiatrically hospitalized cohort would suggest that these adolescents might, as a group, manifest poorer emotion-regulatory capacities such as affect tolerance and affect modulation as compared with normal controls. Using growth curve modeling, we also found that emotion-regulatory capacities showed a linear increase from ages 14 to 16, suggesting that they are linked to developmental maturation.

As expected, emotion-regulatory capacities were highly relevant to adolescents' behaviors during interactions with their parents. The capacity to modulate emotion expression and to tolerate greater negative affect was linked significantly in the expected directions with adolescents' typical levels of facilitating behavior. That is, adolescents with stronger emotion-regulatory capacities displayed more facilitating behaviors in the discussions of moral dilemmas. As predicted, hierarchical linear modeling analyses of covariation over time indicated that across the three family interactions, when parents displayed the most hostility toward each other, their adolescent children displayed the most hostility toward their parents. More interparental hostility also covaried, but only at a trend level across the three family discussions, with more attempts by adolescents to engage positively in the family's assigned task of discussing moral dilemmas. More importantly, emotion-regulatory capacities moderated these within-family links between interparental hostility and adolescent behavior toward parents. Compared with adolescents who were judged as less able to experience and acknowledge negative feelings, those who were seen as better able to tolerate a range of feeling states were more likely to show an increase in facilitating behaviors when interparental hostility in their families increased. Adolescents who were judged as better able to modulate their emotional expression and behavior when experiencing negative feelings were less likely than adolescents with difficulties modulating their emotions to show increased hostility when their parents' behavior toward each other became more hostile. Adolescents' capacities for regulating emotions predicted which strategies were more commonly employed.

The findings of this study have implications for our understanding of adolescent development and of the role of emotional regulation in both adolescent and family pathology: We found (1) growth across adolescence in teenagers' capacities for affect tolerance and affect modulation; (2) connections between the lack of these adaptive strategies and psychopathology (less present in the clinical sample); (3) links between these capacities and typical family behaviors; and (4) evidence that these capacities may shape adolescents' responses to a common risk factor—interparental conflict.

Importantly, psychiatric background was not directly linked with variations in adolescents' behavior in the presence of interparental hostility, even though differences in emotion-regulatory abilities did moderate this link. The stronger explanatory power of emotion-regulatory capacities as compared with psychiatric history is of note and may be due to two factors. First, the emotion-regulatory variables used in this study may tap more psychologically meaningful and specific psychological processes than those captured by the fact of psychiatric hospitalization or by specific psychiatric diagnoses. Second, the predictive strength of our emotion-regulatory variables may also be due to our rigorous measurement strategy of combining interview-based assessments of coping and defending strategies from three separate years to capture an enduring characteristic of the adolescents. In contrast, adolescents' psychiatric history may reflect a less stable marker of functioning.

Understanding the defenses that adolescents rely on to manage emotion in challenging situations may offer clinically useful insights that differ from the information gained by delineation of particular syndromes. The moderating effects of the two emotion-regulatory variables provide support for considering affect tolerance and modulation of emotion expression as important mechanisms for managing stress that have behavioral consequences in interpersonal relationships. When faced with an emotionally challenging situation, greater comfort with experiencing a range of affective states may give adolescents access to a broader repertoire of coping strategies and allow them to remain engaged with others in positive ways (Dodge, 1991). The ability to modulate behavioral and expressive reactions associated with negative emotional arousal may be necessary to inhibit an impulsive tendency to react to interpersonal conflict with an aggressive response.

How do these capacities for emotion regulation relate to more traditionally defined defense mechanisms? As noted above, affect tolerance is one of the core ego functions in Kernberg's (1967, 2004) conceptualization of neurotic, borderline, and psychotic levels of psychopathology. Borderline individuals suffer from low anxiety tolerance and resort to primitive (i.e., maladaptive) defenses to allay anxiety. Modulation of affect can thus be understood as the capacity to employ defenses in the service of managing potentially threatening emotion.

EARLY ADULTHOOD: DEFENSIVE FUNCTIONING IN MEN WHO EXHIBIT INTIMATE PARTNER VIOLENCE

Managing hostile impulses that inevitably arise in intimate relationships is crucial to relationship functioning. Understanding the factors that promote adaptive regulatory responses to anger is essential to the prevention and treatment of partner violence, which affects more than 25% of intimate relationships (Tjaden & Theonnes, 2000). Because intimate partner violence (IPV) is not a psychiatric diagnosis but a specific behavior, it cuts across the entire spectrum of psychopathology. Accordingly, researchers have looked for transdiagnostic psychological characteristics that distinguish those who are physically aggressive toward their partners from those who are not. Not surprisingly, defenses and their relation to capacities for regulation of emotions and impulses have been of particular interest. For example, in his studies of male batterers, Dutton (1993, 1998) found a preponderance of borderline personality pathology with attendant use of maladaptive (primitive) defenses. Xu, Wang, Xie, and Sun (2002) found greater use of immature defenses among men who were violent toward intimate partners compared with those who were not. Similarly, Porcerelli, Cogan, Kamoo, and Leitman (2004) found that the use of projection, as scored from the Thematic Apperception Test (TAT), was significantly correlated with more severe violent behavior in men with histories of IPV.

While the previous study discussed in this chapter illustrated the most common approach to capturing defensive processes—the use of narratives derived from individual interviews to identify the use of particular defenses—in this study we used a more novel source of data for identifying defense mechanisms. Individuals' verbal and nonverbal behaviors during videotaped couple discussions of marital conflicts were carefully coded using a well-validated system for rating defenses—the Defense Mechanism Rating Scale (DMRS; Perry & Ianni, 1998). To our knowledge, no previous studies have examined links between IPV and men's use of defenses as scored from actual interactions with their partners. We studied a sample of couples in which men had histories of physical aggression toward their partners ranging from no aggression to severe violence. Our goal was to examine links between men's histories of IPV and both the overall adaptiveness of their defenses and the use of particular types of defenses.

We examined defensive functioning in 57 men with and without histories of recent IPV. The men were part of a sample of heterosexual couples recruited from the community to participate in a study of couple communication (for details, see Waldinger & Schulz, 2006). Recruitment focused on younger, urban, ethnically and socioeconomically diverse couples, with oversampling of couples with a history of domestic violence or childhood sexual abuse. Eligible couples were required to be living together in a committed relationship (but not necessarily married) for a minimum of 12 months. Fifty-seven men were chosen randomly from the larger study sample of 109 men to arrive at approximately equal groups of violent and nonviolent men for this study. Their mean age was 32.2 years ($SD = 8.4$). The average length of relationship for the couples was 3.5 years ($SD = 4.0$), 30% were married, and 58% did not have children. The ethnic make-up of the sample was 53% Caucasian, 35% African American, 5% Hispanic, 2% Asian or Pacific Islander, and 5% Native American. The median family income per year was between $30,000 and $45,000, and participants varied widely in their educational experience.

Intimate partner violence was assessed using the Conflict Tactics Scale, Version 2 (CTS-2; Straus, Hamby, Boney-McCoy, & Sugarman, 1996). The CTS-2 is a 78-item self-report questionnaire asking about the frequency and severity of participants' aggressive behaviors toward partners in the past year. Physical aggression includes acts that range in severity from slapping or shoving to using a knife or gun.

Psychological aggression includes acts involving verbally intimidating, demeaning, or humiliating the partner. The CTS-2 has demonstrated good reliability and good discrimination and construct validity (Straus et al., 1996). The CTS-2 physical and psychological aggression subscales were used as continuous variables in all analyses. We used the highest score reported by either partner for each individual's aggression score to counter underreporting that is more socially desirable (Archer, 1999; Schafer, Caetano, & Clark, 2002).

Defenses were rated by coders who reviewed videotapes of a couple interaction task in which men discussed areas of disagreement with their partners (for details, see Schulz & Waldinger, 2004; Waldinger & Schulz, 2006). In the interaction sessions, participants were asked independently to identify an incident in the past month or two in which their partner did something that frustrated, disappointed, upset, or angered them. Each participant recorded on audiotape a one- or two-sentence statement summarizing the incident and reaction. The couple was then brought together and, in counterbalanced order, discussed one incident identified by the man and one identified by the woman. The audiotaped summary of each incident was played to initiate discussions, and participants were told to discuss the identified incidents and to try to come to a better understanding of what occurred.

Coders rated participants for adaptiveness of defenses using the DMRS (Perry & Ianni, 1998). The DMRS employs a manual with definitions of 27 defense mechanisms. Each defense is defined, including a description of its psychological function as well as a list of its "near neighbors" and how to distinguish one from the other. Raters identified each defense as it occurred during videotaped discussions, transcribing portions of the interview that illustrated the defense coded. Two raters scored each interview and then met for discussion to arrive at consensus ratings. The number of times each defense was present was divided by the total number of defenses scored to get a proportional score for each defense. These were then multiplied by the weighting of that defense on a scale from 1 (*least mature*) to 7 (*most mature*). This hierarchy of defenses has been empirically validated in a number of studies (Perry et al., 1998; Vaillant, 1992; Vaillant, Bond, & Vaillant, 1986). Weighted scores were then summed to arrive at an overall defensive functioning score, with higher scores denoting a higher proportion of more adaptive defenses. Scores ranged from 2.8 to 7.0, $M = 4.6$ ($SD = 1.3$).

As expected, we found that overall defensive functioning ratings were negatively linked with the severity of the men's recent violence toward their partners ($r = -.26$, $p < .05$). There was an even stronger link between men's overall defensive functioning and the severity of psychological aggression toward their partner ($r = -.40$, $p = .002$). We also found links between the severity of men's physical and psychological aggression and their use of specific types of defenses. The frequency of minor image-distorting defenses (in particular, devaluation, idealization, and omnipotence) was linked with the severity of physical and psychological aggression ($rs = .25$ and $.40$, respectively, $ps < .05$).

These findings are consistent with clinical observations that men who are violent toward intimate partners tend to devalue their partners and display behaviors that suggest wishes for omnipotent control (Dutton, 1998). It is also not surprising that we found negative links between men's use of obsessional defenses (intellectualization, isolation of affect, and undoing) and their levels of physical and psychological aggression at the trend level (rs = −.23 and −.24, respectively, ps < .10). These defenses regulate discomforting affect by banishing it from awareness, a strategy that would reduce the likelihood of physical violence resulting from anger. As with the study of adolescents described in the previous section, defenses that involve more adaptive emotion regulation were linked with more socially acceptable and affiliative behaviors. This connection confirms the underlying assumption that difficulties in emotion regulation contribute to intimate partner aggression.

LATE LIFE: DEFENSES AS PREDICTORS OF OCTOGENARIAN WELL-BEING

Older adults report higher levels of emotional well-being than their younger counterparts (Carstensen, Pasupathi, Mayr, & Nesselroade, 2000). One source of this greater well-being may be that older adults are better than younger adults at regulating emotions (Birditt & Fingerman, 2005). A prominent theory of emotion regulation in aging, socioemotional selectivity theory (Carstensen, Isaacowitz, & Charles, 1999), suggests that this regulatory advantage is related to a preferential attention to and memory for positively valenced rather than negatively valenced aspects of reality. In contrast to this adaptive view of positively biased attention and memory processes, clinical and theoretical understandings of defense mechanisms posit that the adaptiveness of defensive strategies depends on the extent to which they impair the user's ability to engage with reality (Haan, 1977; Vaillant, 1971). Theories about defense mechanisms propose that engaging directly with distressing or discomforting affects and experiences is adaptive, especially in the long run. By contrast, socioemotional selectivity theory predicts that, at least in older adults, selectively attending to positive rather than negative aspects of experience is beneficial. The latter view is echoed in other literatures, including developments in positive psychology (Fredrickson & Carstensen, 1998; Seligman, 2002).

In this study, we explored the tensions between a traditional view of defenses that emphasizes the adaptive benefits of directly engaging with one's distress and the view outlined more recently in socioemotional selectivity theory that selective attention to and memory for the positive over the negative leads to enhanced well-being. Using data from a 70-year longitudinal study of adult development, we examined empirical links between these two conceptualizations of adaptive emotion regulation and the ability of these theories to predict emotional well-being in late life (Waldinger & Schulz, in press).

Study participants were drawn from a cohort of men recruited initially between 1939 and 1942 for a study of adult development (for details, see Waldinger & Schulz, 2010). A university health service recruited 268 male college sophomores (aged 18–19 years) for an intensive multidisciplinary study (Vaillant, 2002) that has continued for 70 years. Participants were originally selected because college entrance examinations revealed no mental or physical health problems, and their deans perceived them as likely to become successful adults. In adult life, most participants worked in high-level, white-collar jobs. Participants completed questionnaires every 2 years, and they were interviewed by study staff on intake and at approximately ages 25, 30, and 50.

Surviving men (n = 93) were asked to participate in home assessments between 2004 and 2008, when they were in their mid-80s. The sample for the current study consisted of 61 men whose mean age was 86.1 years (SD = 1.5). To be eligible to participate, men had to score above 25 (indicating minimal or no cognitive impairment) on the Telephone Interview for Cognitive Status (Brandt, Spencer, & Folstein, 1988) and be in sufficient physical health to be able to complete the in-home procedures described later.

To assess preferential memory for positively valenced visual images as an index of the positivity effect, men were asked to view positive, negative, and neutral images from the International Affective Picture System (Ito, Cacioppo, & Lang, 1998), which is a standardized set of images rated on a number of dimensions including emotional valence (positive vs. negative) and emotional arousal. In a protocol similar to that used by Charles, Mather, and Carstensen (2003), participants viewed a series of 60 positive, 60 negative, and 60 neutral pictures, each for 3 seconds (Bradley, Lang, Coan, & Allen, 2007). Participants were asked to view the series of pictures as if they were watching TV. They were not told that there would be a subsequent test of memory for these images. After 30 minutes, they were again presented with these images intermixed with new ones. Participants were asked to indicate whether each picture was an "old" picture (viewed previously) or a "new" picture.

Memory bias was assessed using these data. Corrected recognition scores for positive, negative, and neutral images were calculated by subtracting the number of images that were incorrectly identified as previously studied ("false alarms") from those that were correctly identified as previously studied ("hits"). *Positivity scores* were calculated for each participant by subtracting his corrected recognition score for negative images from (1) his corrected recognition score for positive images and (2) his corrected recognition score for neutral images. Scores greater than zero indicate bias toward remembering positively valenced images, and scores less than zero indicate preferential memory for negatively or neutrally valenced images.

Defenses in early and midadulthood were rated from interviews with participants conducted at three points in time. During college, a staff psychiatrist conducted eight one-hour interviews with each man. At age 30, men were interviewed by a trained anthropologist for approximately 2 hours. Interviews at ages 45–50 were conducted by a psychiatrist or social worker, lasted 2–3 hours, and took place in participants' homes or at their workplaces. Interview protocols were designed to focus on challenges in participants' relationships, physical health, and work. Interviewers took notes during the interviews and wrote extensive summaries immediately following each meeting. Interviewers were instructed to elucidate but not label the behaviors that participants reported using to cope with their difficulties (Vaillant, 1992).

Defenses were assessed using ratings of the occurrence of specific defenses by three independent raters who were blind to other information about participants. From all available interview summaries, raters identified vignettes illustrating defenses during challenging times. The number of identified vignettes per participant ranged from

10 to 30 per interview. Coders gave each vignette a single rating for the best-fitting defense using a coding manual developed by Vaillant (1977). Defenses were recategorized for this study based on the degree to which the defense represented avoidance or engagement with threatening or stressful phenomena. Avoidant defenses reflected emotion-regulatory strategies that were directed at avoiding both upsetting emotions and the source of stress. These included most of the defenses labeled "immature" or "neurotic" in Vaillant's hierarchy of defenses: acting out, displacement, dissociation, hypochondriasis, isolation of affect, passive aggression, projection, reaction formation, and repression. Engaging defenses were those in which individuals appeared to be making efforts to manage uncomfortable emotions without disengaging from the painful or stressful source of those emotions. With the exception of altruism, engaging defenses included all those labeled "mature" in the Vaillant hierarchy: anticipation, humor, sublimation, and suppression.

Overall scores for avoidant and engaging defenses were calculated by summing the ratings reflecting the number of times these defenses appeared in interview vignettes. In addition, because both the number of vignettes analyzed and the number of defenses identified varied across participants, the percentage of total defenses that were engaging defenses was also computed (= engaging defenses divided by the sum of engaging plus avoidant defenses) and used in analyses.

Life satisfaction was measured using the Satisfaction With Life Scale (Diener, Emmons, Larsen, & Griffin, 1985). This self-administered questionnaire asks participants to rate how much they agree or disagree with five life satisfaction statements on a 7-point Likert-type scale. Scores are summed to generate a total score that ranges from 5 to 35.

We found that participants were rated as using avoidant defenses at twice the rate of engaging defenses when they were aged 19–50. Men who displayed a higher percentage of engaging defenses in midlife reported greater late-life satisfaction ($r = .34$, $p = .008$). We also found a significant link between frequency of avoidant defenses displayed in midlife and lower life satisfaction in late life ($r = -.32$, $p = .01$). The links between defenses and life satisfaction remained significant and were of similar magnitude even after controlling for IQ at age 19 and for family of origin socioeconomic status using Hollingshead–Redlich classifications (Hollingshead & Redlich, 1958), suggesting that these links were not due to differences in verbal fluency or advantages associated with intelligence or higher socioeconomic status. By contrast, in this sample, there were no significant links between positivity bias (i.e., scores for corrected recognition of positive, negative, or neutral images) and concurrent life satisfaction.

The findings of strong links *across more than 30 years* between predominant modes of defense and subjective well-being are impressive. The fact that more frequent use of engaging defenses in midlife predicted greater life satisfaction in old age suggests that, at least over time, facing life's uncomfortable aspects more squarely may enhance one's appreciation of life rather than detract from it. The advantages of defensive strategies that involve more direct engagement with a source of challenge or distress have been highlighted in two other literatures. Research arising out of behavioral traditions has established behavioral avoidance as a risk factor for multiple kinds of psychopathology, including depression and anxiety (Harvey, Watkins, Mansell, & Shafran, 2004; Hayes, Wilson, Gifford, Follette, & Strosahl, 1996). Investigations of different coping styles have found that strategies involving relatively more direct engagement with a stressful challenge rather than avoidance are more closely linked with adaptation (Holahan & Moos, 1991).

Examining links between midlife defenses and late-life memory, we found moderate to strong negative links between the total number of avoidant defenses assessed from midlife vignettes and correct recognition of positive, negative, and neutral images as older men ($rs = -.39$, $-.46$, and $-.33$, respectively, all $ps < .01$). That is, the presence of more avoidant defenses in midlife interviews was associated with less accurate recognition of all types of images in a laboratory-based memory test more than 30 years later. The percentage of all defenses that were engaging was linked with better memory for negative ($r = .28$, $p < .05$) and neutral ($r = .28$, $p < .05$) images, but not for positive ones ($r = .12$, $p = $ ns). Moreover, there was a marginally significant link between the relative predominance of engaging defenses in midlife and the difference in correctly recognized images that were positive versus negative in late life ($r = -.22$, $p = .09$). This trend indicates that individuals rated as displaying proportionately greater use of engaging defenses in midlife displayed less selective memory for positively valenced (as compared with negatively valenced) images in their 80s.

The links between defense styles and later memory for visual images may point to the capacity of defense measures to capture enduring ways of engaging in affectively salient situations. The measures of defenses derived from careful coding of interview material may capture an underlying tendency of not turning away from uncomfortable stimuli and reactions—a tendency that persists and manifests in the ability to attend to and recall all types of information, including unpleasant information, as we age. Conversely, "burying one's head in the sand" by using avoidant defenses to cope with distressing experiences and emotions may manifest as poorer attention to and memory for novel stimuli of any valence in old age.

The study has some important limitations. The 61 men who participated are a subset of the 268 in the original cohort. The fact that all were white males from middle- and upper-class backgrounds of one historical cohort limits the generalizability of our findings. We have used only a single measure of positivity in late life. It is important to recognize that positivity has been operationalized and assessed in multiple ways (e.g., autobiographical memory (Kennedy, Mather, & Carstensen, 2004) that may be differentially associated with well-being. Finally, the conceptualization of defenses used in this study highlights the avoidant and engaging dimensions of these mental mechanisms, and other potentially important dimensions could be highlighted and tested.

More generally, research on defenses continues to face fundamental challenges. Most prominent are definitional issues and problems in measurement. Although there are widely accepted definitions of specific defenses (e.g., repression, reaction formation), there exists no standard lexicon of defenses with definitions that are recognized by all researchers and clinicians. In addition, measurement of defenses remains a highly individual endeavor with few widely used approaches. Self-report instruments measure consciously held views about one's own coping mechanisms. Yet many consider defense mechanisms to operate, by definition, outside of awareness and therefore inaccessible through self-reports. The three research approaches highlighted in this chapter all involved methods designed to account for less conscious aspects of defensive functioning. Qualitative material from interviews or open-ended self-reported vignettes was coded by independent raters using three different valid and reliable coding systems. Such methods are labor-intensive and require considerable time and effort in coder training and determination of interrater reliability. Continued efforts are needed to standardize definitions of defense mechanisms and operationalize their measurement in ways that can be used across multiple studies so that data can be compared and pooled across investigations.

DISCUSSION AND CONCLUSIONS

In each of the studies in this chapter, we took an existing approach to coding defenses and adapted it to index defensive processes. We then examined the adaptive consequences of these defensive processes in developmentally salient situations at particular life stages. One challenge for researchers inclined to study defensive processes is that many conceptualizations of defenses are dated in that they were created 40 years ago, and terminology and conceptualization in the field have continued to grow. But with thoughtful adaptation, these traditional approaches can be applied in productive ways. As Fonagy (1982) and others have noted, it is critical for psychodynamically informed research to use language that is accessible to broader audiences. Conceptualizations of defense have much in common with modern conceptualizations of emotion regulation; however, it is critical for researchers employing constructs of defenses to make this case.

Each of these studies links maturity of defense mechanisms—particularly as they reflect capacities for emotion regulation—to adaptive functioning and psychological well-being. Both clinical and empirical work suggests that defenses typically mature with age (Haan, Millsa, & Hartka, 1986; Vaillant, 1992), and that they are amenable to change in psychotherapy (e.g., Ambresin, de Roten, Drapeau, & Despland, 2007). Further research aimed at understanding an individual's habitual defensive style in managing uncomfortable emotion may point the way to specific psychotherapeutic interventions and in this way complement more traditional diagnostic categorization.

ACKNOWLEDGMENTS

We would like to acknowledge the contributions of Pal Johansen and Bjørn Svendsen, who rated the videotaped couple discussions using the DMRS, and Elizabeth Kensinger, who developed the International Affective Picture System protocol and calculated the memory scores used in Study III.

REFERENCES

Allen, J. P., Hauser, S. T., Eickholt, C., Bell, K. L., & O'Connor, T. G. (1994). Autonomy and relatedness in family interactions as predictors of negative adolescent affect. *Journal of Research on Adolescence, 4,* 535–552.

Ambresin, G., de Roten, Y., Drapeau, M., & Despland, J.-N. (2007). Early change in maladaptive defence style and development of the therapeutic alliance. *Clinical Psychology and Psychotherapy, 14,* 89–95.

Archer, J. (1999). Assessment of the reliability of the conflict tactics scales: A meta-analytic review. *Journal of Interpersonal Violence, 14,* 1263–1289.

Birditt, K. S., & Fingerman, K. L. (2005). Do we get better at picking our battles?: Age group differences in descriptions of behavioral reactions to interpersonal tensions. *Journals of Gerontology: Series B: Psychological Sciences and Social Sciences, 60,* P121–P128.

Bradley, M. M., Lang, P. J., Coan, J. A., & Allen, J. J. B. (2007). The International Affective Picture System (IAPS) in the study of emotion and attention *Handbook of emotion elicitation and assessment* (pp. 29–46). New York: Oxford University Press.

Brandt, J., Spencer, M., & Folstein, M. (1988). The Telephone Interview for Cognitive Status. *Neuropsychiatry, Neuropsychology, and Behavioral Neurology, 1,* 111–117.

Brenner, C. (1981). Defense and defense mechanisms. *Psychoanalytic Quarterly, 50,* 557–569.

Brenner, C. (1994). The mind as conflict and compromise formation. *Journal of Clinical Psychoanalysis, 3,* 473–488.

Brenner, C., & Cooper, A. M. (2006). Conflict, compromise formation, and structural theory *Contemporary psychoanalysis in America: Leading analysts present their work* (pp. 1–20). Arlington, VA: American Psychiatric Publishing.

Brown, T. A., & Barlow, D. H. (2009). A proposal for a dimensional classification system based on the shared features of the DSM-IV anxiety and mood disorders: Implications for assessment and treatment. *Psychological Assessment, 21,* 256–271.

Carstensen, L. L., Isaacowitz, D. M., & Charles, S. T. (1999). Taking time seriously: A theory of socioemotional selectivity. *American Psychologist, 54,* 165–181.

Carstensen, L. L., Pasupathi, M., Mayr, U., & Nesselroade, J. R. (2000). Emotional experience in everyday life across the adult life span. *Journal of Personality and Social Psychology, 79,* 644–654.

Charles, S. T., Mather, M., & Carstensen, L. L. (2003). Focusing on the positive: Age differences in memory for positive, negative, and neutral stimuli. *Journal of Experimental Psychology, 85,* 163–178.

Colby, A., Kohlberg, L., & Candee, D. (1986). *Assessing moral judgements: A manual.* Cambridge, UK: Cambridge University Press.

Cole, P. M., Michel, M. K., & Teti, L. O. D. (1994). The development of emotion regulation and dysregulation: A clinical perspective. In N. A. Fox (Ed.), *The development of emotion regulation: Biological and behavioral considerations* (Vol. 59, pp. 73–100). Chicago: University of Chicago Press.

Costa, P. T., Jr., Zonderman, A. B., McCrae, R. R., Cummings, E. M., Greene, A. L., & Karraker, K. H. (1991). Personality, defense, coping, and adaptation in older adulthood *Life-span developmental psychology: Perspectives on stress and coping* (pp. 277–293). Hillsdale, NJ: Erlbaum.

Cramer, P. (2008). Seven pillars of defense mechanism theory. *Social and Personality Psychology Compass, 2,* 1963–1981.

Crockenberg, S., & Langrock, A. (2001). The role of specific emotions in children's responses to interparental conflict: A test of the model. *Journal of Family Psychology, 15,* 163–182.

Crockenberg, S. B., & Forgays, D. (1996). The role of emotion in children's understanding and emotional reactions to marital conflict. *Merrill-Palmer Quarterly, 42,* 22–47.

Davies, P. T., Forman, E. M., Rasi, J. A., & Stevens, K. I. (2002). Assessing children's emotional security in the interparental relationship: The security in the Interparental Subsystem Scales. *Child Development, 73*, 544–562.

Diener, E., Emmons, R. A., Larsen, R. J., & Griffin, S. (1985). The Satisfaction With Life Scale. *Journal of Personality Assessment, 49*, 71–75.

Dodge, K. A. (1991). Emotion and social information processing. In J. Garber & K. A. Dodge (Eds.), *The development of emotion regulation and dysregulation.* New York: Cambridge University Press.

Dutton, D. G. (1993). Borderline personality in perpetrators of psychological and physical abuse. *Violence and Victims, 8*, 327–337.

Dutton, D. G. (1998). *The abusive personality: Violence and control in intimate relationships.* New York: Guilford Press.

Fonagy, P. (1982). The integration of psychoanalysis and experimental science: A review. *International Journal of Psychoanalysis, 9*, 125–145.

Fraley, R. C., Garner, J. P., & Shaver, P. R. (2000). Adult attachment and the defensive regulation of attention and memory: Examining the role of preemptive and postemptive defensive processes. *Journal of Personality and Social Psychology, 79*, 816–826.

Fredrickson, B. L., & Carstensen, L. L. (1998). Choosing social partners: How old age and anticipated endings make people more selective. In M. P. Lawton & T. A. Salthouse (Eds.), *Essential papers on the psychology of aging: Essential papers in psychoanalysis* (pp. 511–538). New York: New York University Press. (Original work published 1894)

Freud, A. (1936). *The ego and the mechanisms of defense.* New York: International Universities Press.

Freud, S. (1997). The defence neuro-psychoses: An endeavor to provide a psychological theory of acquired hysteria, many phobias and obsessions, and certain hallucinatory psychoses. In D. J. Stein & M. H. Stone (Eds.), *Essential papers on obsessive–compulsive disorder.* (pp. 33–44). New York: New York University Press.

Gross, J. J., & Thompson, R. A. (2007). Emotion regulation: Conceptual foundations. In J. J. Gross (Ed.), *Handbook of emotion regulation* (pp. 3–24). New York: Guilford Press.

Haan, N. (1977). *Coping and defending: Processes of self–environment organization.* New York: Academic Press.

Haan, N., Millsa, R., & Hartka, E. (1986). As time goes by: Change and stability in personality over fifty years. *Psychology and Aging, 1*, 220–232.

Harvey, A. G., Watkins, E., Mansell, W., & Shafran, R. (2004). *Cognitive behavioral processes across psychological disorders: A transdiagnostic approach to research and treatment.* New York: Oxford University Press.

Hauser, S., Houlihan, J., Powers, S., Jacobson, A., Noam, G., Weiss-Perry, B., et al. (1991). Adolescent ego development within the family: Family styles and family sequences. *International Journal of Behavioral Development, 14*, 165–193.

Hauser, S., Powers, S., Weiss-Perry, B., Follansbee, D., Rajapark, D., Greene, W., et al. (1992). *Constraining and enabling coding system.* Boston: Harvard Medical School.

Hauser, S. T. (1978). *Semi-structured interview for adolescents.* Unpublished interview protocol.

Hauser, S. T., Powers, S., & Noam, G. (1991). *Adolescents and their families: Paths of ego development.* New York: Free Press.

Hayes, S. C., Wilson, K. G., Gifford, E. V., Follette, V. M., & Strosahl, K. (1996). Experiential avoidance and behavioral disorders: A functional dimensional approach to diagnosis and treatment. *Journal of Consulting and Clinical Psychology, 64*, 1152–1168.

Holahan, C. J., & Moos, R. H. (1991). Life stressors, personal and social resources, and depression: A 4-year structural model. *Journal of Abnormal Psychology, 100*, 31–38.

Hollingshead, A., & Redlich, F. (1958). *Social class and mental illness: A community study.* New York: Wiley.

Insel, T., Cuthbert, B., Garvey, M., Heinssen, R., Pine, D. S., Quinn, K., et al. (2010). Research domain criteria (RDoC): Toward a new classification framework for research on mental disorders. *American Journal of Psychiatry, 167*, 748–751.

Ito, T. A., Cacioppo, J. T., & Lang, P. J. (1998). Eliciting affect using the International Affective Picture System: Trajectories through evaluative space. *Personality and Social Psychology Bulletin, 24,* 855–879.

Katz, L. F., & Gottman, J. M. (1995). Vagal tone protects children from marital conflict. *Development and Psychopathlogy, 7,* 83–92.

Katz, L. F., & Woodin, E. M. (2002). Hostility, hostile detachment, and conflict engagement in marriages: Effects on child and family functioning. *Child Development, 73,* 636–652.

Keck, P. E., Jr., McElroy, S. L., Strakowski, S. M., Bourne, M. L., & West, S. A. (1997). Compliance with maintenance treatment in bipolar disorder. *Psychopharmacology Bulletin, 33,* 87–91.

Kennedy, Q., Mather, M., & Carstensen, L. L. (2004). The role of motivation in the age-related positivity effect in autobiographical memory. *Psychological Science, 15,* 208–214.

Kernberg, O. F. (1967). Borderline personality organization. *Journal of the American Psychoanalytic Association, 15,* 641–685.

Kernberg, O. F. (2004). Borderline personality disorder and borderline personality organization: Psychopathology and psychotherapy. In J. J. Magnavita (Ed.), *Handbook of personality disorders: Theory and practice* (pp. 92–119). Hoboken, NJ: Wiley.

Kring, A. M. (2010). The future of emotion research in the study of psychopathology. *Emotion Review, 2,* 225–228.

Lazarus, R. S. (1983). The costs and benefits of denial. In S. Breznitz (Ed.), *The denial of stress* (pp. 1–30). New York: International Universities Press.

Lazarus, R. S. (2000). Toward better research on stress and coping. *American Psychologist, 55,* 665–673.

Luyten, P., Blatt, S. J., & Corveleyn, J. (2005). Introduction. In J. Corveleyn, P. Luyten, & S. J. Blatt (Eds.), *The theory and treatment of depression: Toward a dynamic interactionism model* (pp. 5–15). Leuven, Belgium: University of Leuven Press.

McWilliams, N. (2004). *Psychoanalytic psychotherapy: A practitioner's guide.* New York: Guilford Press.

Perry, J., & Ianni, F. F. (1998). Observer-rated measures of defense mechanisms. *Journal of Personality, 66,* 993–1024.

Perry, J. C., Hoglend, P., Shear, K., Vaillant, G. E., Horowitz, M., Kardos, M. E., et al. (1998). Field trial of a diagnostic axis for defense mechanisms for DSM-IV. *Journal of Personality Disorders, 12,* 56–68.

Porcerelli, J. H., Cogan, R., Kamoo, R., & Leitman, S. (2004). Defense mechanisms and self-reported violence toward partners and strangers. *Journal of Personality Assessment, 82,* 317–320.

Schafer, J., Caetano, R., & Clark, C. L. (2002). Agreement about violence in U.S. couples. *Journal of Interpersonal Violence, 17,* 457–470.

Schulz, M. S., & Lazarus, R. S. (2012). Emotion regulation during adolescence: A cognitive-mediational conceptualization. In P. K. Kerig, M. S. Schulz, & S. T. Hauser (Eds.), *Adolescence and beyond: Family processes and development* (pp. 19–42). New York: Oxford University Press.

Schulz, M. S., & Waldinger, R. J. (2004). Looking in the mirror: Participants as observers of their own and their partners' emotions in marital interactions. In P. Kerig & D. Baucom (Eds.), *Couple observational coding systems* (pp. 259–272). Hillsdale, NJ: Erlbaum.

Schulz, M. S., Waldinger, R. J., Hauser, S. T., & Allen, J. P. (2005). Adolescents' behavior in the presence of interparental hostility: Developmental and emotion regulatory influences. *Development and Psychopathology, 17,* 489–507.

Seligman, M. E. P. (2002). *Authentic happiness: Using the new positive psychology to realize your potential for lasting fulfillment.* New York: Free Press.

Shapiro, D. (1965). *Neurotic styles.* New York: Basic Books.

Straus, M. A., Hamby, S. L., Boney-McCoy, S., & Sugarman, D. B. (1996). The revised Conflict Tactics Scales (CTS2): Development and preliminary psychometric data. *Journal of Family Issues, 17,* 283–316.

Strodtbeck, F. L. (1958). Husband–wife interaction and revealed differences. *American Sociological Review, 16,* 468–473.

Tjaden, P., & Theonnes, N. (2000). Extent, nature, and consequences of intimate partner violence. Washington, DC: U.S. Department of Justice Offie of Justice Programs.

Vaillant, G. E. (1971). Theoretical hierarchy of adaptive ego mechanisms. *Archives of General Psychiatry, 24,* 107–118.

Vaillant, G. E. (1977). *Adaptation to life.* Boston: Little, Brown.

Vaillant, G. E. (1992). *Ego mechanisms of defense: A guide for clinicians and researchers.* Washington, DC: American Psychiatric Press.

Vaillant, G. E. (2000). Adaptive mental mechanisms: Their role in a positive psychology. *American Psychologist, 55,* 89–98.

Vaillant, G. E. (2002). The study of adult development. In E. Phelps, A. Colby, & J. F. Furstenberg (Eds.), *Looking at lives.* New York: Russell Sage Foundation.

Vaillant, G. E., Bond, M., & Vaillant, C. O. (1986). An empirically validated heirarchy of defense mechanisms. *Archives of General Psychiatry, 43,* 786–794.

Waldinger, R. J., & Schulz, M. S. (2006). Linking hearts and minds in couple interactions: Intentions, attributions and overriding sentiments. *Journal of Family Psychology, 20,* 494–504.

Waldinger, R. J., & Schulz, M. S. (2010). Facing the music or burying our heads in the sand?: Adaptive emotion regulation in mid- and late-life. *Research in Human Development, 7,* 292–306.

Xu, L., Wang, X., Xie, Y., & Sun, Y. (2002). Controlled study on defense mechanisms in male violent offenders. *Chinese Mental Health Journal, 16,* 841–842.

Zuroff, D. C., Mongrain, M., & Santor, D. A. (2004). Commentary on Coyne and Whiffen (1995). *Psychological Bulletin, 130,* 489–511.

PART II

PSYCHOPATHOLOGY IN ADULTS

CHAPTER 7

Depression

Sidney J. Blatt

Depression is a dysphoric affect state ranging from mild and transient experiences to profoundly disabling disorders involving intensely depressed mood, distorted thoughts, and neurovegetative disturbances, including sleep disruption and loss of energy, weight, and sexual desire. It is an extensive public health issue, being one of the most frequent mental health disorders (Murray & Lopez, 1996), with a lifetime prevalence of approximately 15% (Blazer, Kessler, McGonagle, & Swartz, 1994). It has a major impact on the psychological and interpersonal functioning of depressed patients and their families, especially their children (Blatt & Homann, 1992; Goodman & Gotlib, 2002), effects that can extend over many years. Depression also has major economic consequences, including the cost of treatment and impaired productivity that has been estimated to account for 175.3 million years lived with disability worldwide in 2010 (Whiteford et al., 2013).

Depression, frequently viewed as the "common cold" of psychiatric disorders, can be a recurrent, chronic, disabling disorder with substantial relapse rates (e.g., Judd, 1997; Kupfer & Frank, 2001; Segal, Pearson, & Thase, 2003). It is often comorbid with personality disorders (e.g., Mulder, 2002), contributing to depression being a treatment-resistant disorder in many patients (e.g., Luyten, Corveleyn, & Blatt, 2005; Westen, Novotny, & Thompson-Brenner, 2004).

This chapter presents a psychodynamic view of depression and its treatment—a view that focuses not on the symptoms of depression, but on the everyday life experiences that are central in depression: feelings of loss and of being abandoned and unloved on the one hand, and feelings of worthlessness, failure, and guilt on the other. First, I present extensive evidence supporting the central role of these two experiences in depression as well as their implications for the treatment of depression. I then present an overview of how this psychodynamic perspective on depression contributes to understanding treatment response in depression, using further analyses of the extensive and comprehensive randomized clinical trial in the outpatient treatment of serious depression, the National Institute of Mental Health (NIMH)-sponsored Treatment of Depression Collaborative Research Program (TDCRP) as an example. In closing, I consider the implications of these formulations and findings about the nature and treatment of depression for understanding personality development and psychopathology more generally, as well as for understanding the mechanisms of therapeutic action.

CLASSIFICATION AND DIAGNOSIS

Much of the effort to understand and treat depression has been dominated by psychiatry's fundamental approach to mental illness, which focuses on the symptoms of disorders. Numerous attempts to differentiate types of depression based on its symptoms, however, have been relatively unproductive, including the more recent distinction between psychotic depression, accompanied by hallucinations and delusions, and severe and milder forms of nonpsychotic melancholia (e.g., Parker et al., 2010). Differentiating subtypes of depression on the basis of symptoms has been relatively unproductive because of the remarkable heterogeneity of symptoms in both clinical and nonclinical samples. As noted by Cicchetti and Rogosch (1996), the same symptoms can appear in different disorders (multifinality), and different symptoms can characterize the same disorder (equifinality).

In contrast, psychodynamic efforts have differentiated types of depression on the basis of everyday life experiences associated with depression. This approach to differentiating types of depressive experiences has a long tradition in psychodynamic thought rooted in Freud's (1915/1957) articulation of so-called oral dependent and superego dynamics in depression, which provided the basis for identifying two independent sources of depression that derive from different life issues central to depression—on the one hand, intense feelings of being unloved, unwanted, uncared for, and abandoned, and on the other, intense concerns about self-worth manifesting in feelings of guilt and failure (Blatt, 1974, 1998; Luyten & Blatt, 2011). This distinction is also useful in understanding the nature of manic defenses against depression. Depressed feelings of being unloved can result in extensive seeking of nurturance and care in exaggerated ways, while intense feelings of failure and worthlessness can result in exaggerated efforts at overcompensation (e.g., Blatt, 1974; Blatt, Quinlan, Chevron, McDonald, & Zuroff, 1982).

This psychodynamic differentiation of two dimensions in depressive experiences—one focused on the quality of interpersonal relatedness (e.g., dependency) and the other on experiences of self-definition (e.g., self-criticism)—has been supported by extensive empirical investigation (e.g., Blatt, D'Affilitti, & Quinlan, 1976; Blatt et al., 1982; see summary in Blatt, 2004; Blatt & Zuroff, 1992) and subsequently elaborated and supported by clinicians and investigators from other theoretical perspectives (i.e., cognitive-behavioral [e.g., Beck, 1983] and interpersonal [e.g., Arieti & Bemporad, 1978, 1980]). These empirical and clinical investigations indicate that these two types of depressive experiences evolve from relatively different early caretaking experiences (e.g., Blatt & Homann, 1992), have different clinical expressions (e.g., Blatt et al., 1982), and respond differently to different therapeutic interventions (Blatt, Zuroff, Hawley, & Auerbach, 2010).

PSYCHODYNAMIC APPROACHES TO DEPRESSION

Blatt and colleagues (Blatt, 1974, 2004; Blatt et al., 1976, 1982; Blatt, Quinlan, & Chevron, 1990), integrating relational, ego psychoanalytic, and cognitive developmental perspectives, differentiated an "anaclitic" (dependent) and an "introjective" (self-critical) dimension in depression. Prototypically, anaclitic or dependent depression is characterized by feelings of loneliness, helplessness, and weakness, and intense and chronic fears of being abandoned and left unprotected and uncared for. Anaclitic depressed individuals have deep, unfulfilled longings to be loved, nurtured, and protected. Because of their inability to internalize experiences of gratification or qualities of the individuals who provided satisfaction, they value others primarily for the immediate care, comfort, and satisfaction they can provide. Separation from others and interpersonal loss create considerable anxiety, fear, and apprehension and are often dealt with by denial and/or a desperate search for alternative sources of gratification and support (Blatt, 1974). Depression is often precipitated by object loss. Anaclitically depressed individuals often express their depression in somatic complaints and frequently seek the care and concern of others, including physicians (Blatt & Zuroff, 1992). These individuals can also seek attention by making suicide attempts, often by overdosing on their prescribed antidepressant medication (Blatt et al., 1982).

Introjective or self-critical depressed individuals, by contrast, are characterized by feelings of unworthiness, inferiority, failure, and guilt. These individuals engage in harsh self-scrutiny and evaluation, and have a chronic fear of criticism and of losing the approval of others. They often strive for excessive achievement and perfection, are frequently highly competitive, work hard, and make extensive demands on themselves—often achieving a great deal but with little lasting satisfaction. Because of their intense competitiveness, they can also be critical of and attacking toward others. Through overcompensation, they constantly strive to achieve and maintain approval and recognition (Blatt, 2004). This focus on issues of self-worth, self-esteem, failure, and guilt can be particularly insidious. Individuals who are highly self-critical and feel guilty and worthless can be at considerable risk for suicide (Beck, 1983; Blatt, 1974; Blatt et al., 1982; Fazaa & Page, 2003). Numerous clinical reports as well as accounts in the public media (e.g., Blatt, 1995a) illustrate the considerable suicidal potential of highly talented, ambitious, and successful individuals who are plagued by intense self-scrutiny, self-doubt, and self-criticism. Powerful needs to succeed and to avoid public criticism, humiliation, and the appearance of being "defective" force some individuals to incessantly seek to achieve and accomplish, but at the same time these individuals are profoundly vulnerable to the criticism of others and to their own self-scrutiny and judgment (Blatt, 1995a).

Arieti and Bemporad (1978, 1980), from a psychodynamic interpersonal perspective, similarly distinguished two types of depression: a "dominant other" and a "dominant goal" depression. When the dominant other is lost or the dominant goal is not achieved, depression can result. Arieti and Bemporad (1978) discussed two intense and basic wishes in depression in this context: "to be passively gratified by the dominant other" and "to be reassured of one's own worth, and to be free of the burden of guilt" (p. 167). In the dominant other depression, the individual desires to be passively gratified by developing a relationship that is clinging, demanding, and dependent. In the dominant goal depression, the individual seeks to be reassured of his or her worth and to be free of guilt by directing every effort toward a goal that has become an end in itself.

Congruent with these earlier psychoanalytic formulations of depression, Beck (1983), from a cognitive-behavioral perspective, distinguished between "sociotropic" (socially dependent) and "autonomous" types of depression. Sociotropy, according to Beck, "refers to the person's investment in positive interchange with other people . . . including passive–receptive wishes (acceptance, intimacy, understanding, support, guidance)" (p. 273). Highly sociotropic individuals are "particularly concerned about the possibility of being disapproved of by others, and they often try to please others and maintain their attachments" (Robins & Block, 1988, p. 848). Depression is most likely to occur in these individuals in response to perceived loss or rejection in social relationships. In contrast, individuality (autonomy), according to Beck, refers to the person's "investment in preserving and increasing his independence, mobility, and personal rights; freedom of choice, action, and expression; protection of his domain . . . and attaining meaningful goals" (p. 272). An autonomously depressed individual is "permeated with the theme of defeat or failure," blaming "himself continually for falling below his standards" and being "specifically self-critical for having 'defaulted' on his obligations" (p. 276). Highly autonomous, achievement-oriented individuals are very concerned about the possibility of personal failure and often try to maximize their control over their environment to reduce the probability of failure and criticism. Depression most often occurs in these individuals in response to perceived failure to achieve or lack of control over the environment.

Research suggests that some patients may have a mixture of both dependent and self-critical issues and that these individuals are more intensely depressed (Blatt et al., 1982) but may be more responsive to long-term intensive psychodynamic treatment (Shahar, Blatt & Ford, 2003) than most other patients who have primarily one or the other type of depression.

EMPIRICAL FINDINGS

Most research on these psychological dimensions in depression has relied on self-report questionnaires to assess these two depressive vulnerabilities. The four major scales include the Dysfunctional Attitude Scale (DAS; Weissman & Beck, 1978), the Depressive Experiences Questionnaire (DEQ; Blatt et al., 1976; Blatt, D'Afflitti, & Quinlan, 1979), the Sociotropy–Autonomy Scale (Beck, 1983), and the Personal Styles Inventory (Robins et al., 1994). All four scales measure an interpersonal dimension variously labeled as dependency, sociotropy, or need for approval, and a self-definitional dimension variously labeled as self-criticism, autonomy, or perfectionism (Blaney & Kutcher, 1991).

Extensive empirical investigations with these and similar scales consistently indicate differences in the current and early life experiences of these two types of depressed individuals (Blatt & Homann, 1992) as well as in their relational and attachment styles (Luyten, Blatt, & Corveleyn, 2005), in the clinical expression of their depression (Blatt, 2004; Blatt et al., 1982), and in their response to therapy (Blatt, 2004; Blatt & Zuroff, 2005; Blatt et al., 2010). These differences are also found in postpartum depression (Besser, Vliegen, Luyten, & Blatt, 2008), supporting the view that it is more productive to focus on the underlying personality dynamics and the experiences that contribute to depression as the basis for understanding depression than on the manifest symptoms of the disorder.

The Anaclitic Dimension of Depression

Research findings (see extensive discussion of these findings cited below in Blatt, 2004) indicate that individuals with elevated scores on the interpersonal dimension of depression (i.e., elevated DEQ Dependency Factor) tend to be more agreeable and have more frequent and constructive interpersonal interactions that are harmonious, stable, and secure. These individuals tend to be more submissive, placating, and attentive to the feelings of others. They tend to seek social support, have an anxious-preoccupied attachment style, and are usually located in the friendly-submissive quadrant of the interpersonal circumplex (Leary, 1957).

More intense interpersonal concerns are associated with less cognitive differentiation, feelings of helplessness, and high levels of anxiety about loss of support. In terms of clinical symptoms, elevated Dependency is associated with somatic concerns, excessive oral behavior, substance abuse—especially with amphetamines and alcohol—and antisocial acts involving a search for nurturance. These individuals tend to make suicidal gestures that are often attempts to communicate their distress and solicit the concern of others, without serious intent to harm themselves. Dependent individuals tend to have intense levels of anxiety, with chronic fears of being abandoned and left unprotected and uncared for because they feel unable to cope with stress.

Research findings (e.g., Blatt, Zohar, Quinlan, Luthar, & Hart, 1996; Blatt, Zohar, Quinlan, Zuroff, & Mongrain, 1995; Bornstein, 1995; Pincus, 2005; Rude & Burnham, 1995) indicate, however, that it is important to differentiate levels or types of interpersonal concerns, to distinguish a more desperate neediness (e.g., dependency) from more mature and adaptive interpersonal relatedness. The Neediness subfactor within the DEQ Dependency factor, but not the Connectedness subfactor, is associated with prior episodes of depression in young adult outpatients, and with feelings of insecurity and fears of being abandoned and hurt (Zuroff, Mongrain, & Santor, 2004). Further research is needed, however, to explore the suggestion that the Connectednesss subfactor, in contrast, is associated with the capacity to develop warm, intimate relationships.

As noted, much of this research on the interpersonal dimension has been based on data derived from questionnaires with nonclinical samples, although several studies have been based on clinical observations (Blatt & Shichman, 1981; Lidz, Lidz, & Rubenstein, 1976), empirical data derived from clinical records (Blatt et al., 1982), and experimental research. Yet, more research is needed, exploring levels of inter-personal relatedness (including dependency) in both clinical and nonclinical samples.

The Introjective Dimension of Depression

Research evidence (see detailed summary in Blatt, 2004) indicates that individuals with intense concerns about self-worth and self-definition (e.g., with elevated scores on the DEQ Self-criticism factor) are more introverted, resentful, irritable, critical of self and others, and isolated and distant, often with unpleasant and hostile inter-personal interactions. Although concerned about achievement, they are apprehensive about failure and are usually less agentic. As college students, they are more often rejected by their roommates, have a fearful–avoidant attachment style, and are usu-ally located in the hostile-submissive quadrant of the interpersonal circumplex.

The convergence of several measures of introjective personality features (i.e., DEQ Self-criticism factor, the Perfectionism factor of the DAS, and the Socially Prescribed Perfectionism Scale [Hewitt & Flett, 1991]) suggests that this construct should be labeled Self-Critical Perfectionism, a personality quality related to low self-esteem and depressive symptoms, substance abuse (especially opiate addiction), eating disorders, excessive worry, intense negative and less positive affect, and a tendency to assume blame and to be critical of oneself and of others. DEQ Self-criticism is related to Neuroticism and to low Agreeableness on the Five-Factor Model (e.g., Wig-gins, 1991). Self-critical individuals are sensitive to criticism and ridicule; they have formal, reserved, distant, cold interpersonal relationships, avoid close relationships, are dissatisfied, distant, and distrustful of others, and use flattery and deception to manipulate others. They have an avoidant attachment style and perceive others as critical and unsupportive. They respond to stress with guilt, self-blame, and hope-lessness, and with maladaptive, avoidant coping strategies. They can exert consider-able effort in trying to compensate for painful feelings of inadequacy and failure by getting excessively involved in activities to inflate their sense of self-worth, but often overextend themselves, resulting in further feelings of being less agentic and a failure.

Self-critical individuals have unrealistic goals and standards and react strongly to any implications of personal failure or loss of control. They are easily provoked to anger, studies suggest, which can be directed toward the self or others, and can be self-destructive and suicidal. Their suicide attempts usually have much greater levels of lethality than those of anaclitic (dependent) individuals, and are often in response to feelings of failure.

Self-critical individuals often generate stressful life events involving rejection and confrontation and do not generate much social support, and thus do not turn to others because they have negative expectations. They make fewer requests for social support and feel distant from their peers. Self-critical women are experienced by oth-ers as less loving, more hostile, and uncooperative. They have fewer friends, are less liked by peers, are competitive and quarrelsome, and select their romantic partners more on the basis of the partner's power and success rather than his or her capacity for intimacy and affection (Zuroff & de Lorimier, 1989).

Many of these maladaptive, self-critical, introjective personality qualities seem to derive from early experiences with highly critical, judgmental, demanding, disapproving, punitive parents whose excessively high standards lead the child to have negative representations of self and others. Studies of early mother–infant interaction (e.g., Beebe et al., 2007) suggest that these self-critical characteristics begin to be transmitted by the mother's caring patterns very early in the infant's life, as early as 4 months of age. Research also indicates that both anaclitic and introjective personality characteristics are transmitted over the generations (Besser & Priel, 2005).

PSYCHODYNAMIC TREATMENT OF DEPRESSION

Brief and long-term psychodynamically oriented treatments for depression that emphasize supportive and expressive techniques focus on recurring relationship patterns, with the goal that insight into these recurrent patterns will contribute to the development of more adaptive and personally fulfilling relationships (Blagys & Hilsenroth, 2000). Extensive research and various meta-analytic studies (for a summary, see Abbass et al., 2006; Driessen et al., 2010; Luyten & Blatt, 2012) indicate that all bona fide treatments of depression are equally effective—that comparisons of different types of psychotherapy, including (brief) psychodynamic therapy, yield essentially equivalent levels of symptom reduction at the termination of treatment. Furthermore, essentially the same level of therapeutic gain is achieved with antidepressant medication—the classic "Dodo bird" effect (Luborsky, Singer, & Luborsky, 1975). Indications suggest, however, that relapse rates are somewhat higher with medication than with psychotherapy (e.g., Cuijpers, van Straten, van Oppen, & Andersson, 2008; Driessen et al., 2010; Shea et al., 1992). Some findings (e.g., Leichsenring & Rabung, 2008) suggest that long-term psychodynamic therapy and psychoanalysis are particularly effective for depressed patients with comorbid conditions, especially personality disorders, with lower relapse rates than briefer treatments (Knekt et al., 2008, 2011) and a substantial reduction in subsequent medical costs (Abbass & Katzman, 2013).

The frequent finding of the Dodo bird effect among bona fide brief treatments for depression raises important questions about whether the equivalent effectiveness of various forms of brief treatment (including medication) is a function of the focus on symptom reduction as the primary criterion of therapeutic effectiveness. A large proportion of the reduction in symptoms usually occurs early in the treatment process, often with relatively limited interventions. The equivalence of various forms of intervention also suggests that these different interventions may share common factors that account for their therapeutic effectiveness. Extensive research on the psychotherapeutic process consistently indicates that the patient's participation in the therapeutic alliance is likely this common factor (e.g., Krupnick et al., 1996; Wampold, 2002; Zuroff & Blatt, 2006), indicating that the patient has engaged with the therapist in ways that facilitate experiencing themselves in new ways with a significant other. But multilevel modeling of the TDCRP data, discussed in more detail below, reveals a significant between-therapist rather than a within-therapist effect, indicating that a patient's participation in the therapeutic alliance is primarily the consequence of the therapist's capacity to establish a constructive relationship with patients (Zuroff, Kelly, Leybman, Blatt, & Wampold, 2010).

The Importance of Patient and Therapist Characteristics and the Therapeutic Alliance

Over the years, colleagues and I have examined the role of patient features, and the introjective and anaclitic personality features specifically, in the treatment of depression, in interaction with therapist features and the quality of the therapeutic alliance. Our further analyses of data from the extensive randomized clinical trial sponsored by NIMH, the Treatment of Depression Collaborative Research Program (TDCRP), which compared the efficacy of cognitive-behavioral therapy (CBT) and interpersonal psychotherapy (IPT) with that of medication (imipramine [IMI] and a double-blind placebo (PLA]), has played a key role in our realization of the importance of patient and therapist factors—and their interactions—in the treatment of depression, across a number of treatments. It is often difficult to study these various factors simultaneously because randomized clinical trials typically focus only on symptom reduction across different treatments and frequently lack a comprehensive assessment of the contributions of the patient and the therapist to the treatment process. Although more research is needed to replicate and extend our findings, the extensive data gathered in the TDCRP enabled us to discover important findings about the contributions of the patient and the therapist to the treatment process.

The Patient's Contribution to the Treatment Process

Initial findings from the TDCRP (e.g., Elkin, 1994) indicated little difference in the effectiveness of the three forms of treatment (the usual Dodo bird effect) and that these different forms of treatment, especially medication, were relatively ineffective in producing sustained therapeutic gain when assessed 18 months after termination of treatment (e.g., Shea et al., 1992). Colleagues and I (e.g., Blatt, Quinlan, Pilkonis, & Shea, 1995; Blatt, Zuroff, et al., 1996) introduced the anaclitic/dependent/sociotropic and introjective/self-critical/autonomous distinction in depression into further analysis of the extensive TDCRP data set. We assumed that a major obstacle to the investigation of therapeutic change has been the assumption of a uniformity or homogeneity among patients—that patients at the start of treatment are more alike than different, and that all patients experience the therapeutic process and change in similar ways. Many psychotherapy investigators and research methodologists (e.g., Beutler, 1976, 1979; Colby, 1964; Cronbach, 1953) have stressed the need to abandon this homogeneity myth and, instead, to incorporate relevant differences among patients into research designs in order to address more complex questions about whether different types of patients are responsive to different aspects of the therapeutic process and change in different ways (Blatt & Felsen, 1993; Paul, 1967). Thus, significant differences in sustained therapeutic change might occur, in a variety of treatment interventions, as a function of interactions between differences in patients' pretreatment personality organization and aspects of the treatment process, especially the quality of the therapeutic relationship. Including a differentiation among patients in research designs and data analytic strategies could provide a fuller understanding of the processes that lead to sustained therapeutic change.

Cronbach (1953; Edwards & Cronbach, 1952) not only emphasized the need to examine the complex patient × treatment and patient × outcome interactions that lead to therapeutic change; he also stressed that these explorations need to be based on a comprehensive theoretical framework of personality development and psychopathology that identified patient personality characteristics relevant to the therapy process. As Edwards and Cronbach noted in 1952, and as many other commentators have amplified since (e.g., Beutler, 1991; Cronbach, 1975; Smith & Sechrest, 1991; Snow, 1991), the identification of relevant personality dimensions in psychotherapy research requires a theoretically comprehensive and empirically supported theory of personality development and organization in order to avoid entering a "hall of mirrors" (Beutler, 1991; Cronbach, 1953, 1975). Consistent with other object relations approaches to the treatment process (e.g., Blatt & Shahar, 2005; Høglend et al., 2008; Piper, Joyce, McCallum, Azim, & Ogrodniczuk, 2002), we introduced the distinction between a preoccupation with issues of interpersonal relatedness and of self-definition into the analysis of the TDCRP data set. Multiple findings suggested that these patient pretreatment personality dimensions might be relevant to the treatment of depression, including prior findings (e.g., Blatt & Ford, 1994; Blatt & Shahar, 2004; Vermote et al., 2010) that these two basic personality dimensions differentiate two groups of patients who respond to different aspects of the treatment process (patient × treatment interaction) in different but equally desirable ways (patient × outcome interaction).

Empirical findings (e.g., Blatt, 1992; Blatt & Ford, 1994; Blatt & Shahar, 2004; Vermote et al., 2010) had already demonstrated that these two groups of patients could be reliably differentiated and that they experience the therapeutic process differently, in both brief and long-term intensive treatment, both as outpatients and as inpatients. Relatedness-preoccupied (anaclitic) patients were responsive primarily to the supportive interpersonal or relational dimensions of therapy, while self-definitional (introjective) patients were responsive primarily to the interpretive or explorative aspects of the treatment process, and they changed in ways congruent with their basic personality organization.

The TDCRP had randomly assigned 250 initially screened patients to one of the four treatment groups. Eighteen psychiatrists and 10 PhD-level clinical psychologists (with mean clinical experience of 11 years) saw patients at one of three treatment sites. Overall, 239 patients had at least one treatment session and were evaluated extensively at intake, at 4-week intervals throughout treatment to termination at 16 weeks, and in three follow-up assessments at 6, 12, and 18 months after the termination of treatment.

Five primary outcome measures were available in the TDCRP: (1) the interview-based Hamilton Depression Rating Scale (HAM; Hamilton, 1960), (2) the self-report Beck Depression Inventory (BDI; Beck & Steer, 1993), (3) the clinician-rated Global Assessment Scale (GAS; Endicott, Spitzer, Fleiss, & Cohen, 1976), the forerunner of the Global Assessment of Functioning (American Psychiatric Association, 1987, 1994), (4) the self-report Symptom Checklist-90 (SCL-90; Derogatis, 1983), and (5) the Social Adjustment Scale (SAS; Weissman & Paykel, 1974). Analysis (Blatt, Zuroff, et al., 1996) indicated that the residualized gain scores of these five outcome measures at termination formed a common factor, which Blatt and colleagues (1996) labeled a "Maladjustment" factor.

Findings by the TDCRP research team (e.g., Elkin, 1994) indicated that the medication group showed a significantly more rapid decline in symptoms at midtreatment (at session 8), but no significant differences were found among the three active treatment conditions at termination—the classic Dodo bird effect. Shea and colleagues (1992), in an analysis of the follow-up evaluations at 18 months posttreatment, considered approximately 35% of the patients to be recovered because they had had minimal or no symptoms for at least 8 consecutive weeks following treatment (39% in CBT, 34% in IPT, 32% in IMI plus clinical management [IMI-CM], and 25.8% in PLA plus clinical management [PLA-CM]). However, approximately 40% of these recovered patients had relapsed by the 18-month evaluation (39% in CBT, 33% in IPT, 50% in IMI-CM, and 37.5% in PLA-CM). Thus, only approximately 20% of the 239 patients who participated in the TDCRP were considered to be "fully recovered" 18 months after the termination of treatment (23.7% in CBT, 23.3% in IPT, 15.8% in IMI-CM, and 16.1% in PLA-CM). In sum, the TDCRP found no significant differences among the three active treatments at termination and at follow-up, and all three active treatment conditions were relatively ineffective in producing therapeutic gain that was sustained through the follow-up period.

The TDCRP investigators had included the DAS in their basic assessment battery. The two factors of the DAS, Self-Critical Perfectionism (SC-PFT) and Need for Approval (NFA), allowed us to introduce introjective (self-critical) and anaclitic (dependent) pretreatment personality dimensions into the analysis of treatment outcome at termination and at the 18-month follow-up evaluation. We also explored, as noted, the processes through which a negative view of self (SC-PFT) impacted the treatment process, interfering with sustained therapeutic change, and we examined how the patient's participation in the therapeutic relationship contributed to the reduction of this negative self-schema, which, in turn, led to sustained symptom reduction.

Pretreatment levels of SC-PFT, as measured by the DAS, significantly interfered with treatment outcome at termination, across all four treatment conditions on all five primary outcome measures in the TDCRP (i.e., HAM, BDI, GAS, SCL-90, and SAS), as well as by the composite maladjustment factor derived from these five measures (Blatt, Quinlan, et al., 1995). Analysis of therapeutic gain over the five assessments conducted during the treatment process (at intake and after 4, 8, 12, and 16 weeks of treatment) indicated that the pretreatment level of SC-PFT interfered dramatically with therapeutic gain, primarily in the latter half of the treatment process, beginning in the ninth treatment session. Patients with high or moderate levels of SC-PFT failed to make additional therapeutic progress after the eighth treatment session. Only patients with lower levels of SC-PFT had significant therapeutic gain as they approached termination. It seems that therapeutic progress in patients with higher levels of SC-PFT was disrupted in the latter half of the treatment process by their anticipation of the forced termination after the 16th treatment session.

It is noteworthy, in contrast, that the Dependency (Need for Approval) factor of the DAS tended ($p = .11$) to be associated with better therapeutic outcome. This result was consistent with findings that preoccupation with interpersonal concerns has both adaptive and maladaptive features (e.g., Blatt, Zohar, et al., 1995; Rude & Burnham, 1995).

Pretreatment levels of SC-PFT were also associated with poor therapeutic outcome at the final 18-month follow-up evaluation as assessed by independent PhD-level clinical evaluators who rated patients' current clinical condition and degree of therapeutic change. The level of pretreatment SC-PFT correlated significantly ($p < .01$) with ratings of a poorer clinical condition at the 18-month follow-up. Patients also rated their current clinical condition, satisfaction with their treatment, and degree of therapeutic change. All three of these ratings at the 18-month follow-up were negatively correlated ($p < .05$ to $< .001$) with pretreatment levels of SC-PFT (Blatt, Zuroff, Bondi, & Sanislow, 2000).

Patients in the follow-up assessments also rated, on 7-point Likert scales, eight items that measured the degree to which they thought their treatment had improved their interpersonal relationships and their ability to cope with their symptoms, feelings, and attitudes associated with depression—which Zuroff and Blatt (2006) labeled Enhanced Adaptive Capacities (EAC). Prior analyses (Zuroff, Blatt, Krupnick, & Sotsky, 2003) of this EAC measure during the follow-up period indicated that these ratings were associated with a capacity to manage life stress. Thus, it is noteworthy that pretreatment levels of SC-PFT were also significantly associated with reduced levels of EAC at all three follow-up assessments, especially at the final follow-up evaluation 18 months after treatment termination (Blatt et al., 2000; Zuroff et al., 2003).

To evaluate the clinical significance of these effects of SC-PFT on therapeutic outcome, effect-size correlations for some of the major results were calculated. Cohen (1988) characterized $r = .10$ as a small effect, $r = .30$ as a medium effect, and $r = .50$ as a large effect. The majority of the reported effects fell in the small, .10–.30, range. For example, the effect-size correlations for SC-PFT were .16 in predicting change in the maladjustment index (Blatt, Zuroff, Bondi, Sanislow, & Pilkonis, 1998) and .21 in predicting EAC at the 18-month follow-up (Blatt et al., 2000), effect sizes not much lower than those found in meta-analyses of the therapeutic alliance and therapeutic outcome (e.g., Horvath & Symonds, 1991; Martin, Garske, & Davis, 2000). Psychotherapy is a complex process with an outcome determined by multiple factors, so a single variable may account for only a limited amount of the variance in outcome, yet still have great practical significance for the individuals receiving or needing psychotherapy.

Do Changes in Personality Explain Changes in Symptoms?

To evaluate more fully the role of SC-PFT in the treatment process, Hawley, Moon-Ho, Zuroff, and Blatt (2006), using latent difference score (LDS) analysis, a structural equation modeling technique that combines features of latent growth and cross-lagged regression models, evaluated temporal effects in coupled change processes in the reduction of both symptoms and personality vulnerability (SC-PFT). Univariate LDS results indicated that depressive symptoms diminish rapidly early in the treatment process with relatively little therapeutic intervention. In contrast,

SC-PFT diminished very gradually throughout treatment. Despite the remarkably rapid decrease in depressive symptoms early in the treatment process, significant unidirectional longitudinal coupling indicated that a patient's level of SC-PFT predicted the rate of decline in symptoms of depression throughout the treatment. In other words, the lack of sustained therapeutic gain in the TDCRP seems to be the consequence of the failure in treatment to address personality vulnerability factors in depression.

How Does Personality Influence Treatment Outcome?

Based on these findings of the importance of a reduction of SC-PFT in the treatment process, colleagues and I sought to examine the mechanisms through which pretreatment SC-PFT affects the therapeutic process. Treatment sessions in the TDCRP had been videotaped, and Krupnick and colleagues (1996), using recordings of sessions 3, 9, and 15, rated the contributions of patients and therapists to the therapeutic alliance on the Vanderbilt Therapeutic Alliance Scale (VTAS; Hartley & Strupp, 1983). They found that the contributions of patients to the therapeutic alliance, but not the contributions of therapists, significantly predicted therapeutic outcome at termination. Zuroff and colleagues (2000), using these ratings, found that pretreatment SC-PFT significantly interfered with patients' participation in the therapeutic alliance, primarily in the second half of the treatment process, thereby limiting their capacity to gain further from this therapy.

Despite these significant mediating effects of patients' contribution to the therapeutic alliance on treatment outcome at termination (Zuroff et al., 2000), a substantial portion of the variance in the relationship of pretreatment SC-PFT to therapeutic outcome remained unexplained. Thus, Shahar, Blatt, Zuroff, Kuperminc, and Sotsky (2004) examined the mediation of patients' perceived level of social support and found a strikingly similar mediational effect of social relationships on therapeutic outcome. Both increases in perceived social support and participation in the therapeutic alliance, as a consequence of lower pretreatment SC-PFT, significantly mediated therapeutic outcome at termination. This accounted for almost all of the variance between pretreatment SC-PFT and treatment outcome at termination. Thus, pretreatment SC-PFT significantly interfered with therapeutic outcome in the TDCRP by disrupting the patient's participation in the therapeutic alliance as well as the patients' general social relationships, indicating the importance of interpersonal factors in the therapeutic process and the need to explore further the role of the therapeutic relationship in the treatment process.

Based on these findings, Zuroff and Blatt (2006) assessed the quality of the therapeutic relationship in the TDCRP with the Barrett-Lennard Relationship Inventory (B-L RI; Barrett-Lennard, 1962, 1985), which had been administered at the end of the second treatment session. Barrett-Lennard, using Carl Rogers's (e.g., 1957, 1959) specification of the necessary and sufficient conditions of effective therapy, developed a scale to assess patients' experience of the therapeutic relationship with regard to therapist empathy (e.g., "Therapist wanted to understand how I saw things"), positive regard (e.g., "He respected me as a person"), and congruence (e.g.,

"I felt he was real and genuine with me"). Substantial research (e.g., Gurman, 1977a, 1977b) has demonstrated the relationship of the B-L RI to treatment outcome. The B-L RI administered in the TDCRP was significantly related to therapeutic gain, as measured by all five outcome measures (HAM, BDI, GAS, SCL-90, and SAS) and the composite maladjustment factor at termination and at 18-month follow-up (Zuroff et al., 2000). The B-L RI was also significantly related to a decline in SC-PFT over the course of treatment and to the level of EAC at follow-up. Consistent with findings by Kim, Wampold, and Bolt (2006), these results, across all four treatment conditions, indicate that the quality of the therapeutic relationship is more important in determining outcome in the brief treatment of depression than the type of treatment. Additionally, the two psychotherapy conditions in the TDCRP (CBT and IPT), compared with the medication condition (IMI), led to significantly greater EAC (Blatt et al., 2000; Zuroff et al., 2003) and significantly greater reduction of stress reactivity (Hawley, Moon-Ho, Zuroff, & Blatt, 2007; Zuroff et al., 2003) in the follow-up evaluations.

What Is the Precise Role of the Therapeutic Alliance?

Although these findings clearly indicate the importance of the therapeutic relationship, questions still remain about how the therapeutic relationship leads to reduction in the negative self-schema and to therapeutic gain. To assess further the mediating factors in the treatment process, Hawley and colleagues (2006), using an LDS analysis of the ratings by Krupnick and colleagues (1996) of patients' contributions on the VTAS to the therapeutic alliance in the third treatment session in the TDCRP, found that the strength of patients' early participation in the therapeutic alliance significantly influenced change in SC-PFT—a development that, as noted earlier, significantly influenced the reduction of depressive symptoms. These findings indicate the importance of the patient's willingness to participate in the therapeutic process, participation that facilitates the reduction of the patient's negative self-schema. The reduction in negative self-schema in the TDCRP is consistent with theoretical formulations in certain varieties of cognitive-behavioral theory (e.g., Beck, 1996; Young, 1999) and in psychodynamic theories (e.g., Blatt, 1974, 1995b; Bowlby, 1988; Horowitz, 1998; Kernberg & Caligor, 2005) about the role of relatively stable, complex, cognitive-affective interpersonal schemas in psychological disturbance and in the treatment process. Both psychodynamic and cognitive-behavioral formulations suggest that distorted representations of self and significant others underlie most forms of psychopathology, including depression. For example, patients with anaclitic or dependent depression often represent themselves as helpless or needy and significant others as absent, neglectful, or abandoning (Blatt, 1974). On the other hand, patients with introjective or self-critical depression usually represent themselves as unworthy or bad and significant others as intrusive, controlling, judgmental, or punitive and critical (Blatt, 2008). These negative feelings about the self and others, possibly including the therapist, may explain the difficulties that introjective, self-critical patients have in participating in the therapeutic alliance and making substantial therapeutic gains in brief treatment.

Although research makes it clear that SC-PFT is a primary vulnerability factor in the etiology of depression (e.g., Blatt, Quinlan, et al., 1995) and that it is very disruptive in the brief treatment of depression, it is noteworthy that personality vulnerability factors are usually not the focus of most treatment manuals or for investigations of the treatment of depression, endeavors that usually focus on clinical symptoms. These findings thus suggest that progress in psychotherapy occurs through the therapist empathically entering the subjective representational world of the patient (e.g., Blatt, 2013), thereby providing experiences of how one engages with others—how to understand one's own thoughts and feelings as well as those of others. These empathic experiences in the therapeutic relationship result in changes in the content and the developmental level of the cognitive structural organization of patients' representation (cognitive-affective schema) of self and others, as well as changes in patients' level of mentalizing (reflective functioning: e.g., Fonagy & Luyten, 2009). The therapist provides the patient with extensive experiences, sometimes involving important and intense personal issues, in which the therapist facilitates the patient experiencing being understood and appreciated by another, eventually encouraging and enabling the patient to understand and appreciate not only their own feelings and thoughts, but also the thoughts and feelings of others—that is, to establish reciprocal, mutually facilitating, intersubjective, interpersonal relationships (e.g., Blatt et al., 2010).

Although these results of our analyses of the TDCRP data indicate that self-critical, perfectionistic, introjective patients do relatively poorly in brief treatment and seem to be disrupted by the imposition of an arbitrary termination of such treatment, it is noteworthy that self-definitional (introjective) patients do relatively well in long-term intensive treatment (Blatt, 1992; Blatt & Shahar, 2005; Vermote et al., 2010). In sum, the results of studies of brief as well as long-term intensive treatment document the validity of the distinction between anaclitic and introjective patients and the value of this distinction in studying patient × treatment and patient × outcome interactions. This is further reinforced by studies indicating the value of differentiating the issues of interpersonal relatedness and self-definition in psychopathology more generally. Indeed, as discussed in more detail elsewhere (see Blatt & Luyten, 2009; Blatt & Shichman, 1983, and in Luyten & Blatt, Chapter 5, and Meehan & Levy, Chapter 15, this volume), although originally developed in the context of depression, Blatt and Shichman (1983) observed that, based on an expanded version of Erik Erikson's (1950) epigenetic psychosocial developmental model, personality development can be conceptualized, from infancy to senescence, as occurring through a synergistic dialectic transaction between two fundamental developmental processes—the development of the capacity to establish meaningful reciprocal interpersonal relationships and the formation of a coherent and integrated self-definition or identity. The differentiation of these two developmental lines creates a theoretical matrix of personality development that establishes continuities among variations in adaptive personality development, in severe disruptions of normal personality development expressed in various types of psychopathology, including depression and personality disorders, as well as the mechanisms or processes involved in personality change in the therapeutic process (Blatt & Shichman, 1983).

CONCLUSIONS AND FUTURE DIRECTIONS

The psychodynamic perspective on depression presented in this chapter has had a major impact on psychological approaches to depression, resulting, over the past 40 years, in literally hundreds of clinical and research contributions elucidating the characteristics of depression, as well as etiological and treatment implications. But much research remains to be done, examining, for example, the implications of gender differences in the occurrence of anaclitic (dependent) and introjective (self-critical) depression and its treatment, especially in gender-incongruently depressed individuals (i.e., anaclitic depressed males and introjective depressed females; see, e.g., Smith, O'Keeffe, & Jenkins, 1988). Future research is also needed to examine the interactions between types of depression and response to medication used to treat the symptoms of depression—that is, whether response to medication is augmented by neediness in anaclitic depression or suppressed by self-loathing in introjective depression.

In terms of the implications of this psychodynamic approach for psychopathology more broadly, it is noteworthy that investigators (e.g., Blatt, Zohar, et al., 1995, 1996; Rude & Burnham, 1995) have differentiated a more and a less mature level of interpersonal relatedness (i.e., "relatedness" and "neediness," respectively) in the dependency factor of the DEQ, and that Blatt and Shahar (2004) have shown that the second and third factors of the DEQ (Self-criticism and Efficacy) respectively delineate a more maladaptive and adaptive level of self-definition. Future research on psychopathology may well be facilitated by noting these and other differences in the developmental level in adaptive and maladaptive dimensions in personality organization. These various developmental levels in personality organization are likely to be accompanied by differences in the organizational structure of associated cognitive-affective interpersonal schemas of self and of others, differences that could further augment and enrich the investigation of various forms of maladaptive personality organization, including depression, from a psychodynamic perspective. Finally, as Luyten and Blatt (2013) observe, the identification of the two fundamental developmental processes of self-definition and interpersonal relatedness in personality development provides a basis for exploring the impact of cultural and neurobiological factors in adaptive and maladaptive personality development.

REFERENCES

Abbass, A. A., Hancock, J. T., Henderson, J., & Kisely, S. R. (2006). Short-term psychodynamic psychotherapies for common mental disorders. *Cochrane Database of Systematic Reviews*, Issue 7 (Article No. CD004687), DOI: 10.1002/14651858.CD004687.pub4.
Abbass, A. A., & Katzman, J. W. (2013). The cost-effectiveness of intensive short-term dynamic psychotherapy. *Psychiatric Annals, 43*, 496–501.
American Psychiatric Association. (1987). *Diagnostic and statistical manual of mental disorders* (3rd ed., rev.). Washington, DC: Author.
American Psychiatric Association. (1994). *Diagnostic and statistical manual of mental disorders* (4th ed.). Washington, DC: Author.

Arieti, S., & Bemporad, J. (1978). *Severe and mild depression: The therapeutic approach.* New York: Basic Books.

Arieti, S., & Bemporad, J. (1980). The psychological organization of depression. *American Journal of Psychiatry, 137,* 1360–1365.

Barrett-Lennard, G. T. (1962). Dimensions of therapist responses as causal factors in therapeutic change. *Psychological Monographs, 76* (43), 1–36.

Barrett-Lennard, G. T. (1985). The Relationship Inventory now: Issues and advances in theory, method, and use. In L. S. Greenberg & W. M. Pinsof (Eds.), *The psychoanalytic process: A research handbook* (pp. 439–476). New York: Guilford Press.

Beck, A. T. (1983). Cognitive therapy of depression: New perspectives. In P. J. Clayton & J. E. Barrett (Eds.), *Treatment of depression: Old controversies and new approaches* (pp. 265–290). New York: Raven.

Beck, A. T. (1996). Beyond belief: A theory of modes, personality, and psychopathology. In P. M. Salkovskis (Ed.), *Frontiers of cognitive therapy* (pp. 1–25). New York: Guilford Press.

Beck, A. T., & Steer, R. A. (1993). *Beck Depression Inventory manual.* San Antonio, TX: Psychological Corporation.

Beebe, B., Jaffe, J., Buck, K., Chen, H., Cohen, P., Blatt, S. J., et al. (2007). Six-week postpartum maternal self-criticism and dependency predict 4-month mother-infant self- and interactive regulation. *Developmental Psychology, 43,* 1360–1376.

Besser, A., & Priel, B. (2005). The apple does not fall far from the tree: Attachment styles and personality vulnerability to depression in three generations of women. *Personality and Social Psychology Bulletin, 31,* 1052–1073.

Besser, A., Vliegen, N., Luyten, P., & Blatt, S. J. (2008). A psychodynamic perspective on depression. In W. Hansson & E. Olsson (Eds.), *New perspectives on women and depression* (pp. 15–62). Hauppauge, NY: Nova Science Press.

Beutler, L. E. (1976, June). *Psychotherapy: What works with whom?* Paper presented at the annual meeting of the Society for Psychotherapy Research, San Diego, CA.

Beutler, L. E. (1979). Toward specific psychological therapies for specific conditions. *Journal of Consulting and Clinical Psychology, 47,* 882–897.

Beutler, L. E. (1991). Have all won and must all have prizes?: Revisiting Luborsky et al.'s verdict. *Journal of Consulting and Clinical Psychology, 59,* 226–232.

Blagys, M. D., & Hilsenroth, M. J. (2000). Distinctive features of short-term psychodynamic-interpersonal psychotherapy: A review of the comparative psychotherapy process literature. *Clinical Psychology: Science and Practice, 7,* 167–188.

Blaney, P. H., & Kutcher, G. S. (1991). Measures of depressive dimensions: Are they interchangeable? *Journal of Personality Assessment, 56,* 502–512.

Blatt, S. J. (1974). Levels of object representation in anaclitic and introjective depression. *Psychoanalytic Study of the Child, 29,* 107–157.

Blatt, S. J. (1992). The differential effect of psychotherapy and psychoanalysis on anaclitic and introjective patients: The Menninger Psychotherapy Research Project revisited. *Journal of the American Psychoanalytic Association, 40,* 691–724.

Blatt, S. J. (1995a). The destructiveness of perfectionism: Implications for the treatment of depression. *American Psychologist, 50,* 1003–1020.

Blatt, S. J. (1995b). Representational structures in psychopathology. In D. Cicchetti & S. Toth (Eds.), *Rochester Symposium on Developmental Psychopathology: Vol. 6. Emotion, cognition, and representation* (pp. 1–33). Rochester, NY: University of Rochester Press.

Blatt, S. J. (1998). Contributions of psychoanalysis to the understanding and treatment of depression. *Journal of the American Psychoanalytic Association, 46,* 723–752.

Blatt, S. J. (2004). *Experiences of depression: Theoretical, clinical and research perspectives.* Washington, DC: American Psychological Association.

Blatt, S. J. (2008). *Polarities of experience: Relatedness and self-definition in personality development, psychopathology, and the therapeutic process.* Washington, DC: American Psychological Association Press.

Blatt, S. J. (2013). The patient's contribution to the therapeutic process: A Rogerian-psychodynamic perspective. *Psychoanalytic Psychology, 30,* 139–166.

Blatt, S. J., D'Afflitti, J. P., & Quinlan, D. M. (1976). Experiences of depression in normal young adults. *Journal of Abnormal Psychology, 85,* 383–389.

Blatt, S. J., D'Afflitti, J., & Quinlan, D. M. (1979). *Depressive Experiences Questionnaire (DEQ).* Unpublished research manual. New Haven, CT: Yale University.

Blatt, S. J., & Felsen, I. (1993). "Different kinds of folks may need different kinds of strokes": The effect of patients' characteristics on therapeutic process and outcome. *Psychotherapy Research, 3,* 245–259.

Blatt, S. J., & Ford, R. (1994). *Therapeutic change: An object relations perspective.* New York: Plenum Press.

Blatt, S. J., & Homann, E. (1992). Parent–child interaction in the etiology of dependent and self-critical depression. *Clinical Psychology Review, 12,* 47–91.

Blatt, S. J., & Luyten, P. (2009). A structural-developmental approach to psychopathology: Two polarities of experience across the lifespan. *Development and Psychopathology, 21,* 793–814.

Blatt, S. J., Quinlan, D. M., & Chevron, E. (1990). Empirical investigations of a psychoanalytic theory of depression. In J. Masling (Ed.), *Empirical studies of psychoanalytic theories* (Vol. 3, pp. 89–147). Hillsdale, NJ: Analytic Press.

Blatt, S. J., Quinlan, D. M., Chevron, E. S., McDonald, C., & Zuroff, D. (1982). Dependency and self-criticism: Psychological dimensions of depression. *Journal of Consulting and Clinical Psychology, 50,* 113–124.

Blatt, S. J., Quinlan, D. M., Pilkonis, P. A., & Shea, T. (1995). Impact of perfectionism and need for approval on the brief treatment of depression: The National Institute of Mental Health Treatment of Depression Collaborative Research Program revisited. *Journal of Consulting and Clinical Psychology, 63,* 125–132.

Blatt, S. J., & Shahar, G. (2004). Psychoanalysis: For what, with whom, and how: A comparison with psychotherapy. *Journal of the American Psychoanalytic Association, 52,* 393–447.

Blatt, S. J., & Shahar, G. (2005). A dialectic model of personality development and psychopathology: Recent contributions to understanding and treating depression. In J. Corveleyn, P. Luyten, & S. J. Blatt (Eds.), *The theory and treatment of depression: Towards a dynamic interactionism model* (pp. 137–162). Leuven, Belgium: University of Leuven Press.

Blatt, S. J., & Shichman, S. (1981). Antisocial behavior and personality organization. In S. Tuttman, C. Kaye, & M. Zimmerman (Eds.), *Object and self: A developmental approach: Essays in honor of Edith Jacobson* (pp. 325–367). Madison, CT: International Universities Press.

Blatt, S. J., & Shichman, S. (1983). Two primary configurations of psychopathology. *Psychoanalysis and Contemporary Thought, 6,* 187–254.

Blatt, S. J., Zohar, A., Quinlan, D. M., Luthar, S. S., & Hart, B. (1996). Levels of relatedness within the dependency factor of the Depressive Experiences Questionnaire for Adolescents. *Journal of Personality Assessment, 67,* 52–71.

Blatt, S. J., Zohar, A. H., Quinlan, D. M., Zuroff, D. C., & Mongrain, M. (1995). Subscales within the dependency factor of the Depressive Experiences Questionnaire. *Journal of Personality Assessment, 64,* 319–339.

Blatt, S. J., & Zuroff, D. C. (1992). Interpersonal relatedness and self-definition: Two prototypes for depression. *Clinical Psychology Review, 12,* 527–562.

Blatt, S. J., & Zuroff, D. C. (2005). Empirical evaluation of the assumptions in identifying evidence based treatments in mental health. *Clinical Psychology Review, 25,* 459–486.

Blatt, S. J., Zuroff, D. C., Bondi, C. M., & Sanislow, C. A. (2000). Short and long-term effects of medication and psychotherapy in the brief treatment of depression: Further analyses of data from the NIMH TDCRP. *Psychotherapy Research, 10,* 215–234.

Blatt, S. J., Zuroff, D. C., Bondi, C. M., Sanislow, C., & Pilkonis, P. A. (1998). When and how perfectionism impedes the brief treatment of depression: Further analyses of the NIMH TDCRP. *Journal of Consulting and Clinical Psychology, 66,* 423–428.

Blatt, S. J., Zuroff, D. C., Hawley, L., & Auerbach, J. S. (2010). The impact of the two-configurations model of personality development and psychopathology on psychotherapy research: Rejoiner to Beutler and Wolf. *Psychotherapy Research, 20,* 65–70.

Blatt, S. J., Zuroff, D. C., Quinlan, D. M., & Pilkonis, P. A. (1996). Interpersonal factors in brief treatment of depression: Further analyses of the National Institute of Mental Health Treatment of Depression Collaborative Research Program. *Journal of Consulting and Clinical Psychology, 64,* 162–171.

Blazer, D., Kessler, R., McGonagle, K., & Swartz, M. (1994). The prevalence and distribution of major depression in a national community sample: The National Comorbidity Survey. *American Journal of Psychiatry, 151,* 979–986.

Bornstein, R. F. (1995). Active dependency. *Journal of Nervous and Mental Disease, 183,* 64–77.

Bowlby, J. (1988). Developmental psychology comes of age. *American Journal of Psychiatry, 145,* 1–10.

Cicchetti, D., & Rogosch, F. A. (1996). Equifinality and multifinality in developmental pscyhopathology. *Development and Psychopathology, 8,* 597–600.

Cohen, J. (1988). *Statistical power analysis for the behavioral sciences* (2nd ed.). Hillsdale, NJ: Erlbaum.

Colby, K. M. (1964). Psychotherapeutic processes. *Annual Review of Psychology, 15,* 347–370.

Cronbach, L. J. (1953). Correlation between persons as a research tool. In O. H. Mowrer (Ed.), *Psychotherapy: Theory and research* (pp. 376–389). New York: Ronald Press.

Cronbach, L. J. (1975). Beyond the two disciplines of scientific psychology. *American Psychologist, 30,* 116–127.

Cuijpers, P., van Straten, A., van Oppen, P., & Andersson, G. (2008). Are psychological and pharmacologic interventions equally effective in the treatment of adult depressive disorders?: A meta-analysis of comparative studies. *Journal of Clinical Psychiatry, 69,* 1675–1685.

Derogatis, L. R. (1983). *SCL-90-R Manual II: Administration, scoring and procedures.* Towson, MD: Clinical Psychometric Research.

Driessen, E., Cuijpers, P., de Maat, S. C. M., Abbass, A. A., de Jonghe, F., & Dekker, J. J. M. (2010). The efficacy of short-term psychodynamic psychotherapy for depression: A meta-analysis. *Clinical Psychology Review, 30,* 25–36.

Edwards, A. L., & Cronbach, L. J. (1952). Experimental design for research in psychotherapy. *Journal of Clinical Psychology, 8,* 51–59.

Elkin, I. (1994). The NIMH Treatment of Depression Collaborative Research Program: Where we began and where we are now. In A. E. Bergin & S. L. Garfield (Eds.), *Handbook of psychotherapy and behavior change* (4th ed., pp. 114–135). New York: Wiley.

Endicott, J., Spitzer, R. L., Fleiss, J. L., & Cohen, J. (1976). The Global Assessment Scale: A procedure for measuring overall severity of psychiatric disturbance. *Archives of General Psychiatry, 33,* 766–771.

Erikson, E. (1950). *Childhood and society* (2nd ed.). New York: Norton.

Fazaa, N., & Page, S. (2003). Dependency and self-criticism as predictors of suicidal behavior. *Suicide and Life-Threatening Behavior, 33,* 172–185.

Fonagy, P., & Luyten, P. (2009). A developmental, mentalization-based approach to the understanding and treatment of borderline personality disorder. *Development and Psychopathology, 21,* 1355–1381.

Freud, S. (1915). Mourning and melancholia. In J. Strachey (Ed. & Trans.), *The standard edition of the complete psychological works of Sigmund Freud* (Vol. 14, pp. 237–258). London: Hogarth Press.

Goodman, S., & Gotlib, I. (2002). *Children of depressed parents. Mechanisms of risk and implications of treatment.* Washington, DC: American Psychological Association.

Gurman, A. S. (1977a). The patient's perception of the therapeutic relationship. In A. S. Gurman & A. M. Razin (Eds.), *Psychotherapy: A handbook of research* (pp. 503–543). New York: Pergamon Press.

Gurman, A. S. (1977b). Therapist and patient factors influencing the patient's perception of facilitative therapeutic conditions. *Psychiatry, 40,* 218–231.

Hamilton, M. A. (1960). A rating scale for depression. *Journal of Neurology, Neurosurgery and Psychiatry, 6,* 56–62.

Hartley, D. E., & Strupp, H. H. (1983). The therapeutic alliance: Its relationship to outcome in brief psychotherapy. In J. Masling (Ed.), *Empirical studies of psychoanalytic theories* (Vol. 1, pp. 1–27). Hillsdale, NJ: Analytic Press.

Hawley, L. L., Moon-Ho, R. H., Zuroff, D. C., & Blatt, S. J. (2006). The relationship of perfectionism, depression, and therapeutic alliance during treatment for depression: Latent difference score analysis. *Journal of Consulting and Clinical Psychology, 74,* 930–942.

Hawley, L. L., Moon-Ho, R. H., Zuroff, D. C., & Blatt, S. J. (2007). Stress reactivity following brief treatment for depression: Differential effects of psychotherapy and medication. *Journal of Consulting and Clinical Psychology, 75,* 244–256.

Hewitt, P. L., & Flett, G. L. (1991). Perfectionism in the self and social contexts: Conceptualization, assessment, and association with psychopathology. *Journal of Personality and Social Psychology, 60,* 456–470.

Høglend, P., Bogwald, K.-P., Amlo, S., Marble, A., Ulberg, R., Sjaastad, M., et al. (2008). Transference interpretations in dynamic psychotherapy: Do they really yield sustained effects? *American Journal of Psychiatry, 165,* 763–771.

Horowitz, M. J. (1998). *Cognitive psychodynamics: From conflict to character.* New York: Wiley.

Horvath, A. O., & Symonds, B. D. (1991). Relation between working alliance and outcome in psychology: A meta-analysis. *Journal of Counseling Psychology, 24,* 240–260.

Judd, L. L. (1997). The clinical course of unipolar major depressive disorders. *Archives of General Psychiatry, 54,* 989–991.

Kernberg, O. F., & Caligor, E. (2005). A psychoanalytic theory of personality disorders. In M. F. Lenzenweger & J. F. Clarkin (Eds.), *Major theories of personality disorder* (2nd ed., pp. 114–156). New York: Guilford Press.

Kim, D. M., Wampold, B. E., & Bolt, D. M. (2006). Therapist effects in psychotherapy: A random-effects modeling of the National Institute of Mental Health Treatment of Depression Collaborative Research Program data. *Psychotherapy Research, 16,* 161–172.

Knekt, P., Lindfors, O., Harkanen, T., Valikoski, M., Virtala, E., Laaksonen, M. A., et al. (2008). Randomized trial on the effectiveness of long-and short-term psychodynamic psychotherapy and solution-focused therapy on psychiatric symptoms during a 3-year follow-up. *Psychological Medicine, 38,* 689–703.

Knekt, P., Lindfors, O., Laaksonen, M. A., Renlund, C., Haaramo, P., Harkanen, T., et al. (2011). Quasi-experimental study on the effectiveness of psychoanalysis, long-term and short-term psychotherapy on psychiatric symptoms, work ability and functional capacity during a 5-year follow-up. *Journal of Affective Disorders, 132,* 37–47.

Krupnick, J. L., Sotsky, S. M., Simmens, S., Moyer, J., Elkin, I., Watkins, J., et al. (1996). The role of the therapeutic alliance in psychotherapy and pharmacotherapy outcome: Findings in the NIMH Treatment of Depression Collaborative Research Program. *Journal of Consulting and Clinical Psychology, 64,* 532–539.

Kupfer, D. J., & Frank, E. (2001). The interaction of drug- and psychotherapy in the long-term treatment of depression. *Journal of Affective Disorders, 62,* 131–137.

Leary, T. (1957). *The interpersonal diagnosis of personality.* New York: Ronald Press

Leichsenring, F., & Rabung, S. (2008). Effectiveness of long-term psychodynamic psychotherapy: A meta-analysis. *Journal of the American Medical Association, 300,* 1551–1565.

Lidz, T., Lidz, R. W., & Rubenstein, R. (1976). An anaclitic syndrome in adolescent amphetamine addicts. *Psychoanalytic Study of the Child, 31,* 317–318.

Luborsky, L., Singer, B., & Luborsky, L. (1975). Is it true that "everyone has won and all must have prizes"? *Archives of General Psychology, 32,* 995–1008.

Luyten, P., & Blatt, S. J. (2011). Psychodynamic approaches to depression: Whither shall we go? [Editorial]. *Psychiatry: Interpersonal and Biological Processes, 74,* 1–3.

Luyten, P., & Blatt, S. J. (2012). Psychodynamic treatment of depression. *Psychiatric Clinics of North America, 35,* 111–129.

Luyten, P., & Blatt, S. J. (2013). Interpersonal relatedness and self-definition in normal and disrupted personality development: Retrospect and prospect. *American Psychologist, 68,* 172–183.

Luyten, P., Blatt, S. J., & Corveleyn, J. (2005). Towards integration in the theory and treatment of depression. In J. Corveleyn, P. Luyten, & S. J. Blatt (Eds.), *The theory and treatment of depression: Towards a dynamic interactionism model* (pp. 253–284). Leuven, Belgium: University of Leuven Press.

Luyten, P., Corveleyn, J., & Blatt, S. J. (2005). The convergence and psychodynamic and cognitive-behavioral theories of depression: A critical review of empirical research. In J. Corveleyn, P. Luyten, & S. J. Blatt (Eds.), *The theory and treatment of depression: Towards a dynamic interactionism model* (pp. 91–136). Leuven, Belgium: University of Leuven Press.

Martin, D. J., Garske, J. P., & Davis, M. K. (2000). Relation of the therapeutic alliance with outcome and other variables: A meta-analytic review. *Journal of Consulting and Clinical Psychology, 68,* 438–450.

Mulder, R. T. (2002). Personality pathology and treatment outcome in major depression: A review. *American Journal of Psychiatry, 159,* 359–371.

Murray, C. J. L., & Lopez, A. D. (1996). *The global burden of disease: A comprehensive assessment of mortality and disability from diseases, injuries and risk factors in 1990 and projected to 2020.* Cambridge, MA: Harvard University Press.

Parker, G., Fink, M., Shorter, E., Taylor, M. A., Akiskal, H., Berrios, G., et al. (2010). Issues for DSM-5: Whither melancholia?: The case for its classification as a distinct mood disorder. *American Journal of Psychiatry, 167,* 745–747.

Paul, G. L. (1967). Strategy of outcome research in psychotherapy. *Journal of Consulting Psychology, 31,* 109–118.

Pincus, A. L. (2005). A contemporary integrative interpersonal theory of personality disorders. In M. F. Lenzenweger & J. F. Clarkin (Eds.), *Major theories of personality disorder* (2nd ed., pp. 282–311). New York: Guilford Press.

Piper, W. E., Joyce, A. S., McCallum, M., Azim, H. F., & Ogrodniczuk, J. S. (2002). *Interpretive and supportive psychotherapies: Matching therapy and patient personality.* Washington, DC: American Psychological Association.

Robins, C. J., & Block, P. (1988). Personal vulnerability, life events, and depressive symptoms: A test of a specific interactional model. *Journal of Personality and Social Psychology, 54,* 847–852.

Robins, C. J., Ladd, J., Welkowitz, J., Blaney, P. H., Diaz, R., & Kutcher, G. (1994). The Personal Style Inventory: Preliminary validation studies of new measures of sociotropy and autonomy. *Journal of Psychopathology and Behavioral Assessment, 16,* 277–300.

Rogers, C. R. (1957). The necessary and sufficient conditions of therapeutic personality change. *Journal of Consulting Psychology, 21,* 95–103.

Rogers, C. R. (1959). A theory of therapy, personality, and interpersonal relationships as developed in the client-centered framework in psychology: A study of science. In S. Koch (Ed.), *Formulations of the person and the social context* (pp. 184–256). New York: McGraw-Hill.

Rude, S. S., & Burnham, B. L. (1995). Connectedness and neediness: Factors of the DEQ and SAS dependency scales. *Cognitive Therapy and Research, 19,* 323–340.

Segal, Z. V., Pearson, J. L., & Thase, M. E. (2003). Challenges in preventing relapse in major depression: Report of a National Institute of Mental Health Workshop on state of the science of relapse prevention in major depression. *Journal of Affective Disorders, 77,* 97–108.

Shahar, G., Blatt, S. J., & Ford, R. Q. (2003). Mixed anaclitic-introjective psychopathology in treatment-resistant inpatients undergoing psychoanalytic psychotherapy. *Psychoanalytic Psychology, 20,* 84–102.

Shahar, G., Blatt, S. J., Zuroff, D. C., Kuperminc, J., & Sotsky, S. M. (2004). Perfectionism impedes social relations and response to brief treatment of depression. *Journal of Social and Clinical Psychology, 23,* 140–154.

Shea, M. T., Elkin, I., Imber, S. D., Sotsky, S. M., Watkins, J. T., Collins, J. F., et al. (1992). Course of depressive symptoms over follow-up: Findings from the National Institute of Mental Health treatment of depression collaborative research program. *Archives of General Psychiatry, 49,* 782–787.

Smith, B., & Sechrest, L. (1991). Treatment of aptitude × treatment interactions. *Journal of Consulting and Clinical Psychology, 59,* 233–244.

Smith, T. W., O'Keeffe, J. C., & Jenkins, M. (1988). Dependency and self-criticism: Correlates of depression or moderators of the effects of stressful events? *Journal of Personality Disorders, 2,* 160–169.

Snow, R. E. (1991). Aptitude–treatment interactions as a framework for research on individual differences in psychotherapy. *Journal of Consulting and Clinical Psychology, 59,* 205–216.

Vermote, R., Lowyck, B., Luyten, P., Vertommen, H., Corveleyn, J., Verhaest, Y., et al. (2010). Process and outcome in psychodynamic hospitalization-based treatment for patients with a personality disorder. *Journal of Nervous and Mental Disease, 198,* 110–115.

Wampold, B. E. (2002). An examination of the bases of evidence-based interventions. *School Psychology Quarterly, 17,* 500–507.

Weissman, A. N., & Beck, A. T. (1978, August–September). *Development and validation of the Dysfunctional Attitudes Scale: A preliminary investigation.* Paper presented at the 86th annual convention of the American Psychological Association, Toronto, Ontario, Canada.

Weissman, M. M., & Paykel, E. S. (1974). *The depressed woman: A study of social relationships.* Chicago: University of Chicago Press.

Westen, D., Novotny, C. M., & Thompson-Brenner, H. (2004). The empirical status of empirically supported psychotherapies: Assumptions, findings, and reporting in controlled clinical trials. *Psychological Bulletin, 130,* 631–663.

Whiteford, H. A., Degenhardt, L., Rehm, J., Baxter, A. J., Ferrari A. J., Erskine, H. E., et al. (2013). Global burden of disease attributable to mental and substance abuse disorders: Findings from the Global Burden of Disease Study 2010. *Lancet, 382,* 1575–1586.

Wiggins, J. (1991). Agency and communion as conceptual coordinates for the understanding and measurement of interpersonal behavior. In W. W. Grove & D. Cicchetti (Eds.), *Thinking clearly about psychology: Vol. 2. Personality and psychotherapy* (pp. 89–113). Minneapolis: University of Minnesota Press.

Young, J. E. (1999). *Cognitive therapy for personality disorders: A schema-focused approach* (3rd ed.). Sarasota, FL: Professional Resource Press.

Zuroff, D. C., & Blatt, S. J. (2006). The therapeutic relationship in the brief treatment of depression: Contributions to clinical improvement and enhanced adaptive capacities. *Journal of Consulting and Clinical Psychology, 47,* 130–140.

Zuroff, D. C., Blatt, S. J., Krupnick, J. L., & Sotsky, S. M. (2003). Enhanced adaptive capacities after brief treatment for depression. *Psychotherapy Research, 13,* 99–115.

Zuroff, D. C., Blatt, S. J., Sotsky, S. M., Krupnick, J. L., Martin, D. J., Sanislow, C. A., et al. (2000). Relation of therapeutic alliance and perfectionism to outcome in brief outpatient treatment of depression. *Journal of Consulting and Clinical Psychology, 68,* 114–124.

Zuroff, D. C., & de Lorimier, S. (1989). Ideal and actual romantic partners of women varying in dependency and self-criticism. *Journal of Personality, 57,* 825–846.

Zuroff, D. C., Kelly, A. C., Leybman, M. J., Blatt, S. J., & Wampold, B. E. (2010). Between-therapist and within-therapist differences in the quality of the therapeutic relationship: Effects on maladjustment self-critical perfectionism. *Journal of Clinical Psychology, 66,* 1–17.

Zuroff, D. C., Mongrain, M., & Santor, D. A. (2004). Conceptualizing and measuring personality vulnerability to depression: Commentary on Coyne and Whiffen (1995). *Psychological Bulletin, 130,* 489–511.

CHAPTER 8

Generalized Anxiety Disorder and Other Anxiety Disorders

Fredric N. Busch and Barbara L. Milrod

In this chapter, we describe the psychodynamic theoretical background, clinical approaches, and psychodynamic research on generalized anxiety disorder (GAD). In addition, we describe a psychodynamic approach to panic disorder (PD) that has demonstrated efficacy, as well as its potential application to a broader range of anxiety disorders, including GAD. Also, proposed changes in the diagnostic system for anxiety disorders and their potential impact on psychodynamic treatments are discussed. A new paradigm for psychiatric diagnosis, deriving from emerging genetic and neuroscience research, has led to a reconsideration of the current classification of anxiety and other mental disorders (Insel & Wang, 2010). The National Institute of Mental Health (NIMH) is undertaking an initiative to reclassify mental disorders based on neurobiological spectra, referred to as Research Domain Criteria (RDoC; NIMH, 2008) in which some anxiety disorders would be categorized as "disorders of fear circuitry" (Andrews, Charney, Sirovatka, & Regier, 2009). This effort will necessarily have an impact on diagnosis of GAD and other disorders such as PD.

CLASSIFICATION AND DIAGNOSIS

GAD was defined in DSM-IV-TR (American Psychiatric Association [APA], 2000), with few changes in DSM-5 (APA, 2013), in terms of excessive anxiety and worry. Cognitive-behavioral treatments and medication have been studied extensively for GAD, and both have demonstrated efficacy in multiple clinical trials (see Huppert & Sanderson, 2010; Van Ameringen, Mancini, Patterson, Simpson, & Truong, 2010).

Despite these significant and encouraging results, many patients with GAD continue to experience symptoms of the disorder after receiving these treatments

(Leichsenring et al., 2009). Reviews indicate that an average of about 50% respond to cognitive-behavioral therapy (CBT) (Huppert & Sanderson, 2010); pharmacotherapy outcomes have been comparable (Mitte, 2005). These rates are complicated by disagreement about definitions of response (Milrod, 2009). Side effects of medication are a significant problem and are associated with an approximately 25% average dropout rate in studies, compared with approximately 9% in CBT studies (Mitte, 2005). Studies of GAD are confounded by high rates of comorbidity, reportedly as high as 91% (Sanderson & Barlow, 1990). Many clinical trials for GAD have treated a relatively less ill population of patients, as GAD with comorbidity has generally been excluded (Van Ameringen et al., 2010). Psychodynamic psychotherapy for GAD has received little systematic study, and results of these studies have been mixed (Crits-Christoph, Connolly, Azarian, Crits-Christoph, & Shappell, 1996; Crits-Christoph, Connolly Gibbons, Narducci, Schamberger, & Gallop, 2005; Leichsenring et al., 2009). Moreover, the forms of psychodynamic treatment studied have differed.

Beginning with DSM-III (APA 1980), the official diagnostic manual of psychiatry made an effort to eschew theory and etiology and focus on observational bases for classification of disorders. Psychoanalysts became concerned that the diagnostic system was constructed in a way that discouraged psychodynamic considerations and added to its marginalization from general psychiatry (see also Luyten & Blatt, Chapter 5; Meehan & Levy, Chapter 15; and Mayes, Luyten, Blatt, Fonagy, & Target, Chapter 25, this volume). More contemporary critiques from the psychiatric and neuroscience communities have focused on the inadequacies of a diagnostic system that classifies disorders based on the clustering of particular phenomenological symptoms and the time course of the illness, as determined by clinical assessments, which are known to fluctuate. These concerns, as well as some of the findings from neuroscience research, are leading to another paradigm shift in psychiatric diagnosis that is designed to incorporate neuroscience and genetic findings and physiological and behavioral measures (Insel & Cuthbert, 2009; NIMH, 2008). This will necessarily have an impact on the diagnosis of disorders with disordered fear circuitry, such as GAD.

Current neuroscience research includes an ongoing effort to develop endophenotypes (genetically measurable traits or characteristics) that can link or distinguish the biological and behavioral components of normal functioning and mental disorders. In this context, the NIMH initiated a plan to develop, for research purposes, new ways of classifying mental disorders based on dimensions of observable behavior and neurobiological measures, referred to as the RDoC project (Insel et al., 2010; NIMH, 2008).

A domain highly relevant to anxiety disorders is that of fear circuitry (Andrews et al., 2009). Neuroimaging and biochemical studies have suggested a series of brain structures and neurotransmitters that are involved in development of the fear response (Gorman, Kent, Sullivan, & Coplan, 2000). Various anxiety disorders may be understood as correlating with overactivity of the subcortical fear system, with lack of adequate inhibitory control by cortical structures. These mechanisms are currently being defined for various anxiety disorders and will likely lead to a reclassification of these diagnoses based on fear circuitry. GAD may well be found to overlap

with other anxiety disorders, and these symptoms and accompanying endophenotypes may lead to new diagnostic categories in which GAD is no longer considered
adequately descriptive.

Developments in diagnostic assessment based on neuroscience and genetics
research do not indicate that psychodynamic psychotherapy will be be seen as a less
important treatment intervention. In fact, defining these factors might help to better understand the various mechanisms by which psychotherapies are effective on a
neurophysiological level. For example, a study of cognitive-behavioral treatment of
PD has shown a shift in the pattern posttreatment to increased activity in the medial
prefrontal cortex and decreased activity in the subcortical fear circuitry (Sakai et al.,
2006). Similarly, studies are underway to identify shifts with psychodynamic treatment of PD (A. J. Gerber, Junior NARSAD Award: Neuroimaging study of three
psychotherapies for patients with panic disorder, awarded 2008). A recent neuroimaging study of GAD indicated the potential relevance of unconscious implicit factors
in problems with emotional regulation (Etkin, Prater, Hoeft, Menon, & Schatzberg,
2010). The authors found that patients with GAD, when presented with an emotional
conflict generated out of awareness, were unable to mobilize the pregenual anterior
cingulate cortex in diminishing amygdalar activity. The study suggests that neuroimaging could be useful in identifying the types of emotional conflicts involved in GAD
and the types of psychodynamic interventions that can aid in relief of symptoms.

PSYCHODYNAMIC APPROACHES TO GAD

Although psychoanalytic theories relating to the genesis and persistence of anxiety
abound, few theorists have developed an overarching psychodynamic formulation
for GAD. Crits-Christoph, Wolf-Palacio, Fichter, and Rudick (1995) suggested a formulation based on research showing insecure or conflicted attachments and/or a history of traumatic events in individuals who develop GAD. According to this theory,
individuals develop a set of core beliefs and fears that obtaining what they need
from significant others, including protection, security, and love, will be difficult and
uncertain. Individuals with GAD become so fearful that they avoid others because
of these worries in relationships. Worries become displaced onto current concerns or
somatic preoccupations. Internalized expectations and representations of relationships, referred to as core conflictual relationship themes (CCRTs; Luborsky, 1984),
in GAD involve, for example, the wish to be cared for by others, with an expected
response that others will not be protective or trustworthy. Individuals with GAD
have a response of anxiety with a fear of disrupted attachments.

Though useful in articulating certain psychodynamic aspects of GAD, the Crits-
Christoph and colleagues (1995) formulation could easily apply to many forms of
anxiety other than GAD. Drawing from this formulation, a literature review (Busch,
Milrod, & Shear, 2010), and our own clinical experience, we propose that people
with GAD fantasize that they must maintain control and be vigilant at all times, or
catastrophe will ensue. This hypervigilant state can develop from a persistent fear of
conscious emergence of unacceptable feelings and fantasies, and an associated fear

of loss of control. In GAD, defenses have been relatively ineffective in neutralizing or disguising unconscious wishes, leading to a sense of ongoing threat and struggle with unacceptable feelings and fantasies that frequently emerge. For instance, in the case of Ms. C described below, rather than denying her feelings, the patient experienced persistent jealousy and anger that contributed to her anxiety. Alternatively, somatization and worry may operate as defenses against unacceptable feelings and fantasies.

As noted by Crits-Christoph and colleagues (1995), chronic worrying can also be derived in response to early relationships that form an internal psychological template in which attachments are experienced as fragile or easily disrupted. This template can include perceptions that the child will be rejected by the parent, cannot depend on the parent for care, or must take care of a fragile or an incompetent parent (Cassidy, Lichtenstein-Phelps, Sibrava, Thomas, & Borkovec, 2009). Based on this insecure attachment, anxiety can be triggered by hostile wishes operating unconsciously, with fears of being rejected by significant others for anger. The presence of insecure attachments within formative relationships intensifies patients' struggle between dependency wishes and the need to separate and become more autonomous. There is a conflict between wishes for closeness in relationships with loved attachment figures, and fears of engulfment and loss of identity. Based on a sense of the caregiver's emotional fragility (Cassidy et al., 2009), individuals can develop a sense of needing to protect their caregiver in order to maintain the relationship. The need to maintain control, chronic fears of disruption in attachments, and defenses against important emotional cues have an adverse impact on current interpersonal relationships, exacerbating chronic worries.

Investigators from various backgrounds have arrived at conclusions that overlap with this psychodynamic formulation (Cassidy et al., 2009). Studies have found that patients with GAD show high levels of emotional avoidance (see Borkovec, Alcaine, & Behar, 2004), and Cassidy and colleagues (2009) suggest that worrying is a means of avoiding emotions that are even more difficult to tolerate. In addition, studies have shown that people with GAD have unusually intense negative affects and difficulty regulating and identifying their emotions. Mennin, Heimberg, Turk, and Fresco (2005) studied two groups: (1) college students with GAD compared with college students without GAD, and (2) patients presenting to a clinic and found to have GAD compared with a control sample recruited from the community who did not meet criteria for any Axis I diagnosis. In each study they found that, compared with controls, college students and patients with GAD "reported heightened intensity of emotions, poorer understanding of emotions, greater negative reactivity to emotional experience, and less ability to self-soothe after negative emotions" (p. 1281). Worry is employed as a less than adaptive attempt to regulate negative emotions. Due to these pressures, these patients lack adequate access to interpersonal cues because of their constant preoccupations, leading to greater problems in their relationships. Cassidy and colleagues suggest that these difficulties develop from insecure attachment, leading to problems in affect regulation and fears about dangers in interpersonal relationships. They found evidence of insecure attachment in GAD patients compared with a nonanxious control group, including a significantly higher level of maternal rejection/neglect and role reversal (feeling that they needed to take care of their caregiver), using the Perceptions of Adult Attachment Questionnaire (Lichtenstein & Cassidy, 1991). These persistent fears and emotional difficulties lead to ineffective attempts to obtain a sense of security from others.

Although these lines of evidence suggest a dynamic formulation consistent with the one proposed here, this formulation has not been directly tested. In addition, as discussed below, psychodynamic treatments have not demonstrated efficacy in the treatment of GAD. Thus, further testing of both the psychodynamic model and the psychodynamic treatment of GAD is necessary.

PSYCHODYNAMIC TREATMENT OF GAD

Crits-Christoph and colleagues (1995) describe a psychodynamic treatment based on addressing the core conflictual relationship themes relevant to GAD. CCRT is a focused way of describing perceptions of relationships, which are considered to be distorted in GAD based on early relationship experiences. Its elements include a wish, the anticipated response of the other, and the response of the self. The therapist aids the patient in identifying these themes and the link between CCRT patterns and symptoms and maladaptive coping responses. Changes in the CCRT, or the expression of it, are believed to be the key component of a successful supportive/expressive (S/E) treatment, including relief of symptoms and new expectations of self and others (Crits-Christoph & Luborsky, 1990). Accuracy of the CCRT interpretation was found to correlate with clinical outcome (Crits-Christoph, Cooper, & Luborsky, 1988).

Setting therapeutic goals and developing a positive therapeutic alliance are considered important aspects of the early phase of treatment. The therapist begins formulating a CCRT, which in GAD often involves wishes to be cared for or protected with an anticipated negative response from others, triggering anxiety and worry. The CCRT is developed by examining relationship episodes, or interactions between oneself and others. In the middle phase, the therapist identifies how the CCRT is linked with past and current relationships, and with symptoms, with opportunities for revising these perceptions. In the termination phase, the anticipated loss of the therapist is linked to the CCRT and the patient's fears of not obtaining what is needed from others. During this phase, the therapist provides a clear summary of the CCRT.

An alternative psychodynamic approach to GAD is based on principles that underlie Panic-Focused Psychodynamic Psychotherapy (PFPP), a symptom-focused treatment developed for patients with PD (Milrod, Busch, Cooper, & Shapiro, 1997), being extended to a transdiagnostic range of anxiety disorders (PFPP-eXtended Range; Busch, Milrod, Singer, & Aronson, 2012, discussed further below). In an effort to make the patient's emotional reactions more understandable, the therapist explores the content of the patient's specific worries, with the goal of determining particular threatening unconscious fantasies that the patient is avoiding with overwhelming anxiety. Early-life relationships and traumatic experiences, as well as conflictual wishes, are examined to determine underpinnings as to why the patient views the world as being so unsafe. The therapist works with the patient to identify the need for control and to explore specific fantasized dangers of loss of control if vigilance is not maintained at all times. Precipitants of worsening GAD symptoms are discussed, including particular intrapsychic and interpersonal conflicts. The therapist identifies defenses, including somatization, which are often triggered when conflicts are experienced as being so unacceptable that they cannot be tolerated or considered consciously in verbal form. Exploration of these defenses allows the patient and therapist to better understand what the patient needs to protect him- or herself against so vigorously.

Clues as to the underlying significance of anxiety can be obtained from the nature of the presentation of the original anxiety, ongoing anxiety as treatment unfolds, and experiences of anxiety in the transference. The therapy provides a safe atmosphere in which frightening unconscious wishes and conflicts can emerge, including those in the relationship with the therapist, and can be rendered less threatening. Even in the safe atmosphere of a psychotherapy, patients with GAD can feel anxious in the therapeutic relationship. This experience provides an opportunity to examine more directly the patient's fears of loss of control and the interpersonal aspects of the anxiety. Conflicts relating to separation and attachment, addressed throughout therapy, frequently intensify and can become a focus during the termination process.

EMPIRICAL FINDINGS

Crits-Christoph and colleagues studied a modification of Luborsky's general S/E psychotherapy targeting GAD symptoms, initially in an open trial of 26 patients (Crits-Christoph et al., 1996). Patients met either (1) DSM-III-R criteria (SCID-P; Spitzer, Williams, Gibbon, & First, 1990) for GAD (n = 21) or (2) DSM-III-R (APA 1987) criteria for Anxiety Not Otherwise Specified and DSM-IV (APA, 1994) criteria for GAD (n = 5). The treatment consisted of 16 weekly sessions of S/E psychotherapy, followed by three monthly booster sessions. Outcome measures included the Hamilton Anxiety Rating Scale (HAM-A; Hamilton, 1959), Hamilton Rating Scale for Depression (Hamilton, 1960), Beck Anxiety Inventory (Beck, Epstein, Brown, & Steer, 1988), Beck Depression Inventory (BDI; Beck, Steer, & Garbin, 1988), and Penn State Worry Questionnaire (Meyer, Miller, Metzger, & Borkovec, 1990). Results indicated a significant reduction in symptoms across outcome measures. At termination, 79% of patients no longer met the criteria for GAD as determined by the SCID-P (Spitzer et al., 1990). In a follow-up pilot study, Crits-Christoph and colleagues (2005) studied 31 patients with primary DSM-IV (SCID-IV; First, Spitzer, Gibbon, & Williams, 1994) GAD treated in a randomized, controlled trial with either manualized S/E GAD-specific treatment (n = 15) or a manualized supportive psychotherapy for GAD (Borkovec & Matthews 1988) (n = 16). They found the S/E treatment to be superior to supportive psychotherapy in remission rates of GAD, defined as a HAM-A score of less than 7.

Leichsenring and colleagues (2009) studied an adaptation of the Crits-Christoph and colleagues (1995) manual that featured an exposure component in comparison to a manualized CBT treatment for patients with primary GAD diagnosed on the Structured Clinical Interview for DSM-IV (SCID-I and SCID-II; Sass, Wittchen,

& Zaudig, 2000; Wittchen, Zaudig, & Fydrich, 1997). Treatments lasted up to 30 sessions. Both treatment groups showed significant improvements in measures of anxiety and depression. No differences were found between groups on the HAM-A (Hamilton, 1959), the Beck Anxiety Inventory (Beck, Epstein, et al., 1988), the Hospital Anxiety and Depression Scale (Zigmond & Snaith, 1983), and the Inventory of Interpersonal Problems (Horowitz, Alden, Wiggins, & Pincus, 2000). CBT was superior to S/E therapy on measures of trait anxiety (State-Trait Anxiety Inventory; Spielberger, Gorsuch, & Lushene, 1970), worry (Penn State Worry Questionnaire; Meyer et al., 1990), and depression (BDI; Beck, Ward, & Mendelson, 1961). In her review of this study, Milrod (2009) noted that the psychodynamic treatment may not have adequately targeted GAD dynamics and symptoms, and therefore may not provide a full evaluation of whether or not other forms of psychodynamic treatment could be efficacious for GAD.

Our group has also explored a potential mediator of the impact of these treatments, panic-specific reflective functioning (PSRF; Rudden, Milrod, Target, Ackerman, & Graf, 2006), which measures awareness of how emotional experience and anxiety symptoms are linked. Rudden and colleagues (2006) examined the role of reflective functioning and specifically PSRF in the PFPP efficacy study described earlier (Milrod et al., 2007). Patients treated with PFPP demonstrated a significant improvement in PSRF from baseline to posttreatment, but those receiving applied relaxation training (ART) did not. This study, which was underpowered, did not demonstrate a correlation between degree of change in PSRF and change in panic severity. Yet, because of these encouraging results, PSRF is being examined as a potential mediator in a recently completed two-site study comparing PFPP with CBT and ART (B. Milrod and J. P. Barber, National Institute of Mental Health Grant No. R01 MH070918/01).

CLINICAL ILLUSTRATION

Ms C. was a 36-year-old executive secretary who suffered from chronic worries regarding her health and social relationships. Her primary worries included recurring concerns about having a serious illness whenever she experienced minor somatic symptoms, and anxiety about being rejected by her friends.

Ms C. developed panic attacks and a worsening of her chronic GAD symptoms in the context of her inability to become pregnant. She felt deprived, angry and jealous of women she knew who were having children. She felt guilty about these feelings and was concerned that she would say something that would reveal her envy, potentially disrupting her relationships. Getting together with a friend who was pregnant or who had a small child triggered her anger and jealousy, along with panic attacks. Arranging a baby shower for a pregnant friend led to facial sensations that she interpreted as possible signs of a brain tumor, creating intense anxiety that slowly resolved after the shower was over.

Exploration of Ms C.'s background shed light on the dynamisms with which she struggled. She described her mother as "wonderful" and her father as demanding, temperamental, controlling, and critical. She said her father had warned her never to make a mistake. He had yelled at her for many things, including forgetting her backpack and missing the school bus. Ms C. was particularly distraught that he had routinely become enraged at her whenever the bus was late arriving home, something over which she had no control. She came to believe she needed to do everything perfectly, or catastrophe would follow. She had felt safe in the company of her mother, but she experienced her father looming in the background in a frightening and disruptive way. A source of relief from her fears was her social relationships, in which she had routinely played the role of being the center of attention, in charge and a leader of her group of girlfriends. She had felt safe being the one to make decisions about the group's activities.

As an adult, Ms C. continued to feel it was essential to be the leader in her group of female friends, but she found this role increasingly difficult, as her friends gradually became less responsive to her efforts to control activities. One significant source of her worries was the threat of not being the center of attention, which she experienced as equivalent to being rejected. For example, she became angry and anxious when two members of the group planned a birthday party for a third member and did not include her in the planning phase. She believed that in becoming closer to each other, her friends would ultimately ignore or exclude her in an ongoing way. In therapy, it gradually emerged that her social group represented a link to the safety of her mother. Threatened disruption of her role in the group symbolically represented her terror of falling into her father's control, thereby losing her source of protection and stability.

With her closest friends in the group, she believed that if things were not perfect, she would lose their friendship. This mindset left little room to negotiate or tolerate even routine tensions. If a conflict with a close friend intensified, she would develop increasing worries about her body; for example, she would focus on headaches or gastrointestinal distress as signs of possible cancer. For example, when her closest friend, J., did not agree to a plan she had arranged for the group to get together weekly for dinner, she became furious with her and then fearful that she would be seen as "mean," leading to worries about rejection. She believed J. was getting together with a friend of J.'s, who was not part of the group, at the same time, and that J. was therefore rejecting her. As her struggle with this friend persisted, she became preoccupied with the thought that her ongoing neck pain might be a sign of cancer. Her jealousy of women with children in her group of friends intensified her perceived threat of disruption in her relationships, flooded as she was with rage and envy.

Ms C. was intensely guilty about her anger, particularly, her frequent fury at her father. When she became angry with him, she felt guilty about criticizing him, and she experienced an urgent need to make up for her thoughts or comments. The guilt was heightened by a sense that her father was in fact vulnerable and that her sister and mother had much greater tolerance for him. For example, she became enraged when her father repeatedly criticized her for keeping the air conditioning at too high a level in her house when her parents visited. When she complained to her mother, her father expressed a fear that Ms C. would turn her mother against him; this intensified her guilt and her sense that her anger was unacceptable and dangerous. In addition, when she felt or expressed anger at her father or others, she worried that she was behaving like her father and so became unrealistically self-critical. At these points, she began to recognize that she expected others to respond to her requests just as her father did with her. Her identification with her father made it difficult for her to experience any angry feelings without feeling guilty and anxious about losing control over her hostile fantasies and impulses.

In addition, it emerged that Ms C. was unaware that she routinely behaved in ways that expressed her anger indirectly, provoking others' angry reactions to her. These angry reactions were unexpected and only intensified her feelings of hurt and wishes to retaliate. This pattern increased her anxiety and caused further disruption of relationships. For example, Ms C. was dismissive of J.'s wish to get together but then was surprised when J. became angry at her, despite her intense emotional reactions when J. acted in the same way. Becoming aware of this covert hostility, though frightening for Ms C., reduced her sense of helplessness and provided a better understanding of why her feelings and relationships felt unmanageable.

The therapist and Ms C. gained further understanding of her anxiety through a detailed focus on the feelings and situations in which it arose. For example, the therapist was able to identify the pattern of increasing fears of having a serious health condition after she experienced angry feelings or jealousy, such as would occur after visiting friends who were pregnant or had small children. These fears were linked to the threat Ms C. felt that she would be criticized or rejected if her negative feelings were revealed. Another related trigger the therapist and patient were able to recognize was the danger of potential disruption of a relationship, either in fantasy or reality. Fears that her feelings of dizziness meant she was having a stroke developed after a girlfriend threatened to end their relationship, signifying her own anger at the friend and a neediness that she found difficult to control.

Ms C.'s worries about illness represented a compromise formation that served several functions. Her symptoms were emotionally understandable in part as a defensive maneuver when her fantasies and fears reached intolerable levels, as it emerged that it was less disorganizing for Ms C. to imagine dangers to her health than being abandoned by friends. The pain and distress caused by her somatic preoccupations also functioned as a self-punishment for her envy of friends and the anger that she routinely felt toward them, and for behaving, in her mind, like her father. Additionally, her somatic preoccupations and panic attacks permitted her to feel she was helpless or potentially disabled (a victim) rather than an angry threat to others.

Despite the fact that Ms C. presented to therapy with what she described as a strong desire to have a child, it emerged in therapy that she also had fears about how a baby might negatively affect her life. She imagined that the baby's behavior would be reminiscent of her father's, constantly demanding and "at her" to get his or her needs met. She feared a baby would damage her body, a fantasy in part related to her fears of the baby/her father's aggression. She felt guilty about ascribing these threats to a baby and worried how she would handle being angry at a baby. She wanted to be the perfect mother, to compensate for these thoughts and feelings, and she worried that a wrong decision or attitude would ruin her child.

Ms C.'s feelings of helplessness and lack of control in a variety of situations and her need for total control everywhere she went were linked to her conflicted feelings and fears regarding her relationship with her father, as well as her identification with him. Her need to control others and to aim toward forming what she imagined were "perfect" relationships were understood as compensatory efforts to minimize the danger of her aggression in this context. The therapist pointed out to Ms C. that her perfectionism was bound to fail and would inevitably leave her further disappointed, frustrated, and frightened. The therapist noted that perfection was neither possible nor necessary for relationships to work. Ms C. began to acknowledge that people could have conflicts and express strong feelings without necessarily experiencing the kinds of threats and criticism she had had with her father. She became more direct in her communications with others rather than keeping her feelings at a great distance from her own awareness.

Several of these themes and dynamics were identified and explored in the transference, providing an opportunity to address these concerns more directly. For example, Ms C. felt that if the therapist was not perfect, it was likely he was hostile and uncaring. Ms C. was angry at the therapist because she did not have full resolution of her anxiety. She believed that he could not fully reassure her about her hypochondriacal fears. She felt guilty about expressing her disappointment and anger at him, and she worried he would release her as a patient. She also feared the therapist would criticize her as her father did—in this case, for not getting better or for not being a good patient. For example, she believed the therapist would be very angry with her if, after improving significantly, she wanted to decrease the frequency of her visits from twice to once weekly, even though the therapist had agreed that this reduction should be considered.

Over the course of therapy, Ms C.'s worries diminished in intensity and frequency, and her panic attacks steadily resolved. She increasingly recognized the link between her worries and her conflicts about anger, jealousy, and her neediness as it had initially surfaced in her relationship with her father and did now with friends and the therapist. She became better able to identify her somatic preoccupations as signals of increased emotional conflict, to observe her own anxiety and moods, and to explore why her worries intensified when they did. In addition, improved access to her feelings allowed her to address tensions more directly with her friends. Ms C. subsequently became pregnant, easing her jealousy, and her fears of bodily damage were diminished by her having understood the link between pregnancy, her relationship to her baby in fantasy, and these fears.

CONCLUSIONS AND FUTURE DIRECTIONS

Psychoanalysts and researchers have made only limited efforts to identify specific dynamics and psychodynamic treatment approaches for GAD, and few research studies have been conducted on GAD-focused psychodynamic treatment. Therefore, limited information is available to make judgments about the utility of psychodynamic interventions for GAD. Further development of psychoanalytic outcome research studies is essential in this regard. These studies should include randomized controlled trials comparing manualized psychodynamic treatments of GAD to a comparator treatment, possibly ART, and also to CBT. Such studies could follow the model of the efficacy for psychodynamic treatment of PD described above. In these efforts, it is important to monitor the shifting approach to GAD diagnosis. The development and testing of transdiagnostic treatment approaches (Busch et al., 2012) may expand the utility and exportability of these psychodynamic approaches.

REFERENCES

American Psychiatric Association. (1980). *Diagnostic and statistical manual of mental disorders* (3rd ed.). Washington, DC: Author.

American Psychiatric Association. (2000). *Diagnostic criteria for diagnostic and statistical manual of mental disorders* (4th ed., text rev.). Washington, DC: Author.

American Psychiatric Association. (2013). *Diagnostic and statistical manual of mental disorders* (5th ed.). Arlington, VA: Author.

Andrews, G., Charney, D. S., Sirovatka, P. J., & Regier, D. A. (2009). *Stress-induced and fear circuitry disorders: Advancing the research agenda for DSM-V*. Washington, DC: American Psychiatric Publishing.

Beck, A. T., Epstein, N., Brown, G., & Steer, R. A. (1988). An inventory for measuring clinical anxiety: Psychometric properties. *Journal of Consulting and Clinical Psychology, 56*, 893–897.

Beck, A. T., Steer, R. A., & Garbin, M. G. (1988). Psychometric properties of the Beck Depression Inventory: Twenty-five years later. *Clinical Psychology Review, 8*, 77–100.

Beck, A. T., Ward, C., & Mendelson, M. (1961). Beck Depression Inventory (BDI). *Archives of General Psychiatry, 4*, 561–571.

Borkovec, T. D., Alcaine, O. M., & Behar, E. (2004). Avoidance theory of worry. In R. G. Heimberg, C. L. Turk, & D. S. Mennin (Eds.), *Generalized anxiety disorder: Advances in research and practice* (pp. 77–108). New York: Guilford Press.

Borkovec, T. D., & Mathews, A. M. (1988). Treatment of nonphobic anxiety disorders: A comparison of nondirective, cognitive, and coping desensitization therapy. *Journal of Consulting and Clinical Psychology. 56*, 877–884.

Busch, F. N., Milrod, B. L., & Shear, M. K. (2010). Psychodynamic concepts of anxiety. In D. J. Stein, E. Hollander, & B. Rothbaum (Eds.), *Textbook of anxiety disorders* (pp. 117–128). Arlington, VA: American Psychiatric Press.

Busch, F. N., Milrod, B. L., Singer, M., & Aronson, A. (2012). *Manual of panic-focused psychodynamic psychotherapy, eXtended range*. London: Routledge.

Cassidy, J., Lichtenstein-Phelps, J., Sibrava, N. J., Thomas, C. L., Jr., & Borkovec, T. D. (2009). Generalized anxiety disorder: Connections with self-reported attachment. *Behavior Therapy, 40*, 23–38.

Crits-Christoph, P., Connolly, M. B., Azarian, K., Crits-Christoph, K., & Shappell, S. (1996). An open trial of brief supportive-expressive psychotherapy in the treatment of generalized anxiety disorder. *Psychotherapy, 33*, 418–430.

Crits-Christoph, P., Connolly Gibbons, M. B., Narducci, J., Schamberger, M., & Gallop, R. (2005). Interpersonal problems and the outcome of interpersonally oriented psychodynamic treatment of GAD. *Psychotherapy: Theory, Research, Practice, Training, 42*, 211–224.

Crits-Christoph, P., Cooper, A., & Luborsky, L. (1988). The accuracy of therapists' interpretations and the outcome of psychotherapy. *Journal of Consulting and Clinical Psychology, 56*, 490–495.

Crits-Christoph, P., & Luborsky, L. (1990). Changes in CCRT pervasiveness during psychotherapy. In L. Luborsky & P. Crits-Christoph (Eds.), *Understanding transference: The CCRT method* (pp. 133–146). New York: Basic Books.

Crits-Christoph, P., Wolf-Palacio, D., Fichter, M., & Rudick, D. (1995). Brief supportive-expressive psychodynamic therapy for generalized anxiety disorder. In J. P. Barber & P. Crits-Christoph (Eds.), *Dynamic therapies for psychiatric disorders (Axis I)* (pp. 43–83). New York: Basic Books.

Etkin, A., Prater, K. E., Hoeft, F., Menon, V., & Schatzberg, A. F. (2010). Failure of anterior cingulate activation and connectivity with the amygdala during implicit regulation of emotional processing in generalized anxiety disorder. *American Journal of Psychiatry, 167,* 545–554.

First, M. B., Spitzer, R. L., Gibbon, M., & Williams, J. B. W. (1994). *Structured clinical interview for Axis I DSM–IV Disorders—Patient Edition.* Washington, DC: American Psychiatric Press.

Gorman, J. M., Kent, J. M., Sullivan, G. M., & Coplan, J. D. (2000). Neuroanatomical hypothesis of panic disorder, revised. *American Journal of Psychiatry, 157,* 493–505.

Hamilton, M. A. (1959). The assessment of anxiety states by rating. *British Journal of Medical Psychology, 32,* 50–55.

Hamilton, M. A. (1960). A rating scale for depression. *Journal of Neurological and Neurosurgical Psychiatry, 23,* 56–62.

Horowitz, L. M., Alden, L. E., Wiggins, J. S., & Pincus, A. L. (2000). *Inventory of interpersonal problems manual.* San Antonio, TX: Psychological Corp.

Huppert, J. D., & Sanderson, W. C. (2010). Psychotherapy for generalized anxiety disorder. In D. J. Stein, E. Hollander, & B. Rothbaum (Eds.), *Textbook of anxiety disorders* (pp. 219–238). Arlington, VA: American Psychiatric Press.

Insel, T., Cuthbert, B., Garvey, M., Heinssen, R., Pine, D. S., Quinn, K., et al. (2010). Research domain criteria (RDoC): Toward a new classification framework for research on mental disorders. *American Journal of Psychiatry, 167,* 748–751.

Insel, T. R., & Cuthbert, B. N. (2009). Endophenotypes: Bridging genomic complexity and disorder heterogeneity. *Biological Psychiatry, 66,* 988–989.

Insel, T. R. & Wang, P. S. (2010). Rethinking mental illness. *Journal of the American Medical Association, 303,* 1970–1971.

Leichsenring, F., Salzer, S., Jaeger, U., Kächele, H., Kreische, R., Leweke, F., et al. (2009). Short-term psychodynamic psychotherapy and cognitive-behavioral therapy in generalized anxiety disorder: A randomized, controlled trial. *American Journal of Psychiatry, 166,* 875–881.

Lichtenstein, J., & Cassidy, J. (1991, April). *The Inventory of Adult Attachment: Validation of a new measure.* Paper presented at the biennial meeting of the Society for Research in Child Development, Seattle, WA.

Luborsky, L. (1984). *Principles of psychoanalytic psychotherapy: A manual for supportive-expressive (SE) treatment.* New York: Basic Books.

Mennin, D. S., Heimberg, R. G., Turk, C. L., & Fresco, D. M. (2005). Preliminary evidence for an emotion dysregulation model of generalized anxiety disorder. *Behavior Research and Therapy, 43,* 1281–1310.

Meyer, T. J., Miller, M. L., Metzger, R. L., & Borkovec, T. D. (1990). Development and validation of the Penn State Worry Questionnaire. *Behaviour Research and Therapy, 28,* 487–495.

Milrod, B. (2009). Psychodynamic psychotherapy outcome for generalized anxiety disorder. *American Journal of Psychiatry, 166,* 841–844.

Milrod, B., Busch, F., Cooper, A., & Shapiro, T. (1997). *Manual of panic-focused psychodynamic psychotherapy.* Washington, DC: American Psychiatric Press.

Milrod, B., Leon, A. C., Busch, F., Rudden, M., Schwalberg, M., Clarkin, J., et al. (2007). A randomized controlled clinical trial of psychoanalytic psychotherapy for panic disorder. *American Journal of Psychiatry, 164,* 265–272.

Mitte, K. (2005). Meta-analysis of cognitive-behavioral treatments for generalized anxiety disorder: A comparison with pharmacotherapy. *Psychological Bulletin, 131,* 785–795.

National Institute of Mental Health. (2008). *The National Institute of Mental Health Strategic Plan.* Bethesda, MD: National Institute of Mental Health. NIH Publication 08-6368. Retrieved from *www.nimh.nih.gov/about/strategic-planning-reports/index.shtml.*

Rudden, M., Milrod, B., Target, M., Ackerman, S., & Graf, E. (2006). Reflective functioning in panic disorder patients: A pilot study. *Journal of the American Psychoanalytic Association 54,* 1339–1343.

Sakai, Y., Kumano, H., Nishikawa, M., Sakano, Y., Kaiya, H., Imabayashi, E., et al. (2006). Changes in cerebral glucose utilization in patients with panic disorder treated with cognitive-behavioral therapy. *NeuroImage, 33,* 218–226.

Sanderson, W. C., & Barlow, D. H. (1990). A description of patients idangosed with DSM-III-R generalized anxiety disorder. *Journal of Nervous and Mental Disease, 178,* 588–591.

Sass, H., Wittchen, H.-U., & Zaudig, M. (2000). *Diagnostisches und statistisches manual psychischer störungen DSM-IV* [Diagnostic and statistical manual of mental disorders DSM-IV]. Bern, Switzerland: Verlag Hans Huber.

Spielberger, C. D., Gorsuch, R. C., & Lushene, R. E. (1970). *Manual for the State–Trait Anxiety Inventory.* Palo Alto, CA: Consulting Psychologist Press.

Spitzer, R. L., Williams, J. B. W., Gibbon, M., & First, M. B. (1990). *Users' guide for the structured clinical interview for DSM-III-R: SCID.* Washington, DC: American Psychiatric Association.

Van Ameringen, M., Mancini, C., Patterson, B., Simpson, W., & Truong, C. (2010). Pharmacotherapy for Generalized Anxiety Disorder. In D. J. Stein, E. Hollander, & B. Rothbaum (Eds.), *Textbook of anxiety disorders* (pp. 193–218). Arlington, VA: American Psychiatric Press.

Wittchen, H.-U., Zaudig, M., & Fydrich, T. (1997). *Strukturiertes klinisches interview für DSM-IV* [Structured clinical interview for DSM-IV]. Goettingen, Germany: Hogrefe.

Zigmond, A. S., & Snaith, R. P. (1983). The Hospital Anxiety and Depression Scale. *Acta Psychiatrica Scandinavica, 67,* 361–370.

CHAPTER 9

Trauma

Jon G. Allen and Peter Fonagy

Notwithstanding an extremely rich clinical literature, the evidence base for psychodynamic treatment of posttraumatic reactions largely must be sought elsewhere, simply because of the relative paucity of psychodynamic research on trauma and its treatment (Roth & Fonagy, 2005; Schottenbauer, Glass, Arnkoff, & Gray, 2008). As is true of the practice of psychotherapy more generally, psychodynamically oriented therapists are treating traumatized patients in the context of the hegemony of cognitive-behavioral approaches inasmuch as these are the most extensively researched (Resick, Monson, & Gutner, 2007; Roth & Fonagy, 2005) and thus are recognized in current treatment guidelines (Foa, Keane, Friedman, & Cohen, 2009) as being effective for the most conspicuous trauma-related disorder, posttraumatic stress disorder (PTSD). Yet there are significant limitations to the effectiveness of accepted treatments for PTSD (Bradley, Greene, Russ, Dutra, & Westen, 2005): A substantial minority of patients continue to meet full criteria after termination; those who no longer meet the criteria may nevertheless be hampered by residual symptoms; long-term follow-up data are sparse; a complete history of trauma exposure often is not well documented; and exclusion criteria limit generalizability. Moreover, PTSD is merely one of myriad disorders for which traumatized patients seek treatment; comorbidity is the rule (Keane, Brief, Pratt, & Miller, 2007; Magruder et al., 2005; Najavits et al., 2009).

Yet, in the face of extensive comorbidity, administering multiple, disorder-specific therapies is not feasible. Accordingly, this chapter is based on the core premise that multifaceted trauma-related psychopathology requires a fundamental shift in perspective—that is, a move from a *disorder-centered* to a *person-centered* approach to treatment (Luyten, Vliegen, Van Houdenhove, & Blatt, 2008), or "a life history perspective" (p. 41) that aspires to "map the myriad complex pathways from early childhood to later adaptive or maladaptive development which can then form the basis for interventions for both preventing and treating disorders" (p. 29).

This review is limited to carving out the territory most pertinent to psychodynamic psychotherapy, namely, adulthood psychopathology to which childhood maltreatment makes a substantial contribution. Throughout, we employ the attachment-related concept of *mentalizing* (Fonagy, 1989), that is, attending to mental states in self and others and interpreting behavior accordingly—in short, holding the mind in mind. The concept of mentalizing is particularly useful here in exploiting the evidence base garnered for cognitive-behavioral approaches: Focusing on mentalizing addresses the natural convergence of cognitive-behavioral and psychodynamic approaches (Allen, 2008a), including the treatment of trauma (Stein & Allen, 2007). This is our simple orienting thesis: *The experience of being left psychologically alone in unbearable emotional states is potentially traumatic owing in part to the absence of mentalizing, and treatment entails creating a secure attachment context conducive to mentalizing in which previously unbearable emotional states can be experienced, expressed, understood, and reflected upon—and thus rendered once again meaningful and bearable.* This review summarizes research bearing on this thesis.

This chapter proceeds in the following steps: (1) We review the current diagnostic controversy pertaining to trauma-related disorders as a context for the need to go beyond narrowly focused, empirically supported treatments; (2) we explore the most favorable niche for psychodynamic psychotherapy, namely, complex developmental psychopathology associated with traumatic attachment relationships in childhood and the potential reenactment of these relationship patterns in adulthood; (3) we employ the concept of experiential avoidance to link our mentalizing approach with eclectic cognitive-behavioral interventions; (4) we present a case example to illustrate the importance of restoring mentalizing in treating trauma; and (5) we identify areas for future research, focusing on putative mechanisms of change.

CLASSIFICATION AND DIAGNOSIS

Trauma is a fuzzy target for treatment. The term is used ambiguously to refer to exposure to potentially traumatic (i.e., extremely stressful) *events* and to the traumatic *effects* of such exposure (i.e., in the sense of having been *traumatized*). Although DSM-IV (American Psychiatric Association [APA], 2000) included subjective experience in the definition of traumatic stress (i.e., feelings of fear, helplessness, or horror), DSM-5 refers only to objective events; see the DSM-5 discussion (APA, 2013, p. 271) about exposure to specific types of death, injury, or violence. This revision is consistent with prior criticism that the subjective criterion focused too narrowly on fear to the exclusion of a host of emotions that also contribute to PTSD, including shame, guilt, anger, and disgust (Brewin, 2003; Friedman, Resick, & Keane, 2007). In addition, some persons develop PTSD without experiencing extreme distress at the time of trauma. Moreover, subjective distress is a weak predictor of PTSD and has little bearing on estimates of prevalence (Friedman & Karam, 2009). The validity of the objective criterion also has been debated, with disagreement about whether it should be broadened or narrowed (Friedman & Karam, 2009; Spitzer, First, & Wakefeld, 2007). We contend that the focus on physical injury that remains in DSM-5 is too narrow: Psychological or emotional abuse (e.g., being sadistically tormented, terrorized, humiliated) can be profoundly damaging (Bifulco, Moran, Baines, Bunn, & Stanford, 2002), as can psychological neglect (Erickson & Egeland, 1996).

Ironically, although PTSD is among a small subset of DSM-5 psychiatric diagnoses that specify a traumatic or stress-related etiology, the etiological role of trauma in PTSD is anything but simple. First, ample evidence indicates that exposure to objectively defined traumatic events is not sufficient to produce PTSD; the vast majority of exposed persons do not develop PTSD (Rosen & Lilienfeld, 2008), although some types of trauma carry a far higher risk than others (e.g., sexual assaults versus automobile accidents). Second, albeit the exception rather than the rule, the symptom cluster of PTSD is sometimes evident in the absence of objectively defined (i.e., criterion A) traumatic events. For example, gauged by responses to symptom checklists—which admittedly lend themselves to overreporting (McHugh & Treisman, 2007)—the PTSD syndrome has been observed in relation to common stressors such as family or romantic relationship problems, occupational stress, parental divorce, and serious illness or death of a loved one (Gold, Marx, Soler-Baillo, & Sloan, 2005; Mol et al., 2005). Regardless of the type of trauma, there is robust evidence for a dose–response relationship: The more severe the stressor, the greater the likelihood of developing PTSD (Friedman et al., 2007; Vogt, King, & King, 2007). Yet, as the foregoing implies, the relationship between severity of stress and illness is by no means monotonic (Rosen & Lilienfeld, 2008); this raises appropriate questions about the precise etiological role of the traumatic event (the "T") in PTSD.

A number of clinicians have proposed diagnosing a broader pattern of trauma-related psychopathology than PTSD. Herman (1992a, 1992b) initially formulated the concept of *complex PTSD* to include a multitude of symptoms, relationship and identity disturbance, as well as patterns of self-harming behavior that can stem from repeated and severe trauma, including childhood abuse and neglect. She proposed that this amalgam of symptoms and personality disturbance be diagnosed as disorders of extreme stress not otherwise specified (Herman, 1993). More recently, van der Kolk (2005) proposed a childhood counterpart of complex PTSD, developmental trauma disorder. Trauma that occurs in the context of attachment relationships plays a significant role in the etiological component of these formulations, and an explicit focus on attachment is central to the concepts of betrayal trauma (DePrince & Freyd, 2007; Freyd, 1996) and attachment trauma (Adam, Sheldon Keller, & West, 1995; Allen, 2001), both of which are potentially associated with extensive developmental psychopathology. Friedman and Karam (2009) reported that the DSM-IV Task Force held a "spirited discussion" (p. 18) about the inclusion of complex PTSD; they stated that the proposal was not adopted because the vast majority (92%) of persons with complex PTSD met the criteria for PTSD, rendering the proposed new diagnosis superfluous. They argued that complex PTSD could merit a niche in the extreme end of a dimensionalized formulation of PTSD. DSM-5 has broadened the diagnostic criteria to include widespread alterations in cognition and mood, added specification for dissociative symptoms, and incorporated problems with emotion regulation and interpersonal functioning among the associated features.

Building on prior conceptualizations, Ford and Courtois (2009) reviewed the range of proposals for characterizing complex PTSD, and their formulation is representative. They define *complex psychological trauma* as "resulting from exposure to severe stressors that (1) are repetitive or prolonged, (2) involve harm or abandonment by caregivers or other ostensibly responsible adults, and (3) occur at developmentally vulnerable times in the victim's life, such as early childhood or adolescence" (p. 13). They construe the multifaceted sequelae as *complex traumatic stress disorders*, namely, "the changes in mind, emotions, body, and relationships experienced following complex psychological trauma, including severe problems with dissociation, emotion dysregulation, somatic distress, or relational or spiritual alienation" (p. 13). Hence complex traumatic stress disorders potentially entail extensive comorbidity, including a range of symptoms and clinical syndromes as well as personality disorders—not to mention existential-spiritual concerns that transcend psychiatry.

Plainly, when we refer to "trauma-related disorders," we must not slip into the single pathogen–single disorder mode of thinking. Rather, we must view these as disorders to which traumatic stress makes some substantial—albeit individually variable—contribution, in conjunction with a host of other etiological factors. This is often true for "simple" PTSD as well as complex PTSD.

PSYCHODYNAMIC APPROACHES TO PTSD

Over the past years, we have advocated an attachment and mentalizing approach to the understanding of trauma. In our usage, the focus on attachment has two senses: (1) referring to trauma that occurs in the context of an attachment relationship and (2) referring to the ensuing disruption of the capacity to develop secure attachments that often results from any type of trauma, with the concomitant impairment of mentalizing and emotion-regulation capacities. We recognize that attachment relationships can be traumatic in adulthood as well as childhood, as battering relationships exemplify (Walker, 1979). Yet, owing to their potentially shaping effects on development, traumatic attachments in childhood merit particular attention. Fonagy and Target (1997) proposed a *dual liability* stemming from childhood traumatic attachments: These relationships not only evoke extreme distress but also impair the development of capacities to regulate emotional distress—in part through compromising the development of mentalizing. More recently, Fonagy proposed a third liability associated with compromised mentalizing, namely, closing the mind to social influence; this liability has profoundly adverse implications for responsiveness to psychotherapy (Allen & Fonagy, 2014).

Attachment and Trauma

Extensive research relates security of infant attachment to caregiver behavior (Ainsworth, Blehar, Waters, & Wall, 1978; Sroufe, Egeland, Carlson, & Collins, 2005;

Weinfield, Sroufe, Egeland, & Carlson, 2008). Sensitively responsive caregivers exemplify mentalizing, being disposed to understand the psychological complexity of their infant, for example, as being autonomous and also in need of care (Sroufe et al., 2005). Hence, they are aware of their infant's signals, interpret them accurately, and respond to them promptly and appropriately. They accept a wide range of emotion, and they are cooperative in adapting their actions to their infant's mood and interests rather than intruding and interfering. Thus, securely attached infants are maintaining not only physical proximity but also psychological proximity to the mentalizing caregiver, who provides both physical and psychological availability (Erickson & Egeland, 1996).

Attachment disruptions, by contrast, typically result in patterns of insecurity, that is, avoidant and ambivalent/resistant (see also Mikulincer & Shaver, Chapter 2, this volume). In the Strange Situation, avoidant infants appear indifferent to their mother: They focus their attention inflexibly on the environment, they do not engage in affective sharing, and they ignore their mother's departure and return. Hence, they do not seek proximity or contact with their mother upon reunion, but rather may turn away or wish to be put down if picked up. This behavior is an adaptive effort to maintain proximity at some distance in response to the caregiver's proclivity to reject attachment behavior: Mothers of avoidant infants tend to be relatively unemotional, tense, irritable, unresponsive to crying, unaffectionate, and aversive to physical contact. Accordingly, the infant *deactivates attachment behavior* and minimizes attachment needs to avoid eliciting further rejection. Avoidant children tend to be relatively distant and isolated, having relationships that are relatively superficial. They are also liable to be hostile, aggressive, and bullying toward other children such that they are disliked. Being inclined to victimize other children, they are likely to elicit control and rejection from teachers.

In the Strange Situation, ambivalent/resistant infants are wary and maintain proximity to their mother to the relative exclusion of play—even before separation. Distressed upon separation, they are not easily calmed upon reunion: They may fuss, cry, squirm, and show anger, pushing away after seeking to be held. Alternatively, they may be passive, crying but not making any effort to seek contact. Their caregivers are likely to be psychologically unaware as well as inconsistently or erratically responsive to their bids for comfort. Accordingly, ambivalent infants *strive to elicit predictable care* by amplifying their emotions; they maximize or hyperactivate attachment needs. In childhood, they are likely to be anxious and distress prone, subject to emotional contagion, and overtly dependent (e.g., seeking proximity to teachers to the exclusion of peer relationships). Concomitantly, they are relatively passive and helpless as well as vulnerable to victimization; accordingly, they are not prone to persistence in problem solving, such that they fall short in developing social or cognitive competence.

These two insecure patterns are adaptive strategies adopted to cope with less-than-optimal caregiving, that is, rejection or inconsistent availability. Yet, there is no straightforward adaptive strategy for meeting attachment needs when the caregiver is frightening. Main and Solomon (1990) developed a way of classifying anomalous infant behaviors in the Strange Situation that were not encompassed within

Ainsworth's three categories; in addition to coding the best-fitting organized strategy, these infants were classified as disorganized-disoriented. The infants' anomalous behavior included simultaneous approach–avoidance (e.g., screaming when the parent left the room and silently moving away from the parent on reunion, or backing toward the parent); direct expression of fear of the parent; odd postures and stereotypical behaviors; and dissociative, trance-like—hence disoriented—states (e.g., freezing, stilling, dazed expressions).

Main and colleagues (Main & Hesse, 1990; Main, Hesse, & Kaplan, 2005) rapidly identified maltreatment as the instigator of fear but also came to recognize that the parent's fearfulness was associated with infant disorganization. Thus, the parent might be frightening or frightened. Such parental behavior was associated with unresolved loss or trauma, such that the frightened parent could be viewed as traumatized but not maltreating. Accordingly, frightening and frightened behavior includes being directly threatening (and abusive) to the child, as well as appearing timid, disorganized, or being in a dissociative state. Paralleling Main's frightening–frightened pattern, Lyons-Ruth and Jacobvitz (1999) identified two patterns of maternal behavior associated with attachment disorganization: hostile intrusiveness and helpless withdrawal. These authors subsequently (Lyons-Ruth & Jacobvitz, 2008) proposed that frightening–frightened behavior is a subset of a broader pattern of *disrupted parental affective communication* associated with infant disorganization; this pattern includes negative-intrusive behavior, role confusion, withdrawal, affective communicative errors, and disorientation. George and Solomon (2008) have further broadened the understanding of parenting related to infant disorganization in referring to a "disabled caregiving system" (p. 846) that includes abdication of care and reflects a potentially wide range of "assaults to the caregiving system" (p. 848). These assaults include parental divorce, child disability, prematurity, perinatal loss of a child, and living in a violent environment (e.g., a war zone).

Infant disorganization frequently develops into an organized strategy by childhood, namely, controlling behavior toward caregivers (Main et al., 2005); this behavior can be either punitive or caregiving (i.e., solicitous). Although disorganized attachment is not a form of psychopathology, it portends a high-risk pathway compared to the organized insecure patterns: Disorganization is associated with both internalizing and externalizing problems from infancy into school age (Lyons-Ruth & Jacobvitz, 2008) and, as we will discuss later in this section, it is predictive of psychopathology into adulthood.

Attachment, Mentalizing, and the Intergenerational Transmission of Trauma

Studies have generally found that infant security of attachment is associated with secure-autonomous parental Adult Attachment Interview (AAI) classification. This classification is associated most directly with narrative coherence (Main, Hesse, & Goldwyn, 2008). These parents' narratives meet linguistic requirements for ideally rational and cooperative conversation, namely: being truthful and providing evidence for statements made; being succinct yet complete; maintaining relevance to the topic at hand; and being clear and orderly. Security is indicated by freedom to explore painful experiences, valuing of attachment, objectivity, forgiveness, ease with imperfections in self and parents, as well as appreciation for the impact of attachment on development and functioning (Hesse, 2008).

Insecure AAI discourse entails different kinds of compromise in coherent discourse that relate to different patterns of infant insecurity (Hesse, 2008; Main et al., 2005, 2008). Avoidant infant attachment is associated with the *dismissing* parental AAI classification, evident in idealization (or devaluation) of attachment, coupled with lack of memory for specific experiences along with minimizing the value of attachment and portraying the self as strong and independent. Ambivalent infant attachment is associated with the *preoccupied* parental AAI classification, characterized by ongoing (e.g., angry) preoccupation with early attachment experiences; responses to questions are long, rambling, vague, and blaming toward parents or self. Infant disorganization is associated with the parental unresolved/disorganized AAI classification, which shows lapses of attention or reasoning in conjunction with discussions of loss and abuse. Infant disorganization also is associated with interviews that cannot be classified, for example, owing to a contradictory intermingling of different attachment classifications.

To underscore the power of mental representations of attachment experience, Fonagy and colleagues (Fonagy, Steele, & Steele, 1991) demonstrated that mothers' attachment security in relation to their parents assessed *prior to the birth* of their infant predicted their infant's security of attachment with them at 12 months. This finding was replicated subsequently for fathers (Steele, Steele, & Fonagy, 1996). A substantial body of research has supported a straightforward transmission model: Parents' working models of attachment are associated with their sensitive caregiving behavior, which, in turn, is associated with the security of their infant's attachment to them (van IJzendoorn, 1995). Yet, this same research reveals a *transmission gap* insofar as sensitive parenting behaviors account for a relatively small proportion of the relation between parental representations and infant attachment.

Research on mentalizing and related constructs is aspiring to narrow the transmission gap. Fonagy, Steele, Steele, Moran, and Higgitt (1991) developed a new scoring system to quantify the level of reflective functioning (mentalizing) in the AAI, an assessment constituting a refinement of Main's (1991) conception of metacognitive monitoring as a contributor to coherent discourse. Fonagy's research demonstrated that reflective functioning and coherence of transcript were highly correlated; yet, in the context of a maternal trauma history, reflective functioning bore a stronger relation to infant attachment security than narrative coherence.

In related research, Slade and colleagues (Slade, 2005; Slade, Grienenberger, Bernbach, Levy, & Locker, 2005) found that mothers' mentalizing capacity in relation to their own attachment history predicted their mentalizing of their 10-month-old infant in a 90-minute Parental Development Interview; their capacity to mentalize in the interview, in turn, predicted their infant's attachment security at 14 months. In contrast to this "offline" mentalizing of the infant in an interview, Meins and colleagues (Meins, 1997; Meins, Fernyhough, Fradley, & Tuckey, 2001) found that mothers' mind-minded commentary during interactions with their 6-month-old infant—indicative of their psychological attunement—predicted their infant's attachment security at 12 months. Arnott and Meins (2007) investigated the entire transmission model for mothers and fathers and found that the parents' security of attachment related positively to mentalizing regarding those attachments; security of attachment and mentalizing related to mind-minded commentary in interaction with their 6-month-old infant; and their mind-minded commentary predicted infant security at 12 months. They identified two developmental pathways: Parental secure attachment was linked to infant security through a high level of parental mind-mindedness, whereas parental insecurity was linked to infant insecurity through a low level of mind-mindedness.

To summarize, attachment research has shown how security of attachment and mentalizing are intertwined in an intergenerational transmission process, for better (parental security and mentalizing capacity, mentalizing interactions, and child security) or worse (parental insecurity and compromised mentalizing capacity, nonmentalizing-traumatizing interactions, and child insecurity). The final link in this chain also is critical: Infant attachment security predicts subsequent child mentalizing capacity (Fonagy, Gergely, & Target, 2008). Meins and colleagues (Meins, 1997; Meins, Fernyhough, Russell, & Clark-Carter, 1998), for example, demonstrated that infant security predicted performance on theory-of-mind tasks at age 4. Yet, subsequent research revealed that mentalizing interactions in infancy, rather than secure attachment per se, are most predictive of subsequent childhood mentalizing capacities (Meins et al., 2002, 2003). Hence, the development of mentalizing capacity can be understood broadly with a simple principle: *mentalizing begets mentalizing.* Conversely, as Fonagy and colleagues have reviewed (Fonagy, Gergely, & Target, 2007; Fonagy et al., 2008), nonmentalizing begets nonmentalizing, as is evident in compromised child mentalizing associated with maltreatment and disorganized attachment. This mentalizing impairment is evident in poorer performance on theory-of-mind tasks, disturbances in mental representations of self and parents, limited capacity to talk about mental states, difficulty understanding emotions and accurately perceiving emotional expressions, empathic failures in relation to other children's distress, and compromised emotion-regulation capacity.

The intergenerational transmission of mentalizing in the context of secure attachment relationships can be understood straightforwardly in the context of pedagogy (Gergely & Csibra, 2005): By mentalizing, parents teach their children to mentalize. Yet, they must do so in the context of emotionally charged interactions that consciously or unconsciously stimulate their own mental representations of attachment and the associated emotions. At worst, with a parental history of trauma, the child's expression of attachment needs—or frustration of these needs—can be a reminder of trauma, evoking a PTSD-like parental response of compromised mentalizing and traumatizing behavior (Allen, 2001). This, too, is a form of teaching that is potentially self-perpetuating. The catch-22s are: We most need to mentalize when we are least able to do it, and, paradoxically, as Main and colleagues (2005) proposed, children most need security (and mentalizing) when they are being frightened, maltreated, or psychologically abandoned.

In comparison with the organized-insecure patterns, disorganized attachment is a far more potent risk factor for psychopathology, in part owing to the substantial link between early maltreatment and attachment disorganization. Indeed, the combination of attachment disorganization with early and prolonged trauma may present the greatest risk for psychopathology (Melnick, Finger, Hans, Patrick, & Lyons-Ruth, 2008). For example, disorganized attachment in infancy increased the risk for PTSD in childhood following trauma exposure (MacDonald et al., 2008). Attesting to its potential long-range developmental impact, Sroufe and colleagues (2005) found disorganized attachment in infancy to be the strongest predictor of global psychopathology at age 17.5 years (i.e., number and severity of diagnoses). As Lyons-Ruth and Jacobvitz (2008) summarized, "attachment disorganization is likely to index a broad relational contribution to maladaptation and psychopathology that cuts across conventional diagnostic categories and interacts with individual biological vulnerability to contribute to a range of psychiatric disorders" (p. 689).

Yet, some specificity exemplifying phenotypic similarity (Dozier, Stovall-McClough, & Albus, 2008) has been shown in the relatively robust relation between infant disorganization and subsequent dissociative pathology. Among the findings of the Minnesota longitudinal study employing teacher ratings, diagnostic interviews, and self-report measures, Carlson (1998) found that disorganization in infancy related to dissociative experiences in elementary and high school as well as at age 19. In another longitudinal study, although Lyons-Ruth and colleagues did not find a direct link between disorganization and later dissociation, they did find maternal disrupted communication in the laboratory (a contributor to disorganization) to be related to dissociation in young adulthood. Notably, a low level of maternal positive emotion, as well as flat affect, was associated with later dissociation (Lyons-Ruth & Jacobvitz, 2008).

Paralleling longitudinal studies relating early attachment to later psychopathology, researchers have investigated the relation been concurrent assessments of adult attachment and trauma. Stovall-McClough, Cloitre, and McClough, (2008), for instance, reported AAI findings for a sample of 150 women with a history of severe physical, sexual, and emotional abuse by a caregiver before age 18, coupled with trauma-related symptoms for which they sought psychotherapy. Remarkably, about 50% of the patients were rated as secure (primarily or secondarily); 38% were preoccupied, and 12% were dismissing. Yet, 52% were unresolved in relation to loss or abuse, and 43% were unresolved regarding abuse. Notably, being unresolved with regard to abuse was associated with a 7.5-fold increase in the likelihood of a PTSD diagnosis (and especially with avoidance symptoms). Moreover, loss of unresolved status with treatment was associated with improvement in PTSD, and exposure treatment was more effective than skills training in promoting resolution. Hence, coming to terms more directly with traumatic experiences is associated with resolution.

Borderline Personality Disorder and Trauma

Borderline personality disorder (BPD) is particularly germane to this chapter: BPD is an exemplar of complex traumatic stress disorders insofar as the symptomatology is multifaceted and typically intertwined with a range of comorbid disorders. Moreover, childhood maltreatment is well established as one of many potential contributors to the etiology of BPD (Ball & Links, 2009), although maltreatment is neither necessary nor sufficient for development of the disorder (Gabbard, 2000). Indeed, Paris (1994) has outlined the sheer complexity and diversity of the etiology of BPD, with potential contributing factors including not only multiple forms of abuse and neglect but also family psychopathology and disturbance as well as broader social disintegration. Although childhood sexual abuse may play a particularly prominent role in the development of BPD (Paris, 2001), it is often intertwined with a broader pattern of family disturbance, such that Zanarini and colleagues (1997) concluded that "childhood sexual abuse reported by borderline patients may represent a *marker of the severity of the familial dysfunction* they experienced, as well as being a traumatic event or series of events in itself" (p. 1104, emphasis added). Moreover, these authors also commented that parental neglect puts the child at increased risk for extrafamilial sexual abuse "by making it clear to the potential perpetrators that no one will notice or care if the child is abused" (p. 1105).

Much of the research on the relation between BPD and childhood maltreatment has relied on retrospective reports, such that more recent prospective studies are providing more solid footing for developmental conclusions. Johnson and colleagues (2006) conducted a series of assessments of family members and their offspring spanning age 6 to 33 and found that low levels of parental affection and nurturing, as well as aversive parental behaviors such as harsh punishment, were associated with later BPD (although they were not specific to BPD). Lyons-Ruth, Yellin, Melnick, and Atwood (2005) found that disrupted maternal communication in infancy correlated significantly with symptoms of borderline pathology assessed at age 18; notably, the total amount of abuse over the lifetime reported in adolescence also contributed to borderline pathology. Disrupted maternal communication and later abuse have been found to make independent and additive contributions to pathology associated with BPD (Melnick et al., 2008).

Carlson, Egeland, and Sroufe (2009) reported on results from the Minnesota study that correlated extensive assessments from infancy onward with BPD symptom counts from structured interviews at age 28. The following early developmental observations related to borderline personality symptoms: attachment disorganization (12–18 months), maltreatment (12–18 months), maternal hostility and boundary dissolution (42 months), family disruption related to father presence (12–64 months), and family life stress (3–42 months). Several precursors of BPD were evident at 12 years: attentional disturbance, emotional instability, behavioral instability, and relational disturbance. The results suggested that disturbances in self-representation in early adolescence may mediate the link between attachment disorganization and personality disorder, based on findings from narrative projective tasks administered at age 12 that included intrusive violence related to the self, unresolved feelings of guilt or fear, and bizarre images related to the self. As these authors noted, "representations and related *mentalizing* processes are viewed as the carriers of experience" (p. 1328, emphasis added) that link early attachment to later psychopathology. Fonagy and colleagues (1996) established the link between mentalizing and BPD more directly, based on assessments of mentalizing capacity (reflective functioning) in the

AAI: 97% of patients with a history of maltreatment coupled with impaired mentalizing capacity met the criteria for BPD, whereas only 17% of the patients reporting abuse in the group with preserved mentalizing satisfied the criteria.

Sroufe and colleagues (2005) commented that an unanticipated finding regarding childhood treatment in their longitudinal study "was the devastating consequences of 'psychological' maltreatment. The pattern of parental psychological unavailability had wide-ranging consequences from early childhood into adulthood" (p. 301). This finding is particularly apt for the development of BPD. As we concluded previously, "the central factor that predisposes the child to BPD is *a family environment that discourages coherent discourse concerning mental states*" (Allen, Fonagy, & Bateman, 2008, p. 274, original emphasis). As Fonagy and Bateman (2008) elaborated, trauma plays a prominent role in shaping the development of BPD by undermining mentalizing. Yet, "the impact of trauma is most likely to be felt as part of a more general failure of consideration of the child's perspective through neglect, rejection, excessive control, unsupportive relationship, incoherence, and confusion" (p. 14).

The core problem in BPD pertains to a collapse of explicit, internal, and cognitive aspects of mentalizing in the context of the activation of the attachment system and associated arousal of emotional distress mediated by automatic, implicit mentalizing (Fonagy & Luyten, 2009). This collapse undermines the person's capacity to maintain self–other differentiation, and thus increases vulnerability to escalating vicious circles of emotional contagion in response to experiences of rejection, misattunement, or abandonment in attachment relationships. The core failure of caregiving that lays the foundation for the development of BPD is the absence of mentalizing in the context of the child's heightened need or distress—that is, the caregiver's response of either emotional withdrawal or emotional contagion.

This mentalizing failure is the context for disorganized and anxious-ambivalent attachment. Coupled with such psychological unavailability, other forms of trauma (e.g., frightening and hostile-intrusive behavior) in early as well as subsequent attachment relationships may lead to chronic, unresolved activation of the attachment system, which is liable to be exacerbated rather than mitigated in attachment relationships—including psychotherapy. Avoidant attachment entails greater capacity to preserve explicit, internal, and cognitive aspects of mentalizing under conditions of emotional arousal. Yet, avoidance offers only limited protection: Not only does avoidance limit the development of a range of secure attachment relationships, but also it is associated with vulnerability, insofar as increasingly intense levels of arousal are liable to result in a collapse of mentalizing with potential flooding of emotion.

Reenactments in Attachment Relationships

Reenactments of previous experience in attachment relationships begin early in life; they are generalizations to new situations of what one has learned previously. In this generic sense, Ainsworth's Strange Situation capitalizes on the likelihood that attachment patterns established in the home will be reenacted by parents and infants in the laboratory. Clinicians treating adult patients with a history of childhood maltreatment have pointed to the cardinal importance of addressing reenactments of traumatic attachment relationships (Chu, 1992; Davies & Frawley, 1994; van der Kolk, 1989). We have made the simple point that reminders of past trauma notoriously evoke symptoms of PTSD, and it is thus futile to desensitize patients to traumatic memories if reenactments of past trauma in current relationships are continually evoking such reminders—in effect, keeping the past trauma alive in relationships and in the mind (Allen, 2005). The obvious strength of a psychodynamic approach is in its attention to attachment relationships in general and the therapeutic use of reenactments in the treatment relationship in particular (Pearlman & Courtois, 2005).

Van der Kolk (1989) pointed to revictimization as a common form of reenactment; for example, childhood sexual abuse can set the stage for participating in pornography and prostitution. A careful prospective study showed that all forms of court-documented maltreatment (sexual and physical abuse as well as neglect) were associated with increased risk of exposure to rape in adulthood (Widom, 1999). Exploring the likelihood of revictimization, Cloitre, Scarvalone, and Difede (1997) contrasted adult sexual assault victims with and without a history of childhood abuse. Those with an early abuse history were more likely to have had multiple sexual and non-rape assaults in adulthood, including assaults by an acquaintance; they also showed more severe psychopathology coupled with pervasive interpersonal problems. The extreme of traumatic attachment in adulthood is exemplified by traumatic bonding, such as in battering relationships (Walker, 1979). These seemingly paradoxical attachments, also evident in infancy, can be understood as reflecting the fact that abuse heightens distress and thereby escalates attachment needs. Such heightened needs thus cement the relationship, particularly when other avenues of attachment are blocked, for example, by an abusive and jealously possessive husband (Allen, 2001). In effect, Main's (Main & Hesse, 1990) formulation of disorganized/disoriented attachment exemplifies the pattern of traumatic bonding in infancy, insofar as the infant with a frightening/frightened caregiver is placed in a profound approach–avoidance conflict that entails fright without solution.

Although we must pay due attention to reenactment of abuse, we should not overlook the equally problematic reenactment and reexperiencing of neglect. As we have proposed, the conjunction of unbearable states with the sense of being psychologically alone is potentially most traumatizing. Hence, these traumatized individuals have become sensitized not only to abuse but also to emotional neglect—what Egeland (1997) aptly termed *psychological unavailability*, a form of mentalizing failure. Such patients respond with extreme dysphoria and often self-destructive behavior to misunderstandings and misattunement as well as objectively mild separations, rejections, and conflicts. In this context, we can think of the "frantic efforts to avoid real or imagined abandonment" characteristic of BPD (APA, 2013, p. 633) as indicative of the posttraumatic reexperiencing of psychological neglect (Allen, 2001). Escalating cycles of reenactment and reexperiencing of neglect are common in conjunction with nonsuicidal self-injury. Responding to an experience of rejection or betrayal, the patient expresses pain through action (e.g., self-cutting or overdosing); the partner potentially responds with parallel unbearable emotional states (e.g., helplessness, fear, anger, shame), which promote distancing; at worst, the partner becomes disgusted and fed up; then the patient's reexperiencing of early traumatic psychological neglect increases further, not infrequently culminating in a suicide attempt. Psychotherapists are not immune to these reenactments, nor are they immune to nonmentalizing responses (e.g., becoming coercive or withdrawing).

Perhaps of greatest concern are reenactments of childhood maltreatment in caregiving relationships. Research linking unresolved/disorganized AAI classifications to infant disorganization in the Strange Situation has made the intergenerational transmission of trauma all too plain. As we discussed earlier, the reasons for such abdication of care are many, reexperiencing and reenactment being among them. That is, the infant's emotional stress and associated attachment needs may constitute a reminder of past trauma for the mother (e.g., her caregiver's psychological unavailability), such that she repeats the behavior of her caregiver in relation to her child.

Neurobiological Contributions

A broad understanding of the biological substrate of stress and trauma in attachment relationships helps to illuminate the sheer extent of the challenges psychotherapists face in striving to promote a mentalizing process.

Coan (2008) elegantly conceptualized the role of attachment in emotion regulation from a neurobiological perspective. He started from the premise: "One of the striking things about humans (and many other mammals) is how well *designed* we are for affiliation" (p. 247, emphasis in original). More specifically, the attachment system is "primarily concerned with the social regulation of emotion responding" (p. 251). As Luyten, Mayes, Fonagy, and van Houdenhove (2015) also have delineated, social contact provides powerful positive reinforcement (in its reward value) and, concomitantly, negative reinforcement (in reducing distress). These reinforcers are mediated, in part, by social cues activating the release of oxytocin and vasopressin in the ventral tegmental area and nucleus accumbens, which, in turn, stimulates dopaminergic and endogenous opioid activity.

Animal research dramatically demonstrates that disruption and trauma in early attachment relationships compound the challenges of distress regulation. Focusing on research with rats, Polan and Hofer (2008) note that the adaptive function of attachment goes far beyond providing protection from predators, as Bowlby (1982) initially proposed: Attachment processes influence neurobiological development in ways that shape basic emotion regulation and adaptive strategies. Specifically, high levels of maternal stimulation immediately after birth, including licking and grooming, lead to toned-down stress reactivity into adulthood, coupled with a proclivity toward exploration and learning. Conversely, low levels of stimulation and interaction (e.g., as associated with prolonged separations) are associated with high levels of fear, defensiveness, and avoidance, along with lower levels of exploratory activity. The biological mechanisms, down to the level of the influence of rearing patterns on gene expression affecting stress-response systems, are being elucidated (Weaver et al., 2004).

Simpson and Belsky (2008) spelled out the putative evolutionary function of these contrasting adaptive patterns: The fearful-defensive (insecure) pattern prepares the animal for a harsh environment with few resources, whereas the converse (secure) pattern prepares the animal for exploratory learning in a stable, resource-rich environment. By extension, resource-rich environments in which the caregiver has sufficient energy resources to have the child's mind in mind generate a sense of trust that promotes the development of mentalizing. In effect, these early rearing experiences are predictive of future environmental conditions to which the animal's stress-response systems and behavior will be adapted. Hence, these adaptive patterns, mediated by epigenetic mechanisms, constitute a form of "soft inheritance" (Polan & Hofer, 2008, p. 167) inasmuch as they are passed on intergenerationally from mothers through their daughters—an animal model of reenactment in attachment relationships.

Research on the long-range impact of early trauma on the emotion-regulation capacities in animals underscores the concerns about the neurobiological effects of childhood maltreatment. More specifically, stress sensitization and associated impairment of emotion-regulation capacities can contribute to trauma-related psychiatric disorders in adults—most notably, depression and PTSD (Nemeroff et al., 2006). Consistent with animal models, Ford (2009) reviewed the literature and suggested that brain development can be skewed toward a focus on either survival or learning. Of particular concern is the possibility of adverse impact on brain development during sensitive periods (Alter & Hen, 2009).

Reviewing the adverse effects of trauma on brain development, De Bellis, Hooper, and Sapia (2005) stated: "PTSD in maltreated children may be regarded as a complex environmentally induced developmental disorder" (p. 168). They cited evidence for a dose–response relationship insofar as earlier onset and longer duration of abuse, as well as severity of PTSD symptoms, have the greatest impact on development. They pointed to dysregulation in the sympathetic nervous system and hypothalamic–pituitary–adrenal axis stress-response systems as well as evidence for smaller brain volumes in multiple areas, including the prefrontal cortex. They also noted indications of compromised neuronal integrity in the anterior cingulate region of the medial prefrontal cortex, which is particularly significant here, given the prominent role of this region in mentalizing (Frith & Frith, 2003).

Our cursory overview of developmental research is intended merely to draw attention to the neurobiological side of the dual liability of attachment trauma that we noted earlier, namely, the combination of evoking extreme distress while simultaneously undermining the development of the capacity to regulate that distress (Fonagy & Target, 1997). Notwithstanding inevitable inconsistencies in research findings, there is considerable convergence on an "amygdalocentric" model of PTSD (Rauch & Drevets, 2009). With its emphasis on the prominent role of the prefrontal cortex, this model is highly pertinent to our concern with trauma-related compromise of mentalizing. Although the circuitry is extremely complex, a broad reciprocity exists between activity of the amygdala (which is activated in response to threat, mediates fear conditioning, and orchestrates many components of the fear response) and the medial prefrontal cortex (which plays a role in extinction and top-down regulation of fear responses): "individuals with anxiety disorders exhibit intrinsically exaggerated amygdala hyperresponsiveness and/or deficient top-down modulation of the amygdala response due to deficiencies in function within mPFC [medial prefrontal cortex] and/or the hippocampus" (p. 219).

This view of PTSD corresponds to what we construe as the broad reciprocity between mentalizing and defensive responding. Owing to what can be construed as a neurochemical switch (Arnsten, 1998; Mayes, 2000), patterns of brain functioning can shift from flexible but relatively slow, prefrontal executive functions to relatively rapid, automatic, and habitual responses mediated by posterior cortical and limbic structures. In effect, mentalizing goes offline as defensive (fight–flight–freeze) responses come online. Although this reciprocity has the adaptive value of promoting rapid responses to imminent danger (e.g., traumatic events), it is maladaptive in less dire interpersonal situations, such as ordinary conflicts in attachment relationships, that call for complex social problem solving (i.e., mentalizing). As Mayes (2000) pointed out, the thresholds for switching from flexible to automatic defensive responding may be permanently altered by exposure to early stress and trauma. As discussed earlier, BPD exemplifies this problem (Fonagy & Luyten, 2009). Yet, different patterns of attachment insecurity—deactivating versus hyperactivating strategies most notably—are associated with different thresholds for switching, consistent with considerable variability in neurobiological patterns of stress regulation associated with individual differences in attachment (Luyten, Mayes et al., 2015).

In sum, research on PTSD is consistent with a broad line of research that contrasts bottom-up emotion generation via limbic structures with top-down emotion regulation via prefrontal structures (Ochsner & Gross, 2005). Mentalizing-focused treatment of trauma, as well as psychotherapeutic treatment more generally, is directed toward promoting top-down regulation. Plainly, trauma-related hypofunctioning of the prefrontal cortex is a major treatment target for mentalizing interventions. Yet, overcontrol of emotion, such as characterizes the dissociative subtype of PTSD, also presents a target for mentalizing interventions, which entail mentalizing emotion or mentalized affectivity (Fonagy, Gergely, Jurist, & Target, 2002; Jurist, 2005), namely, feeling and thinking about feeling simultaneously. Of course, both extremes of underregulation and overregulation of emotion compromise the capacity for mentalizing emotion (i.e., implicitly and explicitly, simultaneously). The catch-22 for psychotherapeutic treatment here is: Mentalizing is most needed when it is least available.

PSYCHODYNAMIC TREATMENT OF TRAUMA

Evidence Base in Treatment Effectiveness

Cognitive-behavioral therapies alone are widely recognized in treatment guidelines for PTSD (Foa et al., 2009). Level A ratings (i.e., based on randomized, well-controlled trials) have been accorded to exposure therapy (Foa & Rothbaum, 1998), stress inoculation therapy (Meichenbaum, 1994; Meichenbaum & Novaco, 1985), and cognitive therapies such as cognitive processing therapy (Resick & Schnicke, 1992, 1993), which combines elements of exposure and cognitive restructuring. Eye movement desensitization and reprocessing (EMDR) also qualifies as an A-level treatment (Foa et al., 2009), notwithstanding the failure of dismantling studies to demonstrate that the eye movements or other bilateral stimuli contribute significantly to its effectiveness (Friedman, Cohen, Foa, & Keane, 2009; Spates, Koch, Cusack, Pagoto, & Waller, 2009). Research has failed to demonstrate a general advantage for any of these A-level therapies in comparison with any other (Bradley et al., 2005; Cahill, Rothbaum, Resick, & Follette, 2009; Resick et al., 2007).

With research failing to favor any single approach, one might make a case for exposure therapy as the first-line intervention—in effect, the one to beat: Exposure therapy is by far the best researched, with a wide range of populations (Cahill et al., 2009). Yet, even in standard form, the empirically supported cognitive-behavioral therapies for trauma are necessarily somewhat eclectic insofar as they typically entail some combination of exposure and cognitive restructuring. Cognitive restructuring, for example, involves writing about the traumatic event(s) and reading the account to the therapist (Resick & Schnicke, 1992). Conversely, prolonged exposure therapy is not administered in pure form. Foa and Kozak (1991) acknowledged, "In effect, we practice informal cognitive therapy during exposure, in that we help clients to examine ways in which they evaluate threat and to develop inferential process that lead to more realistic conclusions" (p. 45). Foa and colleagues (Foa, 1997; Foa, Huppert, & Cahill, 2006) have proposed that recovery through emotional processing of trauma hinges on three factors: emotional engagement with the trauma memory, alterations of trauma-related cognitions (i.e., that the world is extremely dangerous and the self completely incompetent), and creation of a coherent narrative. From our perspective, all these factors entail mentalizing. Emotional engagement entails *mentalized affectivity* (Fonagy et al., 2002), that is, mentalizing in the context of emotional arousal. Revising trauma-related cognitions entails mentalizing about self and others; in the context of attachment trauma, the dangerousness of the world pertains to attachment relationships. Hence, exposure therapy entails revising internal working models of self and others. Most notably, the emphasis on narrative coherence dovetails with mentalizing in the context of attachment security, as we discussed earlier. Yet, in exposure therapy, as in cognitive-behavioral therapy more generally, the patient–therapist relationship is in the background, although the quality of the relationship is beginning to garner more attention in outcome studies (Resick et al., 2007). To reiterate, we emphasize the importance of developing a coherent trauma narrative in the context of a secure attachment relationship. As Foa and colleagues (2006) acknowledge, exposure therapy is merely one of many possible contexts in which this might occur: "Emotional processing can occur as a result of everyday experiences . . . or in the context of psychosocial treatment, such as cognitive and behavioral therapies or psychodynamic therapy" (p. 8).

Psychodynamic Psychotherapy

Since its inception in *Studies in Hysteria* (Breuer & Freud, 1895/1957), psychodynamic psychotherapy has long been a method for facilitating emotional processing of traumatic experience. Yet, controlled trials on the efficacy of psychodynamic treatment for PTSD are noteworthy for their rarity (Kudler, Krupnick, Blank, Herman, & Horowitz, 2009; Schottenbauer et al., 2008), such that the exceptions are noteworthy. Brom, Kleber, and Defares (1989) compared Horowitz's (1997) approach to psychodynamic psychotherapy for trauma with systematic desensitization and hypno-therapy, and they also included a wait-list control group. All three active treatments were effective compared to the control group; there were only small differences among them, although the psychodynamic treatment showed greater improvement at follow-up, suggesting the mobilization of an ongoing change process (Kudler et al., 2009). However, the traumas treated varied widely in severity and included bereavements. A pilot study of interpersonal therapy for PTSD (Bleiberg & Markowitz, 2005) is also noteworthy as an investigation of a nonexposure-based intervention that focused on the interpersonal sequelae of PTSD such as distrust and the adverse effects of trauma-related symptoms on current relationships. The treatment not only decreased PTSD symptoms but also diminished depression and anger, while improving interpersonal functioning. Although some of the patients had a history of childhood abuse, only a small proportion showed personality disturbance; moreover, active substance abuse was an exclusion criterion. Hence, neither of these studies of psychodynamic treatment addressed complex traumatic stress disorders.

Given the overlap between complex traumatic stress disorders and BPD (Herman, 1992b), coupled with the frequent contribution of attachment trauma to the development of BPD, research on psychodynamic treatments for BPD is pertinent to the evidence base for psychodynamic approaches to treating trauma. Two random-ized controlled studies of transference-focused psychotherapy (TFP), wherein focus on the patient–therapist relationship is central to the treatment, have been shown to be more effective in some domains than comparison groups, that is, compared to dialectical behavior therapy (DBT) and supportive treatment (Clarkin, Levy, Lenzenweger, & Kernberg, 2007), as well as to treatment by experienced community psychotherapists (Doering et al., 2010). Psychodynamically informed psychotherapy coupled with medication management has also been found to be equivalent in effectiveness to DBT for the treatment of BPD (McMain et al., 2009).

Most pertinent to our concerns, mentalization-based treatment (MBT; Bateman & Fonagy, 2006) was developed in the context of a psychoanalytically oriented, mul-tifaceted partial hospitalization program for treating BPD. A randomized controlled trial has shown MBT to be more effective than treatment as usual in a series of studies (Bateman & Fonagy, 1999, 2001), culminating in an 8-year follow-up study (Bateman & Fonagy, 2008), the longest follow-up in controlled research on treatment of BPD reported to date (Levy, 2008). In addition, a purer form of MBT—that is, an intensive outpatient program consisting of weekly individual and group psycho-therapy sessions—has been shown to be superior in effectiveness to structured clini-cal management that focused on support and problem solving (Bateman & Fonagy, 2009). In this context, Herman (2009) noted that such recent clinical advances in the treatment of BPD are encouraging in relation to the treatment of complex PTSD. Herman commented that the 8-year follow-up study of MBT "may ultimately define a new standard of care for BPD" (p. xvi), and she went on, "It leads me to won-der about developing similarly intensive, multimodal treatment models for complex PTSD" (pp. vi–xvii). The effectiveness of the intensive outpatient treatment program (Bateman & Fonagy, 2009), however, suggests that it is not so much the intensity of the treatment but rather the focus and duration that might be crucial. Moreover, the addition of group treatment to individual psychotherapy may be especially valuable in the treatment of complex PTSD, given emerging evidence on the effectiveness of various forms of group psychotherapy for treating trauma (Ford, Fallot, & Harris, 2009; Shea, McDevitt-Murphy, Ready, & Schnurr, 2009).

Narrowly construed, as in cognitive-behavioral approaches, trauma treatment desensitizes the patient to painful intrusive memories, which are the cardinal symptom of PTSD (i.e., intrusion symptoms). Yet, the couplet of fear and avoidance are central to anxiety disorders more generally (Andrews, McEvoy, & Slade, 2009), and avoidance is the main target of exposure treatments for anxiety disorders, including trauma. Reexperiencing and avoidance were the central focus of Horowitz's (1997) psychodynamic approach to treating grief and trauma.

It is ironic that cognitive-behavioral therapies targeting avoidance have become preeminent, inasmuch as avoidance of painful emotion, and the defenses and resistances that abet avoidance, have been the target of psychodynamic treatment since its inception. The convergence of cognitive-behavioral and psychodynamic treatments associated with the focus on emotional avoidance has become most evident in third-generation, metacognitive approaches (Brewin, 2006; Hayes, 2004), the successors to (first-generation) behavior therapy and the earlier (second-generation) versions of cognitive therapy. These metacognitive approaches converge with our interest in mentalizing (Allen, 2008a; Bjorgvinsson & Hart, 2006) by shifting the focus from changing the *content* of cognition (i.e., the nature of various cognitive distortions) to working with mental *processes,* namely, the way individuals relate to their thoughts and emotions. For example, rather than countering the thought, "I'm worthless," with evidence to the contrary, the patient is encouraged to adopt a more reflective and nonjudgmental stance toward such thoughts, perhaps with awareness: "I think I'm worthless when I'm depressed." Accordingly, mindfulness practice, intended to promote this stance, is increasingly being incorporated into cognitive-behavioral approaches and has shown promise, for example, in preventing relapse in major depression (Segal, Williams, & Teasdale, 2002).

The contrast between situational and experiential avoidance (Hayes, Strosahl, Bunting, Twohig, & Wilson, 2004) is particularly apt in the treatment of trauma. Situational avoidance is relatively straightforward: The traumatized person avoids situations similar to that in which the trauma occurred (e.g., avoiding parking garages after having been assaulted in one; avoiding driving after a car wreck). Accordingly, *in vivo* exposure targets situational avoidance. Experiential avoidance, by contrast, entails avoiding one's own mind. Experiential avoidance tends to backfire, as research on ironic mental processes attests (Wegner, 1994, 1997): One must remain alert to the avoided mental content in order to avoid having it come to mind. Accordingly, as has long been evident to psychodynamic psychotherapists, experiential avoidance serves to maintain symptoms.

Traumatized persons commonly maintain experiential avoidance by negatively reinforcing (i.e., distress-reducing) actions such as substance abuse, non-suicidal self-injury, as well as bingeing and purging (Nock, 2009; Roemer & Orsillo, 2009). Such actions exemplify one nonmentalizing mode of experience (Fonagy et al., 2002), namely, the *teleological mode,* wherein mental states are expressed in concrete goal-directed actions instead of in explicit mental representations such as words (e.g., as in the patient who communicates emotional pain through cuts on the arms). The *pretend mode* is another nonmentalizing form of experiential avoidance, wherein mental states are decoupled from reality (Fonagy et al., 2002). As we have noted earlier, states of dissociative detachment (e.g., depersonalization and derealization) are common concomitants of trauma, and these states are akin to the pretend mode: Mental contents lose emotional ties to reality and, in that sense, become meaningless.

Experiential avoidance is a natural defense in relation to a third nonmentalizing mode of experience, namely, *psychic equivalence* (Fonagy et al., 2002). In the psychic-equivalence mode, the person equates mental contents with external reality, losing the sense of mental states as *representations* of external reality. Dreaming best exemplifies psychic equivalence: The dreamer experiences the dream as being real; waking up, recognizing, "it was only a dream," reflects the reinstatement of mentalizing. Paranoid delusions also exemplify psychic equivalence; ironically, wondering, "Am I being paranoid?" exemplifies mentalizing. Posttraumatic flashbacks, like dreams, dramatically show psychic equivalence: Reliving the trauma as if it were happening again in the present takes the place of remembering the trauma; the experience of remembering as such reflects mentalizing. Thus, one patient aptly referred to her flashbacks as "daymares." Plainly, psychic equivalence, as evident in paranoid states, nightmares, and flashbacks, can be terrifying. Little wonder that experiential avoidance is such a pervasive problem when one considers the possibility of being terrorized by one's own mind.

As we construe it, the counterpart to psychic equivalence in the current theory of cognitive-behavioral therapy is *cognitive fusion*, "an important cornerstone of the [Acceptance and Commitment Therapy] model" (Hayes, Strosahl, & Wilson, 1999, p. 74). Cognitive fusion refers to the failure to distinguish mental events from the reality they more or less arbitrarily represent. Cognitive fusion reflects a failure to be aware of the mental process that generates the mental content. Accordingly, the content is taken at face value—in short, there is a "fusion of the symbol and the event" (Hayes et al., 1999, p. 73). Akin to psychic equivalence, such fusion fuels experiential avoidance insofar as mental events are experienced as too real, often overwhelmingly so. Hence, parallel to mentalizing, interventions aim to promote cognitive *defusion*, shifting attention from mental content to mental process.

As already noted, mindfulness practice is being adopted widely as an intervention to target experiential avoidance in conjunction with its application to an increasingly wide range of stress-related disorders (Roemer & Orsillo, 2009). Noting the convergence, we have characterized mentalizing as *mindfulness of mind* (Allen, 2006), exemplified in the *mentalizing stance,* namely, an open-minded attitude of curiosity and inquisitiveness about mental states (Bateman & Fonagy, 2006). More specifically, mindful attentiveness to mental states in self and others is a necessary precondition for reflective (explicit) mentalizing (Allen, 2013). Furthermore, as we have noted elsewhere, the mentalizing stance has an ethical dimension (Allen, 2008b; Allen et al., 2008); hence, in the overlap between mindfulness and mentalizing, we see a rather remarkable convergence of two divergent traditions: the ethical-philosophical foundations of Buddhism as contrasted with the psychoanalytic and attachment-theory-based foundations of developmental psychopathology. Their kinship lies not only in their overlapping views of mental phenomena but also in their melioristic aspirations of relieving suffering—not by avoiding it, but rather by embracing it through mindfulness or mentalizing.

The overlap between mentalizing and mindfulness, as we have construed it, implies that mindfulness practice has the potential to promote mentalizing—especially the form of insight meditation that draws attention to mental states (Goldstein & Kornfield, 1987; Kornfield, 2009). Accordingly, with the aim of promoting emotion regulation, Linehan (1993) has incorporated mindfulness practice into DBT. Yet, we caution that mentalizing (mindfully) is a dynamic skill: Particularly with a history of attachment trauma, being mindful of one's emotional state while sitting quietly in a safe environment is a far cry from remaining mindful in the midst of emotional conflict in a primary attachment relationship—especially when such conflict resonates with prior trauma. Hence, mindfulness practice could be a helpful adjunct to psychotherapy, but it is no substitute for it.

CLINICAL ILLUSTRATION

Evelyn was referred for psychodynamic psychotherapy in the context of several weeks of intensive inpatient treatment. This treatment was precipitated by incapacitating symptoms of dizziness and fainting for which she had an extensive medical workup, but it revealed no associated general medical condition. Psychiatric treatment was recommended. Although the symptoms had abated somewhat, Evelyn was badly shaken by the experience and sought additional intensive treatment.

Implicitly, Evelyn presented for psychotherapy with a mentalizing agenda inasmuch as she accepted the premise of a psychiatric disorder with the principle that her somatic symptoms had a psychological basis, but she had no specific psychological understanding. She talked about the terrifying experience that her "unconscious mind" had taken control over her body. She feared that, if she could not address the psychological problems, her symptoms would recur. Hence, she was highly motivated to collaborate in psychotherapy, and, in the first session, she agreed to investigate the psychological basis of her symptoms. In effect, her fainting spells exemplify the nonmentalizing teleological mode of expressing conflict in action rather than narrative. With a mentalizing focus, a central theme evolved in the psychotherapy: being "rendered unconscious" by fear in the context of traumatic sexual experiences.

Evelyn had a virtually life-long history of anxiety and social isolation. She grew up in a family that was in continual turmoil. Both parents drank heavily and fought with each other as well as with Evelyn's much older brother, who intimidated and bullied the entire family. Evelyn found refuge in school: She described herself as an "average student" who thrived in competitive sports, which provided her with a much-needed source of self-esteem. But she remained distant from peers and was ashamed to invite anyone to her home. Moreover, she was isolated even within her home, confining herself to her bedroom where she was somewhat insulated from the continual fighting. She remained deeply resentful that her parents never divorced. She finished high school and then worked her way through college, ultimately earning a degree in geology. Apart from work and school, she remained socially isolated; she rarely dated, and she did not develop close friendships or confiding relationships. Yet she maintained a long-term relationship with her college roommate, with whom she said she felt "comfortable at a distance" (i.e., emotional distance).

After completing her education, Evelyn embarked on a satisfying career in oil and gas exploration. She traveled extensively, and, in the interim between trips, she lived with her former roommate, who was happy to have her occasional companionship. In the years prior to her hospitalizations, however, she became progressively more withdrawn and remote when living with her friend. Feeling a need for more space, she rented an apartment. Around the same time, she lost her job in the context of a corporate merger, and then she was entirely on her own. She became increasingly despondent, and her health deteriorated. She developed insomnia and, in a "desperate" effort to sleep, she took an overdose of anti-anxiety medication. She said that she was not suicidal; rather, "I just wanted to knock myself out." Yet, when she awakened, she was afraid that she could have killed herself, and she admitted herself to an acute psychiatric hospital.

In the acute hospital, Evelyn's physical condition and mood improved. Yet, when plans for discharge were being formulated, she panicked about being alone again, and she became incapacitated by dizziness and fainting spells. After an extensive workup revealed no neurological basis for her "spells," intensive inpatient psychiatric treatment was recommended. With the prospect of further care and support, her somatic symptoms gradually abated, but she remained frightened of further inexplicable episodes.

As the psychotherapy process evolved in the longer-term hospitalization, it quickly became evident that Evelyn's somatic symptoms were part and parcel of a broader pattern of trauma-related dissociative symptoms rooted in sexual trauma. Evelyn had never talked about this traumatic experience; it was largely unmentalized, as she had coped through situational and experiential avoidance. Exemplifying the core of traumatic experience, Evelyn had endured prolonged periods of being psychologically alone in the context of unbearably painful emotional states. The loss of her occupation and the superficial social connections it provided, coupled with her disconnecting from her one enduring friendship, brought this painful psychological aloneness to a crisis point. She rallied during the acute hospitalization but—at the point of discharge with the prospect of further disconnection—she became panicky, triggering the somatic symptoms.

A mentalizing narrative that provided a psychological context for her somatic symptoms gradually unfolded over the course of the intensive psychotherapeutic treatment. In the months prior to the loss of her job, Evelyn had been highly distressed by sexual comments and innuendo by a junior coworker, which she was unable to "shrug off" as her other coworkers had done. She had felt unable to protest or cope, merely aspiring to ignore the coworker and "tune him out." This experience reverberated with sexual trauma in her early adult life, in which a neighbor in her apartment complex forced himself on her repeatedly over the course of several years. She reported being utterly passive in that situation, submitting without protest. Indeed, she stated that she "spaced out" during sexual activity, feeling disconnected from her body. She felt as if she were "weightless, floating in space." She recalled times during intercourse when she could not will herself to move, as if she were "losing consciousness." We thus came to understand how she had continually "escaped" in the context of unwanted sexual experiences. Moreover, as the psychotherapy progressed, Evelyn revealed an earlier history of being sexually molested by her bullying older brother, sometimes accompanied by one of his friends. She said that her memory for this sexual abuse was limited, but she recalled similar experience of feeling detached from her body and "spacing out" mentally.

The psychotherapy did not go smoothly. As Evelyn remembered and talked about her trauma history in psychotherapy and in other treatment relationships in the hospital, she contended with an escalation of intrusive memories and dissociative defenses. Notably, the inherently time-limited nature of the intensive inpatient treatment constituted pressure to work quickly, yet it was crucial for Evelyn not to be overwhelmed in the process. She and the therapist endeavored to pace the work, using the metaphor of putting on the brakes in alternation with (gently) stepping on the accelerator. Moreover, the therapist discussed with Evelyn the impact of talking about these traumatic sexual experiences with a man. She acknowledged inhibition but said that she felt relatively safe, given the professional nature of the relationship. As the work progressed, she was surprised and pleased with her ability to talk openly with a man. But it was not easy.

As Evelyn talked about her history of sexual trauma in the psychotherapy, she struggled with ongoing dissociative symptoms, that is, feeling detached and spacing out—not only in the psychotherapy sessions but also to some degree in the hospital more generally, whenever she felt anxious. Thus, bringing to mind the painful and frightening memories, even without going into detail, reinstated the dissociative defenses that she had employed to cope at the earlier time. Evelyn worked hard in the psychotherapy to remain engaged in the face of her proclivity to dissociate. "Grounding" strategies were employed to counter her detachment, for example, paying keen attention to current experience in various sensory modalities, including meditative focus on her breathing. Most importantly, the therapist worked to help her maintain eye contact and to stay engaged in conversation when she was in states of distress. In addition to learning how to employ grounding techniques, Evelyn also used imagery to diffuse the intrusive traumatic memories. She had associated dissociation with "disappearing," and she put this metaphor to constructive use, imagining that those who abused her were disappearing into the clouds over the horizon. In psychotherapy sessions, she practiced deliberately bringing traumatic images to mind and then putting them out of mind using this imagery. Thus, as contrasted with becoming immersed in memories in the psychic-equivalence mode (i.e., blurring memory with current reality), she was able to mentalize in the sense of recognizing that the images were a reflection of mental states that she could influence.

Not surprisingly, being beset by posttraumatic symptoms and dissociation, Evelyn had difficulty consistently remaining engaged in a highly structured inpatient treatment program that involved attendance and active participation in therapeutic groups and activities as well as an expectation of ongoing, open communication with staff members. Throughout her history, Evelyn had coped with innumerable sources of stress by withdrawing and isolating; naturally, she repeated this pattern in the hospital. Albeit through passivity, she became involved in a battle of wills with her male psychiatrist, who reminded her of her older brother. She feared that she would be discharged, started to struggle with dizziness again, and at this point was able to link the symptom to her previous traumatic experience of being overpowered as well as fearing being alone. This conflict marked a turning point in Evelyn's treatment: The therapy helped her to speak up about her feelings regarding what she perceived as impossible demands; she did so, negotiating with her psychiatrist on the basis of what she felt capable of doing. Hence, as we discussed in the psychotherapy, she moved from a position of being passively traumatized and spaced out to active coping.

Early in life, Evelyn had learned to remain silent about abuse, and, as just illustrated, much of the treatment entailed helping Evelyn to speak up and recover her voice. Albeit hesitantly and ambivalently, she had spoken up about her trauma history in psychotherapy. She took the initiative to write a narrative about her experience of trauma and healing, which she read aloud in the psychotherapy session. Her narrative was thorough, emotional, articulate, and forceful. She had moved from passive dissociation to assertive engagement. Perhaps most striking was Evelyn's shift over the course of treatment from emotional remoteness to a feeling of warm engagement, which was evident in the psychotherapy as well as in her evolving relationships with her peers.

Evelyn was apprehensive about terminating the psychotherapy, given the feeling of safety she had come to associate with the relationship and especially her prior history of becoming incapacitated in the context of discharge from a hospital. With support, she was able to make the transition to intensive outpatient treatment. She had come to understand her previously bewildering symptoms. The therapist also viewed her somatic symptoms as serving the unconscious strategic function of forcing caregiving, although he did not make this interpretation. Evelyn also overcame her psychological incapacitation in being able to speak out about present interpersonal conflicts and problems as well as about past trauma—without spacing out. Having developed an understanding of the psychological basis of her symptoms, she ended this episode of treatment without fear that her unconscious mind would take over her body. Mentalizing in the context of safe relationships was the key psychological process.

CONCLUSIONS AND FUTURE DIRECTIONS

At the end of a psychoeducational group session on trauma conducted by one of us (Jon Allen), a patient presented him with the following quotation from Chekhov's *Cherry Orchard*: "If many remedies are prescribed for an illness, you may be certain that the illness has no cure." She had come across a paraphrase; the original (in translation) reads, "You know, when people suggest all sorts of cures for some disease or other, it means it's incurable. I keep thinking, racking my brains, and I come up with plenty of solutions, plenty of remedies, and basically, that means none—not one" (Chekhov, 1998, pp. 25–26). We have a spate of treatments for PTSD, BPD, and now complex PTSD. Perhaps we should not be surprised that we have so many remedies and no cures for the multifarious effects of problematic childrearing that extend across generations. And it should not be surprising that, despite dramatic progress, no one is sanguine about the extent of effectiveness of treatments for psychiatric disorders in general, much less the multifaceted developmental psychopathology we put under the broad umbrella of complex traumatic stress disorders.

Although we have emphasized how the conceptual foundations of cognitive-behavioral and psychodynamic approaches to trauma overlap, psychodynamic treatments have not been well researched, especially in relation to complex traumatic stress disorders. Given their overlap with BPD, one place to begin would be incorporating assessments of trauma history and trauma-related disorders (i.e., PTSD and dissociative disorders) into research on the treatment of BPD; standardized assessment tools abound (Briere & Spinazzola, 2009). More to the point, as Schottenbauer and colleagues (2008) advocated, is the development of manuals for psychodynamic approaches to trauma treatment and research on their effectiveness. As described earlier, eclectic treatments for complex trauma that are compatible with psychodynamic psychotherapy are being researched, but head-to-head comparisons with viable alternatives have not been conducted. A fundamental question might be: What elements must be added to exposure therapy for complex traumatic stress disorders to achieve substantial added benefit? More specifically, from a psychodynamic and attachment perspective, what is the added benefit of addressing attachment relationships, including reenactments of traumatic attachment patterns inside and outside psychotherapy?

Yet, with treatment manuals proliferating, we must wonder: Do we need more therapies—and more acronyms? Evidence for the benefits of secure attachment relationships is legion in childhood (Berlin, Cassidy, & Appleyard, 2008; Sroufe et al., 2005), adolescence (J. P. Allen, 2008) and in adulthood (Feeney, 2008; Mikulincer & Shaver, 2007), and there is no dearth of methods for assessing security of attachment in adults (Crowell, Fraley, & Shaver, 2008; Mikulincer & Shaver, 2007). Plainly, incorporating assessments of attachment security into a range of treatment approaches for complex trauma would be valuable. Would exposure-based interventions suffice to enhance attachment security? Would transference-focused interventions also be required?

Although MBT's effectiveness has been established, research on the impact of psychotherapy on mentalizing capacity is limited. Ironically, much of the existing data comes from treatments other than MBT, although research on mentalizing changes in MBT is underway. Clarkin and colleagues (2007) compared the effects of TFP for BPD with those of DBT and supportive psychotherapy. Over the course of a one-year period of multiple assessments, all three treatments were associated with improvement across a number of domains, although TFP was associated with a wider array of changes. Most pertinent for present purposes, using the AAI, Levy and colleagues (2006) found that TFP—but not DBT or supportive psychotherapy—increased reflective functioning (mentalizing capacity) along with narrative coherence and security of attachment. Unexpectedly, improvement in mentalizing and narrative coherence did not lead to changes in resolution of trauma, perhaps because these treatments focused primarily on current relationships and not on exploring past trauma. As the authors state, however, it is left to future research to demonstrate a relationship between these putative mechanisms of change and improvement in interpersonal relationships, self-regulation, and symptomatology.

Toth, Rogosch, and Cicchetti (2008) also assessed changes in reflective functioning in mothers engaged in a year-long course of toddler–parent psychotherapy. This intervention is modeled after Fraiberg and colleagues' (Fraiberg, Adelson, & Shapiro, 1975) clinical approach to increasing maternal attunement, in part by fostering mothers' awareness of the impact of their prior relationships on their current interactions with their child. Mothers with a history of major depression were randomized to an intervention and control group, and they were compared with nondepressed mothers. Results showed the greatest gains in the intervention group; specifically, 49% of mothers in the depressed intervention group moved from low to high reflective functioning, as compared with 28% in the depressed control group and 24% in the normal control group. Security of toddler attachment, assessed at pre- and postintervention points, revealed far higher rates of insecurity in both groups of depressed mothers compared to controls prior to the intervention. Rates of security increased dramatically with treatment for the depressed intervention group (from 17 to 67%) but not for the depressed control group (from 22% to 17%). Concomitantly, rates of disorganized attachment decreased dramatically for the intervention group (from 38 to 11%) compared to the depressed control group (41% at both points). Yet, despite concomitant improvement in maternal reflective functioning and toddler attachment security, the authors found no evidence that the changes in security could be attributed to improvement in reflective functioning. They proposed that such a relation would more likely emerge if mentalizing regarding the mother–toddler relationship were assessed, rather than mentalizing in relation to the mothers' childhood attachments (i.e., in the AAI).

Toth and colleagues' proposal is consistent with the findings of research we reviewed earlier on the relation between mentalizing interactions and infant attachment security: Mentalizing is relationship-specific. Accordingly, future research on the treatment of attachment trauma ideally would assess the level of mentalizing patients display over the course of treatment and the relation of positive changes in mentalizing to treatment outcomes, including quality of representations of self and others, attachment security, and emotion-regulation capacities. Such research should be complemented by assessment of therapists' mentalizing capacities, which are likely to vary between therapists as well as within therapists among patients, and across sessions within patients (Diamond, Stovall-McClough, Clarkin, & Levy, 2003; Fonagy & Luyten, 2009). Such research would test our assumption that mentalizing enables the reworking of internal working models of self and attachment relationships, which Bowlby (1982) viewed as perpetuating attachment patterns, for better or for worse. As Bretherton (2005) summarized, the function of internal working models is "to make the relational world more predictable, shareable, and meaningful" (p. 36), and this function is optimized in secure attachment relationships. Yet, consistent with the variability of mentalizing across relationships, internal working models are to a considerable degree relationship-specific (Bretherton & Munholland,

2008). Furthermore, given its relationship-specific and dynamic nature (Fonagy & Target, 1997), mentalizing capacity will vary not only across relationships but also within a relationship according to the activation of the attachment system, coupled with the individual's degree of attachment security in that particular relationship. The same will be true of relationships with psychotherapists.

A psychodynamic approach to psychotherapy for trauma would seem optimal for lessening defensive processes that block awareness of internal working models and thus impede their revision and updating, particularly with the opportunity to examine patient–therapist interactions toward this end. We assume that a systematic mentalizing focus in psychodynamic psychotherapy is most likely to promote the ongoing capacity to revise working models in accordance with current reality. But the extent to which psychodynamic psychotherapy achieves this aim in treating trauma, whether it does so more thoroughly than other approaches such as exposure therapy, and the extent to which enhanced mentalizing mediates this process in any approach to trauma treatment are empirical questions.

REFERENCES

Adam, K. S., Sheldon Keller, A. E., & West, M. (1995). Attachment organization and vulnerability to loss, separation, and abuse in disturbed adolescents. In S. Goldberg, R. Muir, & J. Kerr (Eds.), *Attachment theory: Social, developmental, and clinical perspectives* (pp. 309–341). Hillsdale, NJ: Analytic Press.

Ainsworth, M. D. S., Blehar, M. C., Waters, E., & Wall, S. (1978). *Patterns of attachment: A psychological study of the Strange Situation*. Hillsdale, NJ: Erlbaum.

Allen, J. G. (2001). *Traumatic relationships and serious mental disorders*. Chichester, UK: Wiley.

Allen, J. G. (2005). *Coping with trauma: Hope through understanding* (2nd ed.). Washington, DC: American Psychiatric Publishing.

Allen, J. G. (2006). Mentalizing in practice. In J. G. Allen & P. Fonagy (Eds.), *Handbook of mentalization-based treatment* (pp. 3–30). Chichester, UK: Wiley.

Allen, J. G. (2008a). Mentalizing as a conceptual bridge from psychodynamic to cognitive-behavioral therapy. *European Psychotherapy, 8*, 103–121.

Allen, J. G. (2008b). Psychotherapy: The artful use of science. *Smith College Studies in Social Work, 78*, 159–187.

Allen, J. G. (2013). *Mentalizing in the development and treatment of attachment trauma*. London: Karnac.

Allen, J. G., & Fonagy, P. (2014). Mentalizing in psychotherapy. In R. E. Hales, S. C. Yudofsky, & L. Roberts (Eds.), *Textbook of psychiatry* (6th ed., pp. 1095–1118). Washington, DC: American Psychiatric Publishing.

Allen, J. G., Fonagy, P., & Bateman, A. (2008). *Mentalizing in clinical practice*. Washington, DC: American Psychiatric Publishing.

Allen, J. P. (2008). The attachment system in adolescence. In J. Cassidy & P. R. Shaver (Eds.), *Handbook of attachment: Theory, research, and clinical applications* (2nd ed., pp. 419–435). New York: Guilford Press.

Alter, M. D., & Hen, R. (2009). Serotonin, sensitive periods, and anxiety. In G. Andrews, D. S. Charney, P. J. Sirovatka, & D. A. Reiger (Eds.), *Stress-induced and fear circuitry disorders: Refining the research agenda for DSM-V* (pp. 159–173). Arlington, VA: American Psychiatric Publishing.

American Psychiatric Association. (2000). *Diagnostic and statistical manual of mental disorders* (4th ed., text rev.). Washington, DC: Author.

American Psychiatric Association. (2013). *Diagnostic and statistical manual of mental disorders* (5th ed). Arlington, VA: Author.

Andrews, G., McEvoy, P., & Slade, T. (2009). Concluding remarks. In G. Andrews, D. S. Charney, P. J. Sirovatka, & D. A. Reiger (Eds.), *Stress-induced and fear circuitry disorders: Refining the research agenda for DSM-V* (pp. 283–300). Arlington, VA: American Psychiatric Publishing.

Arnott, B., & Meins, E. (2007). Links between antenatal attachment representations, postnatal mind-mindedness, and infant attachment security: A preliminary study of mothers and fathers. *Bulletin of the Menninger Clinic, 71*, 132–149.

Arnsten, A. F. T. (1998). The biology of being frazzled. *Science, 280*, 1711–1712.

Ball, J. S., & Links, P. S. (2009). Borderline personality disorder and childhood trauma: Evidence for a causal relationship. *Current Psychiatry Reports, 11*, 63–68.

Bateman, A., & Fonagy, P. (1999). Effectiveness of partial hospitalization in the treatment of borderline personality disorder: A randomized controlled trial. *American Journal of Psychiatry, 156*, 1563–1569.

Bateman, A., & Fonagy, P. (2001). Treatment of borderline personality disorder with psychoanalytically oriented partial hospitalizaiton: An 18-month follow-up. *American Journal of Psychiatry, 158*, 36–42.

Bateman, A., & Fonagy, P. (2006). *Mentalization based treatment for borderline personality disorder: A practical guide.* New York: Oxford University Press.

Bateman, A., & Fonagy, P. (2008). 8-year follow-up of patients treated for borderline personality disorder: Mentalization-based treatment versus treatment as usual. *American Journal of Psychiatry, 165*, 631–638.

Bateman, A., & Fonagy, P. (2009). Randomized controlled trial of outpatient Mentalization-Based Treatment versus structured clinical management for borderline personality disorder. *American Journal of Psychiatry, 166*, 1355–1364.

Berlin, L. J., Cassidy, J., & Appleyard, K. (2008). The influence of early attachments on other relationships. In J. Cassidy & P. R. Shaver (Eds.), *Handbook of attachment: Theory, research, and clinical applications* (2nd ed., pp. 333–347). New York: Guilford Press.

Bifulco, A., Moran, P. M., Baines, R., Bunn, A., & Stanford, K. (2002). Exploring psychological abuse in childhood II: Association with other abuse and adult clinical depression. *Bulletin of the Menninger Clinic, 66*, 241–258.

Bjorgvinsson, T., & Hart, J. (2006). Cognitive behavioral therapy promotes mentalizing. In J. G. Allen & P. Fonagy (Eds.), *Handbook of mentalization-based treatment* (pp. 157–170). Chichester, UK: Wiley.

Bleiberg, K. L., & Markowitz, J. C. (2005). A pilot study of interpersonal psychotherapy for post-traumatic stress disorder. *American Journal of Psychiatry, 162*, 181–183.

Bowlby, J. (1982). *Attachment and loss: Vol. I. Attachment* (2nd ed.). New York: Basic Books.

Bradley, R., Greene, J., Russ, E., Dutra, L., & Westen, D. (2005). A multidimensional meta-analysis of psychotherapy for PTSD. *American Journal of Psychiatry, 162*, 214–227.

Bretherton, I. (2005). In pursuit of the internal working model construct and its relevance to attachment relationships. In K. E. Grossman, K. Grossman, & E. Waters (Eds.), *Attachment from infancy to adulthood: The major longitudinal studies* (pp. 13–47). New York: Guilford Press.

Bretherton, I., & Munholland, K. A. (2008). Internal working models in attachment relationships: Elaborating a central construct in attachment theory. In J. Cassidy & P. R. Shaver (Eds.), *Handbook of attachment: Theory, research, and clinical applications* (2nd ed., pp. 102–127). New York: Guilford Press.

Breuer, J., & Freud, S. (1957). *Studies on hysteria.* New York: Basic Books. (Original work published 1895)

Brewin, C. R. (2003). *Post-traumatic stress disorder: Malady or myth?* New Haven, CT: Yale University Press.

Brewin, C. R. (2006). Understanding cognitive behaviour therapy: A retrieval competition account. *Behaviour Research and Therapy, 44*, 765–784.

Briere, J., & Spinazzola, J. (2009). Assessment of the sequelae of complex trauma: Evidence-based measures. In C. A. Courtois & J. D. Ford (Eds.), *Treating complex traumatic stress disorders: An evidence-based guide* (pp. 104–123). New York: Guilford Press.

Brom, D., Kleber, R. J., & Defares, P. B. (1989). Brief psychotherapy for posttraumatic stress disorders. *Journal of Consulting and Clinical Psychology, 57,* 607–612.

Cahill, S. P., Rothbaum, B. O., Resick, P. A., & Follette, V. M. (2009). Cognitive-behavioral therapy for adults. In E. B. Foa, T. M. Keane, M. J. Friedman, & J. A. Cohen (Eds.), *Effective treatments for PTSD: Practice guidelines from the International Society for Traumatic Stress Studies* (2nd ed., pp. 139–222). New York: Guilford Press.

Carlson, E. A. (1998). A prospective longitudinal study of attachment disorganization/disorientation. *Child Development, 69,* 1107–1128.

Carlson, E. A., Egeland, B., & Sroufe, L. A. (2009). A prospective investigation of the development of borderline personality symptoms. *Development and Psychopathology, 21,* 1311–1334.

Chekhov, A. (1998). *The cherry orchard* (S. Mulrine, Trans.). London: Nick Hern.

Chu, J. A. (1992). The therapeutic roller coaster: Dilemmas in the treatment of childhood abuse survivors. *Journal of Psychotherapy: Practice and Research, 1,* 351–370.

Clarkin, J. F., Levy, K. N., Lenzenweger, M. F., & Kernberg, O. F. (2007). Evaluating three treatments for borderline personality disorder: A multiwave study. *American Journal of Psychiatry, 164,* 922–928.

Cloitre, M., Scarvalone, P., & Difede, J. (1997). Posttraumatic stress disorder, self- and interpersonal dysfunction among sexually retraumatized women. *Journal of Traumatic Stress, 10,* 437–452.

Coan, J. A. (2008). Toward a neuroscience of attachment. In J. Cassidy & P. R. Shaver (Eds.), *Handbook of attachment: Theory, research, and clinical applications* (2nd ed., pp. 241–265). New York: Guilford Press.

Crowell, J. A., Fraley, R. C., & Shaver, P. R. (2008). Measurement of individual differences in adolescent and adult attachment. In J. Cassidy & P. R. Shaver (Eds.), *Handbook of attachment: Theory, research, and clinical applications* (2nd ed., pp. 599–634). New York: Guilford Press.

Davies, J. M., & Frawley, M. G. (1994). *Treating the adult survivor of childhood sexual abuse.* New York: Basic Books.

De Bellis, M. D., Hooper, S. R., & Sapia, J. L. (2005). Early trauma exposure and the brain. In J. J. Vasterling & C. R. Brewin (Eds.), *Neuropsychology of PTSD: Biological, cognitive, and clinical perspectives* (pp. 153–177). New York: Guilford Press.

DePrince, A. P., & Freyd, J. J. (2007). Trauma-induced dissociation. In M. J. Friedman, T. M. Keane, & P. A. Resick (Eds.), *Handbook of PTSD: Science and practice.* New York: Guilford Press.

Diamond, D., Stovall-McClough, C., Clarkin, J. F., & Levy, K. N. (2003). Patient–therapist attachment in the treatment of borderline personality disorder. *Bulletin of the Menninger Clinic, 67,* 227–259.

Doering, S., Horz, S., Rentrop, M., Fischer-Kern, M., Schuster, P., Benecke, C., et al. (2010). Transference-focused psychotherapy v. treatment by community psychotherapists for borderline personality disorder: Randomised controlled trial. *British Journal of Psychiatry, 196,* 389–395.

Dozier, M., Stovall-McClough, K. C., & Albus, K. E. (2008). Attachment and psychopathology in adulthood. In J. Cassidy & P. R. Shaver (Eds.), *Handbook of attachment: Theory, research, and clinical applications* (2nd ed., pp. 718–744). New York: Guilford Press.

Egeland, B. (1997). Mediators of the effects of child maltreatment on developmental adaptation in adolescence. In D. Cicchetti & S. L. Toth (Eds.), *Developmental perspectives on trauma: Theory, research, and intervention* (Vol. 8, pp. 403–434). Rochester, NY: University of Rochester Press.

Erickson, M. F., & Egeland, B. (1996). Child neglect. In J. Briere, L. Berliner, J. A. Bulkley, C.

Jenny, & T. Reid (Eds.), *The APSAC handbook on child maltreatment* (pp. 4–20). Thousand Oaks, CA: Sage.

Feeney, J. A. (2008). Adult romantic attachment: Developments in the study of couple relationships. In J. Cassidy & P. R. Shaver (Eds.), *Handbook of attachment: Theory, research, and clinical applications* (2nd ed., pp. 456–481). New York: Guilford Press.

Foa, E. B. (1997). Psychological processes related to recovery from a trauma and effective treatment for PTSD. In R. Yehuda & A. C. McFarlane (Eds.), *Psychobiology of posttraumatic stress disorder* (Vol. 823, pp. 410–424). New York: New York Academy of Sciences.

Foa, E. B., Huppert, J. D., & Cahill, S. P. (2006). Emotional processing theory: An update. In B. O. Rothbaum (Ed.), *Pathological anxiety: Emotional processing in etiology and treatment.* New York: Guilford Press.

Foa, E. B., Keane, T. M., Friedman, M. J., & Cohen, J. A. (Eds.). (2009). *Effective treatments for PTSD: Practice guidelines from the International Society for Traumatic Stress Studies* (2nd ed.). New York: Guilford Press.

Foa, E. B., & Kozak, M. J. (1991). Emotional processing: Theory, research, and clinical implications for anxiety disorders. In J. D. Safran & L. S. Greenberg (Eds.), *Emotion, psychotherapy, and change* (pp. 21–49). New York: Guilford Press.

Foa, E. B., & Rothbaum, B. O. (1998). *Treating the trauma of rape: Cognitive-behavioral therapy for PTSD.* New York: Guilford Press.

Fonagy, P. (1989). A child's understanding of others. *Bulletin of the Anna Freud Centre, 12,* 91–115.

Fonagy, P., & Bateman, A. (2008). The development of borderline personality disorder: A mentalizing model. *Journal of Personality Disorders, 22,* 4–21.

Fonagy, P., Gergely, G., Jurist, E. L., & Target, M. (2002). *Affect regulation, mentalization, and the development of the self.* New York: Other Press.

Fonagy, P., Gergely, G., & Target, M. (2007). The parent–infant dyad and the construction of the subjective self. *Journal of Child Psychology and Psychiatry, 48,* 288–328.

Fonagy, P., Gergely, G., & Target, M. (2008). Psychoanalytic constructs and attachment theory and research. In J. Cassidy & P. R. Shaver (Eds.), *Handbook of attachment: Theory, research, and clinical applications* (2nd ed., pp. 783–810). New York: Guilford Press.

Fonagy, P., Leigh, T., Steele, M., Steele, H., Kennedy, R., Mattoon, G., et al. (1996). The relation of attachment status, psychiatric classification, and response to psychotherapy. *Journal of Consulting and Clinical Psychology, 64,* 22–31.

Fonagy, P., & Luyten, P. (2009). A developmental, mentalization-based approach to the understanding and treatment of borderline personality disorder. *Development and Psychopathology, 21,* 1355–1381.

Fonagy, P., Steele, H., & Steele, M. (1991). Maternal representations of attachment during pregnancy predict the organization of infant–mother attachment at one year of age. *Child Development, 62,* 891–905.

Fonagy, P., Steele, M., Steele, H., Moran, G. S., & Higgitt, A. C. (1991). The capacity for understanding mental states: The reflective self in parent and child and its significance for security of attachment. *Infant Mental Health Journal, 12,* 201–218.

Fonagy, P., & Target, M. (1997). Attachment and reflective function: Their role in self-organization. *Development and Psychopathology, 9,* 679–700.

Ford, J. D. (2009). Neurobiological and developmental research: Clinical implications. In C. A. Courtois & J. D. Ford (Eds.), *Treating complex traumatic stress disorders: An evidence-based guide* (pp. 31–58). New York: Guilford Press.

Ford, J. D., & Courtois, C. A. (2009). Defining and understanding complex trauma and complex traumatic stress disorders. In C. A. Courtois & J. D. Ford (Eds.), *Treating complex traumatic stress disorders: An evidence-based guide* (pp. 13–30). New York: Guilford Press.

Ford, J. D., Fallot, R. D., & Harris, M. (2009). Group therapy. In C. A. Courtois & J. D. Ford (Eds.), *Treating complex traumatic stress disorders: An evidence-based guide* (pp. 415–440). New York: Guilford Press.

Fraiberg, S., Adelson, E., & Shapiro, V. (1975). Ghosts in the nursery: A psychoanalytic approach ot the problems of impaired infant–mother relationships. *Journal of the American Academy of Child Psychiatry, 14*, 387–421.

Freyd, J. J. (1996). *Betrayal trauma: The logic of forgetting childhood abuse.* Cambridge, MA: Harvard University Press.

Friedman, M. J., Cohen, J. A., Foa, E. B., & Keane, T. M. (2009). Integration and summary. In E. B. Foa, T. M. Keane, M. J. Friedman, & J. A. Cohen (Eds.), *Effective treatments for PTSD: Practice guidelines from the International Society for Traumatic Stress Studies* (2nd ed., pp. 617–642). New York: Guilford Press.

Friedman, M. J., & Karam, E. G. (2009). Posttraumatic stress disorder. In G. Andrews, D. S. Charney, P. J. Sirovatka, & D. A. Regier (Eds.), *Stress-induced and fear circuitry disorders: Refining the research agenda for DSM-V* (pp. 3–29). Arlington, VA: American Psychiatric Publishing.

Friedman, M. J., Resick, P. A., & Keane, T. M. (2007). Key questions and an agenda for future research. In M. J. Friedman, T. M. Keane, & P. A. Resick (Eds.), *Handbook of PTSD: Science and practice* (pp. 540–561). New York: Guilford Press.

Frith, U., & Frith, C. D. (2003). Development and neurophysiology of mentalizing. *Philosophical Transactions of the Royal Society of London, Series B, Biological Sciences, 358*, 459–473.

Gabbard, G. O. (2000). *Psychodynamic psychiatry in clinical practice* (3rd ed.). Washington, DC: American Psychiatric Press.

George, C., & Solomon, J. (2008). The caregiving system: A behavioral systems approach to parenting. In J. Cassidy & P. R. Shaver (Eds.), *Handbook of attachment: Theory, research, and clinical applications* (2nd ed., pp. 833–856). New York: Guilford Press.

Gergely, G., & Csibra, G. (2005). The social construction of the cultural mind: Imitative learning as a mechanism of human pedagogy. *Interaction Studies, 6*, 463–481.

Gold, S. D., Marx, B. P., Soler-Baillo, J. M., & Sloan, D. M. (2005). Is life stress more traumatic than traumatic stress? *Journal of Anxiety Disorders, 19*, 687–698.

Goldstein, J., & Kornfield, J. (1987). *Seeking the heart of wisdom: The path of insight meditation.* Boston: Shambhala.

Hayes, S. C. (2004). Acceptance and commitment therapy and the new behavior therapies: Mindfulness, acceptance, and relationship. In S. C. Hayes, V. M. Follette, & M. M. Linehan (Eds.), *Mindfulness and acceptance: Expanding the cognitive-behavioral tradition* (pp. 1–29). New York: Guilford Press.

Hayes, S. C., Strosahl, K. D., Bunting, K., Twohig, M., & Wilson, K. G. (2004). What is acceptance and commitment therapy? In S. C. Hayes & K. D. Strosahl (Eds.), *A practical guide to acceptance and commitment therapy* (pp. 3–29). New York: Springer.

Hayes, S. C., Strosahl, K. D., & Wilson, K. G. (1999). *Acceptance and commitment therapy: An experiential approach to behavior change.* New York: Guilford Press.

Herman, J. L. (1992a). Complex PTSD: A syndrome in survivors of prolonged and repeated trauma. *Journal of Traumatic Stress, 5*, 377–391.

Herman, J. L. (1992b). *Trauma and recovery.* New York: Basic Books.

Herman, J. L. (1993). Sequelae of prolonged and repeated trauma: Evidence for a complex posttraumatic syndrome (DESNOS). In J. R. T. Davidson & E. B. Foa (Eds.), *Posttraumatic stress disorder: DSM-IV and beyond* (pp. 213–228). Washington, DC: American Psychiatric Press.

Herman, J. L. (2009). Foreword. In C. A. Courtois & J. D. Ford (Eds.), *Treating complex traumatic stress disorders* (pp. xiii–xvii). New York: Guilford Press.

Hesse, E. (2008). The Adult Attachment Interview: Protocol, method of analysis, and empirical studies. In J. Cassidy & P. R. Shaver (Eds.), *Handbook of attachment: Theory, research, and clinical applications* (2nd ed., pp. 552–598). New York: Guilford Press.

Horowitz, M. J. (1997). *Stress response syndromes: PTSD, grief, and adjustment disorders* (3rd ed.). Northvale, NJ: Jason Aronson.

Johnson, J. G., Cohen, P., Chen, H., Kasen, S., & Brook, J. S. (2006). Parenting behaviors associated with risk for offspring personality disorder during adulthood. *Archives of General Psychiatry, 63,* 579–587.

Jurist, E. L. (2005). Mentalized affectivity. *Psychoanalytic Psychology, 22,* 426–444.

Keane, T. M., Brief, D. J., Pratt, E. M., & Miller, M. W. (2007). Assessment of PTSD and its comorbidities in adults. In M. J. Friedman, T. M. Keane, & P. A. Resick (Eds.), *Handbook of PTSD: Science and practice* (pp. 279–305). New York: Guilford Press.

Kornfield, J. (2009). *The wise heart: A guide to the universal teachings of Buddhist psychology.* New York: Random House.

Kudler, H. S., Krupnick, J. L., Blank, A. S., Jr., Herman, J. L., & Horowitz, M. J. (2009). Psychodynamic therapy for adults. In E. B. Foa, T. M. Keane, M. J. Friedman, & J. A. Cohen (Eds.), *Effective treatments for PTSD: Practice guidelines from the International Society for Traumatic Stress Studies* (2nd ed., pp. 346–369). New York: Guilford Press.

Levy, K. N. (2008). Psychotherapies and lasting change. *American Journal of Psychiatry, 165,* 556–559.

Levy, K. N., Meehan, K. B., Kelly, K. M., Reynoso, J. S., Weber, M., Clarkin, J. F., et al. (2006). Change in attachment patterns and reflective function in a randomized control trial of transference-focused psychotherapy for borderline personality disorder. *Journal of Consulting and Clinical Psychology, 74,* 1027–1040.

Linehan, M. M. (1993). *Cognitive-behavioral treatment of borderline personality disorder.* New York: Guilford Press.

Luyten, P., Mayes, L. C., Fonagy, P., & Van Houdenhove, B. (2015). *Attachment and the interpersonal nature of stress regulation: A developmental framework.* Manuscript submitted for publication.

Luyten, P., Vliegen, N., Van Houdenhove, B., & Blatt, S. J. (2008). Equifinality, multifinality, and the rediscovery of the importance of early experiences: Pathways from early adversity to psychiatric and (functional) somatic disorders. *Psychoanalytic Study of the Child, 63,* 27–60.

Lyons-Ruth, K., & Jacobvitz, D. (1999). Attachment disorganization: Unresolved loss, relational violence, and lapses in behavioral and attentional strategies. In J. Cassidy & P. R. Shaver (Eds.), *Handbook of attachment: Theory, research, and clinical applications* (pp. 520–554). New York: Guilford Press.

Lyons-Ruth, K., & Jacobvitz, D. (2008). Attachment disorganization: Genetic factors, parenting contexts, and developmental transformation from infancy to adulthood. In J. Cassidy & P. R. Shaver (Eds.), *Handbook of attachment: Theory, research, and clinical applications* (2nd ed., pp. 666–697). New York: Guilford Press.

Lyons-Ruth, K., Yellin, C., Melnick, S., & Atwood, G. (2005). Expanding the concept of unresolved mental states: Hostile/helpless states of mind on the Adult Attachment Interview are associated with disrupted mother–infant communication and infant disorganization. *Development and Psychopathology, 17,* 1–23.

MacDonald, H. Z., Beeghly, M., Grant-Knight, W., Augustyn, M., Woods, R. W., Cabral, H., et al. (2008). Longitudinal association between infant disorganized attachment and childhood posttraumatic stress symptoms. *Development and Psychopathology, 20,* 493–508.

Magruder, K. M., Frueh, B. C., Knapp, R. G., Davis, L., Hamner, M. B., Martin, R. H., et al. (2005). Prevalence of posttraumatic stress disorder in Veterans Affairs primary care clinics. *General Hospital Psychiatry, 27,* 169–179.

Main, M. (1991). Metacognitive knowledge, metacognitive monitoring, and singular (coherent) vs. multiple (incoherent) model of attachment. In C. M. Parkes, J. Stevenson-Hinde, & P. Marris (Eds.), *Attachment across the life cycle* (pp. 127–159). London: Routledge.

Main, M., & Hesse, E. (1990). Parents' unresolved traumatic experiences are related to infant disorganized attachment status: Is frightened and/or frightening parental behavior the linking mechanism? In M. T. Greenberg, D. Cicchetti, & E. M. Cummings (Eds.), *Attachment in the preschool years: Theory, research, and intervention* (pp. 161–182). Chicago: University of Chicago Press.

Main, M., Hesse, E., & Goldwyn, R. (2008). Studying differences in language usage in recount-ing attachment history: An introduction to the Adult Attachment Interview. In H. Steele & M. Steele (Eds.), *Clinical applications of the Adult Attachment Interview* (pp. 31–68). New York: Guilford Press.

Main, M., Hesse, E., & Kaplan, N. (2005). Predictability of attachment behavior and represen-tational processes at 1, 6, and 19 years of age: The Berkeley Longitudinal Study. In K. E. Grossmann, K. Grossmann, & E. Waters (Eds.), *Attachment from infancy to adulthood: The major longitudinal studies* (pp. 245–304). New York: Guilford Press.

Main, M., & Solomon, J. (1990). Procedures for identifying infants as disorganized/disoriented during the Ainsworth Strange Situation. In M. T. Greenberg, D. Cicchetti, & E. M. Cummings (Eds.), *Attachment in the preschool years: Theory, research, and intervention* (pp. 121–160). Chicago: University of Chicago Press.

Mayes, L. C. (2000). A developmental perspective on the regulation of arousal states. *Seminars in Perinatology, 24,* 267–279.

McHugh, P. R., & Treisman, G. (2007). PTSD: A problematic diagnostic category. *Journal of Anxiety Disorders, 21,* 211–222.

McMain, S. F., Links, P. D., Gnam, W. H., Guimond, T., Cardish, R. J., Korman, L., et al. (2009). A randomized trial of dialectical behavior therapy versus general psychiatric management for borderline personality disorder. *American Journal of Psychiatry, 166,* 1365–1374.

Meichenbaum, D. (1994). *A clinical handbook/practical therapist manual for assessing and treat-ing adults with posttraumatic stress disorder (PTSD).* Waterloo, Ontario, Canada: Institute Press.

Meichenbaum, D., & Novaco, R. W. (1985). Stress inoculation: A preventative approach. *Issues in Mental Health Nursing, 7,* 419–435.

Meins, E. (1997). *Security of attachment and the social development of cognition.* Hove, UK: Psychology Press.

Meins, E., Fernyhough, C., Fradley, E., & Tuckey, M. (2001). Rethinking maternal sensitivity: Mothers' commments on infants' mental processes predict security of attachment at 12 months. *Journal of Child Psychology and Psychiatry, 42,* 637–648.

Meins, E., Fernyhough, C., Russell, J., & Clark-Carter, D. (1998). Security of attachment as a predictor of symbolic and mentalising abilities: A longitudinal study. *Social Development, 7,* 1–24.

Meins, E., Fernyhough, C., Wainwright, R., Clark-Carter, D., Das Gupta, M., Fradley, E., et al. (2003). Pathways to understanding mind: Construct validity and predictive validity of mater-nal mind-mindedness. *Child Development, 74,* 1194–1211.

Meins, E., Fernyhough, C., Wainwright, R., Das Gupta, M., Fradley, E., & Tuckey, M. (2002). Maternal mind-mindedness and attachment security as predictors of theory of mind under-standing. *Child Development, 73,* 1715–1726.

Melnick, S., Finger, B., Hans, S., Patrick, M., & Lyons-Ruth, K. (2008). Hostile–helpless states of mind in the AAI: A proposed additional AAI category with implications for identifying disorganized infant attachment in high-risk samples. In H. Steele & M. Steele (Eds.), *Clinical applications of the Adult Attachment Interview* (pp. 399–423). New York: Guilford Press.

Mikulincer, M., & Shaver, P. R. (2007). *Attachment in adulthood: Structure, dynamics, and change.* New York: Guilford Press.

Mol, S. S. L., Arntz, A., Metsemakers, J. F. M., Dinant, G.-J., Vilters-Van Montfort, P. A. P., & Knottnerus, J. A. (2005). Symptoms of post-traumatic stress disorder after non-traumatic events: Evidence from an open population study. *British Journal of Psychiatry, 186,* 494–499.

Najavits, L. M., Ryngala, D., Back, S. E., Bolton, E., Mueser, K. T., & Brady, K. T. (2009). Treat-ment of PTSD and comorbid disorders. In E. B. Foa, T. M. Keane, M. J. Friedman, & J. A. Cohen (Eds.), *Effective treatments for PTSD: Practice guidelines from the International Society for Traumatic Stress Studies* (2nd ed., pp. 508–535). New York: Guilford Press.

Nemeroff, C. B., Bremner, J. D., Foa, E. B., Mayberg, H. S., North, C. S., & Stein, M. B. (2006).

Posttraumatic stress disorder: A state-of-the-science review. *Journal of Psychiatric Research,* 40, 1–21.

Nock, M. K. (Ed.). (2009). *Understanding nonsuicidal self-injury.* Washington, DC: American Psychological Association.

Ochsner, K. N., & Gross, J. J. (2005). The cognitive control of emotion. *Trends in Cognitive Sciences,* 9, 242–249.

Paris, J. (1994). *Borderline personality disorder: A multidimensional approach.* Washington, DC: American Psychiatric Press.

Paris, J. (2001). Psychosocial adversity. In W. J. Livesley (Ed.), *Handbook of personality disorders: Theory, research, and treatment* (pp. 231–241). New York: Guilford Press.

Pearlman, L. A., & Courtois, C. A. (2005). Clinical applications of the attachment framework: Relational treatment of complex trauma. *Journal of Traumatic Stress, 18,* 449–459.

Polan, H. J., & Hofer, M. A. (2008). Psychobiological origins of infant attachment and its role in development. In J. Cassidy & P. R. Shaver (Eds.), *Handbook of attachment: Theory, research, and clinical applications* (2nd ed., pp. 158–172). New York: Guilford Press.

Rauch, S. L., & Drevets, W. C. (2009). Neuroimaging and neuroanatomy of stress-induced and fear circuitry disorders. In G. Andrews, D. S. Charney, P. J. Sirovatka, & D. A. Reiger (Eds.), *Stress-induced and fear circuitry disorders: Refining the research agenda for DSM-V* (pp. 215–254). Arlington, VA: American Psychiatric Publishing.

Resick, P. A., Monson, C. M., & Gutner, C. (2007). Psychosocial treatments for PTSD. In M. J. Friedman, T. M. Keane, & P. A. Resick (Eds.), *Handbook of PTSD: Science and practice* (pp. 330–358). New York: Guilford Press.

Resick, P. A., & Schnicke, M. K. (1992). Cognitive processing therapy for sexual assault victims. *Journal of Consulting and Clinical Psychology, 60,* 748–756.

Resick, P. A., & Schnicke, M. K. (1993). *Cognitive processing therapy for rape victims: A treatment manual.* London: Sage.

Roemer, L., & Orsillo, S. M. (2009). *Mindfulness- and acceptance-based behavioral therapies in practice.* New York: Guilford Press.

Rosen, G. M., & Lilienfeld, S. O. (2008). Posttraumatic stress disorder: An empirical evaluation of core assumptions. *Clinical Psychology Review, 28,* 837–868.

Roth, A., & Fonagy, P. (2005). *What works for whom?: A critical review of psychotherapy research* (2nd ed.). New York: Guilford Press.

Schottenbauer, M. A., Glass, C. A., Arnkoff, D. B., & Gray, S. H. (2008). Contributions of psychodynamic approaches to treatment of PTSD and trauma: A review of the empirical treatment and psychopathology literature. *Psychiatry, 71,* 13–34.

Segal, Z. V., Williams, J. M. G., & Teasdale, J. D. (2002). *Mindfulness-based cognitive therapy for depression: A new approach to preventing relapse.* New York: Guilford Press.

Shea, M. T., McDevitt-Murphy, M., Ready, D. J., & Schnurr, P. P. (2009). Group therapy. In E. B. Foa, T. M. Keane, M. J. Friedman, & J. A. Cohen (Eds.), *Effective treatments for PTSD: Practice guidelines from the International Society for Traumatic Stress Studies* (2nd ed., pp. 306–326). New York: Guilford Press.

Simpson, J. A., & Belsky, J. (2008). Attachment theory within a modern evolutionary framework. In J. Cassidy & P. R. Shaver (Eds.), *Handbook of attachment: Theory, research, and clinical applications* (2nd. ed., pp. 131–157). New York: Guilford Press.

Slade, A. (2005). Parental reflective functioning: An introduction. *Attachment and Human Development, 7,* 269–281.

Slade, A., Grienenberger, J., Bernbach, E., Levy, D., & Locker, A. (2005). Maternal reflective functioning, attachment, and the transmission gap: A preliminary study. *Attachment and Human Development, 7,* 283–298.

Spates, C. R., Koch, E., Cusack, K., Pagoto, S., & Waller, S. (2009). Eye movement desensitization and reprocessing. In E. B. Foa, T. M. Keane, M. J. Friedman, & J. A. Cohen (Eds.), *Effective treatments for PTSD: Practice guidelines from the International Society for Traumatic Stress Studies* (2nd ed., pp. 279–305). New York: Guilford Press.

Spitzer, R. L., First, M. B., & Wakefield, J. C. (2007). Saving PTSD from itself in DSM-V. *Journal of Anxiety Disorders, 21,* 233–241.

Sroufe, L. A., Egeland, B., Carlson, E. A., & Collins, W. A. (2005). *The development of the person: The Minnesota Study of Risk and Adaptation from Birth to Adulthood.* New York: Guilford Press.

Steele, H., Steele, M., & Fonagy, P. (1996). Associations among attachment classificaitons of mothers, fathers, and their infants. *Child Development, 67,* 541–555.

Stein, H., & Allen, J. G. (2007). Mentalizing as a framework for integrating therapeutic exposure and relationship repair in the treatment of a patient with complex posttraumatic psychopathology. *Bulletin of the Menninger Clinic, 71,* 273–290.

Stovall-McClough, K. C., Cloitre, M., & McClough, J. F. (2008). Adult attachment and posttraumatic stress disorder in women with histories of childhood abuse. In H. Steele & M. Steele (Eds.), *Clinical applications of the Adult Attachment Interview* (pp. 320–340). New York: Guilford Press.

Toth, S. L., Rogosch, F. A., & Cicchetti, D. (2008). Attachment-theory-informed intervention and reflective functioning in depressed mothers. In H. Steele & M. Steele (Eds.), *Clinical applications of the Adult Attachment Interview* (pp. 154–172). New York: Guilford Press.

van der Kolk, B. A. (1989). The compulsion to repeat the trauma: Reenactment, revictimization, and masochism. *Psychiatric Clinics of North America, 12,* 389–411.

van der Kolk, B. A. (2005). Developmental trauma disorder. *Psychiatric Annals, 35,* 401–408.

van IJzendoorn, M. H. (1995). Adult attachment representations, parental responsiveness, and infant attachment: A meta-analysis on the predictive validity of the Adult Attachment Interview. *Psychological Bulletin, 117,* 387–403.

Vogt, D. S., King, D. W., & King, L. A. (2007). Risk pathways for PTSD: Making sense of the literature. In M. J. Friedman, T. M. Keane, & P. A. Resick (Eds.), *Handbook of PTSD: Science and practice* (pp. 99–115). New York: Guilford Press.

Walker, L. E. (1979). *The battered woman.* New York: Harper & Row.

Weaver, I. C. G., Cervoni, N., Champagne, F. A., D'Alessio, A. C., Sharma, S., Seckl, J. R., et al. (2004). Epigenetic programming by maternal behavior. *Nature Neuroscience, 7,* 847–854.

Wegner, D. M. (1994). Ironic processes of mental control. *Psychological Review, 101,* 34–52.

Wegner, D. M. (1997). When the antidote is the poison: Ironic mental control processes. *Psychological Science, 8,* 148–150.

Weinfield, N. S., Sroufe, L. A., Egeland, B., & Carlson, E. (2008). Individual differences in infant–caregiver attachment: Conceptual and empirical aspects of security. In J. Cassidy & P. R. Shaver (Eds.), *Handbook of attachment: Theory, research, and clinical applications* (2nd ed., pp. 78–101). New York: Guilford Press.

Widom, C. S. (1999). Posttraumatic stress disorder in abused and neglected children grown up. *American Journal of Psychiatry, 156,* 1223–1229.

Zanarini, M. C., Williams, A. A., Lewis, R. E., Reich, R. B., Soledad, C. V., Marino, M. F., et al. (1997). Reported pathological childhood experiences associated with the development of borderline personality disorder. *American Journal of Psychiatry, 154,* 1101–1106.

CHAPTER 10

Obsessive–Compulsive Disorder

Guy Doron, Mario Mikulincer, Michael Kyrios,
and Dar Sar-El

Kelly, a 22-year-old woman, steps into Guy Doron's office and describes her problem: "I can't leave my apartment without someone I trust watching over me. I fear having an urge to assault people, especially old women and children or anyone I believe is weaker than me. I feel like a horrible person, I fear myself. It is a terrible way to live." Mike, a 37-year-old man, is preoccupied with different fears: "Two months after the beginning of every relationship, I start doubting how I feel about the other person and whether I actually like them. Eventually the strain of the never-ending questioning gets too much, makes me depressed, anxious, and guilty, and I cannot function without ending the relationship."

Kelly and Mike both suffer from obsessive–compulsive disorder (OCD), a disorder that has been rated as a leading cause of disability by the World Health Organization (1996). OCD is characterized by the occurrence of unwanted and disturbing intrusive thoughts, images, or impulses (obsessions), and by compulsive rituals that aim to reduce distress or to prevent feared events (i.e., intrusions) from occurring (American Psychiatric Association [APA], 2013; Rachman 1997). As can be seen in the examples presented here, the specific manifestation of OCD symptoms may vary widely from patient to patient, making it a highly heterogeneous and complex disorder (Abramowitz, McKay, & Taylor, 2008; McKay et al., 2004). Kelly's symptoms, like those of many others suffering from this disorder, include morality-related worries, feelings, and cognitions, such as perceived violation of moral standards, guilt, and inflated responsibility (e.g., Salkovskis, 1985; Steketee, Quay, & White, 1991). Mike's obsessive–compulsive (OC) symptoms revolve around intimate relationship issues, an obsessional theme that has only recently begun to be systematically investigated (Doron, Derby, & Szepsenwol, 2014; Doron, Derby, Szepsenwol, & Talmor, 2012b).

In this chapter, we present a recent model of OCD suggesting that sensitivity in specific domains of self (e.g., morality and relational domains) may increase the likelihood of developing obsessional preoccupations around issues related to these domains. We further argue that when coinciding with dysfunctions of the attachment system, such sensitivities can disrupt the process of coping with intrusive experiences and therefore contribute to OCD. For people with high attachment anxiety, experiences challenging an important self-domain can increase the accessibility of maladaptive cognitions (e.g., "I'm bad," "I'm not competent") and activate dysfunctional cognitive processes (e.g., an inflated sense of responsibility, catastrophic interpretations of relationship breakup) that result in the development of obsessional preoccupations and disabling compulsive behaviors. This model integrates notions taken from psychodynamic and cognitive-behavioral approaches in an attempt to provide a deeper and richer understanding of the etiology and development of OCD symptoms.

We begin this chapter with a brief description of OCD and current models of the disorder. We then describe the role of dysfunctional self-perceptions and sensitive self-domains—domains of the self that are extremely important for maintaining self-worth (Doron & Kyrios, 2005)—in OCD. Next, we review empirical findings linking attachment insecurities and obsessive–compulsive phenomena and propose a diathesis–stress model whereby experiences challenging sensitive self-domains and attachment insecurities interact to increase vulnerability to OCD. We then look at morality as an important self-domain in OCD and present findings showing that experiences challenging the morality self-domain can lead to OCD symptoms and that this effect is moderated by attachment anxiety. Finally, we present initial data examining a yet unexplored theme of OCD: relationship-centered OC symptoms.

CLASSIFICATION AND DIAGNOSIS

The definition of OCD in DSM-5 is essentially the same as that in DSM-IV, except OCD has been taken out of the anxiety disorders and placed in a new category that embraces a spectrum of related disorders (APA, 2013). Obsessions are unwanted and disturbing intrusive thoughts, images, or impulses. Obsessional themes include contamination fears, pathological doubt, a need for symmetry or order, body-related worries, and sexual or aggressive obsessions, scrupulosity, and relationship-centered preoccupations. Compulsions are deliberate, repetitive, and rigid behaviors or mental acts that people perform in response to their obsessions as a means of reducing distress or preventing some feared outcome from occurring. Common compulsive behaviors include repeated checking, washing, counting, reassurance seeking, ordering behaviors, and hoarding.

A wide range of etiological theories have been proposed for OCD (e.g., psychological, biological, and neuropsychological). For instance, several studies have supported the role of biological and structural brain abnormalities in OCD (e.g., Pigott & Seay, 1998) and the involvement of neuropsychological mechanisms, such as attention, concentration, executive functions, and memory (see Greisberg & McKay, 2003, for a review). However, the findings are inconsistent, and the studies suffer from severe methodological limitations (e.g., lack of control of confounding variables), thereby making interpretation difficult (e.g., Cottraux & Gérard, 1998; Kuelz, Hohagen, & Voderholzer, 2004; Riffkin et al., 2005). For example, neuropsychological deficits related to OCD (e.g., visuospatial memory impairment) may be a reflection and not a cause of OCD symptoms (Nedeljkovic & Kyrios, 2007; Nedeljkovic, Moulding, Kyrios, & Doron, 2009). Impaired performance in memory tasks, for instance, may result from nonspecific factors such as perfectionism and the inability to make decisions rather than from neurological vulnerabilities (e.g., Otto, 1992; Purcell, Maruff, Kyrios, & Pantelis, 1998). In fact, Abramovitch, Dar, Hermesh, and Schweiger (2011) recently suggested a novel "executive overload model" of OCD that illustrates how overflow of obsessive thoughts may cause an overload on the executive system, which, in turn, interferes with neuropsychological functioning. Moreover, whereas some studies report an association between neuropsychological functioning and OCD symptom severity (e.g., Abramovitch, Dar, Schweiger, & Hermesh, 2011; Lacerda et al., 2003), others have failed to document such an association (e.g., Kuelz et al., 2004), while some have found a negative association despite poorer performance among OCD patients relative to controls (Purcell et al., 1998).

Cognitive-behavioral theories have generated a more consistent body of empirical evidence that has led to the development of effective treatments (see Frost & Steketee, 2002, for a review). According to these theories, most of us experience a range of intrusive phenomena that are similar in form and content to clinical obsessions (Rachman & de Silva, 1978), but individuals with OCD misinterpret such intrusions based on dysfunctional beliefs (e.g., inflated responsibility, perfectionism, intolerance for uncertainty, threat overestimation; Obsessive Compulsive Cognitions Working Group [OCCWG], 1997). Moreover, individuals with OCD tend to rely on ineffective strategies for managing intrusive thoughts and reducing anxiety (e.g., thought suppression, compulsive behavior), which, paradoxically, exacerbate the frequency and intensity of intrusions and result in OCD (Clark & Beck, 2010; Salkovskis, 1985).

PSYCHODYNAMIC APPROACHES TO OCD

Self-Sensitivity and OCD

Whereas cognitive models have improved the understanding and treatment of OCD, recent findings suggest that a substantial proportion of individuals with OCD do not exhibit higher levels of dysfunctional beliefs than those recorded in community samples (e.g., Taylor et al., 2006). In addition, findings regarding the specificity of the dysfunctional beliefs related to OCD are equivocal (e.g., OCCWG, 2005; Tolin, Worhunsky, & Maltby, 2006). Cognitive theories have also been criticized for not sufficiently addressing the developmental and motivational bases of the disorder (e.g., Guidano & Liotti, 1983; O'Kearney, 2001). Moreover, although very effective with most clients, a substantial proportion of patients do not respond to cognitive-behavioral therapy (CBT; Fisher & Wells, 2005).

In response to these criticisms, Doron and colleagues (e.g., Doron & Kyrios, 2005; Doron, Kyrios, & Moulding, 2007; Doron, Kyrios, Moulding, Nedeljkovic,

& Bhar, 2007) incorporated theories of the self within existing cognitive models of OCD. Specifically, they proposed that the transformation of intrusive thoughts into obsessions is moderated by the extent to which intrusive thoughts challenge core perceptions of the self. Indeed, Bhar and Kyrios (2007) and Clark and Purdon (1993) had already argued that the appraisal of an intrusive thought as challenging or inconsistent with one's sense of self (i.e., as ego dystonic) contributes to the formation of obsessions.

According to Doron and Kyrios (2005), because of sociocultural and developmental factors (e.g., parental acceptance that is contingent on competence in particular domains, or ambivalent parenting characterized by rejection but camouflaged by an outward expression of devotion; Guidano & Liotti, 1983), specific self-domains become extremely important for defining a person's sense of self-worth ("sensitive self-domains"; Doron & Kyrios, 2005). As a result, perceived competence in these self-domains becomes crucial for maintaining self-worth (Harter, 1998), and people tend to be preoccupied with events that bear on their perceived competence in sensitive self-domains (e.g., Wolfe & Crocker, 2003). In OCD, sensitive self-domains include areas such as morality, job/school performance, and relationship functioning (e.g., Doron, Moulding, Kyrios, & Nedeljkovic, 2008; Doron, Sar-El, Mikulincer, & Kyrios, 2012; Doron et al., 2014).

Possibly due to unrelenting high expectations and perceived punitive consequences for not meeting such unrealistic expectations, individuals with OCD feel a sense of incompetence in these specific domains. It is not sufficient that individuals have a sense of self that is contingent on morality- or competence-based domains in order to be vulnerable to OCD, although having a limited range of self-worth contingencies may place one at general risk (Ahern & Kyrios, 2010; Doron & Kyrios, 2005; Kyrios, 2010). However, a sense of incompetence in contingent domains (i.e., "sensitive self-domains") may constitute vulnerability for OCD (Doron & Kyrios, 2005; Doron et al., 2008).

Doron and Kyrios (2005) further proposed that thoughts or events that challenge sensitive self-domains (e.g., immoral thoughts or behaviors) damage a person's self-worth and activate attempts at repairing the damage and compensating for the perceived deficits. In the case of individuals with OCD, these coping responses may, paradoxically, further increase the occurrence of unwanted intrusions and the accessibility of "feared self" cognitions (e.g., "I'm bad," "I'm immoral," "I'm unworthy") (Aardema, Moulding, Radomsky, Doron, & Allamby, 2013). In this way, for such individuals, common aversive experiences may activate overwhelmingly negative evaluations in sensitive self-domains (Doron et al., 2008). These processes, together with the activation of other dysfunctional thoughts (e.g., an inflated sense of responsibility, threat overestimation), are self-perpetuating and can result in the development of obsessions and compulsions (see Figure 10.1).

The Moderating Role of Attachment Insecurities

Although sensitive self-domains have been implicated in OCD (Doron et al., 2008), it is unlikely that every person experiencing an aversive event that challenges such

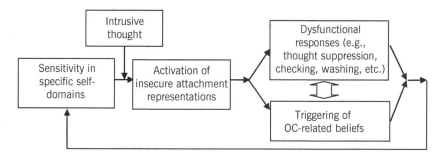

FIGURE 10.1. Hypothesized relationship between self-structures, attachment, and obsessive–compulsive (oc) phenomena.

self-domains will be flooded by negative self-evaluations, dysfunctional beliefs, and obsessions. Some individuals whose sensitive self-domains are challenged by failures and setbacks adaptively protect their self-images from unwanted intrusions and restore emotional equanimity. In fact, for most people, experiences challenging sensitive self-domains would result in the activation of distress-regulation strategies that can dissipate unwanted intrusions, reaffirm the challenged self, and restore emotional composure. The main question here concerns the psychological mechanisms that interfere with this adaptive regulatory process and foster the activation of "feared self" cognitions and the cascade of dysfunctional beliefs that result in OCD symptoms.

In an attempt to respond to this question, Doron, Moulding, Kyrios, Nedeljkovic, and Mikulincer (2009) proposed that attachment insecurities can disrupt the process of coping with experiences that challenge sensitive self-domains and thereby contribute to OCD. According to attachment theory (Bowlby, 1973, 1982; Mikulincer & Shaver, 2007a; see also Mikulincer & Shaver, Chapter 2, this volume), interpersonal interactions with protective others ("attachment figures") are internalized in the form of mental representations of self and others ("internal working models"), which have an impact on close relationships, self-esteem, emotion regulation, and mental health throughout life. Interactions with attachment figures who are available and supportive in times of need foster the development of both a sense of attachment security and positive internal working models of the self and others. When attachment figures are rejecting or unavailable in times of need, attachment security is undermined, and negative models of self and others and attachment insecurities are formed.

Research, beginning with Ainsworth, Blehar, Waters, and Wall (1978) and continuing through recent studies by social and personality psychologists (reviewed by Mikulincer & Shaver, 2003, 2007a), indicates that attachment insecurities are organized around two orthogonal dimensions, attachment-related anxiety, and avoidance (Brennan, Clark, & Shaver, 1998). The first dimension, attachment anxiety, reflects the degree to which a person worries that a partner will not be available or adequately responsive in times of need. The second dimension, avoidance, reflects the extent to which he or she distrusts relationship partners' goodwill and strives to maintain autonomy and emotional distance from them (see also Mikulincer & Shaver, Chapter 2; Luyten & Blatt, Chapter 5; and Steele & Steele, Chapter 20, this volume).

According to attachment theory, a sense of attachment security facilitates the process of coping with, and adjustment to, life's adversities, and the restoration of emotional equanimity following aversive events (Mikulincer & Shaver, 2007a). Moreover, attachment security is associated with heightened perceptions of self-efficacy, constructive distress-regulation strategies, and maintenance of a stable sense of self-worth (e.g., Collins & Read, 1990; Mikulincer & Florian, 1998). Laboratory studies also indicate that experimental manipulations aimed at contextually heightening access to security-enhancing representations (i.e., security priming) restore emotional equanimity after distress-eliciting events and buffer posttraumatic dysfunctional cognitions (see Mikulincer & Shaver, 2007b, for a review).

The sense of attachment security may act, at least to some extent, as a protective shield against OCD-related processes, such as the activation of feared-self cognitions and dysfunctional beliefs following events that challenge sensitive self-domains (Doron et al., 2009). For people who have chronic or contextually heightened mental access to the sense of attachment security, these aversive experiences and the intrusion of unwanted thoughts will result in the activation of effective distress-regulation strategies that dissipate the thoughts, reaffirm the challenged self, and restore well-being.

Conversely, attachment insecurities can impair the process of coping with experiences challenging sensitive self-domains and thereby increase the chances of OCD symptoms. Following these experiences, insecurely attached individuals may fail to find inner representations of security and/or external sources of support, and so may experience a cascade of distress-exacerbating mental processes that can culminate in emotional disorders. For example, anxiously attached individuals tend to react to such failure with catastrophizing, exaggerating the negative consequences of the aversive experience, ruminating on these negative events, and hyperactivating attachment-relevant fears and worries, such as the fear of being abandoned because of one's "bad" self (Mikulincer & Shaver, 2003). Avoidant people tend to react to such aversive events by attempting to suppress distress-eliciting thoughts and negative self-representations. However, these defenses tend to collapse under high emotional or cognitive load (Mikulincer, Dolev, & Shaver, 2004), leaving the avoidant person flooded with unwanted thoughts, negative self-representations, and self-criticism. These kinds of thoughts and feelings tend to perpetuate threat overestimation, lead to overwhelming, uncontrollable distress, and exacerbate unwanted thought intrusions and negative self-views, thereby contributing to the development of obsessions.

EMPIRICAL FINDINGS

Self-Sensitivity and Attachment

There is growing evidence for the role of self-structures in the transformation of intrusive thoughts into OCD symptoms. For example, Rowa, Purdon, Summerfeldt, and Antony (2005) found that individuals with OCD rated more upsetting obsessions as more meaningful and contradictory of valued aspects of the self than less upsetting obsessions. Bhar and Kyrios (2007) found that individuals with OCD exhibited higher levels of self-ambivalence (i.e., worry and uncertainty about their self-concept) than nonclinical controls, although they did not differ from individuals suffering from other anxiety disorders. Doron and colleagues (2007) found that young adults who reported higher sensitivity to morality-related self-domains, social acceptability, and job/school competence (overvaluing a domain while feeling incompetent in that domain) were more likely to report OCD-related cognitions and symptoms. In another study, Doron and colleagues (2008) found that individuals with OCD reported higher levels of self-sensitivity in the domains of morality and job competence than individuals with other anxiety disorders.

There is also evidence supporting the involvement of attachment insecurities in vulnerability to OCD. First of all, both attachment anxiety and avoidance are associated with dysfunctional cognitive processes similar to those included in current cognitive models of OCD (OCCWG, 2005). For instance, attachment anxiety is associated with exaggerated threat appraisals (e.g., Mikulincer & Florian, 1998), perfectionism (e.g., Wei, Mallinckrodt, Russell, & Abraham, 2004), difficulties in suppressing unwanted thoughts (e.g., Mikulincer et al., 2004), rumination on these thoughts (e.g., Mikulincer & Florian, 1998), and self-devaluation in aversive situations (Mikulincer, 1998). Similarly, avoidant attachment is associated with setting high, unrealistic, and rigid personal standards of excellence (Mikulincer & Shaver, 2003, 2007a), self-criticism, maladaptive perfectionism, and intolerance of uncertainty, ambiguity, and personal weaknesses (Mikulincer & Shaver, 2007a). Moreover, avoidant people tend to overemphasize the importance of maintaining control over undesirable thoughts and suppressing thoughts of personal inadequacies and negative personal qualities (Mikulincer et al., 2004).

Recently, Doron and colleagues (2009) provided direct evidence for a link between attachment insecurities and OCD symptoms. They showed that attachment insecurities, both anxiety and avoidance, predicted dysfunctional OCD-related beliefs (e.g., perfectionism and overestimation of threat) and OCD symptoms. Moreover, the contribution of attachment anxiety and avoidance to OCD symptoms was fully mediated by OCD-related beliefs, and remained significant even after statistically controlling for depression symptoms.

Moral Sensitivity and OCD

Morality is one of the sensitive self-domains most frequently involved in the development and maintenance of OCD. The idea that moral preoccupation is related to OCD has been a part of the psychiatric literature since the beginning of the 20th century. For example, Freud (1909/1987) suggested that persistent unwanted aggressive, horrific, or sexual thoughts accompanied by ritualistic behaviors are the result of unsuccessful defense mechanisms (characteristic of the anal-sadistic psychosexual developmental stage) against potential violations of moral standards. Individuals with OCD tend to suffer from unconscious conflicts between unacceptable, immoral sexual or aggressive impulses and the demands of the superego (moral conscience). They attempt to resolve this conflict by relying on undoing (i.e., defensively neutralizing unacceptable ideas by compulsive acts) and reaction formation (i.e., unconsciously developing attitudes and behaviors opposite to the unacceptable repressed impulses).

More recent object relations theories emphasize the role of mental representations or cognitive-affective schemas of self and others in the development of OCD (Blatt, Auerbach, & Levy, 1997; Levy, Blatt, & Shaver, 1998). According to this view, the same psychic structures (ego, superego, and id) and conflicts exist in nonpathological and pathological psychological functioning (Blatt & Shichman, 1983). However, the capacity to integrate and balance these conflictual aspects of the ego system in individuals with OCD is compromised (Kempke & Luyten, 2007). As a result, these individuals tend to hold negative representations of the self, self-criticism, hypermorality, and negative views of others as critical and punishing. This seems to lead to difficulties commonly associated with OCD, such as ambivalence, intolerance of personal imperfections, and strong need for control and autonomy (e.g., Blatt & Shichman, 1983; Mallinger, 1984; Shapiro, 1965).

Cognitive theories of OCD have also implicated morality concerns in the maintenance of OCD. For instance, Rachman and Hodgson (1980) argued that individuals with OCD are of "tender conscience," and Salkovskis, Shafran, Rachman, and Freeston (1999) suggested that individuals suffering from OCD exhibit "dedication to work and an acute sense of social obligation" (p. 1060). Salkovskis (1985) argued that an overinflated sense of personal responsibility, defined as the tendency to believe that one may be pivotally responsible for causing or failing to prevent harm to oneself or others, is one of the core beliefs leading to the transformation of common intrusive thoughts into obsessions. Beliefs about the importance of thoughts have also been suggested to have an important moral element, such as the belief that having a negative thought is as bad as performing a negative act (moral thought-action fusion; Shafran, Thordarson, & Rachman, 1996).

Research has also linked morality-relevant emotions such as guilt, shame, and disgust with obsessive–compulsive phenomena. For instance, stronger feelings of guilt and shame (i.e., negative emotional reactions to social or moral transgressions) have been associated with OCD, anxiety, and depression (see Tangney & Dearing, 2002, for a review). Disgust, which has been theoretically and empirically linked with OCD symptoms (e.g., Olatunji, Lohr, Sawchuk, & Tolin, 2007; Rachman, 2004), has been found to be provoked by violations of moral standards (e.g., Miller, 1997; Rozin, Haidt, & McCauley, 2000) and to elicit the need to physically cleanse (Zhong & Liljenquist, 2006). Finally, there are indications that obsessive–compulsive phenomena are associated with religious denomination and strength of religiosity (e.g., Sica, Novara, & Sanavio, 2002). Highly religious individuals exhibit OCD-related beliefs and symptoms with religious themes, such as praying or washing away one's sins (e.g., Abramowitz, Deacon, Woods, & Tolin, 2004; Rasmussen & Tsuang, 1986; Steketee et al., 1991).

More recently, research has provided evidence of the association between OCD and sensitivity in the morality self-domain (e.g., Doron et al., 2008). For example, Ferrier and Brewin (2005) reported that, compared to individuals with other clinical anxiety disorders, as well as normal controls, individuals with OCD were more likely to draw negative moral inferences about themselves from their intrusive thoughts (e.g., perception of self as dangerous by virtue of being bad, immoral, or insane). Ahern and Kyrios (2010) reported that, compared to individuals who experienced distressing reactive obsessions, those experiencing moral/sexual intrusions were significantly more likely to appraise their intrusive thoughts as ego dystonic, to report greater self-ambivalence, and to use avoidant cognitive techniques (e.g., distracting themselves with an activity, replacing the thought with a more pleasant thought, telling themselves to stop). However, Franklin, McNally, and Riemann (2009) failed to find an association between moral reasoning and OCD. Specifically, OCD patients and controls were asked to choose one of two undesirable courses of action (both involving loss of life) in a series of hypothetical moral dilemmas. No group difference was found in the choice of options and latencies to resolve the moral dilemmas. Hence, the relationship between OCD symptoms and morality may not be extended to moral reasoning but is limited to the emotional and self-relevant aspects of moral concerns.

In three experimental studies using subtle cues of threat to the morality self-domain, Doron, Sar-El, and Mikulincer (2012) have shown that this threat led to heightened reported urge to act and likelihood of acting in response to contamination-related scenarios in a nonclinical sample. These effects were specific to cues that were ascribed as self-relevant, baring negative undertone and targeting the morality domain (versus a morality-irrelevant domain). These effects were not related to preexisting variations in self-esteem, stress, anxiety, or depression, and were not accounted for by mood fluctuations. It seems that even subtle threats to the morality self-domain can increase OC-related behavioral tendencies.

Intimate Relationships and OCD

One OCD theme that has only recently begun to be systematically explored is OC symptoms centering on romantic relationships (ROCD; Doron, Derby, Szepsenwol, & Talmor, 2012a; Doron, Derby, et al., 2012b; Doron, Talmor, Szepsenwol, & Derby, 2012). Previous research has indicated that, compared with the general population, OCD patients often report disturbances in relationship functioning, including lower likelihood of marrying and increased marital distress (e.g., Emmelkamp, de Haan, & Hoogduin, 1990; Rasmussen & Eisen, 1992; Riggs, Hiss, & Foa, 1992). Doron, Derby, and colleagues (2012a, 2012b), however, proposed that OC phenomena are likely to affect relationships more directly when the main focus of the symptoms is the relationship itself. One such ROCD presentation is obsessions and compulsions focused on the individual's feelings toward his or her partner (e.g., "Do I really love my partner?"), the partner's feelings toward the individual (e.g., "Does my partner really love me?"), or the "rightness" of the relationship experience (e.g., "Is this relationship the right one?") can directly erode relationship quality and contribute to relationship termination.

Recently, Doron, Derby, and colleagues (2012b) conducted two independent studies using nonclinical cohorts to assess relationship-centered OC phenomena and their links with related constructs. In the first study, Doron and colleagues (2012) constructed a 12-item self-report scale tapping relational OCD—the Relationship Obsessive Compulsive Inventory (ROCI). This scale assesses the severity of obsessive thoughts (e.g., preoccupation and doubts) and compulsive behaviors (e.g., checking and reassurance seeking) on three relational dimensions: one's feelings toward one's partner (e.g., "I continuously reassess whether I really love my partner"), the partner's feelings toward the individual (e.g., "I continuously doubt my partner's love for me"), and the "rightness" of the relationship ("I check and recheck whether my relationship feels right"). A confirmatory factor analysis supported the three-factor structure of the ROCI, and the three subscales revealed high reliability scores (ranging from .84 to .89).

In the second study, Doron and colleagues (2012b) found that higher ROCI scores were associated with higher levels of common OCD symptoms and cognitions, negative mood, low self-esteem, relationship ambivalence, and attachment insecurities. Findings also showed that ROCI scores significantly predicted relationship dissatisfaction and depression, over and above common OCD symptoms, relationship ambivalence, negative mood, low self-esteem, and attachment insecurities. These findings indicate that the ROCI captures a relatively distinct theoretical construct and has unique predictive value.

Findings revealed moderate associations between relationship-centered OC symptoms and other cognitive dysfunctional beliefs, suggesting that additional factors may contribute to the development and maintenance of relationship-centered OC phenomena. Since effective treatment of particular OCD presentations involves improved understanding of both common OCD mechanisms and more specific mechanisms that are adjusted to each manifestation (e.g., Abramowitz, Huppert, Cohen, Tolin, & Cahill, 2002; McKay et al., 2004), further exploration should be devoted to the unique etiological processes involved in the formation and preservation of relationship-centered OC symptoms.

We believe that self-sensitivity in the romantic domain, catastrophic relationship beliefs, and attachment insecurities may be particularly important in the development and maintenance of relationship-centered OC phenomena. Specifically, perceptions of incompetence in the romantic domain may enhance sensitivity to intrusions challenging self-perceptions in this relational domain (e.g., "I do not feel right with my partner at the moment"). Such intrusions may then trigger catastrophic relationship appraisals (e.g., being in a relationship I am not sure about will make me miserable forever") and other maladaptive appraisals (e.g., "I shouldn't have such doubts regarding my partner"), followed by neutralizing behaviors (e.g., reassurance-seeking and checking).

Attachment insecurities, and especially attachment anxiety, may exacerbate this cascade of unpleasant mental events in several important ways. The hypervigilance of anxiously attached individuals toward real or imagined relationship threats may make them especially vulnerable to intrusions challenging self-perceptions in the relational domain. Moreover, their reliance on hyperactivating strategies, such as insistent, repetitive attempts to obtain love from relationship partners (Mikulincer & Shaver, 2007a), may predispose such individuals to compulsive reassurance-seeking and checking behaviors, particularly in the context of intimate relationships.

Insecurely attached individuals may also fail to find inner representations of security or external sources of support, and may therefore experience a cascade of distress-exacerbating mental processes following negative relational events (e.g., disapproval, rejection, criticism, betrayal). For instance, anxiously attached individuals tend to react to such events with catastrophizing, exaggerating the negative consequences of the aversive experience, ruminating on the negative event and its consequences, and hyperactivating attachment-relevant fears and worries, such as the fear of being abandoned because of one's "bad" self (Mikulincer & Shaver, 2003). In addition, since attachment figures in adulthood are likely to be one's romantic partners, the tendency to search for physical, emotional, or cognitive proximity to attachment figures in times of need may refocus insecurely attached individuals on their aversive relational experience (i.e., the initial trigger of intrusions and compulsions), thereby exacerbating rather than inhibiting the obsessional cycle.

Indeed, recent findings indicate that contingency of self in the relational domain and attachment anxiety jointly contribute (i.e., double-relationship vulnerability) to the development and maintenance of ROCD symptoms (Doron, Szepsenwol, Karp, & Gal, 2013). In one study, attachment anxiety was linked with more severe ROCD symptoms mainly among individuals whose self-worth was strongly dependent on their relationship. Subtle hints of incompetence in the relational self-domain were found to increase ROCD tendencies in the second study, but mainly among individuals high in both attachment anxiety and relationship-contingent self-worth. Thus, coinciding self-vulnerability in the relational self-domain and attachment anxiety may result in increased susceptibility to relationship-related obsessive doubts and worries.

On this basis, we suggested that self-sensitivity in the relational domain and attachment insecurities contribute to the development of relationship-centered obsessions by, on the one hand, increasing insecure individuals' vigilance to relationship threats, and, on the other, impairing their capacity for adaptive coping with such challenging experiences.

CONCLUSIONS AND FUTURE DIRECTIONS

In our view, some individuals perceive themselves as incompetent in domains that they view as extremely important for self-worth (i.e., sensitive self-domains), such as the domains of morality and intimate relationships. Experiences challenging such self-domains (e.g., doubts about one's capacity to provide others with help, not being sure about one's partner's love) may lead to an increase in negative self-cognitions (e.g., "I'm bad," "I'm incompetent") and lead to the development of obsessive intrusions. Attachment insecurities can exacerbate this cascade of unpleasant mental events by impairing adaptive coping. Conversely, attachment security may protect a person against the adverse effects of these experiences.

In this chapter, we reviewed both correlational and experimental findings that support the hypothesized roles of morality concerns and attachment insecurities in OCD. We then proposed that such mechanisms may be involved in a yet little explored area of OCD—relationship-centered OC symptoms. Taken together, the reviewed findings expand our understanding of the ways in which self-sensitivity and attachment insecurities are involved in the development and maintenance of OCD. Intrusions are more likely to activate dysfunctional beliefs and trigger OCD symptoms in insecurely attached individuals who are sensitive in a specific self-domain.

Though consistent with our theoretical model, this new body of research has several limitations. First, many studies have been conducted with nonclinical samples. Although nonclinical individuals experience OCD-related beliefs and symptoms, they may differ from clinical patients in the type and severity of symptoms and the resulting degree of impairment. Future research on self-sensitivity, attachment insecurities, and OCD symptoms should include clinical samples. Examining different clinical groups would facilitate the identification of specific factors associated with particular kinds of OCD symptoms. Second, laboratory studies conducted with clinical and nonclinical samples should further examine whether dispositional attachment insecurities intensify the adverse effects of experimental inductions challenging self-perceptions in the morality and relational domains. These studies should also examine the extent to which experimentally induced attachment security (security priming) buffers the adverse effects of dispositional attachment insecurities and events challenging self-perceptions in the morality or relational domains on OCD-related behavioral tendencies.

Despite these limitations, and pending further replication of the reviewed findings, particularly with clinical samples, our findings may have important implications for the understanding and treatment of OCD. We believe that OCD-related assessments and interventions focused on sensitive self-domains and attachment insecurities can improve therapeutic outcomes. When dealing with individuals presenting with OCD, therapists should consider expanding their conceptualization of OCD to include the evaluation of a patient's self-sensitivities and his or her attachment working models (Doron & Moulding, 2009). Patients may, for example, have a rigid and limited perception of morality (e.g., believing they should be free of sexual urges before marriage), such that any urge or thought that challenges their moral standards leads to self-criticism, morbid rumination, and compulsions. Similarly, other patients may have rigid views of competence in the romantic relationship domain (e.g., the behavior, feelings, and thoughts they should have when in an intimate relationship), such that any intrusion threatening their competence in this domain could result in the development of morbid preoccupations (Doron & Derby, in press).

When a client has this kind of limiting self-view, special emphasis should be placed on expanding his or her self-concept. This could be done by identifying and bolstering other self-domains, increasing the client's skills in other domains, or challenging the rigidity and boundaries of the sensitive self-domain (e.g., "What does being moral mean to you?"; "What does it mean to be a good relationship partner?"). The contingency of self-worth in the sensitive domain could also be explicitly explored, such that the client understands the relation between anxiety and perceptions of failure in that self-domain. This would help the clinician with case formulation, particularly in understanding why specific mental intrusions lead to heightened emotional reactions or avoidance behavior.

In a similar way, "attachment-based CBT" (Doron & Moulding, 2009) addresses issues regarding trust and heightened fear of abandonment, and explores attachment-related internal models within the therapeutic context. It is common for OCD symptoms to be associated with strong attachment-related fears (e.g., horrific images of a partner having an accident followed by making repeated phone calls). In such cases, fear of abandonment can be addressed by challenging dysfunctional perceptions, exploring the relation between relationship fears and OCD, and devising behavioral experiments aimed at increasing tolerance for ordinary separations. This may reduce a client's tendency to interpret relationship experiences, including the therapeutic relationship, in frightening terms, improve therapeutic efficacy, and possibly reduce dropout and relapse rates compared with those for traditional CBT.

REFERENCES

Aardema, F., Moulding, R., Radomsky, A. S., Doron, G., & Allamby, J. (2013). Fear of the self and obsessionality: Development and validation of the Fear of Self Questionnaire. *Journal of Obsessive–Compulsive and Related Disorders, 3,* 306–315.

Abramovitch, A., Dar, R., Hermesh, H., & Schweiger, A. (2011). Comparative neuropsychology of adult obsessive–compulsive disorder and attention deficit/hyperactivity disorder: Implications for a novel executive overload model of OCD. *Journal of Neuropsychology, 6,* 161–191.

Abramovitch, A., Dar, R., Schweiger, A., & Hermesh, H. (2011). Neuropsychological impairments and their association with obsessive-compulsive symptom severity in obsessive–compulsive disorder. *Archives of Clinical Neuropsychology, 26,* 364–376.

Abramowitz, J. S., Deacon, B. J., Woods, C. M., & Tolin, D. F. (2004). Association between Protestant religiosity and obsessive–compulsive symptoms and cognitions. *Depression and Anxiety, 20,* 70–76.

Abramowitz, J. S., Huppert, J. D., Cohen, A. B., Tolin, D. F., & Cahill, S. P. (2002). Religious obsessions and compulsions in a non-clinical sample: The Penn Inventory of Scrupulosity (PIOS). *Behaviour Research and Therapy, 40,* 825–838.

Abramowitz, J. S., McKay, D., & Taylor, S. (2008). *Clinical handbook of obsessive–compulsive disorder and related problems.* Baltimore: Johns Hopkins University Press.

Ahern, C., & Kyrios, M. (2010, July). *The role of self-ambivalence and contingent self-worth in the experience of unwanted intrusive thoughts.* Paper presented at the 27th International Congress of Applied Psychology, Melbourne, Australia.

Ainsworth, M. D., Blehar, M. C., Walters, E., & Wall, S. (1978). *Patterns of attachment: A psychological study of the strange situation.* Hillsdale, NJ: Erlbaum.

American Psychiatric Association. (2000). *Diagnostic and statistical manual of mental disorders* (4th ed., text rev.). Washington, DC: Author.

American Psychiatric Association. (2013). *Diagnostic and statistical manual of mental disorders* (5th ed.). Arlington, VA: Author.

Bhar, S., & Kyrios, M. (2007). An investigation of self-ambivalence in obsessive–compulsive disorder. *Behaviour Research and Therapy, 45,* 1845–1857.

Blatt, S. J., Auerbach, J. S., & Levy, K. N. (1997). Mental representations in personality development, psychopathology, and the therapeutic process. *Review of General Psychology, 1,* 351–374.

Blatt, S. J., & Shichman, S. (1983). Two primary configurations of psychopathology. *Psychoanalysis and Contemporary Thought, 6,* 187–254.

Bowlby, J. (1973). *Attachment and loss: Vol. 2. Separation: Anxiety and anger.* New York: Basic Books.

Bowlby, J. (1982). *Attachment and loss: Vol. 1. Attachment* (2nd ed.). New York: Basic Books.

Brennan, K. A., Clark, C. L., & Shaver, P. R. (1998). Self-report measurement of adult attachment. In J. A. Simpson & W. S. Rholes (Eds.), *Attachment theory and close relationships* (pp. 46–76). New York: Guilford Press.

Clark, D. A., & Beck, A. T. (2010). *Cognitive therapy of anxiety disorders: Science and practice.* New York: Guilford Press.

Clark, D. A., & Purdon, C. (1993). New perspectives for a cognitive theory of obsessions. *Australian Psychologist, 28,* 161–167.

Collins, N. L., & Read, S. J. (1990). Adult attachment, working models, and relationship quality in dating couples. *Journal of Personality and Social Psychology, 58,* 644–663.

Cottraux, J., & Gérard, D. (1998). Neuroimaging and neuroanatomical issues in obsessive–compulsive disorder: Toward an integrative model—perceived impulsivity. In R. P. Swinson, M. M. Antony, S. Rachman, & M. A. Richter (Eds.), *Obsessive–compulsive disorder: Theory, research, and treatment* (pp. 154–180). New York: Guilford Press.

Doron, G., & Derby, D. (in press). Assessment and treatment of relationship-related OCD symptoms (ROCD): A modular approach. In J. S. Abramowitz, D. McKay, & E. A. Storch (Eds.), *Handbook of obsessive–compulsive disorder across the lifespan.* Hoboken, NJ: Wiley.

Doron, G., Derby, D., & Szepsenwol, O. (2014). Relationship obsessive–compulsive disorder (ROCD): A conceptual framework. *Journal of Obsessive–Compulsive and Related Disorders, 3,* 169–180.

Doron, G., Derby, D., Szepsenwol, O., & Talmor. D. (2012a). Flaws and all: Exploring partner-focused obsessive–compulsive symptoms. *Journal of Obsessive–Compulsive and Related Disorders, 1,* 234–243.

Doron, G., Derby, D., Szepsenwol, O., & Talmor. D. (2012b). Tainted love: Exploring relationship-centered obsessive compulsive symptoms in two non-clinical cohorts. *Journal of Obsessive–Compulsive and Related Disorders, 1,* 16–24.

Doron, G., & Kyrios, M. (2005). Obsessive compulsive disorder: A review of possible specific internal representations within a broader cognitive theory. *Clinical Psychology Review, 25,* 415–432.

Doron, G., Kyrios, M., & Moulding, R. (2007). Sensitive domains of self-concept in obsessive–compulsive disorder (OCD): Further evidence for a multidimensional model of OCD. *Journal of Anxiety Disorders, 21,* 433–444.

Doron, G., Kyrios, M., Moulding, R., Nedeljkovic, M., & Bhar, S. (2007). "We do not see things as they are, we see them as we are": A multidimensional world-view of obsessive compulsive disorder (OCD). *Journal of Cognitive Psychotherapy, 21,* 221–235.

Doron, G., & Moulding, R. (2009). Cognitive behavioral treatment of obsessive compulsive disorder: A broader framework. *Israel Journal of Psychiatry and Related Science, 46,* 257–263.

Doron, G., Moulding, R., Kyrios, M., & Nedeljkovic, M. (2008). Sensitivity of self beliefs in obsessive compulsive disorder (OCD). *Anxiety and Depression, 25,* 874–884.

Doron, G., Moulding, R., Kyrios, M., Nedeljkovic, M., & Mikulincer, M. (2009). Adult attachment insecurities are related to obsessive compulsive phenomena. *Journal of Social and Clinical Psychology, 28,* 1022–1049.

Doron, G., Sar-El, D., & Mikulincer, M. (2012). Threats to moral self-perceptions trigger obsessive compulsive contamination-related behavioral tendencies. *Journal of Behavior Therapy and Experimental Psychiatry, 43,* 884–890.

Doron, G., Sar-El, D., Mikulincer, M., & Kyrios, M. (2012). When moral concerns become a psychological disorder: The case of obsessive compulsive disorder. In M. Mikulincer & P. R. Shaver (Eds.), *Social psychology of morality: Exploring the causes of good and evil* (pp. 293–310). Washington, DC: American Psychological Association.

Doron, G., Szepsenwol, O., Karp, E., & Gal, N. (2013). Obsessing about intimate relationships: Testing the double relationship-vulnerability hypothesis. *Journal of Behavior Therapy and Experimental Psychiatry, 44,* 433–440.

Doron, G., Talmor, D., Szepsenwol, O., & Derby, S. D. (2012). Relationship-centered obsessive compulsive phenomena. *Psicoterapia Cognitiva e Comportamentale, 18,* 79–90.

Emmelkamp, P. M., de Haan, E., & Hoogduin, C. A. (1990). Marital adjustment and obsessive–compulsive disorder. *British Journal of Psychiatry, 156*, 55–60.

Ferrier, S., & Brewin, C. (2005). Feared identity and obsessive compulsive disorder. *Behaviour Research and Therapy, 43*, 1363–1374.

Fisher, P. L., & Wells, A. (2005). How effective are cognitive and behavioral treatments for obsessive–compulsive disorder?: A clinical significance analysis. *Behaviour Research and Therapy, 43*, 1543–1558.

Franklin, S. A., McNally, R. J., & Riemann, B. C. (2009). Moral reasoning in obsessive–compulsive disorder. *Journal of Anxiety Disorders, 23*, 575–577.

Freud, S. (1987). Notes upon a case of obsessional neurosis ("the Rat Man"). In A. Richards (Ed.), *Case histories II: The "Rat Man," Schreber, the "Wolf Man," a case of female homosexuality* (Vol. 9, pp. 33–128). Harmondsworth, UK: Penguin Books. (Original work published 1909)

Frost, R. O., & Steketee, G. (Eds.). (2002). *Cognitive approaches to obsessions and compulsions: Theory, assessment, and treatment.* Amsterdam: Pergamon/Elsevier.

Greisberg, S., & McKay, D. (2003). Neuropsychology of obsessive–compulsive disorder: A review and treatment implications. *Clinical Psychology Review, 23*, 95–117.

Guidano, V. F., & Liotti, G. (1983). *Cognitive processes and emotional disorders.* New York: Guilford Press.

Harter, S. (1998). The development of self-representations. In W. Damon & N. Eisenberg (Eds.), *Handbook of child psychology* (5th ed., Vol. 3, pp. 553–617). Hoboken, NJ: Wiley.

Kempke, S., & Luyten, P. (2007). Psychodynamic and cognitive-behavioral approaches of obsessive–compulsive disorder: Is it time to work through our ambivalence? *Bulletin of the Menninger Clinic, 71*, 291–311.

Kuelz, A. K., Hohagen, F., & Voderholzer, U. (2004). Neuropsychological performance in obsessive–compulsive disorder: A critical review. *Biological Psychology, 65*, 185–236.

Kyrios, M. (2010, July). *The self in obsessive–compulsive disorder.* Invited address at the 27th International Congress of Applied Psychology, Melbourne, Australia.

Lacerda, A. L., Dalgalarrondo, P., Caetano, D., Haas, G. L., Camargo, E. E., & Keshavan, M. S. (2003). Neuropsychological performance and regional cerebral blood flow in obsessive–compulsive disorder. *Progress in Neuro-Psychopharmacology and Biological Psychiatry, 27*, 657–665.

Levy, K. N., Blatt, S. J., & Shaver, P. R. (1998). Attachment styles and parental representations. *Journal of Personality and Social Psychology, 74*, 407–419.

Mallinger, A. E. (1984). The obsessive's myth of control. *Journal of the American Academy of Psychoanalysis, 12*, 147–165.

McKay, D., Abramowitz, J. S., Calamari, J. E., Kyrios, M., Radomsky, A., Sookman, D., et al. (2004). A critical evaluation of obsessive–compulsive disorder subtypes: Symptoms versus mechanisms. *Clinical Psychology Review, 24*, 283–313.

Mikulincer, M. (1998). Adult attachment style and affect regulation: Strategic variations in self-appraisals. *Journal of Personality and Social Psychology, 75*, 420–435.

Mikulincer, M., Dolev, T., & Shaver, P. R. (2004). Attachment-related strategies during thought suppression: Ironic rebounds and vulnerable self-representations. *Journal of Personality and Social Psychology, 87*, 940–956.

Mikulincer, M., & Florian, V. (1998). The relationship between adult attachment styles and emotional and cognitive reactions to stressful events. In J. A. Simpson & W. S. Rholes (Eds.), *Attachment theory and close relationships* (pp. 143–165). New York: Guilford Press.

Mikulincer, M., & Shaver, P. R. (2003). The attachment behavioral system in adulthood: Activation, psychodynamics, and interpersonal processes. In M. P. Zanna (Ed.), *Advances in experimental social psychology* (Vol. 35, pp. 53–152). New York: Academic Press.

Mikulincer, M., & Shaver, P. R. (2007a). *Attachment in adulthood: Structure, dynamics, and change.* New York: Guilford Press.

Mikulincer, M., & Shaver, P. R. (2007b). Boosting attachment security to promote mental health, prosocial values, and inter-group tolerance. *Psychological Inquiry, 18*, 139–156.

Miller, W. I. (1997). The anatomy of disgust. Cambridge, MA: Harvard University Press.

Nedeljkovic, M., & Kyrios, M. (2007). Confidence in memory and other cognitive processes in obsessive–compulsive disorder. *Behaviour Research and Therapy, 45,* 2899–2914.

Nedeljkovic, M., Moulding, R., Kyrios, M., & Doron, G. (2009). The relationship of cognitive confidence to OCD symptoms. *Journal of Anxiety Disorders, 23,* 463–468.

O'Kearney, R. (2001). Motivation and emotions in the cognitive theory of obsessive–compulsive disorder: A reply to Salkovskis and Freeston. *Australian Journal of Psychology, 53,* 7–9.

Obsessive Compulsive Cognitions Working Group. (1997). Cognitive assessment of obsessive–compulsive disorder. *Behaviour Research and Therapy, 35,* 667–681.

Obsessive Compulsive Cognitions Working Group. (2005). Psychometric validation of the Obsessive Beliefs Questionnaire: Factor analyses and testing of a brief version. *Behaviour Research and Therapy, 43,* 1527–1542.

Olatunji, B. O., Lohr, J. M., Sawchuk, C. N., & Tolin, D. F. (2007). Multimodal assessment of disgust in contamination-related obsessive–compulsive disorder. *Behaviour Research and Therapy, 45,* 263–276.

Otto, M. W. (1992). Normal and abnormal information processing: A neuropsychological perspective on obsessive compulsive disorder. *Psychiatric Clinics of North America, 15,* 825–848.

Pigott, T. A., & Seay, S. M. (1998). Biological treatments for obsessive–compulsive disorder: Literature review. In P. R. Swinson, M. M. Antony, S. Rachman, & M. A. Richter (Eds.), *Obsessive–compulsive disorder: Theory, research, and treatment.* New York: Guilford Press.

Purcell, R., Maruff, P., Kyrios, M., & Pantelis, C. (1998). Neuropsychological deficits in obsessive–compulsive disorder: A comparison with unipolar depression, panic disorder, and normal controls. *Archives of General Psychiatry, 55,* 415–423.

Rachman, S. (1997). A cognitive theory of obsessions. *Behaviour Research and Therapy, 35,* 793–802.

Rachman, S. (2004). Fear of contamination. *Behaviour Research and Therapy, 42,* 1227–1255.

Rachman, S., & de Silva, P. (1978). Abnormal and normal obsessions. *Behaviour Research and Therapy, 16,* 233–248.

Rachman, S., & Hodgson, R. J. (Eds.). (1980). *Obsessions and compulsions.* Englewood Cliffs, NJ: Prentice-Hall.

Rasmussen, S. A., & Eisen, J. L. (1992). The epidemiology and clinical features of obsessive compulsive disorder. *Psychiatric Clinics of North America, 15,* 743–758.

Rasmussen, S. A., & Tsuang, M. T. (1986). Clinical characteristics and family history in DSM-III obsessive–compulsive disorder. *American Journal of Psychiatry, 143,* 317–322.

Riffkin, J., Yücel, M., Maruff, P., Wood, S. J., Soulsby, B., Olver, J., et al. (2005). A manual and automated MRI study of anterior cingulate and orbito-frontal cortices, and caudate nucleus in obsessive–compulsive disorder: Comparison with healthy controls and patients with schizophrenia. *Psychiatry Research: Neuroimaging, 138,* 99–113.

Riggs, D. S., Hiss, H., & Foa, E. B. (1992). Marital distress and the treatment of obsessive compulsive disorder. *Behavior Therapy, 23,* 585–597.

Rowa, K., Purdon, C., Summerfeldt, L. J., & Antony, M. (2005). Why are some obsessions more upsetting than others? *Behaviour Research and Therapy, 43,* 1453–1465.

Rozin, P., Haidt, J., & McCauley, C. R. (2000). Disgust. In M. Lewis & J. M. Haviland-Jones (Eds.), *Handbook of emotions* (2nd ed., pp. 637–653). New York: Guilford Press.

Salkovskis, P. M. (1985). Obsessional-compulsive problems: A cognitive-behavioral analysis. *Behaviour Research and Therapy, 23,* 571–583.

Salkovskis, P. M., Shafran, R., Rachman, S., & Freeston, M. H. (1999). Multiple pathways to inflated responsibility beliefs in obsessional problems: Possible origins and implications for therapy and research. *Behaviour Research and Therapy, 37,* 1055–1072.

Shafran, R., Thordarson, D. S., & Rachman, S. (1996). Thought-action fusion in obsessive compulsive disorder. *Journal of Anxiety Disorders, 10,* 379–390.

Shapiro, D. (1965). *Neurotic styles.* New York: Basic Books.

Sica, C., Novara, C., & Sanavio, E. (2002). Religiousness and obsessive–compulsive cognitions and symptoms in an Italian population. *Behaviour Research and Therapy, 40,* 813–823.

Steketee, G., Quay, S., & White, K. (1991). Religion and guilt in OCD patients. *Journal of Anxiety Disorders, 5,* 359–367.

Tangney, J. P., & Dearing, R. L. (2002). *Shame and guilt.* New York: Guilford Press.

Taylor, S., Abramowitz, J. S., McKay, D., Calamari, J. E., Sookman, D., & Kyrios, M. (2006). Do dysfunctional beliefs play a role in all types of obsessive–compulsive disorder? *Journal of Anxiety Disorders, 20,* 85–97.

Tolin, D. F., Worhunsky, P., & Maltby, N. (2006). Are "obsessive" beliefs specific to OCD?: A comparison across anxiety disorders. *Behaviour Research and Therapy, 44,* 469–480.

Wei, M., Mallinckrodt, B., Russell, D. W., & Abraham, W. (2004). Maladaptive perfectionism as a mediator and moderator between adult attachment and depressive mood. *Journal of Counseling Psychology, 51,* 201–212.

Wolfe, C., & Crocker, J. (2003). What does the self want? Contingencies of self-worth and goals. In S. J. Spencer, S. Fein, M. P. Zanna, & J. M. Olson (Eds.), *Motivated social perception* (pp. 147–170). Mahwah, NJ: Erlbaum.

World Health Organization. (1996). *Global burden of disease: A comprehensive assessment and morbidity from disease, injuries, and risk factors in 1990 and projected to 2020.* New York: Author.

Zhong, C. B., & Liljenquist. K. (2006). Washing away your sins: threatened morality and physical cleansing. *Science, 313,* 1451–1452.

CHAPTER 11

Substance Use Disorders

William H. Gottdiener and Jesse J. Suh

This chapter discusses the etiology, psychology, and treatment of substance use disorders (SUDs) from a contemporary psychodynamic perspective. This discussion is important for two reasons. First, psychodynamically oriented psychotherapists outnumber psychotherapists worldwide despite the growing number of psychotherapists who practice from cognitive-behavioral and other perspectives (Orlinsky et al., 2005). Second, despite the large number of psychodynamic psychotherapists who are available to provide treatment, some people in the psychodynamic community believe that it is not possible to understand or to treat people with an SUD psychodynamically (Levin & Weiss, 1994). We write this chapter with a belief that the available empirical and clinical evidence suggest otherwise.

Our primary goal, therefore, is to describe the theoretical and scientific knowledge about the psychodynamics of SUDs and psychodynamic treatments for SUDs, and to provide a clinical vignette to help clinicians understand that treatment of patients with an SUD requires the same range of supportive and expressive psychodynamic techniques that are used for other clinical problems. We hope to demonstrate that it is possible to understand and treat SUDs psychodynamically. In addition, we hope to stimulate continued interest in scientific research on the psychodynamics of SUDs and on the development of psychodynamic treatments for SUDs (see Gottdiener, 2008).

In order to provide readers with a grounding in the theoretical and empirical literature on the psychodynamics involved in SUD pathology and on psychodynamic psychotherapy for SUDs, we first discuss issues concerning classification, diagnosis and prevalence, and the theoretical underpinnings, with a focus on affect regulation and the self-medication hypothesis (Khantzian & Albanese, 2008). Then we review empirical psychodynamic literature on the etiology of SUDs. We discuss research on ego functioning impairments in people with an SUD, focusing on defense mechanisms because defense mechanisms are the mental mechanisms most responsible for affect regulation (Cramer, 2002; Vaillant, 1993). We then discuss the two major treatment philosophies of SUD treatment—abstinence and harm reduction—and review the empirical research on psychodynamic approaches to treating SUDs, discussing the implications of the self-medication hypothesis for treatment. Next, we discuss how to conduct a psychodynamic diagnosis of SUDs and determine the suitability of psychodynamic treatment for SUDs. Finally, we provide a clinical vignette of psychodynamic treatment for SUD and discuss directions for future research.

CLASSIFICATION AND DIAGNOSIS

In DSM-5 (APA, 2013), the DSM-IV (APA, 2000) criteria for substance abuse and substance dependence have been combined into a single SUD defined in terms of a maladaptive pattern of substance use leading to clinically significant impairment or distress. SUDs are a severe public health problem (Coombs, 2005). In the United States alone, 20.6 million people over the age of 12 were deemed to be diagnosable with alcohol or substance dependence or abuse (Substance Abuse and Mental Health Services Administration, 2012). Furthermore, 18.9 million adults aged over 18 had an SUD, with an estimated 8 million of them meeting the criteria for a comorbid mental illness. Similarly, there were approximately 45 million adults aged 18 and older who had a diagnosable mental illness, of whom approximately 9 million have an SUD.

Treatment utilization among people with an SUD is poor. Although over 20 million people over 12 years of age have an SUD, the most recent research in 2011 found that slightly fewer than 4 million of them actually received treatment (Substance Abuse and Mental Health Services Administration, 2012). Nearly 6 million illicit drug users and 15.5 million alcohol users with a diagnosable SUD did not think (denied) they needed SUD treatment.

The magnitude of the SUD problem has led to a wide range of research and theories that attempt to explain why people develop an SUD and how SUDs should best be treated (see Mee-Lee & Gastfriend, 2008).

PSYCHODYNAMIC APPROACHES TO SUDs

All psychodynamic theories of the development and maintenance of SUDs posit that people abuse psychoactive drugs in order to reduce or eliminate pain and suffering (see Levin & Weiss, 1994; Yalisove, 1997). In "Civilization and Its Discontents," Freud (1930/1961) examined the purpose of human life, our need to prevent pain and to extend pleasure in our lives. The "unpleasurable sensations" are circumvented by intoxicating the self with substances, to "withdraw from the pressure of reality and find refuge in a world" (p. 23). Freud's emphasis on the influence of drives led Rado (1933) to stress the pleasurable and regressive states in SUDs. Although the brief pleasure is followed by suffering, "if the substance and the dose were well chosen, the first pharmacogenic pleasure-effect remains as a rule the most impressive event of its kind in the whole course of the illness" (Rado, 1933, p. 55). Rado also emphasized the significance of each type of substance and the corresponding psychological and pharmacological effects from using the substances. Analgesics, for example, ameliorated psychological pain, and stimulants enhanced and elevated the experience of pleasure. Similarly, Fenichel (1945) also emphasized substance abuse as a means of reducing the experience of pain. He wrote, "They still act as if any tension were dangerous trauma. Their actions are not directed (or are less directed) toward the positive aim of achieving a goal but rather more toward the negative aim of getting rid of tension; their aim is not pleasure but the discontinuance of pain. Any tension is felt as hunger was felt by the infant, that is, as a threat to his very existence" (p. 368).

The central premise that all psychodynamic SUD theories share thus involves the person's capacity to regulate affective experience (for compilations of primary readings of important psychodynamic papers on SUD, see Levin & Weiss, 1994; Shaffer & Burglass, 1981; Yalisove, 1997). Indeed, we view many psychodynamic theories that cover the topic of SUDs as fitting under the rubric of the self-medication hypothesis (Khantzian & Albanese, 2008; Suh, Ruffins, Robins, Albanese, & Khantzian, 2008). Deriving from developmental psychopathology, the self-medication hypothesis posits that problems in affect regulation predispose people to develop an SUD because taking psychoactive drugs enables a person to exert control over his or her affective experiences. In particular, psychoactive drugs enable people to regulate dysphoria.

Disorder of Emotional Functioning

During infancy, facilitated by responsive and supportive parental attachment figures, and the experience of attachment to consistent figures, people develop a capacity for self-organization and affect regulation (Fonagy & Target, 2003). Within the context of human relationships and successive parent–infant interactions, the infant learns to experience different aspects of his or her own internal world. Certain internal feeling states elicit recognition and responses by the environment, and these early experiences form psychological structures that are necessary for organizing internal feeling states (Greenspan, 1977). Such internal qualities during the early years are important, as they can be predictive of later psychopathologies (Caspi, Moffitt, Newman, & Silva, 1996), personalities (Caspi & Silva, 1995), and general health (Moffitt et al., 2011).

Based on empirical research, Fonagy and Target (2003) argued that this interpersonal experience helps develop a person's "mentalizing" capacities—that is, the ability to reflect on the relationship between the internal state and the physical reality, which contributes considerably to a person's understanding of the self as a mental agent. Through the interaction with "benign, reflective and sufficiently attuned" (Fonagy & Target, 2003, p. 271) caregivers, the child arrives at a conclusion that his or her feelings, beliefs, and wishes determine the caregiver's reactions, and so the child establishes a "core sense of selfhood." The child begins to consider the self as a regulating agent. Gradually, adequate doses of affect-regulating mirroring allow the child to distinguish between the internal world and the external one, and he or she experiences once-unmanageable feelings as indestructible of the outer world (Fonagy & Target, 2003). The child learns to modulate those previously overwhelming affects in the relationship.

When the intersubjective attunement between caregiver and child becomes incongruent or pathological, such affect mirroring can disrupt mentalizing, and the defects in affective capacity may manifest in the form of psychopathology. According to the framework proposed by Fonagy and Target (2003), the caregiver's misperception of the infant's emotion may bring about the child's internalization of misidentified primary emotional state and bring forth the subsequent experience of emptiness and false selfhood. Another possibility is that the caregiver's amplified attunement to the child's affective states may challenge the child's ability to undertake reflective functioning, which allows affect regulation to develop. The child's failure to engage in reflective functioning results in problems with affect regulation. Fonagy and Target suggested that these affect-regulating modes are the prelude to adult patients presenting narcissistic personality disorder and borderline personality disorder. Therefore, in the presence of environmental inconstancy, trauma, and neglect, major developmental flaws, defects, or distortions occur in character structure, such that emotional-regulatory mechanisms are dysfunctional (Treece & Khantzian, 1986). Insel (2003) argued that the drive for attachment occurs along the same neural pathways as the drive to engage in addictive behaviors, including substance abuse. Suchman and colleagues (Suchman, DeCoste, Castiglioni, Legow, & Mayes, 2008; Suchman, McMahon, Zhan, Mayes, & Luthar, 2006) have developed a treatment for substance-abusing mothers and their infants that is based on the idea that addictions are a form of attachment disorder (discussed later in this chapter).

Such an impairment in a person's ability to regulate feelings, to establish and maintain a healthy regard for one's self, and to care for one's self influences coping with inevitable life disappointments and tensions, tolerating distress, or finding relief from suffering. Brown (1993), illustrating the connection between affective development and psychopathology in a review of past empirical studies, concluded that adults with borderline personality organization experience intense affects but fail to modulate them. Among people with a neurotic level of personality organization, unacceptable or uncomfortable affects often remain unconscious through the successful use of defenses such as repression and dissociation. Kohut (1977) refers to these more serious impairments as "defects in the self" and hypothesized that psychoactive drug abuse is often used as a remedy for them.

The Self-Medication Hypothesis

The self-medication hypothesis maintains that people develop SUDs in order to cope with unbearable dysphoria that is borne from early and persistent problems with affect regulation (Khantzian & Albanese, 2008). Furthermore, specific types of psychoactive drugs are chosen because they help people regulate (and cope with) specific emotions (e.g., using opiates to cope with experiences of rage; Suh et al., 2008).

However, the most recent iteration of the self-medication hypothesis specifies neither the source of the substance abuser's dysphoria nor the reason for a person to experience difficulties coping with dysphoria. Dysphoria and the ability to cope with it could be caused by trauma, inborn ego deficits, unresolved intrapsychic conflicts, poor self-object relations and attachments, and psychopathology, or a combination of these (see also Director, 2002; Dodes, 2003; Gottdiener & Suh, 2012; Morgenstern & Leeds, 1993).

Furthermore, once a person becomes drug dependent, the reason for continued use becomes partly biologically motivated (Johnson, 2001). Drug dependence leads to alterations in the brain's neurochemistry, which in turn lead people to develop a new biological drive for drugs that is akin to the libidinal and aggressive drives. And, like libido and aggression, the "drug drive" must be gratified. One manifestation of the "drug drive" can be found in the dreams of sober former drug abusers who frequently dream about using drugs (Johnson, 2001). In this way, the drug dream, like any dream, enables the sober person to obtain drive gratification without having to relapse.

EMPIRICAL FINDINGS

The Self-Medication Hypothesis

Does research on the etiology of SUDs support the self-medication hypothesis? A number of longitudinal studies have found that people who later develop an SUD have early problems with affect regulation. Shedler and Block (1990) reported on a cohort of people who were followed from 3 to 18 years of age. They found that, as early as 3 years of age, children could display different abilities of ego control, defined as the sum total of mental processes (Block, 2002). Ego control in this view includes affect regulation and the behavior that ensues from it. Children who had poor ego control at age 3 were likely to have poor ego control as adolescents. Most importantly, those children who had poor ego control at age 3 and in adolescence were most likely to develop an SUD after they had experimented with drugs as adolescents, compared with children who had good ego control at age 3 and in adolescence. Adolescents who had good ego control were unlikely to develop an SUD after experimenting with drugs. Furthermore, parents of people who developed an SUD were observed to have poor-quality interactions with their children when the children were 5 years old.

Other longitudinal studies have found that adolescents who experience trauma that is diagnosable as posttraumatic stress disorder are also significantly more likely to develop an SUD as adults (Chilcoat & Menard, 2003). Additionally, people who develop an SUD manifest considerably greater use of immature defenses compared with those who do not develop an SUD (Bornstein, Gottdiener, & Winarick, 2010; Soldz & Vaillant, 1998). The use of immature and lower-level defense mechanisms is consistent with the finding that potential substance abusers have early problems with affect regulation because defense mechanisms are the mental mechanisms responsible for affect regulation. These empirical studies support the validity of the self-medication hypothesis and highlight the role of affect dysregulation in SUDs. Furthermore, the findings underscore the potential importance of identifying affect dysregulation at an early age. For example, it is possible that preventive interventions could be developed to help people who are at risk for SUDs.

Effects of SUDs on Ego Functioning

Once an SUD develops, how does being a substance abuser effect a person's ego functioning? Ego functioning, which can be defined as higher-order mental processes, object relations/attachments, and defense mechanisms (Akhtar, 2009), has been studied extensively in the psychoanalytic literature, and a sizeable body of research is beginning to accrue in addition to what has been observed clinically. The impact on ego functions requires careful consideration by clinicians who work with substance abusers. For example, assessing which ego functions are impaired and measuring to what degree ego functions change as a result of effective treatment would provide important means by which treatment progress and success could be measured.

Bellak, Hurvich, and Gediman (1973) operationalized the concept of ego functions in a semistructured clinical research interview and derived 12 functions, comprising: (1) reality testing, (2) judgment, (3) sense of reality of the world and of the self, (4) regulation and control of drives, affects, and impulses, (5) object relations, (6) thought processes, (7) adaptive regression in the service of the ego, (8) defensive functioning, (9) stimulus barrier, (10) autonomous functioning, (11) synthetic-integrative functioning, and (12) mastery-competence. A number of studies have been conducted using Bellak and colleagues' ego function assessment interview or the self-report version (Juni & Stack, 2005) in opiate- or stimulant-dependent adults receiving treatment for their SUD (Juni & Stack, 2005), while some studies have reported ego functions of active substance abusers (Milkman & Frosch, 1984). The results indicate that, compared with nonclinical controls, individuals with an SUD showed considerable problems with the 12 ego functions. Additionally, impaired ego functioning paradoxically may itself become a continued reason to abuse psychoactive drugs because intoxication helps people ignore their ego function impairments (Treece, 1984). Questions remain about ego function impairment in people who primarily abuse alcohol, hallucinogens, marijuana, nicotine, or other psychoactive substances. In addition, it is unclear whether SUDs result in long-term ego function impairment in people who become sober; findings in the neuropsychological literature are mixed (Verdejo-Garcia, Lopes-Torrecillas, Gimenez, & Perez-Garcia, 2004). Some research on ego function impairment suggests that people develop a drug of choice to cope with certain types of dysphoria (Milkman & Frosch, 1984), though research supports this conclusion inconsistently (Khantzian & Albanese, 2008). In sum, the literature demonstrates that preexisting problems in affect regulation may predispose individuals to develop SUDs and place them at risk. In addition, an SUD may exacerbate preexisting affect regulation problems by reducing the effectiveness of a person's overall ego functioning.

Self-Deception and Defense Mechanisms in SUDs

Given that people use psychoactive drugs as a way to cope with dysphoria, one goal of SUD treatment would involve helping patients cope with dysphoria more effectively.

The main mental processes used to help people cope with dysphoria are defense mechanisms, which serve to regulate affective experience, protect the self, and reduce the experience of dysphoria (Brenner, 1982; Cramer, 2006; Shapiro, 2000; Vaillant, 1993).

Defense mechanisms have their effects via self-deception (Shapiro, 2000). This is true of so-called immature, neurotic, and mature defense mechanisms (Vaillant, 1993). The smoker who continues to smoke after a laryngectomy (e.g., by placing a cigarette in the stoma in his or her throat to smoke) may use the immature defense of denial by ignoring the serious untoward consequences of smoking. In contrast, an alcoholic writer who could write only inconsistently when intoxicated and who then becomes sober and subsequently writes prolifically is able to do so because he or she suppresses the urge to get drunk, anticipates the consequences of relapsing, and sub-limates his or her desire for intoxication. He or she might be able to write prolifically by turning that desire for intoxication into a creation to be shared with the world; he or she uses mature defense mechanisms of anticipation, suppression, and sublimation (Cramer, 2006; Vaillant, 1993). In addition, patients diagnosed with alcoholism were found to use fewer immature defenses and more mature defenses after 6 weeks of treatment (O'Leary, Donovan, & Kasner, 1975). Thus, one goal of treatment might be to help patients exchange immature defense mechanisms for mature ones (Gottdie-ner, 2013).

PSYCHODYNAMIC TREATMENT OF SUDs

Treatment Principles

For clinicians unfamiliar with the treatment of people with SUDs, it is important to know that treatment is frequently classified into two disparate philosophical camps (Denning, 2004; Tatarsky, 2007). The first of these is considered the more traditional treatment, where abstinence is the immediate goal and sobriety is the only accept-able long-term treatment outcome; the second subscribes to harm reduction. The harm reduction perspective posits that the primary short- and long-term treatment goals should involve helping patients to reduce the potential harms that can occur to themselves and to the people and the environment with which they come into contact. Abstinence and sobriety are viewed as the best ways to reduce potential harms caused by an SUD and are considered germane to and included within the harm reduction treatment philosophy. Distinctive to a harm reduction perspective is the acceptance that immediate abstinence and long-term sobriety might not be possible for any one person and that relapse is the norm for people trying to overcome their SUD.

A harm reduction treatment philosophy is viable and practical when understand-ing (and treating) patients' SUDs from a psychodynamic view. Theoretically speak-ing, given that psychoactive drugs serve defensive purposes, the person will likely relapse because he or she will likely engage in behaviors that are associated with the use of immature defense mechanisms, unless the immature defense mechanism that is the underlying motivation for drug abuse changes and becomes substituted with a more mature one. New compromise formations (i.e., sobriety) can develop only if the underlying defense mechanisms become more mature. In addition, given that an

SUD patient has developed a new psychobiological drive for a drug, it is unrealistic to expect the person to abstain from wanting to gratify his or her drug drive without finding alternative means of gratification. Successful nondrug means of gratifying the drug drive require reduction in the strength of the drive coupled with the use of more mature defense mechanisms so that new compromise formations can be developed. We realize from clinical experience that the development of more mature defense mechanisms might actually be fostered by attempts to be abstinent and sober, although we know of no research that has been conducted to test this clinical observation.

Readers unfamiliar with the literature on the abstinence and harm reduction treatment philosophies should be aware that harm reduction has at times been portrayed as a permissive or carefree perspective on substance abuse. However, clinicians with a harm reduction perspective treat patients with considerable concern regarding how to help them diminish potential harm. The focus of a harm reduction treatment is directed toward how the patient is functioning in the immediate moment. The clinical focus is on how the patients are presenting rather than on talking and behaving in their sessions so that the therapist can help the patients reduce their self-estrangement and become more aware of their desire to use drugs to deny their problems. In addition, therapists frequently integrate focus on self-estrangement with psychoeducation about the potential harms caused by drug abuse (Tatarsky, 2007). When a patient comes for an initial consultation and states loudly and forcefully that "I have to stop drinking! I get nothing out of it!" it is clear that the patient is making a statement to convince him- or herself of something he or she does not believe. In this way, denial is evident because the patient is denying his or her own feelings and intentions in that immediate moment. When the therapist says to the patient that "*Having* to stop using and *getting nothing out* of using are different than *wanting* to stop using," the therapist is guiding the patient to examine his or her defenses. When the same patient says that he or she is as fit and healthy as ever despite drinking, the therapist tells the patient about the wide range of potential health problems that can occur, sometimes unintentionally, due to alcohol abuse, and discusses concrete ways of trying to reduce potential harms and improve the patient's health.

Empirical Research on Psychodynamic Treatments

The topic of harm reduction leads naturally to discussion of effective psychodynamic treatments for SUDs. As noted above, there has been considerable controversy in the psychoanalytic clinical literature regarding the appropriateness of psychodynamic psychotherapies for people with an SUD. Some members of the psychoanalytic community maintain that SUDs cannot be understood or treated psychoanalytically (Levin & Weiss, 1994). Despite the controversy, the results of the first generation of psychotherapy research were encouraging and found that psychodynamic psychotherapies helped improve the functioning of people with addictive disorders; this was consistent with the overall efficacy found for psychodynamic therapies (Smith, Glass, & Miller, 1980).

The modern era of psychotherapy research also finds that psychodynamic psychotherapy is efficacious for a wide range of psychological problems (Shedler, 2010;

see also Leichsenring, Kruse, & Rabung, Chapter 23, this volume) and has seen the development of a number of psychodynamic psychotherapies for SUDs. Although, to date, the number of randomized controlled clinical trials of psychodynamic psychotherapies for SUDs is modest, a small but growing body of empirical research on the efficacy of psychodynamic treatments for SUDs shows promising results and augurs for the further development of these treatments (Gottdiener, 2008; Woody, 2003). We are aware of three different psychodynamic treatments that have been manualized and tested in randomized controlled clinical trials. These interventions are supportive-expressive therapy (SET; Crits-Christoph et al., 2008; Luborsky & Luborsky, 2006); dynamic deconstructive psychotherapy (DDP; Gregory, DeLucia-Deranja, & Mogle, 2010; Gregory, Remen, Soderberg, & Ploutz-Snyder, 2009; Gregory et al., 2008), and combined psychiatric and addictive disorders treatment (COPAD; Rosenthal, 2002). Psychodynamic treatments in all of these studies produced significantly greater improvements in patients' function compared with the comparison treatments.

SET is an individual psychotherapy that has been assessed and shown to be effective for a wide range of psychological problems (Luborsky & Luborsky, 2006) including opiate and cocaine dependence. The results of these studies found that SET significantly reduces drug usage and improves a variety of areas of psychosocial functioning in opiate-dependent patients who simultaneously receive methadone maintenance therapy and adjunctive drug counseling, and in cocaine-dependent patients who also receive adjunctive drug counseling (Crits-Christoph et al., 2008; Woody, 2003).

DDP (Gregory et al., 2008, 2009, 2010) is an individual psychotherapy developed to treat people with borderline personality disorder and comorbid SUD. It has been found to significantly reduce both symptoms of borderline personality disorder and polysubstance abuse.

COPAD (Rosenthal, 2002) is a group psychotherapy that was developed to treat patients who have comorbid schizophrenia and SUDs. It is a supportive psychodynamic psychotherapy that combines group treatment with adjunctive psychosocial and psychiatric treatments. The results of research on COPAD showed significant reductions in patients' psychotic and SUD symptoms. As in the DDP research, participants in the COPAD study used a wide range of drugs.

A further treatment and prevention program called the Mothers and Toddlers Program (MTP) has been developed based on a psychodynamic model of developmental psychopathology (Suchman et al., 2006). MTP was designed to treat substance-abusing mothers who have children between 1 and 3 years of age (Suchman et al., 2008). The aim of MTP treatment is to foster the mothers' capacity to mentalize (Allen, 2003)—to better identify their children's psychological experiences—so that they can more accurately and effectively respond to their children. In this way, MTP serves double duty as a primary treatment for the parent and as a secondary prevention intervention for the child(ren). Parents who have a better ability to mentalize can in turn help their children develop good enough abilities to mentalize. MTP is thus derived from attachment and mentalizing theory. It is possible to view attachment theory as an organizing principle that draws together most, if not all, psychodynamic theories of SUD:

• People have drives for affiliation and attachment, which could be seen as a libidinal variant from ego psychology.

• The ability to develop strong, adaptive attachments leads to the development of a strong therapeutic alliance, which in turn helps patients develop the capacity to tolerate psychological pain and improves the functioning of their defense mechanisms.

• Mentalization is a complex process that involves mental images of self and other and the relationship between the two. This makes attachment theory part of object relations theories because attachment provides the impetus to form mental images of self and other. Along these lines, mentalization can be considered an ego function that is also the basis of self-object relations.

• If therapists view the data that occur (i.e., the transfer of information between patient and therapist) in the clinical situation as a function of the contributions of patient, therapist, and the experiences of both, then the degree to which each person becomes attached to the other will also determine the experiences of the people involved in the treatment, the theories derived from those treatments, and any new treatments or prevention programs that are developed.

• Like all psychodynamic treatments, the development of a strong therapeutic alliance between therapist and patient is essential. Moreover, the parent's strong relationship with the therapist becomes the model the mother uses to develop a strong relationship with her child(ren).

Research on MTP is relatively new, but the results are promising. To date, MTP has been compared with a parent education program (PEP) in which the focus of the intervention was educating parents in how to parent their children better (Suchman et al., 2010). Mothers in the MTP group improved considerably more than mothers in the PEP group on aspects of their mentalizing ability and their caregiving behavior toward their children. More research on this therapy is clearly needed.

The evidence from the above-mentioned studies indicates that psychodynamic psychotherapies may be useful in the treatment of individuals with various SUDs and may improve symptoms associated with severe comorbid psychiatric disorders. The available research evidence suggests that psychodynamic psychotherapy can help people with an SUD and that it is often best used in combination with other adjunctive psychosocial and/or psychiatric treatments, although the effective use of psychodynamic psychotherapy exclusively for the treatment of SUDs has been noted in a number of case studies (see Yalisove, 1997).

Psychodynamic Diagnosis of SUDs and Suitability for Psychodynamic Treatment

As noted above, the self-medication hypothesis posits that the main motive for abusing drugs is the reduction of dysphoria. Although drug abusers use drugs in an effort to improve their affective functioning, drug abuse creates considerable, well-known iatrogenic problems, including an increased likelihood of health problems and premature death. If dysphoria drives drug abuse, by implication, the focus of treatment for people with an SUD would be to reduce their dysphoria by helping them to resolve the conflicts and problems that create their unhappiness. As was the case with the manualized psychodynamic treatments discussed above, psychodynamic psychotherapy would focus on the whole person and not just on the person's drug abuse. In addition, because the sources of dysphoria can be complicated and complex, any adjunctive treatment required could be used to help patients get better.

When a patient comes for an initial consultation, the therapist may note the patient's drug preference because, according to the pharmacospecificity aspect of the self-medication hypothesis, the drug of choice might provide vital clues to the specific painful emotions with which the patient predominantly suffers. Khantzian, Halliday, and McAuliffe (1990) developed a modified psychodynamic psychotherapeutic approach that incorporates supportive, semistructured techniques. While engaging patients with empathy and reflective modes, the therapist allows the patient's inner experience and patterns of psychological defense to unfold. In this reflective space, the patient develops an understanding of his or her painful emotions and the maladaptive defenses involved in his or her SUD, which enables the patient to make changes in his or her behavioral patterns. The discovery of specific psychological and emotional qualities within each substance group can enhance understanding of the dynamics of a patient's SUD and assist the therapist in designing treatment interventions according to the patient's unique characteristics. Treatment goals would involve improving ego functions to ameliorate emotional suffering and/or to enable emotional expression to become less restrictive. A recovering alcohol-dependent patient who is alexithymic would benefit by learning to acknowledge and manage those emotions, hence, improving his or her affect regulation abilities.

The diagnosis of SUD is conducted using clinical interviews, psychological tests, and/or biological tests (Frances, Miller, & Mack, 2005). The diagnostic criteria based on the *Diagnostic and Statistical Manual of Mental Disorders, Fourthth Edition, Text Revision* (DSM-IV-TR; American Psychiatric Association, 2000) are used to assess the behavioral and physical symptoms of SUD. Psychodynamically oriented clinicians should supplement the DSM-IV-TR diagnosis with the criteria listed in the *Psychodynamic Diagnostic Manual* (PDM; PDM Task Force, 2006). The PDM diagnosis of "addictive/substance use disorders" is derived from the self-medication hypothesis and complements the DSM-IV-TR diagnostic criteria by enabling clinicians to gain a better understanding of the phenomenological experience of a person's SUD.

The clinician must decide whether a psychodynamic treatment is suitable for a patient once the diagnosis of SUD has been made. We believe that the range of supportive-expressive therapeutic techniques in psychodynamic treatments, congruent with the evidence reviewed above, is suitable for SUD patients at any level of treatment in various contexts from medical detoxification inpatient to outpatient private practice (Gottdiener, 2001). Research has found that although there are effective treatments for SUDs, no one treatment or set of placement criteria works for all patients (Mee-Lee & Gastfriend, 2008). Thus, clinicians must currently use their best clinical judgment when determining what type of treatment to use.

CLINICAL ILLUSTRATION

In the following case vignette, we aim to show one way in which a psychodynamic clinician can approach the treatment of a person with an SUD. The primary goal is to establish a therapeutic alliance. The secondary goal is to introduce the patient to himself—to his conflicts around his substance abuse—in the language of motivational interviewing, his ambivalence about whether or not to become involved in treatment and reduce his use or stop altogether.

The patient was a college-educated man in his mid-50s working in a professional field. He had experienced a severe life-threatening traumatic event several months before coming to see the therapist. Although only mildly injured physically, the patient was devastated emotionally.

Despite having no developmental history of trauma or even of substance use during adolescence, the patient became an alcoholic in his 20s from the stress of a painful romantic relationship. The patient eventually sought help. He went through alcohol detoxification, a one-month-long inpatient alcohol rehabilitation and then became intensely involved in Alcoholics Anonymous (AA) for 15 years. Although the patient reported that he had stopped attending AA meetings 10 years prior to the near-lethal traumatic event that brought him into therapy, he had not had a drink during that 10-year period. He came to treatment at this time, however, because he had begun to drink again, and to drink heavily.

The patient was casually dressed and appeared neat and clean at the initial consultation. He also appeared lucid but later told the therapist that he had drunk a six-pack of beer approximately 2 hours before coming to the session. It was clear that the discrepancy between the patient's self-report and his sober behavior meant that he was once again alcohol dependent. The patient said, in a matter-of-fact manner, that he drank too much, and then forcefully stated:

PATIENT: I have to stop! I'm weak! I'm pissing my life away from drinking. I need to get back to AA. Alcohol does nothing for me—it's just bad for my health. I gotta do what's right and the only reason I don't is because I'm a lazy bum.

THERAPIST: You sound like you're making a speech. I don't think you're lazy; I think you're just not that interested in stopping drinking. The negative consequences don't seem to outweigh whatever positive benefits you feel you get from the alcohol. If they did, you'd probably stop drinking. It seems that you want to drink and do so continuously.

PATIENT: That's crazy to want to continue drinking—look at all the problems it's creating for me.

THERAPIST: It might be crazy, but it makes sense that you would actually do what you want to do despite the negative consequences.

PATIENT: But I can't help myself. Once I have one drink I have another. I have to stop.

THERAPIST: Having to stop is not the same as wanting to stop. It seems to me that you disapprove of wanting to drink and even of the negative consequences of drinking, but that you want to continue drinking.

PATIENT: So, you're saying that the only way to stop drinking is for me to want to stop drinking?

THERAPIST: Yes.

PATIENT: I want to . . . I guess.

THERAPIST: You "guess"?

PATIENT: (*Smiles and chuckles.*) I do want to drink. I like it. I feel badly after I drink, but nothing helps me forget about the incident like getting drunk. At the same time, I know it's bad for my health and my girlfriend hates me for the way I've been. She's running out of patience and I'm missing work. Something's got to give. How do I stop, Doc? How do I stop myself from picking up the first drink?

THERAPIST: It might help if you actually accept that you want to drink; that you feel like you need a drink to deal with life.

PATIENT: But it's just a weakness.

THERAPIST: Calling it a weakness shows your disapproval of your desire to drink, but it doesn't change that there are times—a lot of times these days—that you want to drink.

PATIENT: (*now teary-eyed*) That's true. I hate myself for it. I used to be so good about not drinking—the pride of my friends and family in recovery—and now look at me. What a bum I've become. . . . I guess I should prepare myself for what's ahead. I know that you therapists like to tell us patients that we should be prepared to use drugs when we feel like crap. I guess I have to summon my willpower for the days ahead.

THERAPIST: Actually, I don't say that to patients, although I know some therapists do. I look at things a bit differently. As I just said, you'll use because you want to, but I think as you feel better—as you are more able to enjoy your life—to feel happier—that you'll be less interested in getting drunk and perhaps eventually not interested at all.

PATIENT: I like that, Doc. That makes sense.

The primary goal in this initial part of the consultation using an open-ended interview style (Miller & Rollnick, 2002) was to establish a therapeutic alliance by empathizing with the patient's difficulties and to begin to introduce to the patient those aspects of himself and attitudes that he wants to avoid knowing (Shapiro, 1989). The focus is on establishing a sound therapeutic alliance because empirical research and clinical observation have found that the quality of the therapeutic alliance is a good predictor of psychotherapy outcome (Horvath & Symonds, 1991). Along these lines, notice that the therapist is not urging the patient to join AA, attend inpatient rehabilitation, go through a detoxification program, or take Antabuse. Although the therapist later asks the patient if he is interested in using these treatment adjuncts, the patient declines.

The above transcript is the initial part of the first session of what became a 2-year treatment. After the initial consultation, the patient returned and reliably came to psychotherapy three times per week. In addition, the therapist suggested that the patient invite an individual whom he trusted to one session per week, in order for the patient to feel more supported in his attempts to cope with his problems. The patient brought his girlfriend into sessions weekly thereafter. The use of a collateral helper to help a patient is formally called network therapy (Galanter, 1999). The person or people in the network also serve as links between the patient and therapist so that they can contact the therapist if problems arise outside of the session and to discuss problems in their weekly session that arose during the previous week.

In addition to the network therapy, the patient also eventually attended a 3-month-long recovery group for traumatized substance abusers. The patient never returned to AA. During the 2-year treatment, the patient went from drinking one six-pack of beer per day to four six-packs of beer per day, including a six-pack that he drank just to quiet his trauma-induced night terrors. Nonetheless, as the patient gained greater connection with his emotions and continued to reduce his self-estrangement, he found himself naturally drinking less and began to realize that he had less interest in getting drunk. By the end of his 2-year treatment, he was drinking one beer per night only three or so days per week. By the end of his treatment, the patient had not gotten drunk in nearly 6 months.

This clinical example demonstrates that psychodynamic psychotherapy may reduce the need for "self-medication" by helping people to become less self-estranged and hence enhance their affect regulation functioning. In addition, the therapist in the vignette viewed individual psychodynamic psychotherapy as the core of treatment but freely incorporated a social network and a short-term trauma group into the treatment. The therapist incorporated what would traditionally be considered insight-oriented and supportive therapeutic interventions into the patient's treatment (see Luborsky & Luborsky, 2006; Rockland, 1989). The clinical example is consistent with the treatment recommendations made by Khantzian and Albanese (2008), which state that for successful treatment, the development of a strong therapeutic alliance is essential; the therapist should view the patient as any other patient; the substance abuse is not a moral failure; and the therapist should be technically flexible in the treatment that is offered; furthermore, psychotherapy with substance abusers is complex and complete cure in the form of sobriety is often not realistic.

CONCLUSIONS AND FUTURE DIRECTIONS

The self-medication hypothesis posits that people abuse psychoactive drugs to help them cope with dysphoria. Research supports the general tenets of the self-medication hypothesis. There is, however, equivocal empirical support for the "drug of choice" aspect, and it is unclear from empirical research whether people choose specific classes of drugs because those drugs help users cope more effectively with certain classes of emotions.

Research on the effects of SUDs on ego functions is limited; not all ego functions in people with an SUD have been studied thoroughly. Nonetheless, the extant research shows that the majority of ego functions are greatly impaired in people with an SUD compared with nonclinical controls. The long-term effects of most psychoactive drugs of abuse on ego functioning remain understudied and unknown, although recent neuropsychological research has found that alcohol abuse leads to long-term cognitive impairments in many alcohol abusers (Moselhy, Georgiou, & Kahn, 2001; Verdejo-Garcia, Lopes-Torrecillas, Gimenez, & Perez-Garcia, 2004).

A number of manualized psychodynamic psychotherapies for SUDs have been tested in randomized controlled clinical trials. All the studies of these treatments show that psychodynamic psychotherapies can be considerably helpful to people with an SUD. However, this body of research is small, and more research needs to be done to further determine for whom, and under what conditions, psychodynamic treatments help patients with SUDs. Nonetheless, the available research, along with clinical experience, should enable therapists to feel confident that a psychodynamic approach can help patients with an SUD and that treatment of patients with an SUD uses the same supportive-expressive psychodynamic interventions used for the treatment of all patients. Indeed, the technical flexibility that psychodynamic psychotherapy provides allows for its use in a wide range of clinical settings (Gottdiener, 2001).

Our main aim in this chapter has been to demonstrate psychodynamic theories and concepts in SUDs. In addition, we wanted to convey the extent of the SUD problem to psychodynamic clinicians; to discuss the self-medication hypothesis of SUD and summarize its research base; to present research findings on the psychodynamics of SUD psychopathology and on results of randomized controlled clinical trials of psychodynamic psychotherapies for SUDs; and to show how a psychodynamic clinician might engage a substance abuser in psychodynamic psychotherapy during the initial consultation. We hope to stimulate new research on the psychodynamics of SUD psychopathology and the development of research on psychodynamic treatments for SUDs. Most of all, we hope to encourage clinicians to engage substance-abusing patients in psychodynamic treatments because psychodynamic psychotherapy can help them.

REFERENCES

Akhtar, S. (2009). *Comprehensive dictionary of psychoanalysis*. London: Karnac.

Allen, J. G. (2003). Mentalizing. *Bulletin of the Menninger Clinic, 67*, 91–112.

American Psychiatric Association (2000). *Diagnostic and statistical manual of mental disorders* (4th ed., text rev.). Washington, DC: Author.

American Psychiatric Association. (2013). *Diagnostic and statistical manual of mental disorders* (5th ed.). Arlington, VA: Author.

Bellak, L., Hurvich, M., & Gediman, H. K. (1973). *Ego functions in schizophrenics, neurotics, and normals: A systematic study of conceptual, diagnostic, and therapeutic aspects*. New York: Wiley.

Block, J. (2002). *Personality as an affect-processing system: Toward an integrative theory.* Mahwah, NJ: Erlbaum.

Bornstein, R. F., Gottdiener, W. H., & Winarick, D. J. (2010). Construct validity of the Relationship Profile Test: Links with defense style in substance abuse patients and comparison with non-clinical norms. *Journal of Psychopathology and Behavioral Assessment, 32,* 293–300.

Brenner, C. (1982). *The mind in conflict.* New York: International Universities Press.

Brown, D. (1993). Affective development, psychopathology, and adaptation. In S. L. Ablon, D. Brown, E. J. Khantzian, & J. E. Mack (Eds.), *Human feelings: Explorations in affect development and meaning* (pp. 5–66). Hillsdale, NJ: Analytic Press.

Caspi, A., Moffitt, T. E., Newman, D. L., & Silva, P. A. (1996). Behavioral observations at age 3 years predict adult psychiatric disorders. *Archives of General Psychiatry, 53,* 1033–1039.

Caspi, A., & Silva, P. A. (1995). Temperamental qualities at age three predict personality traits in young adulthood: Longitudinal evidence from a birth cohort. *Child Development, 66,* 486–498.

Chilcoat, H. D., & Menard, C. (2003). Epidemiological investigations: Comorbidity of posttraumatic stress disorder and substance use disorder. In P. Ouimette & P. J. Brown (Eds.), *Trauma and substance abuse: Causes, consequences, and treatment of comorbid disorders* (pp. 9–28). Washington, DC: American Psychological Association.

Coombs, R. H. (2005). *Addiction counseling review: Preparing for comprehensive, certification, and licensing examinations.* Mahwah, NJ: Erlbaum.

Cramer, P. (2006). *Protecting the self: Defense mechanisms in action.* New York: Guilford Press.

Crits-Christoph, P., Connolly-Gibbons, M. B. Gallop, R., Ring-Kurtz, S., Barber, J. P., Worley, M., et al. (2008). Supportive-expressive psychodynamic therapy for cocaine dependence: A closer look. *Psychoanalytic Psychology, 25,* 483–498.

Denning, P. (2004). *Practicing harm reduction psychotherapy: An alternative approach to addictions.* New York: Guilford Press.

Director, L. (2002). The value of relational psychoanalysis in the treatment of chronic drug and alcohol use. *Psychoanalytic Dialogues, 12,* 551–579.

Dodes, L. M. (2003). *The heart of addiction.* New York: HarperCollins.

Fenichel, O. (1945). *The psychoanalytic theory of neurosis.* New York: Norton.

Fonagy, P., & Target, M. (2003). *Psychoanalytic theories. Perspectives from developmental psychopathology.* New York: Brunner-Routledge.

Frances, R. J., Miller, S. I., & Mack, A. H. (2005). *Clinical textbook of addictive disorders* (3rd ed.). New York: Guilford Press.

Freud, S. (1961). *Civilization and its discontents.* London: Hogarth Press. (Original work published 1930)

Galanter, M. (1999). *Network therapy for alcohol and drug abuse.* New York: Guilford Press.

Gottdiener, W. H. (2001). The utility of individual supportive psychodynamic psychotherapy for substance abusers in a therapeutic community. *Journal of the American Academy of Psychoanalysis, 29,* 469–481.

Gottdiener, W. H. (2008). Introduction to symposium of psychoanalytic research on substance use disorders. *Psychoanalytic Psychology, 25,* 458–460.

Gottdiener, W. H. (2013). Assimilative dynamic addiction psychotherapy. *Journal of Psychotherapy Integration, 23,* 39–48.

Gottdiener, W. H., & Suh, J. J. (2012). Expanding the single-case study: A proposed psychoanalytic research program. *Psychoanalytic Review, 99,* 81–102.

Greenspan, S. I. (1977). Substance abuse: an understanding from psychoanalytic developmental and learning perspectives. In J. D. Blaine & D. A. Julius (Eds.), *Psychodynamics of drug dependence* (pp. 73–87). Northvale, NJ: Jason Aronson.

Gregory, R. J., Chlebowski, S., Kang, D., Remen, A. L., Soderberg, M. G., Stepkovitch, J., et al. (2008). A controlled trial of psychodynamic psychotherapy for co-occurring borderline personality disorder and alcohol use disorder. *Psychotherapy: Theory, Research, Practice, Training, 45,* 28–41.

Gregory, R. J., DeLucia-Deranja, E., & Mogle, J. A. (2010). Dynamic deconstructive psycho-therapy versus optimized community care for borderline personality disorder co-occurring with alcohol use disorders: A 30-month follow-up. *Journal of Nervous and Mental Disease, 198,* 292–298.

Gregory, R. J., Remen, A. L., Soderberg, M., & Ploutz-Snyder, R. J. (2009). A controlled trial of psychodynamic psychotherapy for co-occurring borderline personality disorder and alcohol use disorder: Six-month outcome. *Journal of the American Psychoanalytic Association, 57,* 199–205.

Horvath, A. O., & Symonds, B. D. (1991). Relation between working alliance and outcome in psychotherapy: A meta-analysis. *Journal of Counseling Psychology, 38,* 139–149.

Insel, T. R. (2003). Is social attachment an addictive disorder? *Physiology and Behavior, 79,* 351–357.

Johnson, B. (2001). Drug dreams: A neuropsychoanalytic hypothesis. *Journal of the American Psychoanalytic Association, 49,* 75–96.

Juni, S., & Stack, J. E. (2005). Ego function as a correlate of addiction. *American Journal on Addictions, 14,* 83–93.

Khantzian, E. J., & Albanese, M. J. (2008). *Understanding addiction as self-medication: Finding hope behind the pain.* New York: Rowman & Littlefield.

Khantzian, E. J., Halliday, K. S., & McAuliffe, W. E. (1990). *Addiction and the vulnerable self: Modified dynamic group therapy for substance abusers.* New York: Guilford Press.

Kohut, H. (1977). Preface. In J. D. Blaine & D. A. Julius (Eds.), *Psychodynamics of drug dependence* (pp. vii–ix). Northvale, NJ: Jason Aronson.

Levin, J. D., & Weiss, R. H. (1994). *The dynamics and treatment of alcoholism: Essential papers.* Northvale, NJ: Jason Aronson.

Luborsky, L., & Luborsky, E. (2006). *Research and psychotherapy: The vital link.* Lanham, MD: Jason Aronson.

Mee-Lee, D., & Gastfriend, D. R. (2008). Patient placement criteria. In M. Galanter & H. D. Kleber (Eds.), *The American Psychiatric Publishing textbook of substance abuse treatment* (4th ed.). Arlington, VA: American Psychiatric Publishing.

Milkman, H., & Frosch, W. A. (1984). The drug of choice. In L. Bellak & L. A. Goldsmith (Eds.), *The broad scope of ego function assessment* (pp. 251–267). New York: Wiley.

Miller, W. R., & Rollnick, S. (2002). *Motivational interviewing: Preparing people for change* (2nd ed.). New York: Guilford Press.

Moffitt, T. E., Arseneault, L., Belsky, D., Dickson, N., Hancox, R. J., Harrington, H., et al. (2011). A gradient of childhood self-control predicts health, wealth, and public safety. *Proceedings of the National Academy of Sciences of the United States of America, 108,* 2693–2698.

Morgenstern, J., & Leeds, J. (1993). Contemporary psychoanalytic theories of substance abuse: A disorder in search of a paradigm. *Psychotherapy, 30,* 194–206.

Moselhy, H. F., Georgiou, G., & Kahn, A. (2001). Frontal lobe changes in alcoholism: A review of the literature. *Alcohol and Alcoholism, 36,* 357–368.

O'Leary, M. R., Donovan, D. M., & Kasner, K. H. (1975). Shifts in perceptual differentiation and defense mechanisms in alcoholics. *Journal of Clinical Psychology, 31,* 565–567.

Orlinsky D. E., Ronnestad, M. H., Willutzki., U., Wiseman, H., Botermans, J-F., & SPR Collaborative Research Network. (2005). The prevalence and parameters of personal therapy in Europe and elsewhere. In J. D. Geller, J. C. Norcross, D. E. Orlinsky (Eds.), *The therapist's own psychotherapy: Patient and clinician perspectives* (pp. 177–191). New York: Oxford University Press.

PDM Task Force. (2006). *Psychodynamic diagnostic manual.* Silver Spring, MD: Alliance of Psychoanalytic Organizations.

Rado, S. (1933). The psychoanalysis of pharmacothymia (drug addiction). *Psychoanalytic Quarterly, 2,* 1–23.

Rockland, L. (1989). *Supportive psychotherapy: A psychodynamic approach.* New York: Basic Books.

Rosenthal, R. N. (2002). Group treatment for patients with substance abuse and schizophrenia. In D. W. Brook & H. I. Spitz (Eds.), *The group therapy of substance abuse* (pp. 327–349). New York: Haworth.

Shaffer, H., & Burglass, M. E. (1981). Classic contributions in the addictions. New York: Brunner/Mazel.

Shapiro, D. (1989). *Psychotherapy of neurotic character.* New York: Basic Books.

Shapiro, D. (2000). *Dynamics of character: Self-regulation in psychopathology.* New York: Basic Books.

Shedler, J. (2010). The efficacy of psychodynamic psychotherapy. *American Psychologist, 65,* 98–109.

Shedler, J., & Block, J. (1990). Adolescent drug use and psychological health: A longitudinal inquiry. *American Psychologist, 45,* 612–630.

Smith, M. L., Glass, G. V., & Miller, T. I. (1980). *The benefits of psychotherapy.* Baltimore: Johns Hopkins University Press.

Soldz, S., & Vaillant, G. E. (1998). A 50-year longitudinal study of defense use among inner city men: A validation of the DSM-IV defense axis. *Journal of Nervous and Mental Disease, 186,* 104–111.

Substance Abuse and Mental Health Services Administration. (2012). *Results from the 2011 National Survey on Drug Use and Health: Mental Health Findings.* NSDUH Series H-45, HHS Publication No. (SMA) 12-4725. Rockville, MD: Substance Abuse and Mental Health Services Administration.

Suchman, N. E., DeCoste, C., Castiglioni, N., Legow, N., & Mayes, L. C. (2008). The Mothers and Toddlers Program: Preliminary findings from an attachment-based parenting intervention for substance abusing mothers. *Psychoanalytic Psychology, 25,* 499–517.

Suchman, N., DeCoste, C., Castiglioni, N., McMahon, T., Rounsaville, B., & Mayes, L. (2010). The Mothers and Toddlers Program: An attachment-based parenting intervention for substance-using women: Post-treatment results from a randomized clinical trial. *Attachment and Human Development, 12,* 483–504.

Suchman, N. E., McMahon, T. J., Zhan, H., Mayes, L. C., & Luthar, S. (2006). Substance abusing mothers and disruptions in child custody: An attachment perspective. *Journal of Substance Abuse Treatment, 30,* 197–204.

Suh, J. J., Ruffins, S., Robins, C. E., Albanese, M. J., & Khantzian, E. J. (2008). Self-medication hypothesis: connecting affective experience and drug choice. *Psychoanalytic Psychology, 25,* 518–532.

Tatarsky, A. (2007). *Harm reduction psychotherapy: A new treatment for drug and alcohol problems.* New York: Jason Aronson.

Treece, C. (1984). Assessment of ego function in studies of narcotic addiction. In L. Bellak & L. A. Goldsmith (Eds.), *The broad scope of ego function assessment* (pp. 268–291). New York: Wiley.

Treece, C., & Khantzian, E. J. (1986). Psychodynamic factors in the development of drug dependence. *Psychiatric Clinics of North America, 9,* 399–412.

Vaillant, G. E. (1993). *The wisdom of the ego.* Boston: Harvard University Press.

Verdejo-Garcia, A., Lopes-Torrecillas, F., Gimenez, C. O., & Perez-Garcia, M. (2004). Clinical implications and methodological challenges in the study of the neuropsychological correlates of cannabis, stimulants, and opioid abuse. *Neuropsychology Review, 14,* 1–41.

Woody, G. E. (2003). Research findings on psychotherapy of addictive disorders. *American Journal on Addictions, 12,* S19–S26.

Yalisove, D. (1997). *Essential papers on addictions.* New York: New York University Press.

CHAPTER 12

Eating Disorders

Heather Thompson-Brenner and Lauren K. Richards

This chapter reviews clinical and research data concerning object relations, developmental history, and identity development in patients with eating disorders (EDs). We also focus on alternative classification schemes suggested by research in personality and in affect, and include research regarding object relations and family/developmental history specifically as it pertains to these proposed classification schemes. Classification systems based specifically on object relations functioning and developmental history have not been investigated to date. We also present two clinical vignettes to illustrate a psychodynamic approach to EDs and discuss directions for future research.

CLASSIFICATION AND DIAGNOSIS

Important changes have been made in the classification of EDs. The *Diagnostic and Statistical Manual of Mental Disorders, Fourth Edition, Text Revision* (DSM-IV-TR) ED classification system included two major diagnoses, anorexia nervosa (AN) and bulimia nervosa (BN), as well as the diagnosis of eating disorder not otherwise specified (EDNOS) (American Psychiatric Association [APA], 2000). Additionally, an appendix provided provisional criteria for binge-eating disorder (BED) (i.e., recurrent binge eating without compensatory behavior), a subcategory of EDNOS. These EDs share the distinctive cognitive feature of overconcern with shape, weight, or eating, to a degree that is subjectively distressing and interferes with functioning. The diagnosis of AN included the criteria of weight deliberately maintained below 85% of the ideal for one's height and among women loss of menses. AN had two subtypes: The "restricting" subtype, which includes individuals who are of low weight through restricting caloric intake and exercising, and the "binge/purge" sub-type, which includes those who also binge or purge regularly. BN is characterized by weight above the AN threshold and regular binge eating and purging by vomiting or other compensatory measures, such as driven exercise, fasting, and use of diuretics or laxatives. BN also had two subtypes: The "purging" subtype, which includes those who compensate by vomiting and/or laxative or diuretic use, and the "nonpurging" subtype, which includes those who compensate by fasting or exercising. In addition to BED, EDNOS included other combinations of symptoms currently under investi-gation, such as "chewing and spitting," purging disorder, and night eating syndrome, as well as subthreshold conditions that are significantly distressing and impairing.

The need for changes in the ED classification system has been extensively dis-cussed, quite publicly, among ED researchers (Attia et al., 2009; Frampton, 2010), but has focused to date on the empirical support for the specific cognitive and behavioral symptom-based classification system, as well as the empirical support for the addition of new categories based on related cognitive and behavioral symptoms. A burgeon-ing number of publications and presentations include data from latent class analyses and other methods of grouping individuals with EDs. However, the most influential of these studies (e.g., Clinton & Norring, 2005; Eddy et al., 2010; Sloan, Mizes, & Epstein, 2005) have been based on the positive presence of the symptoms/criteria already included in DSM-IV-TR, as opposed to alternative constructs of interest to psychodynamic classification.

Perhaps the largest problem with the criteria for EDs in DSM-IV-TR is the very large number of EDNOS diagnoses in clinical settings. Over half of individuals seek-ing treatment for EDs are given a diagnosis of EDNOS according to DMS-IV-TR (e.g., Eddy, Celio Doyle, Hoste, Herzog, & Le Grange, 2008), although those indi-viduals do not differ significantly from those who meet full threshold diagnostic criteria (Keel, Brown, Holm-Denoma, & Bodell, 2011). This is largely due to the heterogeneity of this category. Other issues concern the clinical utility of the criteria for established ED diagnoses. For example, there is a lack of empirical support for the clinical utility of the loss of menses criterion in AN (Attia & Roberto, 2009), and it has been consistently argued that the low weight criterion (i.e., < 85% of expected bodyweight) is arbitrary and difficult to define. Furthermore, the language describing motivations for low weight AN (i.e., "refusal to maintain weight") requires inference about the patient's emotions and is unclear. With respect to BN and BED, the largest issue is the frequency threshold of twice-weekly binge and/or purging episodes, as individuals meeting this threshold do not differ significantly on measures of impair-ment or distress from those who binge and/or purge less frequently (e.g., Wilson & Sysko, 2009).

In response, the APA's DSM-5 (2013) has made several changes to the ED diag-nostic system. The Eating Disorders Workgroup utilized targeted literature reviews, data analyses, and professional feedback in order to revise the current criteria to address these issues. While more detailed reviews of these proposed changes can be found elsewhere (Keel, Brown, Holland, & Bodell, 2011; Sysko et al., 2012), some major changes include adding BED as a formal diagnosis, making the language describing the motivations and thresholds for low weight in AN clearer; eliminating the criterion of loss of menses; eliminating the "nonpurging" category of BN; and including more specific syndromes within the current EDNOS category, such as sub-threshold AN, BN, and BED (Attia et al., 2009; Frampton, 2010).

Concurrent with the extensive public review of the cognitive and behavioral symptom-based classification system, important progress has been made in several areas of ED research that are more relevant to psychodynamic constructs and theories of classification. Convergent research indicates patterned heterogeneity in several other areas that ED clinicians and researchers increasingly take into account in clinical decision making. These areas, which we review in this chapter, include (1) research concerning patterned variation in personality styles; (2) research demonstrating the importance of differences in attachment style among individuals with EDs; and (3) within-group variation in characteristic patterns of affective experience and affect regulation. In each area of research—personality, attachment, and affect—early investigations attempted to demonstrate that individuals with EDs as a group differed from normal and clinical controls on the variables of interest, or that individuals with AN differed from those with BN. However, in each case it was noted that substantial within-group variation occurred among individuals with EDs, with some showing personality functioning, attachment style, and affective experience more akin to those of normal controls, excepting the presence of distress associated with the ED, while others showed consistent but varying patterns of more severe and chronic distress. It became apparent that the DSM diagnoses were not sensitive enough to capture additional dimensions of psychopathology crucial to treatment of ED symptoms. Furthermore, it was noted that the same core symptoms—dietary restriction, binge eating, and compensation—might serve different functions based on the personality style or affect-regulation needs of the individual employing the symptom (e.g., Westen & Harnden-Fischer, 2001). Therefore, efforts to create meaningful and useful categories within the population with EDs have resulted and are reviewed here.

PSYCHODYNAMIC APPROACHES TO EDs

Coherent theories regarding the underpinnings of ED symptoms are somewhat more recent than those of other diagnostic categories, given that EDs—particularly BN and variants of EDNOS—were identified as common psychological clinical syndromes more recently than other general categories such as anxiety and depression. Clinicians such as Hilde Bruch (1962), Selvini Palazzoli (1965, 1974), and Salvador Minuchin (Minuchin, Rosman, & Baker, 1978) aggregated their clinical observations and developed theories that were discussed and tested by psychological researchers in the 1970s. However, early theory and research were largely based on comparisons between individuals with EDs and those without EDs, or between those with AN and those with BN, in the effort to find patterns of personality, affect, development, and object relations that explained symptom expression for each diagnostic group. These theories and related research are still influential and inform the research conducted more recently in these areas.

Personality and Defensive Functioning

Some of the earliest psychoanalytic formulations of AN in the 1940s and 1950s interpreted emaciation in accordance with the conflict/drive theories of the time—for
example, rejection of the mature female figure due to conflicts over feminine sexuality
(e.g., Waller, Kaufman, & Deutsch, 1940). Although these conceptualizations were
meaningful to some patients—and some research established evidence for aspects of
these conflicts, for example, in the "maturity fears" subscale of the popular Eating
Disorders Inventory (Garner, Olmstead, & Polivy, 1983)—developments in psychoanalytic ego psychology and academic personality psychology soon led to emphasis
on particular personality traits and defensive functioning common among individuals with particular eating symptoms (see Kernberg, 1980; Steiger & Bruce, 2004).
Individuals with primarily restricting symptoms were noted to have rigid, obsessional, and avoidant defenses (Norman, Blais, & Herzog, 1993), as well as elevated
conscientiousness and emotional inhibition (Casper, Hedeker, & McClough, 1992).
Conversely, individuals with binge/purge traits were noted to have more impulsive,
self-destructive, externalizing, and histrionic traits (e.g., Mitchell, Hatsukami, Pyle,
& Eckert, 1986; see Lilenfeld, Wonderlich, Riso, Crosby, & Mitchell, 2006, for a
review).

Affective Experience and Affect Regulation

Food restriction, binge eating, and purging have long been thought to serve affect-
regulatory purposes (e.g., Herman & Polivy, 1975). Restriction has been theorized to
suppress or avoid affective experience, and alexithymia—associated with the avoidant, rigid, and obsessional defenses noted above—has been frequently described as
a characteristic of individuals with restricting symptoms (Halmi, 1974; Vitousek &
Manke, 1994). Early affect-regulatory theories posited that that negative affect triggers binge eating among dieters, and purging represents an effort to escape the consequent negative emotions following binge eating (Herman & Polivy, 1975). Other
approaches emphasize possible self-regulatory functions of disordered eating, such
as modulation of negative affect or self-soothing (e.g., Esplen, Garfinkel, & Gallop,
2000; Ogden & Wardle, 1991). Alternative theories suggest that disordered eating
may also distract an individual from her worries or mask her distress by giving her
something more tangible and specific to worry about than the initial source of her
distress (see Polivy, Herman, & McFarlane, 1994, for a review). Another theory suggests that concentrating on ingesting large amounts of food may serve as a means of
escape from experiencing the aversive self-awareness brought on by negative mood
states (Heatherton & Baumeister, 1991; Schupak-Neuberg & Nemeroff, 1993).

Object Relations: Family History and Identity

Extensive early theory also focused on competing conceptualizations of object relations functioning characteristic of individuals with EDs. However, within-group differences in object relations and identity have not been typically focused on as the

possible bases for classification schemes. Early observers of self–other processes in AN posited that the central dynamic in AN was a struggle in which the body had been invested with the negative attributes of the maternal object, who was overwhelming and needed to be held in check (Palazzoli, 1965, 1974). Furthermore, overly controlling and intrusive mothers were thought to produce a core sense of helplessness and ineffectiveness in the child (Palazzoli, 1965, 1974). Minuchin and colleagues (1978) observed extreme enmeshment, overprotection, conflict avoidance, and rigidity in families with children with AN, contributing to the maintenance and expression of the disorder. Hilde Bruch also described AN as a developmental problem in which the child failed to individuate and became arrested (or regressed) in a childlike dependency (Bruch, 1978, 1982). Early feeding problems, as well as family styles characterized by enmeshment, high levels of expressed emotion (or criticism), and low levels of warmth were often observed (see Hodes & Le Grange, 1993; Treasure et al., 2008, for a review).

It has been posited that parents may contribute to the development of ED symptoms in children through disrupted attachment (see Ward, Ramsay, & Treasure, 2000), modeling of disordered eating and related attitudes (see Rodgers & Chabrol, 2009), and direct communication regarding the importance of thinness, achievement, perfection, or self-control (Kiang & Harter, 2006). Sexual abuse has long been thought to show relationships to EDs. It has been repeatedly cited as one possible etiological factor in the development of ED symptoms, which may be mediated through low self-esteem, intense negative affect, borderline personality disorder, poor maternal relationships, or other related issues (Everill & Waller, 1995; Wonderlich et al., 2001).

Theorists and clinicians have also identified impoverished sense of identity as an important aspect of object relations among individuals with EDs. Clinicians suggested that patterns of enmeshment, together with difficulty with adolescent individuation, resulted in a lack of a "core" to the child's personality (Bruch, 1978) and a limited set of tools for self-evaluation (Bruch, 1982). Researchers in past decades have focused on a definition of identity disturbance that emphasizes a negative self-concept and elevated self-criticism, relating these problems to the lack of a positive self-representation, an expression of dissatisfaction with the self, and ED behaviors (e.g., Schupack-Neuberg & Nemeroff, 1993). More recently, popular books by clinicians and memoirists have provided descriptions of recovery from EDs that emphasize the development of a sense of self that is separate from the expectations of others, distinct from achievement, and based on an awareness of emotions and desires (e.g., Liu, 2007; Reindl, 2001).

EMPIRICAL FINDINGS

Substantial research has concerned attempts to classify individuals with EDs on the basis of within-group heterogeneity in three overlapping domains: personality style, attachment style, and affective experience/affect regulation. Two major new systems have emerged, each with substantial statistical support—one based on grouping individuals by their personality style and the other based on grouping individuals by the presence or absence of intense negative affect. Each system has amassed evidence suggesting that the subtyping schemes are supported statistically and show indications of validity as a classification system, as evidenced by patterned associations to adaptive functioning, comorbidity, treatment outcome, and long-term course. A smaller set of studies has indicated that attachment style may be an important aspect of personality, predicting treatment response and important clinical process variables such as treatment alliance and reflective functioning (e.g., Skårderud, 2007a, 2007b, 2007c; Tasca et al., 2006; Tasca, Ritchey, & Balfour, 2011). Although the simple presence of intense negative affect is the base of mainstream research efforts to establish subtypes among EDs, a smaller set of preliminary data has been collected using a more multifaceted and psychodynamically informed measure of affect, the Affect Regulation and Experience Q-sort (AREQ; Westen, Muderrisoglu, Fowler, Shedler, & Koren, 1997). Preliminary efforts to group individuals with EDs according to within-group heterogeneity on this measure have yielded intriguing results in need of additional research support.

Personality and Defensive Functioning

As an alternative to cluster analyses including the behavioral and cognitive symptoms already emphasized in DSM-5, a separate set of studies has clustered individuals with mixed ED symptoms on the basis of their personality traits (see also Thompson-Brenner, Weingeroff, & Westen, 2009, for an additional review). The majority of these studies have identified three types, but some studies have identified three to five types, each of which may include individuals with any of the ED diagnoses. Research has consistently suggested the presence of a *high-functioning* type, with minimal personality pathology and mature defenses; an *emotionally dysregulated* type, with borderline and histrionic tendencies (e.g., emotional instability); an *avoidant-insecure* type, with anxious, depressed, and socially avoidant tendencies; and a *constricted-obsessional* type, with obsessional, compulsive, and rigid defenses (Espelage, Mazzeo, Sherman, & Thompson, 2002; Goldner, Srikameswaran, Schroeder, Livesley, & Birmingham, 1999; Thompson-Brenner, Eddy, Franko, et al., 2008; Thompson-Brenner, Eddy, Satir, Boisseau, & Westen, 2008; Thompson-Brenner & Westen, 2005; Westen & Harnden-Fischer, 2001; Wonderlich et al., 2005). In addition, two studies found a *behaviorally dysregulated* type, which showed stimulus-seeking, antisocial, and impulsive dysregulated behavioral traits, rather than symptoms of affective dysregulation (Thompson-Brenner, Eddy, Franko, et al., 2008; Wonderlich et al., 2005).

All the studies in this area using samples with various ED diagnoses suggest that the subtypes do not directly map on to the current diagnostic system, and each subtype includes individuals with all diagnoses. However, the subtypes also show some relation to ED symptoms: Individuals in the constricted-obsessional and avoidant-insecure groups tend to demonstrate higher levels of current or historical anorexic features, while those in the two dysregulated subtypes typically show binge/purge behaviors (Espelage et al., 2002; Thompson-Brenner, Eddy, Satir, et al., 2008; Westen & Harnden-Fischer, 2001; Wonderlich et al., 2005).

Personality subtyping studies suggest substantial group differences in adaptive functioning and comorbid diagnoses. In our own studies of adults with mixed EDs and adults with BN, personality subtype has been strongly related to Global Assessment of Functioning (GAF) scores (Thompson-Brenner, Eddy, Franko, et al., 2008; Thompson-Brenner & Westen, 2005; Westen & Harden-Fischer, 2001). Mean pretreatment GAF score for the high-functioning groups is 10 to 20 points higher than that of the dysregulated group (a statistically significant difference), with the adjustment of the constricted groups falling between them; similarly, histories of hospitalization (for problems other than the ED) are significantly more common for the dysregulated groups and in some cases the avoidant-insecure group as well (Thompson-Brenner, Eddy, Franko, et al., 2008; Thompson-Brenner & Westen, 2005; Westen & Harden-Fischer, 2001). Subjects with EDs and dysregulated personality styles have shown significant comorbidity with posttraumatic stress disorder, substance use disorders, and externalizing disorders in general (Thompson-Brenner, Eddy, Franko, et al., 2008; Thompson-Brenner, Eddy, Satir, et al., 2008; Thompson-Brenner & Westen, 2005; Westen & Harnden-Fischer, 2001; Wonderlich et al., 2005). The constricted-obsessional group has shown substantial comorbidity in the areas of anxiety disorders as well as obsessive–compulsive personality disorder (Thompson-Brenner, Eddy, Satir, et al., 2008; Thompson-Brenner & Westen, 2005; Wonderlich et al., 2005). Those with avoidant personality styles show co-occurring anxiety disorders as well, but are more frequently diagnosed with avoidant personality disorder (Thompson-Brenner, Eddy, Franko, et al., 2008; Thompson-Brenner, Eddy, Satir, et al., 2008). Individuals in the high-functioning group show significantly fewer co-occurring Axis I and Axis II personality disorders across all the studies cited above.

Studies tracing the course of the different personality subtypes have also observed substantial between-group differences in treatment outcome and longitudinal course. Multiple studies suggest that in the short term, individuals with the high-functioning personality style show better outcome than other types (Thompson-Brenner, Eddy, Satir, et al., 2008; Thompson-Brenner & Westen, 2005; Wildes, 2010). Some studies indicate that the constricted-obsessional group shows a short-term treatment outcome that falls between those of the high-functioning and dysregulated groups (Thompson-Brenner & Westen, 2005; Wildes, 2010). A single long-term longitudinal study of all five personality subtypes found that both the dysregulated and avoidant groups showed long-term poor global outcome relative to the other groups; however, the avoidant group in particular showed poor outcome for AN as well as poor global outcome (Thompson-Brenner, Eddy, Franko, et al., 2008). In general, across treatment-outcome and longitudinal studies, global functioning appears to be a somewhat more robust measure of differences between personality groups than specific ED outcome (Thompson-Brenner, Eddy, Franko, et al., 2008). Notably, research concerning clinician countertransference suggests that clinicians respond more negatively to patients from the more psychopathological subtypes than to high-functioning patients, even when perceived improvement and other key variables are controlled for (Satir, Thompson-Brenner, Boisseau, & Crisafulli, 2009).

The research concerning etiological differences in personality subtypes is scarcer, but, several studies have suggested that both genetic factors and early experiences may contribute to the development of different personality subtypes among those with EDs. However, the research in this area is not conclusive. Some studies have indicated that individuals with dysregulated styles have both more externalizing disorders in first-degree relatives and more traumatic childhood experiences (e.g., Thompson-Brenner, Eddy, Satir, et al., 2008; Westen & Harden-Fischer, 2001; Wonderlich et al., 2001). One more recent study of familial risk between personality subtypes indicated that the more constricted-obsessional subtype showed the greatest incidence of shared familial risk for AN in particular (Holliday, Landau, Collier, & Treasure, 2006). Studies specifically concerning differences in genetic markers between subtypes based on personality traits have had mixed results. One as-yet-unpublished study suggests that the shared genetic risk between BN and substance abuse is higher among those from the dysregulated group than among the other personality subtypes (Slane, Burt, & Klump, 2010). Steiger and colleagues found a significant interaction between genetic markers (serotonin transporter genes) and childhood abuse among individuals in the dysregulated subtype (Steiger et al., 2007), as well as an association between the constricted-obsessional type and a particular genetic region of relevance to serotonin transport (Steiger et al., 2009). Wonderlich and colleagues (2005) found no differences in the genetic variations in the serotonin transporter gene between slightly different subtypes identified in another study. However, there is considerable variety in the methods both for identification of subtypes and for analyses of associations with genetic factors, and much additional research is needed in this area in particular.

Attachment Style and Reflective Functioning

Recent research has focused on the utility of assessing and treating patterns of attachment and associated interpersonal functioning as important dimensions of variation among individuals with EDs. In general, studies comparing ED samples with non-psychiatric controls have found, as expected, a higher rate of insecure attachment among ED samples—however, these observations were not specific to EDs relative to other severe psychiatric disorders, and the effect of active ED symptomatology on current attachment style was typically not assessed over time (for reviews, see O'Kearney, 1996; O'Shaughnessey & Dallos, 2009; Tasca et al., 2011; Ward et al., 2000). Most reviewers conclude that, as with personality and defense style, efforts to associate specific attachment styles (e.g., secure, dismissing, preoccupied, unresolved) with specific ED subtypes (e.g., AN and BN) were not conclusive, as attachment style varied significantly within ED subtype (O'Kearney, 1996; O'Shaughnessy & Dallos, 2008; Ward et al., 2000). However, some reviewers have concluded that dismissing attachment is somewhat more characteristic of AN, while preoccupied attachment is somewhat more characteristic of BN (Candelori & Ciocca, 1998), but this pattern is not manifestly true for all individuals with EDs.

Recent research has focused on the important patterns of variation in attachment style within the group of individuals with EDs, as well as relationships between attachment and interpersonal functioning, reflective functioning, and treatment outcome. Two recent cluster-analytic studies that have included both attachment style and ED symptoms in statistical analyses have reported somewhat similar results. Turner, Bryant-Waugh, and Peveler (2009), in their analysis of a mixed ED sample, and Lunn, Poulsen, and Daniel (2012), in their analysis of individuals with BN, each found four groups, three of which had similar features: one group with low attachment insecurity and low ED symptoms overall, one with high attachment insecurity and low ED symptoms overall, and one with low (or average) attachment insecurity but high levels of binge eating and purging. These two studies did not find converging results regarding a pattern of specific attachment or coping styles characteristic of the clusters (Lunn et al., 2012; Turner et al., 2009).

Recent studies focusing on the importance of attachment style to treatment process and outcome have found intriguing results. Studies have shown that attachment anxiety predicts poor outcome from treatment across ED diagnoses (Illing, Tasca, Balfour, & Bissada, 2010); that avoidant attachment predicts less engagement early in treatment, which in turn predicts poor outcome (Illing, Tasca, Balfour, & Bissada, 2011); and that high attachment anxiety predicts poor outcome from cognitive-behavioral therapy (CBT), but good outcome from psychodynamic group treatment (Tasca et al., 2006). Research also suggests that high attachment avoidance predicts premature termination from inpatient treatment among individuals with AN (Tasca, Taylor, Bissada, Ritchie, & Balfour, 2004) and from group CBT for those with BED (Tasca et al., 2006). Furthermore, Tasca and colleagues (2012) found that the strength of the relationship between group alliance ratings and outcome depended on attachment; specifically, the relationship between alliance and outcome was stronger for individuals in the group with higher attachment anxiety.

Attachment researchers suggest that attachment style is an important focus for treatment (e.g., Tasca et al., 2011), as well as an important predictor of other variables that are targets for psychodynamic treatments, such as object relations/interpersonal style (e.g., Lunn et al., 2012) and reflective functioning (e.g., Skårderud, 2007a, 2007b, 2007c; Tasca et al., 2011).

Affective Experience and Affect Regulation

The body of general research on affect in EDs, including research indicating the presence of persistent negative affect and the possible function of ED symptoms to regulate affect, has grown substantially in recent years. The research summarized above concerning personality includes data pertaining to affective experience, given that the different subtypes appear to have different affective experiences—for example, the high-functioning group has less negative affect overall; individuals in the dysregulated group experience intense dysregulated affect that they act to control and eliminate through desperate activity; and the constricted-obsessional and avoidant groups have characteristic ways of eliminating negative affect altogether or avoiding situations that trigger extreme negative affect (e.g., Westen & Harnden-Fischer, 2001). However, there are two other areas of research in addition to the cluster-analytic, personality-based system described above that are highly relevant to the potential classification of EDs based directly on differences in affective experience or affect regulation. These include an alternative subtyping system, simpler than the personality subtyping system described earlier, which would classify individuals based on the presence or absence of intense, long-standing, impairing negative affect; and cluster-analytic research using the AREQ to identify multiple characteristic affective traits among individuals with EDs. Data from these two focused areas are summarized for this review.

Negative Affect/Dietary Subtypes

A substantial body of coordinated research has focused on validating two subtypes of EDs, based on the presence of negative affect versus dietary restriction. Based on the theory presented above, suggesting that negative affect triggers binge eating to provide comfort and distraction, and other research suggesting that both negative affect and dieting behavior longitudinally predict the development of EDs (Stice, 1998; Stice & Agras, 1998), a series of studies were conducted to assess whether a two-type classification system, based on the presence and absence of severe negative affect, was statistically sound, reliable and valid, and related to comorbidity, outcome, and course.

The first set of studies of these possible subtypes used cluster analysis that grouped individuals on the basis of simple, validated measures of dietary restraint, such as the relevant subscale of the Eating Disorders Examination (EDE; Cooper, Cooper, & Fairburn, 1989) and scales measuring current negative affect and self-esteem such as the Beck Depression Inventory (BDI; Beck, Steer, & Garbin, 1988) and the Rosenberg Self-Esteem Scale (Rosenberg, 1979). Results from these cluster analyses supported the presence of two types: one pure dietary subtype, with elevations on multiple measures of dietary restraint, and one mixed negative-affect/dietary (or dietary-depressive) subtype, again with elevations on measures of dietary restraint, but also showing higher levels of current depression and lower levels of self-esteem (Stice & Agras, 1999). Using very similar measures and cluster-analytic techniques, similar findings were later identified in adults with BED (although levels of dietary restraint overall were lower) (Grilo, Masheb, & Wilson, 2001; Stice et al., 2001); in adolescents with ED symptoms on an inpatient unit (although adaptive functioning across the board was low) (Grilo, 2002); in adolescents with BN (Chen & Le Grange, 2007); and in children and adolescents with any type of loss of control over eating (Goldschmidt et al., 2008). In contrast, one additional study from Spain of adult women with mixed EDs, using a slightly different statistical technique but similar measures, found four types, including two dietary and two depressive subtypes, with inconclusive but interesting differences in temperament and co-occurring psychopathology (Peñas-Lledó et al., 2009).

The researchers investigating differences between the dietary-depressive and pure dietary types established a fairly consistent pattern of associated comorbidities and adaptive functioning, with some variation that could be expected based on the samples used (noted above). Across most studies, the dietary-depressive type was associated with lower general functioning, lower interpersonal functioning, and more co-occurring anxiety, mood, and personality disorders (e.g., Chen & Le Grange, 2007; Stice & Agras, 1999; Stice et al., 2001). In some studies, the dietary-depressive group also showed higher levels of ED severity than the pure dietary group (e.g., Chen & Le Grange, 2007; Goldschmidt et al., 2008; Stice et al., 2001). Although the test–retest reliability of the subtyping distinction was reported to be adequate, kappas were reported in the range of .55–.61, indicating some instability, which might be expected based on the known instability in negative affect on the BDI over longer time periods (Grilo et al., 2001; Stice, Bohon, Marti, & Fischer, 2008).

Research evidence suggests that treatment outcome and long-term course also differ between patients with EDs classified in the dietary-depressive and the pure dietary subtypes. The research to date on treatment outcome has concerned outcome and follow-up measurements primarily from short-term psychotherapy, such as CBT, interpersonal psychotherapy (IPT), and inpatient treatment. These studies have found that abstinence rates were significantly lower among the dietary-depressive type immediately following treatment by CBT for BN (Stice & Agras, 1999), and that both eating pathology and general functional impairment were more severe at both 6-month and 3-year follow-up time points (Stice et al., 2008). Following CBT for BED, individuals in the dietary-depressive subtype showed more frequent binge-eating episodes in another study (Masheb & Grilo, 2008). In a study of three treatments for BED (CBT, IPT, and behavioral weight loss), high negative affect predicted less improvement in binge eating, and no significant treatment × negative affect interactions were found (Wilson, Wilfley, Agras, & Bryson, 2010). Similarly, in a previous study (Loeb, Wilson, Gilbert, & Labouvie, 2000), negative affect predicted more posttreatment binge eating in both guided and unguided self-help (based on CBT principles) for binge eating.

Affect Regulation and Experience Q-Sort

Two of our own studies have used the AREQ method to investigate within-group differences among individuals with EDs. One study investigated a sample of adults with AN and BN, using a cluster-analytic technique (which produces groups of individuals, or subtypes), and the other investigated a sample of adolescents with all ED diagnoses, using a factor-analytic technique (which produces identifiable distinct traits). Here we present the results of these as-yet-unpublished analyses to illustrate the nature of more fine-grained analyses of affective experience and affect regulation among EDs, and to inform future researchers in this area.

The AREQ is a Q-sort measure consisting of 98 observer-rated (in these studies, clinician-rated) items aimed at measuring affective experience and regulation dimensions that have shown good convergent, discriminant, and predictive validity (Westen et al., 1997). Factors demonstrated to relate to affective experience and regulation in prior factor analyses include socialized negative affect, positive affect, intense negative affect, goal-focused responses, externalizing defenses, and avoidant defenses (Westen et al., 1997). Good internal validity has been replicated over multiple studies (Löffler-Stastka & Stigler, 2011; Westen et al., 1997), and recent studies indicate good interrater reliability across cross-cultural samples (Löffler-Stastka & Stigler, 2011; Westen et al., 1997).

STUDY 1

The aim of the first study using the AREQ with individuals with EDs was to repli-cate the three-subtype system that had been based to date on personality data. The investigators conceptualized affect regulation as a subcategory of personality and were interested to see whether cluster-analytic techniques focused on affect alone would find similar types. AREQ data were collected from 103 MD- and PhD-level therapists recruited from the registers of the American Psychological Association and the American Psychological Association, who were currently treating adult patients with BN or AN. The patients had been in therapy for a mean of 22 sessions ($SD = 27$). Approximately two-thirds of the patients met the criteria for BN, and approximately one-third for AN; 95% of the sample of patients was Caucasian. Further details concerning the methods of data collection and the sample are given by Westen and Harnden-Fischer (2001).

To examine whether there were identifiable subtypes based on affective experi-ence and affect regulation, we performed a Q-factor analysis using the 98 items from the AREQ. Whereas standard analysis identifies features, or traits composed of mul-tiple items, Q-factor analysis uses the same statistical technique to group individu-als into subgroups whose entire item profile shows statistical similarities (for Q-sort typological methods, see Block, 1978; Caspi, 1998). We applied standard factor-analytic procedures, first entering all patients' profiles into a principal components analysis, specifying eigenvalues ≥ 1. The scree plot suggested a break at three factors; the first five factors cumulatively accounted for 50.0% of the variance. To match the data-analytic procedures used in identifying the three personality subtypes using the personality measure, we subjected the data to varimax (orthogonal) rotations speci-fying three, four, and five factors. All three produced similar solutions with three clear and interpretable factors. We retained the first three factors of the five-factor solution, which cumulatively accounted for 43.0% of the variance. (The advantage of retaining three of five factors is that doing so minimizes "noise" that can occur when the procedure forces items into the last factors.)

Table 12.1 presents the four items concerning affect that were identified empiri-cally as most descriptive of patients in each Q-factor derived from the AREQ. As Table 12.1 shows, Q-factor analysis of the AREQ data identified three coherent styles of regulating and experiencing emotion, with the first characterized by socialized or internalized negative affect as well as adaptive coping, the second by intense negative affect and emotional dysregulation, and the third by asceticism, compulsiveness, and emotional constriction.

The three subtypes identified by cluster analyses of the AREQ showed distinct similarities to those identified through subtyping of the superordinate personality measure. To assess the extent to which this classification maps on to the classifica-tion by personality profiles discussed earlier using the Shedler–Westen Assessment Procedure-200, we assigned category membership to patients who loaded ≥ 0.50 on one of the Q-factors as above and used a coefficient of contingency (scaled from 0 to 1) to assess the extent to which patients classified by one classification were similarly

TABLE 12.1. Affect Regulation and Experience Subtypes

High-functioning/socialized negative affect subtype

• Tends to feel guilty	2.1
• Is able to experience a full range of emotions	2.0
• Tends to feel anxious	1.9
• Is able to use and benefit from help and advice when distressed	1.9

Emotionally dysregulated/undercontrolled affect subtype

• Tends to feel unpleasant emotions (e.g., sadness, anxiety, guilt) intensely	2.3
• Behaves in manifestly self-destructive ways when upset (e.g., fast driving, wrist cutting)	2.1
• Can plunge into deep despair that lasts for several weeks	1.9
• Tends to feel sad or unhappy	1.8

Constricted/overcontrolled affect subtype

• Appears to derive a sense of self-worth and/or moral superiority by denying him- or herself pleasure	2.5
• Tends to display specific obsessions or compulsions when distressed	1.7
• Tends to feel bad or unworthy instead of feeling appropriately angry at others	1.6
• Tends to become anxious when daily routines are altered	1.6

Note. The number to the right of each item is a standardized factor score that indicates how central the item is in defining the prototype (i.e., the number of standard deviations above the mean relative to the other 97 items in the Q-sort).

classified by the other. The results indicated very high concordance (coefficient of contingency = .71).

STUDY 2

The second study using the AREQ aimed to see whether standard factor analysis of the AREQ in a sample of adolescents with EDs produced a factor structure of traits that resembled results from previous factor analyses of the AREQ with other populations (e.g., Westen et al., 1997), or that had distinct features indicative of characteristic affect-regulation strategies among individuals with EDs. AREQ, ED, and family history data were collected from 120 clinicians. The clinicians were drawn from a practice-research network of child/adolescent clinicians with MDs or PhDs and at least five years' postlicensure experience. They were sampled if they were currently treating an adolescent with an ED, aged 15–18, whom they had been seeing for ≥ 6 clinical contact hours but ≤ 1 year (to minimize confounds imposed by personality change with treatment). Additional description of the sample and methods for this study is included in Thompson-Brenner, Eddy, Satir, and colleagues (2008).

Using a principal-axis factor analytic method, our own analyses of AREQ data from adolescents with EDs resulted in six affect-regulation factors, explaining approximately 46% of the variance in the AREQ. Four of these factors were either unique to the ED sample or particularly recognizable as common features of affect regulation and personality structure in EDs, or they explained important variance in aspects of associated variables in ED populations (e.g., Thompson-Brenner, Eddy, Satir, et al., 2008; Thompson-Brenner & Westen, 2005; Weingeroff, Thompson-Brenner, Pratt, Sherry, & Westen, 2007). These four factors were termed *ascetic/driven* (e.g., "Appears to derive a sense of self-worth and/or moral superiority by denying herself pleasure," "Tends to immerse herself in work to avoid distressing feelings or situations"); *socialized/internalizing* (e.g., "Tends to feel guilty," "Tends to feel bad or unworthy instead of feeling appropriately angry at others"); *dysregulated* (e.g., "Behaves in manifestly self-destructive ways when upset," "Emotional expression appears peculiar, inappropriate, or incongruent with content of communications"), and *avoidant/alexithymic* (e.g., "Often seems unaware of own wishes, needs, or feelings," "Has a limited ability to recognize, identify, or label own emotions"). Additional affect-regulation factors identified in our ED sample that very closely resembled affect-regulatory traits from previous factor analyses of the AREQ with other populations (e.g., Westen et al., 1997) included *externalizing* (e.g., "Tends to lash out at others when distressed or angry," "Tends to deny responsibility for her own problems"), and *adaptive/positive* (e.g., "Displays emotion appropriate in quality and intensity to the situation at hand," "Has the ability to reflect and postpone action until emotions are calm").

Preliminary analysis of both the subtype scores (derived from Study 1) and the factor scores (derived from Study 2) indicated that affect regulation shows important relationships to other variables indicative of reliability and validity, although only a limited number of associated variables have been investigated to date. Although this line of investigation is not as advanced as the other two subtyping schemes, affect-regulation style shows significant cross-sectional relationships to adaptive functioning, personality disorder diagnosis, and school and social functioning (Weingeroff et al., 2007).

CLINICAL ILLUSTRATION

In order to illustrate the differences observed among groups of individuals with EDs in personality and affective styles described above, we present two clinical illustrations. Each vignette is drawn from a single session at a critical point in an integrative form of psychotherapy for EDs, in which the first portion of therapy, focused on patterns of eating and symptom remission, had concluded, and a more psychodynamic period, focused on patterns of personality, affect, and interpersonal relationships, was underway. The two cases are intended as contrasts. The session material represented here is based on various recordings, but is thorough altered/disguised to protect clients' confidentiality, as well as edited for ease of presentation.

The first vignette illustrates a session with a 21-year-old female patient. She was successful in her biomedical studies and had skipped several grades growing up. She described having a circle of old friends, but few close friends and no romantic relationships. Her focus was primarily on her studies, and she was young for her graduate program. She described her mother as somewhat rigid, for example, "living by the clock," and her father as "relatively" relaxed. During the early portion of treatment, which was based on cognitive-behavioral principles, she responded well to structured interventions and had been binge/purge-free at the time of this session for 2 months. However, she still struggled with dietary rules and her desires to break them. According to the DSM-IV diagnostic system, she met criteria for a diagnosis of EDNOS (subclinical BN) and no other comorbid DSM-IV diagnoses. Her case is meant to illustrate patterns that would be characteristic of the constricted-obsessional personality type and avoidant/alexithymic affect-regulation factors, and to demonstrate how ED symptoms manifest as expressions of these defenses and affect-regulatory strategies. According to the two-type negative affect-based system, however, she would most likely fall into the pure dietary group, due to the absence of intense negative affect. The vignette is also intended to illustrate how more open-ended psychodynamic psychotherapy may have elicited subtle patterns of affect regulation and personality style in response to the process that might not emerge in a more structured set of interventions.

PATIENT: Last night I had an unusual thought for me. I thought, "I wish I could have a lot of M&Ms."

THERAPIST: So you didn't want just a few M&Ms, you wanted to eat a lot. Did you ask yourself the question, "Why would I want to do that?"?

PATIENT: For a second it actually sounded not so bad.

THERAPIST: Any idea why?

PATIENT: It was approaching a situation where I almost wanted to do it. I wanted to be able to just be looser with what I was eating. In fact I don't want to, because I don't want the consequences of binge eating. But it was strange to wish that I could just be loose.

THERAPIST: What would being loose do for you?

PATIENT: Um (pause) . . . I don't know.

THERAPIST: I'm trying to get to the piece of you that wanted that, despite all the reasons that you've stated you wouldn't do that, right now I'm more interested in the part of you that it still appeals to a little bit.

PATIENT: I understand. (Laughs.) There is the part of me that likes food, of course. But I'm not sure I am trying to get enjoyment out of food exactly—it is like, I'm doing something else.

THERAPIST: What might that be?

PATIENT: Um, last night, I think I was feeling stressed, stress over things being tight—like tight, as opposed to loose. Like I was trying to make plans for today and I was figuring multiple things out for tomorrow, but all my plans seemed to depend on the weather. And I had to, like, go to bed unresolved, because I didn't know if it would snow.

THERAPIST: Uh huh, you felt unresolved.

PATIENT: Yeah . . . that's actually probably a big part of it. 'Cause I, I hate leaving things, like . . . open like that. That is true when I have fights with people. I don't want to get mad in the first place, but I really don't want things to be left like that. I need things to be tied up. Maybe the eating, being loose about eating, maybe that would direct attention away from that unresolved feeling.

THERAPIST: Tell me a little more about how that works in your relationships. Sounds like that could be a theme.

PATIENT: I guess I like to plan things. But otherwise, like, I don't know . . . like, what do you mean, like, in relationships? That's kind of broad I guess.

THERAPIST: It is kind of an unclear question. Kind of uncertain . . . (pause) Are you having a hard time right now? How are you feeling right now? As we are sitting here together?

PATIENT: I always feel a little discomfort here because it is not usual for me to, like, verbalize any of this at all. It feels so strange.

THERAPIST: Yeah. And I also am using kind of this moment even, to get right into what we're talking about. Because it's kind of a little bit uncertain in here right now. I'm not telling you what to do, I'm not even responding that much. I'm just wondering what that might be like for you. We've actually created a kind of space that was like last night, or other times that you couldn't plan, but in this case it is not possible to plan how you are interacting with me.

PATIENT: It's actually pretty tough, I think.

THERAPIST: Tough . . .

PATIENT: Um . . . it is actually, it is hard, just because I never really give myself this much time or freedom to just talk about things. I usually just try to stay away from this stuff. And here, I never really know what I'm going to say so that's really weird, actually. This is a perfect example. That's why it's like tough for me. It's never a simple thing, with you because I can't know how it will go.

Although this patient was not assessed for attachment style or for reflective functioning, it is interesting to consider her clinical process from these important points of view. This patient might be classified as securely attached; however, her self-representation as a perfect child led to a pattern of self-distancing and avoidance of conflict that at times resembled dismissive attachment patterns. This effort to keep relationships conflict-free may have resulted in a reduced ability for reflective functioning—a lack of insight into her own and others' minds—and limited affect-regulatory strategies. As this excerpt shows, her focus on food served the purpose of simplifying her concerns relative to the unpredictable broader world, including the unpredictability and complexity of interpersonal relationships.

The second (contrasting) case vignette also illustrates a part of a session with a 20-year-old female college student with a DSM-IV diagnosis of EDNOS (subclinical BN). This patient, however, also had a co-occurring diagnosis of borderline personality disorder. She described her father as emotionally labile and manipulative, with a history of a violent temper, and reported a pattern of relating to him by "giving him multiple chances to be a better father, but he never learns." In treatment, she observed similar patterns in her current relationship with her romantic partner. She noticed a fear of being rejected by her partner, against which she defended by acting angry and aggressive. This vignette illustrates her work in a later session from integrative treatment, where again the focus had shifted from providing concrete strategies to counteract the behavioral symptoms of her ED to a more dynamic process, with exploration of her emotional dysregulation and relational style. She had stopped binge eating and purging with some difficulty, and reported intense self-hatred associated with her body size. This vignette illustrates similarities and differences in the personality style and emotion regulation of a patient who would be characterized as "dysregulated" in the personality and affect-regulation subtyping systems, and as "dietary-depressive" in the two-type negative affect-based system. She describes emotions that spin out of control and utilizes externalizing defenses as well as projective identification as strategies to help with her emotion regulation.

THERAPIST: So you said you were blaming Aidan for the day going badly. Can you tell me more about that?

PATIENT: I managed not to really lash out at him, but I was a little sharp, pretty aggressive, actually. Like when we were riding the bus. I was really worried we were going to be late. So I was looking for a way to get rid of that anxiety, I guess.

THERAPIST: Let's go back a little further. . . . In that moment, when you were acting like that to him, what were you feeling right before that moment? Before you were being mean to him?

PATIENT: I was really anxious and worried about my work. All the things that I have to do, the things I was behind on, they were piling up. I was thinking we would be late for the meeting, and then late to get back, and I could not even be starting my homework until nine o'clock. So there were so many interrelated time things piling up and seeming overwhelming. So yeah, I guess I just kind of lashed out.

THERAPIST: And what do you think Aidan was thinking, or feeling, and doing?

PATIENT: I think he was just trying to help. He kept saying, "Relax, we are on our way, there's nothing we can do."

THERAPIST: So what do you think you wanted, when you lashed out at him?

PATIENT: Hmm. I guess I was irritated, like it felt like, I am taking this seriously, why aren't you taking it as seriously? Like, wait, is there something wrong with me? Am I making too big a deal of this? And I don't want to admit that I'm wrong because I am in fact upset, and my emotions are real. So, Aiden must be wrong. And if I am mean to him, then he won't be as calm any more, then maybe he'll snap out of it. . . . This might be a little off topic, but it reminds me of something that used to happen in my family. I was an emotional kid. And I would get really upset about things that might seem stupid, like say, there is nothing for dessert when I really wanted it. Say, when I was four or something. And I'd get furious with my mother, like screaming, "I really want cookies!!!" I would have a fit. And she would smile at me, or like kinda laugh, like she thought it was adorable for a four-year-old to be so intense about something. She might have been trying to make me smile, too, but I would do whatever it took to make her angry, like me.

THERAPIST: And how did that make you feel when she would smile or laugh at you?

PATIENT: I felt like she was kind of diminishing my feelings. You know? You are laughing at my distress.

THERAPIST: So you want people to be aggressive and angry when you are?

PATIENT: Yeah. At least upset. Like, negative.

THERAPIST: And how does that work out with Aidan?

PATIENT: He doesn't really get angry . . . usually I think he gets more depressed, more sad when I do that. So, I don't know. The thought of what it would be like if I was dating someone else worries me. If I were with someone who was more volatile. . . . I could have such a dysfunctional relationship. And I feel bad that I upset Aidan. There are people who can handle it, and people who cannot. My mom is good at remaining calm, even when I am at my worst. But my dad? Forget about it. If I'm miserable and I want to make him miserable, it will happen. So, I don't know, that day Aidan was trying to help me out, but I wanted to make him mean and angry, to match me.

THERAPIST: Umm-hmm.

PATIENT: Also, since I was eating, I honestly think in the moment that made me feel better. When we were in rush mode we ran to McDonald's and I was eating on the bus, so when I was doing that and he was trying to calm me down, the two combined did help. That is also I think why I usually binged and purged, to relieve my anxiety. I didn't do that—I couldn't, I was on the bus—but just eating a normal amount made me feel less tense, and I stopped taking it out on Aidan.

CONCLUSIONS AND FUTURE DIRECTIONS

There is substantial research converging on alternative subtyping systems of interest to psychodynamic researchers and clinicians, based on personality style and the presence of intense negative affect, but each system has its own strengths and limitations. Both systems have established that they have validity additional to that of the DSM-IV diagnostic system, as indicated by their power to predict important associated variables such as comorbidity and outcome above and beyond the variability accounted for in ED diagnosis. Additional preliminary research, published in this chapter, has been conducted on a system of classification based on affect regulation as assessed by the AREQ. However, this system seems to strongly resemble the personality-based system and has not been investigated as thoroughly as the other two systems.

The personality subtype system is well supported in that multiple studies, using different methods, have found converging support for the presence of high-functioning/perfectionistic, dysregulated/undercontrolled, and constricted/overcontrolled groups. Individuals in each group, or with high scores on the items most characteristic of the groups, show distinct patterns of personality style, as well as distinct associations with adaptive functioning variables, co-occurring psychopathology, treatment outcome, long-term course, and etiological factors such as genetics and family/developmental history.

The limitations of the research in this area to date are related to the strengths. Because the studies have employed different methods both of assessment and of statistical analysis, there is notable variation in the results. The number of identified subtypes ranges between three and five, and the five-subtype system—which begins to resemble the DSM-5 personality disorder diagnoses—has not been tested for additional utility beyond that of the existing Axis II (or proposed new personality disorder classification) system. Furthermore, the solutions with higher numbers of subtypes are somewhat unwieldy for use in research studies, given both the high number of them and the lack of a validated measure that would definitively identify an individual's subtype without the use of factor or cluster analysis.

Some of the limitations of personality assessment and classification also naturally apply to the personality-based subtyping systems for EDs. Personality assessment is unreliable by self-report, and only a few, highly time-consuming methods of observer report show acceptable levels of reliability. Personality researchers are increasingly moving toward a dimensional, rather than categorical, method of describing personality pathology, and these developments may have implications for ED investigators as well. It remains to be seen whether it is more useful to continue to conduct subtyping/cluster-analytic studies, including multiple different variables (behavioral symptoms, personality style, attachment style, reflective functioning, etc.), resulting in more and more subtypes, or whether it is more useful to assess patients with EDs (and other patients) on the full set of important treatment predictors and fully describe each individual as he or she varies on all these important dimensions.

The research demonstrating and investigating the negative affect/dietary (dietary-depressive) and pure dietary subtypes of EDs has definitely benefited from the coordinated efforts of the researchers involved. Due to the consistency in the methods (in both assessment and statistical analyses), the results have been more consistent and constitute actual replication as opposed to converging results. The simplicity of the system allows for additional power in treatment outcome studies, and the simplicity of assessment does allow people to be categorized relatively easily on the basis of BDI score and Rosenberg Self-Esteem Scale score.

One important limitation to this system, which is highlighted in a comparison with the personality research, is that there is substantial heterogeneity in personality style among the group with high negative affect. The personality subtyping system suggests there are important differences within the negative affect/dietary subtype that may require further delineation. In addition, levels of negative affect are known to vary over time, and a classification based on a BDI score would have severe limitations in test–retest reliability over any extended time period. Finally, research has not been conducted that has linked these types to developmental, genetic, or other possible etiological factors.

Future research might fruitfully compare the two subtyping systems directly and assess whether other important variables, such as object relations functioning, family style, or cognitive functioning and neurobiological variables, show stronger associations with one of the proposed subtyping systems. Furthermore, any longitudinal research that could establish whether issues such as personality predated the development of an ED would be particularly useful. Studies investigating etiological factors would also be most helpful if they assessed the contributions of both genetics and experience, as well as their interaction. Additional fruitful research could establish a reliable and valid measure that was able to designate which subtype an individual belonged to or dimensional measures (subscales) that might establish dimensional scores on the same variables.

The best systems of diagnosis help to inform the effective process of treatment. Research focused on psychodynamic treatment tends to suggest that it has a positive effect on symptoms (see Thompson-Brenner et al., 2009). However, treatment comparing psychodynamic treatment with structured cognitive-behavioral treatments (CBTs) has found limited support for the effect of psychodynamic treatment on symptom functioning relative to CBT (e.g., Poulsen, Lunn, & Daniel, 2011). Given that psychodynamic treatment does not focus as directly on immediate symptom change, this is perhaps not surprising. Psychodynamic research would more usefully focus in several alternative areas, all relevant to psychodynamic diagnosis. First, psychodynamically informed classification systems can help inform the outcomes that should be measured in treatment studies—for example, personality functioning, affect regulation and experience, and attachment anxiety, which may show more improvement in treatments that are focused on these problems. Second, psychodynamically informed subtyping systems may be useful as mediating variables; that is, they may help to identify subgroups that respond differently to different treatment approaches. A few such studies have indicated the promise of this approach. As noted earlier, research investigating psychodynamic group treatment for BED suggests that IPT, which has limited goals of a psychodynamic nature, has the most empirical support with respect to its relationship to personality subtypes. One study has investigated whether the negative affect subtype (in the two-type system) predicted response to CBT and IPT for BED, and failed to show that subtype-mediated treatment response (Wilson, Wilfley, Agras, & Bryson, 2010). However, a reanalysis of existing data, including more variables in the subtyping system, found that one type—the type with both high shape and weight concerns and high negative affect—showed better response to IPT than to CBT, while other types showed more remission with CBT (Sysko, Hildebrandt, Wilson, Wilfley, & Agras, 2010). Other trials are underway investigating other approaches to treating both symptoms and personality functioning by integrating aspects of each (see Richards & Thompson-Brenner, in press) or investigating new psychodynamic approaches that directly target psychodynamic psychopathology and mechanisms of change, such as a trial of mentalization-based treatment currently underway by Paul Robinson and colleagues (unpublished). Psychodynamic researchers should carefully consider the complexities of diagnosis and likely variable treatment response in their treatment outcome design and data-analytic strategy.

REFERENCES

American Psychiatric Association. (2000). *Diagnostic and statistical manual of mental disorders* (4th ed., text rev.). Washington, DC: Author.

American Psychiatric Association. (2013). *Diagnostic and statistical manual of mental disorders* (5th ed.). Arlington, VA: Author.

Attia, E., Becker, A., Bryant-Waugh, R., Hoek, H., Marcus, M., Mitchell, J., et al. (2009, September). *Eating disorders and DSM-V: Current status.* Symposium presentation at the 15th annual meeting of the Eating Disorders Research Society, Brooklyn, NY.

Attia, E., & Roberto, C. (2009). Should amenorrhea be a diagnostic criterion for anorexia nervosa? *International Journal of Eating Disorders, 42,* 581–589.

Beck, A. T., Steer, R. A., & Garbin, M. (1988). Psychometric properties of the Beck Depression Inventory: 25 years of evaluation. *Clinical Psychology Review, 8,* 77–100.

Block, J. (1978). The Q-sort method in personality assessment and psychiatric research. Palo Alto, CA: Consulting Psychologists Press.

Bruch, H. (1962). Perceptual and conceptual disturbances in anorexia nervosa. *Psychosomatic Medicine, 24,* 187–199.

Bruch, H. (1978). *The golden cage.* London: Open Books.

Bruch, H. (1982). Anorexia nervosa: Therapy and theory. *American Journal of Psychiatry, 139,* 1531–1538.

Candelori, C., & Ciocca, A. (1998). Attachment and eating disorders. In P. Bria, A. Ciocca, & S. De Risio (Eds.), *Psychotherapeutic issues in eating disorders; Models, methods and results* (pp. 139–153). Rome, Italy: Universo.

Casper, R. C., Hedeker, D., & McClough, J. F. (1992). Personality dimensions in eating disorders and their relevance for subtyping. *Journal of the American Academy of Child and Adolescent Psychiatry, 31,* 830–840.

Caspi, A. (1998). Personality development across the lifespan. In W. Damon (Ed.) & N. Eisenberg (Vol. Ed.), *Handbook of child psychology: Vol. 3. Social, emotional, and personality development* (pp. 311–388). New York: Wiley.

Chen, E. Y., & Le Grange, D. (2007). Subtyping adolescents with bulimia nervosa. *Behaviour Research and Therapy, 45,* 2813–2820.

Clinton, D., & Norring, C. (2005). The comparative utility of statistically derived eating disorder clusters and DSM-IV diagnoses: Relationship to symptomatology and psychiatric comorbidity at intake and follow-up. *Eating Behaviors, 6,* 403–418.

Cooper, Z., Cooper, P. J., & Fairburn, C. G. (1989). The validity of the Eating Disorder Examination and its subscales. *British Journal of Psychiatry, 154,* 807–812.

Eddy, K. T., Celio Doyle, A., Hoste, R. R., Herzog, D. B., & Le Grange, D. (2008). Eating disorder not otherwise specified in adolescents. *Journal of the American Academy of Child and Adolescent Psychiatry, 47,* 156–164.

Eddy, K. T., Le Grange, D., Crosby, R. D., Hoste, R. E., Doyle, A. C., Smyth, A, et al. (2010). Diagnostic classification of eating disorders in children and adolescents: How does DSM-IV-TR compare to empirically-derived categories? *Journal of the American Academy of Child and Adolescent Psychiatry, 49,* 277–287.

Espelage, D. L., Mazzeo, S. E., Sherman, R., & Thompson, R. (2002). MCMI-II profiles of women with eating disorders: A cluster analytic investigation. *Journal of Personality Disorders, 16,* 453–463.

Esplen, M. J., Garfinkel, P., & Gallop, R. (2000). Relationship between self-soothing, aloneness, and evocative memory in bulimia nervosa. *International Journal of Eating Disorders, 27,* 96–100.

Everill, J. T., & Waller, G. (1995). Reported sexual abuse and eating psychopathology: A review of the evidence for a causal link. *International Journal of Eating Disorders, 18,* 1–11.

Frampton, I. (2010, October). *How can neuropsychology help in eating disorder diagnosis?* Symposium presentation at the 16th annual meeting of the Eating Disorders Research Society, Cambridge, MA.

Garner, D. M., Olmstead, M. P., & Polivy, J. (1983). Development and validation of a multidimensional eating disorders inventory for anorexia and bulimia nervosa. *International Journal of Eating Disorders, 2,* 15–34.

Goldner, E. M., Srikameswaran, S., Schroeder, M. L., Livesley, W. J., & Birmingham, C. L. (1999). Dimensional assessment of personality pathology in patients with eating disorders. *Psychiatry Research, 85,* 151–159.

Goldschmidt, A. B., Tanofsky-Kraff, M., Goossens, L., Eddy, K. T., Ringham, R., Zanovski, S. Z., et al. (2008). Subtyping children and adolescents with loss of control eating by negative affect and dietary restraint. *Behaviour Research and Therapy, 46,* 777–787.

Grilo, C. M. (2002). Recent research of relationships among eating disorders and personality disorders. *Current Psychiatry Reports, 4,* 18–24.

Grilo, C. M., Masheb, R. M., & Wilson, G. (2001) Subtyping binge eating disorder. *Journal of Consulting and Clinical Psychology, 69,* 1066–1072.

Halmi, K. (1974). Anorexia nervosa: Demographic and clinical features in 94 cases. *Psychosomatic Medicine, 36,* 18–26.

Heatherton, T. F., & Baumeister, R. F. (1991). Binge eating as escape from self-awareness. *Psychological Bulletin, 110,* 86–108.

Herman, C. P., & Polivy, J. (1975). Anxiety, restraint, and eating behavior. *Journal of Abnormal Psychology, 84,* 666–672.

Hodes, M., & Le Grange, D. (1993). Expressed emotion in the investigation of eating disorders: A review. *International Journal of Eating Disorders, 13,* 279–288.

Holliday, J., Landau, S., Collier, D., & Treasure, J. (2006). Do illness characteristics and familial risk differ between women with anorexia nervosa grouped on the basis of personality pathology? *Psychological Medicine, 36,* 529–538.

Illing, V., Tasca, G. A., Balfour, L., & Bissada, H. (2010). Attachment insecurity predicts eating disorder symptoms and treatment outcomes in a clinical sample of women. *Journal of Nervous and Mental Disorders, 198,* 653–659.

Illing, V., Tasca, G. A., Balfour, L., & Bissada, H. (2011). Attachment dimensions and group climate growth in a sample of women seeking treatment for eating disorders. *Psychiatry, 74,* 255–269.

Keel, P., Brown, T. A., Holland, L. A., & Bodell, L. P. (2011). Empirical classification of eating disorders. *Annual Review of Clinical Psychology, 8,* 381–404.

Keel, P., Brown, T., Holm-Denoma, J. M., & Bodell, L. (2011). Comparison of DSM-IV vs. proposed DSM-5 diagnostic criteria for eating disorders: Reduction of EDNOS and validity. *International Journal of Eating Disorders, 44,* 553–560.

Kernberg, O. (1980). Foreword. In J. A. Sours (Ed.), *Starving to death in a sea of objects: The anorexia nervosa syndrome* (pp. ix–xi). New York: Jason Aronson.

Kiang, L., & Harter, S. (2006). Sociocultural values of appearance and attachment processes: An integrated model of eating disorder symptomatology. *Eating Behaviors, 7,* 134–145.

Lilenfeld, L. R. R., Wonderlich, S., Riso, L. P., Crosby, R., & Mitchell, J. E. (2006). Eating disorders and personality: A methodological and empirical review. *Clinical Psychology Review, 26,* 299–320.

Liu, A. (2007). *Gaining: The truth about life after eating disorders.* New York: Warner Books.

Loeb, K. L., Wilson, G. T., Gilbert, J. S., & Labouvie, E. (2000). Guided and unguided self-help for binge eating. *Behaviour Research and Therapy, 38,* 259–272.

Löffler-Stastka, H., & Stigler, K. (2011). Der Affektwahrnehmung und Affektregulation

Q-Sort-Test (AREQ): Validierung und Kurzform. [The Affect Experience and Affect Regulation Q-Sort Test (AREQ): Validation and short version.] *Psychotherapie, Psychosomatik, Medizinische Psychologie, 61*, 225–232.

Lunn, S., Poulsen, S., & Daniel, S. I. (2012). Subtypes in bulimia nervosa: The role of eating disorder symptomatology, negative affect, and interpersonal functioning. *Comprehensive Psychiatry, 53*, 1078–1087.

Masheb, R. M., & Grilo, C. M. (2008). Prognostic significance of two sub-categorization methods for binge eating disorder: Negative affect and overvaluation predict, but do not moderate, specific outcomes. *Behavior Research and Therapy, 46*, 428–437.

Minuchin, S., Rosman, B. L., & Baker, L. (1978). *Psychosomatic families: Anorexia nervosa in context.* Cambridge, MA: Harvard University Press.

Mitchell, J. E., Hatsukami, D., Pyle, R. L., & Eckert, E. D. (1986). The bulimia syndrome: Course of the illness and associated problems. *Comprehensive Psychiatry, 27*, 165–170.

Norman, D. K., Blais, D., & Herzog, D. B. (1993). Personality characteristics of eating-disordered patients as identified by the Millon Clinical Multiaxial Inventory. *Journal of Personality Disorders, 14*, 213–218.

O'Kearney, R. (1996). Attachment disruption in anorexia nervosa and bulimia nervosa: A review of theory and empirical research. *International Journal of Eating Disorders, 20*, 115–127.

O'Shaughnessy, R., & Dallos, R. (2009). Attachment research and eating disorders: A review of the literature. *Clinical Child Psychology and Psychiatry, 14*, 559–574.

Ogden, J., & Wardle, J. (1991). Cognitive and emotional responses to food. *International Journal of Eating Disorders, 10*, 297–311.

Palazzoli, M. S. (1965). Interpretation of mental anorexia. In J. E. Meyer & H. Felbdman (Eds.), *Anorexia nervosa.* Stuttgart, Germany: Thieme.

Palazzoli, M. S. (1974). *Self-starvation.* New York: Jason Aronson.

Peñas-Lledó, E., Fernández-Aranda, F., Jiménez-Murcia, S., Granero, R., Penelo, E., Soto A., et al. (2009). Subtyping eating disordered patients along drive for thinness and depression. *Behaviour Research and Therapy, 47*, 513–519.

Polivy, J., Herman, C. P., & McFarlane, T. (1994). Effects of anxiety on eating: Does palatability moderate distress-induced overeating in dieters? *Journal of Abnormal Psychology, 103*, 505–510.

Poulsen, S., Lunn, S., & Daniel, S. I. F. (2011, April). *A randomized controlled trial of psychoanalytic psychotherapy and cognitive behavioral therapy for bulimia nervosa.* Paper presented at the International Conference on Eating Disorders, Miami, FL.

Reindl, S. M. (2001). *Sensing the self.* Cambridge, MA: Harvard University Press.

Richards, L. K., & Thompson-Brenner, H. (in press). An evidence-based case report of the treatment of bulimia nervosa with integrative dynamic therapy. *Psychotherapy.*

Rodgers, R., & Chabrol, H. (2009). Parental attitudes, body image disturbance and disordered eating amongst adolescents and young adults: A review. *European Eating Disorders Review, 17*, 137–151.

Rosenberg, M. (1979). *Conceiving the self.* New York: Basic Books.

Satir, D. A., Thompson-Brenner, H., Boisseau, C. L., & Crisafulli, M. A. (2009). Countertransference reactions to adolescents with eating disorders: Relationships to clinician and patient factors. *International Journal of Eating Disorders, 42*, 511–521.

Schupak-Neuberg, E., & Nemeroff, C. J. (1993). Disturbances in identity and self-regulation in bulimia nervosa: Implications for a metaphorical perspective of "body as self." *International Journal of Eating Disorders, 13*, 335–347.

Skårderud, F. (2007a) Eating one's words, part I: "Concretised metaphors" and reflective function in anorexia nervosa—an interview study. *European Eating Disorders Review, 15*, 163–174.

Skårderud, F. (2007b). Eating one's words, part II: The embodied mind and reflective function in anorexia nervosa—theory. *European Eating Disorders Review, 15*, 243–252.

Skårderud, F. (2007c). Eating one's words, part III: Mentalisation-based psychotherapy for anorexia nervosa—an outline for a treatment and training manual. *European Eating Disorders Review, 15*, 323–339.

Slane, J. D., Burt, S. A., & Klump, K. L. (2010, October). *Eating pathology and alcohol use: shared genetic influences.* Poster presentation at the 16th Annual Meeting of the Eating Disorders Research Society, Cambridge, MA.

Sloan, D. M., Mizes, J. S., & Epstein, E. M. (2005). Empirical classification of eating disorders. *Eating Behaviors, 6*, 53–62.

Steiger, H., & Bruce, K. R. (2004). Personality traits and disorders associated with anorexia nervosa, bulimia nervosa, and binge eating disorder. In T. D. Brewerton (Ed.), *Clinical handbook of eating disorders: An integrated approach* (pp. 209–230). New York: Marcel Dekker.

Steiger, H., Richardson, J., Joober, R., Gauvin, L., Israel, M., Bruce, K. R, et al. (2007). The 5HTTLPR polymorphism, prior maltreatment and dramatic-erratic personality manifestations in women with bulimic syndromes. *Journal of Psychiatry and Neuroscience, 32*, 354–362.

Steiger, H., Richardson, J., Schmitz, N., Joober, R., Israel, M., Bruce, K. R., et al. (2009). Association of trait-defined, eating-disorder sub-phenotypes with (biallelic and triallelic) 5HTTLPR variations. *Journal of Psychiatric Research, 43*, 1086–1094.

Stice, E. (1998). Prospective relation of dieting behaviors to weight change in a community sample of adolescents. *Behavior Therapy, 29*, 277–297.

Stice, E., & Agras, W. S. (1998). Predicting onset and cessation of bulimic behaviors during adolescence: A longitudinal grouping analysis. *Behavior Therapy, 29*, 257–276.

Stice, E., & Agras, W. S. (1999). Subtyping bulimic women along dietary restraint and negative affect dimensions. *Journal of Consulting and Clinical Psychology, 67*, 460–469.

Stice, E., Agras, W. S., Telch, C. F., Halmi, K. A., Mitchell, J. E., & Wilson, G. T. (2001). Subtyping binge eating-disordered women along dieting and negative affect dimensions. *International Journal of Eating Disorders, 30*, 11–27.

Stice, E., Bohon, C., Marti, C. N., & Fischer, K. (2008). Subtyping women with bulimia nervosa along dietary and negative affect dimensions: Further evidence of reliability and validity. *Journal of Consulting and Clinical Psychology, 76*, 1022–1033.

Sysko, R., Hildebrandt, T., Wilson, G. T., Wilfley, D. E., & Agras, W. S. (2010). Heterogeneity moderates treatment response among patients with binge eating disorder. *Journal of Consulting and Clinical Psychology, 78*, 681–690.

Sysko, R., Roberto, C. A., Barnes, R. D., Grilo, C. M., Attia, E., & Walsh, B. T. (2012). Test–retest reliability of the proposed DSM-5 eating disorder diagnostic criteria. *Psychiatry Research, 196*, 302–308.

Tasca, G. A., Ritchie, K., & Balfour, L. (2011). Implications of attachment theory and research for the assessment and treatment of eating disorders. *Psychotherapy, 48*, 249–259.

Tasca, G. A., Ritchie, K., Conrad, G., Balfour, L., Gayton, J., Daigle, V., et al. (2006). Attachment scales predict outcome in a randomized controlled trial of two group therapies for binge eating disorder: An aptitude by treatment interaction. *Psychotherapy Research, 16*, 106–121.

Tasca, G. A., Ritchie, K., Demidenko, N., Balfour, L., Krysanski, V., Weekes, K., et al. (2012). Matching women with binge eating disorder to group treatment based on attachment anxiety: Outcomes and moderating effects. *Psychotherapy Research, 23*, 301–314.

Tasca, G. A., Taylor, D., Ritchie, K., & Balfour, L. (2004). Attachment predicts treatment completion in an eating disorders partial hospital program among women with anorexia nervosa. *Journal of Personality Assessment, 83*, 201–212.

Thompson-Brenner, H., Eddy, K. T., Franko, D. L., Dorer, D. J., Vashchenko, M., Kass, A. E., et al. (2008). A personality classification system for eating disorders: A longitudinal study. *Comprehensive Psychiatry, 49*, 551–560.

Thompson-Brenner, H., Eddy, K. T., Satir, D., Boisseau, C. L., & Westen, D. (2008). Personality subtypes in adolescents with eating disorders: Validation of a classification approach. *Journal of Child Psychology and Psychiatry, 49*, 170–180.

Thompson-Brenner, H., Weingeroff, J., & Westen, D. (2009). Empirical support for psychody-namic psychotherapy for eating disorders. In R. Levy & S. J. Ablon (Eds.), *Handbook of evidence-based psychodynamic psychotherapy: Bridging the gap between science and practice* (pp. 67–92). New York: Humana Press

Thompson-Brenner, H., & Westen, D. (2005). Personality subtypes in eating disorders: Validation of a classification in a naturalistic sample. *British Journal of Psychiatry, 186*, 516–524.

Treasure, J., Sepulveda, A. R., MacDonald, P., Whitaker, W., Lopez, C., Zabala, M., et al. (2008). The assessment of the family of people with eating disorders. *European Eating Disorders Review, 16*, 247–255.

Turner, H., Bryant-Waugh, R., & Peveler, R. (2009). An approach to sub-grouping the eating disorder population: Adding attachment and coping style. *European Eating Disorders Review, 17*, 269–280.

Vitousek, K., & Manke, F.(1994). Personality variables and disorders in anorexia nervosa and bulimia nervosa. *Journal of Abnormal Psychology, 103*, 137–147.

Waller, J. V., Kaufman, M. R., & Deutsch, F. (1940). Anorexia nervosa. *Psychosomatic Medicine, 2*, 3–10.

Ward, A., Ramsay, R., & Treasure, J. (2000). Attachment research in eating disorders. *British Journal of Medical Psychology, 73*, 35–51.

Weingeroff, J., Thompson-Brenner, H., Pratt, E., Sherry, H., & Westen, D. (2007, May). *Affect regulation in adolescent and adult eating disorders.* Paper presented to the International Conference for the Academy of Eating Disorders, Baltimore.

Westen, D., & Harnden-Fischer, J. (2001). Personality profiles in eating disorders: Rethinking the distinction between Axis I and Axis II. *American Journal of Psychiatry, 158*, 547–562.

Westen, D., Muderrisoglu, S., Fowler, C., Shedler, J., & Koren, J. (1997). Affect regulation and affective experience: Individual differences, group differences, and measurement using a Q-sort procedure. *Journal of Consulting and Clinical Psychology, 65*, 429–439.

Wildes, J. E. (2010, October). *Empirically-derived personality subtypes in patients with anorexia nervosa: Validity and clinical utility in a tertiary care center.* Symposium presentation at the 16th annual meeting of the Eating Disorders Research Society, Cambridge, MA.

Wilson, G. T., & Sysko, R. (2009). Frequency of binge eating episodes in bulimia nervosa and binge eating disorder: Diagnostic considerations. *International Journal of Eating Disorders, 42*, 603–610.

Wilson, G. T., Wilfley, D. E., Agras, W. S., & Bryson, S. W. (2010). Psychological treatments of binge eating disorders. *Archives of General Psychiatry, 67*, 94–101.

Wonderlich, S. A., Crosby, R. D., Joiner T., Peterson, C. B., Bardone-Cone, A., Klein, M., et al. (2005). Personality subtyping and bulimia nervosa: Psychopathological and genetic correlates. *Psychological Medicine, 35*, 649–657.

Wonderlich, S. A., Crosby, R. D., Mitchell, J. E., Thompson, K., Smyth, J. M., & Jones-Paxton, M. (2001). Sexual trauma and personality: developmental vulnerability and additive effects. *Journal of Personality Disorders, 15*, 496–504.

CHAPTER 13

Psychosis

Susanne Harder and Bent Rosenbaum

The psychodynamic understanding of psychosis is inherently developmental and interpersonal. Since the 1980s, it has been characterized by strong cross-fertilization and integration between different psychodynamic approaches, and between psychodynamic and other psychological approaches, as well as by an integration of psychological understanding with knowledge from the biological and socio-cultural sciences. The historical development of psychodynamic models of psychosis has followed the general path of development within psychodynamic thinking. The first theoretical models were formulated by Freud in the years 1890–1925. Following his classical descriptions, several lines of thinking developed, of which only the most influential are reviewed here—the ego-psychology models, which explore the dynamics of drive, drive representation and the ego, and the Kleinian and post-Kleinian models, which focus on the dynamics of internal object relations, meaning-making, and symbol formation. We also include a discussion of interpersonal, intersubjective, and self-psychology approaches to psychosis that explore the dynamics of interpersonal relations, self, subjectivity, and intersubjectivity. Finally, we discuss more contemporary psychodynamic models that focus on the dynamics of attachment patterns and of shared emotionality, and on the capacity for self-awareness and mentalization. We review the empirical support for these models, as well as their contribution to the contemporary psychodynamic understanding of psychosis.

CLASSIFICATION AND DIAGNOSIS

Psychosis is a broadly defined category encompassing manifestations of several disorders. The diagnostic systems of the *Diagnostic and Statistical Manual of Mental*

Disorders (DSM; American Psychiatric Association [APA], 2013) and the *International Classification of Diseases* (ICD; World Health Organization [WHO], 1992) separate psychosis into two main diagnostic groups: *affective psychosis*, which includes diagnoses of depression and mania, and the so-called *nonaffective psychosis*, which includes schizophrenia as the most important diagnostic entity. A few other diagnoses, for example, posttraumatic stress disorder and (in DSM-5) borderline personality disorder, may also include psychotic phenomena but to a lesser extent.

This chapter focuses on the schizophrenia-spectrum types of psychoses. It will devote particular attention to the fragmentation of the self and the disorganization of the mind, which, from a psychodynamic perspective, are considered to be core characteristics of psychosis. These characteristics encompass phenomena such as disturbances in self-awareness, self-reflection, and cognitive and affective understanding of self–other relations; delusional sense and understanding of one's thoughts and communication; distorted perceptual experience of one's body and its demarcations and functions; and incoherent or fragmented sense of time and of "being present in the world." Psychotic states within the affective spectrum may to some extent be characterized in the same way, but these states are phenomenologically different and thus different from a theoretical point of view. Affective psychotic states will be mentioned only briefly.

PSYCHODYNAMIC APPROACHES TO PSYCHOSIS

Freud and the Ego-Psychological Approach to Psychosis

On one hand, Freud's understanding of the development of psychotic states of mind resembles his account of the development of disturbed nonpsychotic mental states in its emphasis on the importance of trauma—the blow to the mind that breaches its boundaries and damages its structural organization—and the defenses against the unbearable affects, ideas, and fantasies inherent in the trauma. On the other hand, and unlike neurotic and other nonpsychotic explanatory models, Freud's models of the pathogenesis of psychosis emphasized severe disturbances in the structure of the self and the ego. Freud outlined three pathways to psychosis, as summarized here:

1. Freud proposed a model with three dimensions of presentations (in German, *Vorstellungen*): *thing presentation*, *word presentation*, and *object presentation*. Withdrawal of libido from the unconscious thing presentation (as opposed to the withdrawal of libido from the conscious object presentation) undermined the capacity of the psychic apparatus for symbol formation and thus led to radical changes in the person's attention and relation to the world (Freud & Abraham, 1965). This radical disturbance entailed loss of interest in objects, and destabilization and distortion of the entire process of symbolization. Unconscious fantasies, material from memory traces, and previous perceptions bypassed the preconscious function of meaning-making and thus impinged on the ego's relating to the world in raw and immediate forms.

2. Freud also hypothesized that during development, psychosis-prone individuals suffer from serious problems with regard to autoerotism and narcissism (Freud, 1911/1958), disturbing the development of the social drive and the origin of a group mind (Freud, 1921/1955) in such a way that the individual was unable to make sense of and engage experientially in the social/erotic relations of the oedipal conflict (Rosenbaum, 2005). As a consequence, the individual is constantly struggling with the following: (a) *distinguishing between what is internal and what is external to the body*: ambiguity as to whether sensations and perceptions belong to the internal or the external world, or whether they are good/positive or bad/negative (i.e., manifestations of disturbances in the autoerotic structure); (b) *distinguishing what belongs to the self from what belongs to the other*: severe conflicts concerning whether thoughts and fantasies originate in and belong to one's self or the other (i.e., disturbances in the narcissistic structure).

3. As a result of persistent frustration of the ego in its continuing development, the ego withdraws its investments in the external world, followed by a radical negation/disavowal of the existence of reality as a symbolic world (i.e., a world with symbolic meaning and common sense) (Freud, 1924a/1961a, 1924b/1961b). By doing so, it simultaneously, in part or wholly, disconnects the person's experience of a relationship with reality. Three factors in this process were presumed to play a pathogenic role: (a) *the dynamics of withdrawal*, that is, the extent to which a radical disconnection of unconscious processes from the world takes place; (b) *the phenomenon of regression to a level of psychic primary functioning*, where the distinctions, functions, and use of words, perceptions, sensations, and fantasies become blurred or assume a fragmented appearance; and (c) *"failed" attempts at restitution by creating another worldview*, different from the socially accepted reality which, for the patient, is ambiguous, perplexing, and confusingly frustrating—using fragments of thoughts, fantasies, perceptions, and sensations to create delusional and hallucinatory viewpoints.

Ego psychology expanded these viewpoints. In psychosis, the affected ego functions were primarily seen in the symptoms of serious instability in the capacity for defense, marked vulnerability to stress, impaired reality testing (e.g., capacity to distinguish between perceptions, feelings, and thoughts; ability to discern subjective and objective elements in our judgment of reality), and impaired cognition and thinking. Within ego psychology, an important controversy arose between defense and deficit theory (Frosch, 1983). The defense approach asserted that, as with neurosis, psychosis could be explained in terms of a dynamic conflict of drives and the defense against it. The deficit theory proposed specific defects in the capacity to organize and sustain mental representations, which may be rooted in psychosocial or neurodevelopmental/innate causes. The extent to which these diverse viewpoints can be integrated remains controversial. Bellak, Hurvich, and Gediman (1973) studied various ego functions, such as reality testing, judgment, object relations, and thought processes and other synthesizing functions, which were seen as dependent on good parenting (regardless of who the caretaker was). Traumatic disruptions of ego development, object relations, self–object differentiation, and an appropriate libido–aggression balance were seen as the foundation for the development of basic anxiety, evolving in response to the sensed possibility of disintegration and dissolution of the self.

During the following decades, the investigation of basic anxiety was predominantly conducted from a Kleinian perspective, while interest in further investigating disturbed ego functions declined as the concept of the ego was replaced with the concept of self. Scharfetter (2008), for instance, linked ego pathology with self-fragmentation.

Ego psychology, as discussed in more detail below, was influential in the development of supportive psychotherapy approaches to psychosis (Gunderson et al., 1984). This approach addresses the deficit in ego function, focusing on current interpersonal problems and difficulties in the management of daily living. The approach is supportive, for example, in relation to reality testing, where the therapist will aim at sensitizing the patient to the perception of internal reality (e.g., recognizing anger and anxiety before they are translated into major or minor projections) (Bellak et al., 1973). Group psychotherapy was thought to function as a suitable setting for self-correction of reality testing. Interpretations in supportive psychotherapy are very limited and judiciously paced. The therapy aims to strengthen existing defenses, relieve symptoms, and improve the management of everyday life.

The Klein–Bion Approach

Klein (1946) introduced an object relational perspective on psychosis based on her concept of the mind as composed of relationships between inner objects and the self in the form of unconscious phantasies. Central to her thinking is the concept of two elementary modes of psychic functioning: the *paranoid-schizoid position* and the *depressive position*. These are basic structures of emotional life, each with its own characteristic anxieties (persecutory and annihilation anxiety vs. fear of loss), its own defensive maneuvers (splitting and projective identification vs. reparation), and its own type of object relations (part objects that are either idealized or persecutory vs. whole objects, where the experience of the other is based on the simultaneous presence of both positive and negative aspects). These positions are thought to originate in the very first months of life, but they remain present throughout life as two modes of psychic functioning. The anxieties and defenses of the paranoid-schizoid position (promoted by aggressiveness) were seen as psychosis-prone elements if they dominated the person's experience of self and others. Klein suggests that malignant forms of aggression were innate, but post-Kleinian psychoanalysts in particular have stressed that constitutional tendencies can be transformed by actual experiences with personal relationships.

Klein (1946) also introduced the concept of *projective identification*, an unconscious phantasy by means of which the mind rids itself of overwhelming emotions and fantasies by splitting them from the self-representation and making them belong to the object. Bion (1967) developed the concept of projective identification further. He did not see it solely as a defensive process, but also as a primary form of communication. If primary caregivers were able to understand and contain the projected emotions, this would lead to development of the ego and to the integrative processes of the depressive position. However, when the frustrations and tensions of the mind could not be contained in either the subject (child) or the object (mother), the fears and defenses associated with the paranoid–schizoid position would dominate, and projective identificatory processes would become excessive and lead to what Bion termed "attacks on linking"—that is, the linking of thoughts, affects, and mutuality in interpersonal relationships. This could cause a breakdown in the sense of coherence and the ability to function in an organized way, resulting in psychotic functioning. Bion proposed that the same individual contained both psychotic and nonpsychotic organizations, which could dominate in turn, depending on the degree of decompensation. Klein and Bion thus saw the use of psychotic functioning as dimensional. It dominated in excessive forms in psychotic states, but it was present to a lesser degree outside psychosis.

Bion (1967) outlined two fundamental ways in which the mental apparatus could deal with emotions and perceptions. The first is a transformation of sense impression into mental contents, thoughts, and thinking, as part of a containing process; this characterizes a nonpsychotic mode of thinking. The second is an attempt to get rid of raw emotions and sense impressions either by evacuating them into one's own body, in the form of somatic sensations and hallucinations, or by projecting them into the other's body, which gives rise to delusions (formed by splitting and excessive projective identification). This characterizes the psychotic mode of functioning. The latter processes lay the ground for formation of the psychotic phenomena seen in states of schizophrenia, such as disturbed understanding of self–other relations, delusional understanding of one's thoughts and communication, and distorted perceptions of one's body. Bion's concept of symbolization has much in common with more recent concepts of mentalizing or metacognition (Dimaggio & Lysaker, 2010)—for example, the notion of regulation of affects by use of mental processes for understanding the self and the other. Furthermore, the concepts of splitting and fragmentation of the ego are conceptually related to the concept of dissociation. Mentalizing and dissociation are discussed later in this chapter in relation to attachment theory.

This line of thinking about psychosis, for which the most important initiators were Klein, Bion, and Rosenfeld (1965), has continued to the present day. Several scholars have made important theoretical and clinical contributions, for example, Meltzer (1975), Ogden (1980), and Jackson (2001; Jackson & Williams, 1994). No single, definitive contemporary model of psychosis can be synthesized from these approaches, but they all have made important contributions to a fuller understanding of different aspects of the psychotic modes of functioning.

Robbins (2011) has proposed an integrative model of the psychotic mind based on Freudian views, ego psychology, and object relations theories. He promotes the concept of a mind-state that he calls *primordial mental activity* (PMA). PMA appears to have a distinctive neurological circuitry similar to that of dream processes (involving the forebrain and limbic-paralimbic structures) and to be present from the onset of life. It seems to arise from affect-generating somatic sensing sensory-perceptual areas of the brain that do not differentiate inner from outer. PMA is a normal way in which the mind works, both in learning and in expression, and is qualitatively different from rational, realistic, self-reflective thought. This mode is responsible for dreaming and predominates in infancy and early childhood. Psychoses are understood as maladaptive expressions of PMA caused by developmental circumstances that thwart the development of thought and the integration of thought and PMA. The driving force of psychosis then becomes raw somatic affect (i.e., PMA) rather than identifiable emotions that characterize thought. The affective experiences are amorphous, dysphoric, self-destructive, panic-ridden, and painful. Ordinary rules of logic, causality, time, and space are not appreciated; there is little sense of the passage of time; the moment is everything, and remembered past and anticipated future make little sense as anchor points for one's identity.

Robbins's idea is in line with contemporary neuroscience and neuropsychoanalytic approaches that describe consciousness as functionally and conceptually "two-layered." According to Edelman (1989, 1992), we can talk about a fine-tuned relationship of primary consciousness and higher-order consciousness, while Damasio (2000) has studied the formation of "core consciousness" and "extended consciousness." Damasio asserts that psychotic states of mania, depression, and schizophrenia may be understood as disturbances of the extended consciousness. Edelman points out that schizophrenia may, among other things, be a disease of inappropriate reentrant mappings affecting imaging, categorization and conceptual systems, memory, and symbolic processes. Edelman hypothesizes that the psychotic person attempts with his or her higher-order consciousness to adapt and reintegrate what a dysfunctional primary-consciousness produces. Damasio has proposed analogous ideas about the relation between the autobiographical self (belonging to the extended consciousness) and the core self (part of core consciousness).

With regard to psychotherapy, the concepts of projective identification and containment are central to the modern Kleinian approach. Where early approaches were focused on interpretations, more recent approaches stress the importance of the containing quality of the therapeutic relationship. The emotional exchange and containment are considered essential for establishing a therapeutic alliance, and they are believed to regulate the pace and timing of explorative and interpretive techniques. The role of the psychosocial, external world in the development of psychotic mental functioning is acknowledged in the Kleinian approach, but the main focus is to understand the dynamics of the internal world in psychotic states and how processes of splitting and projective identification form the psychotic patient's emotional life as well as his or her thinking and behavior in relation to external relationships and the outside world in general. The aim of psychotherapy is to help the patient reestablish the capacity to differentiate him- or herself and his or her conflicting desires from those of other people, and to recognize that the reality of his or her inner "imaginative" world is different from the reality of the external "real" world. This involves reducing his or her use of projective identification, withdrawing projections, recovering lost parts of the self, and recognizing and tolerating (containing) unwanted and feared impulses and wishes. The patient can thereby hope to regain or acquire a new and more stable sense of identity and a capacity to think for him- or herself, and ultimately become able to take more responsibility for his or her own mind (Jackson, 2001).

North American Interpersonal–Relational Models

The interpersonal model, originally proposed by Sullivan (1962), traced the developmental roots of psychosis back to the very first years of life. In contrast to the Klein–Bion model, Sullivan discarded the concept of drives and constitutional factors, and focused on the influence of social and interpersonal factors both in his general model of psychic development and in his model of psychosis. In his view, an individual cannot be understood in isolation from his or her social relationships and cultural environment.

At the beginning of life, the infant's emotional needs must be met by a responsive caretaker. The quality of these early relationships determines the degree and the quality of integration of the infant's personality. According to Sullivan, the risk for psychosis is related to mid-infancy, when the infant starts to develop a sense of self and a "self-system" that consists of three different ways of organizing experiences of self-with-other: "good-me," "bad-me," and "not-me." The presence of anxiety is central to bad experiences. Sullivan saw the source of anxiety as entirely relational: If the mother was anxious in relation to the child, this anxiety would be induced in the infant as well. The "not-me" experience is an experience of intense anxiety that takes place in relation to significant others where no solution to the anxiety can be achieved. To defend itself from these emotions, the child splits off this part of the self through dissociation. Psychosis develops as a result of a breakdown of a defensive system of "security operations" and the return of the dissociated, "not-me" part of the personality into consciousness, which causes disorganization. The psychotic breakdown is related to a highly anxiety-provoking experience or a longer series of subjectively difficult adjustment efforts, most often during adolescence, when great demands are placed on the individual's capacity for social transition. In the transition to adulthood, the person must establish his or her position in the social-cultural environment and face the challenges of forming socially and sexually intimate relationships. People with an excessive amount of "not-me" dissociated parts of the personality are at risk of not being able to meet the challenges and make the necessary integration into society. This "dissociation hypothesis" has been further developed in recent work (see below).

The interpersonal therapy model sees the therapist as an active participant-observer in the therapeutic process, who places emphasis on the interpersonal exchanges between patient and therapist. The model focuses on clarifying the patient's difficulties with others by observing and investigating the vicissitudes of the therapeutic relationship. Furthermore, it encourages recall of forgotten memories and investigates the anxiety connected with such recall (Fromm-Reichmann, 1950), but its main focus is on the here and now. Although Fromm-Reichmann believed it was important for patients to gain insight into their affects, Sullivan, like Federn (1952), did not stress this. Instead, he focused on reorganization of the disintegrated personality.

Intersubjective Models

Building on Kohut's self psychology (e.g. Kohut, 1977) emphasizing the role of sub-jective experiences of the self, Stolorow, Brancroft, and Atwood (1995) developed an intersubjective psychodynamic approach to psychosis. This approach also focuses on contributions from interpersonal experiences to the development of psychosis. Cen-tral to their thinking is the idea of a need for validation of subjective experiences in an intersubjective "system of differently organized, interacting subjective worlds" (Stol-orow et al., 1995). Lack of validation during childhood due to absent or unreliable parenting leaves the child's belief in his or her own subjective reality unstable and pre-disposes the child to psychosis. Psychotic states develop when a powerful emotional reaction that creates an urgent need for validation is not validated by another person. The affective reaction then cannot be integrated, and the child feels threatened by disintegration. Delusions are understood as the result of an attempt to maintain psy-chological integrity by elaborating delusional ideas that symbolically concretize the experience, which is losing its subjective reality due to lack of validation.

From a therapeutic perspective, the approach advocated by Stolorow and col-leagues (1995), focuses on the therapist's attempt to comprehend the core of subjective truth symbolically encoded in the patient's delusional ideas and to communicate this understanding in a form that the patient can use. A consistent empathic decoding of the patient's subjective truths gradually establishes the therapeutic bond as an inter-subjective context in which the patient's belief in his or her own personal reality can become more firmly consolidated. This diminishes the need for delusional concreti-zations, which then tend to recede. Whereas this approach focuses on disturbances in intersubjective meaning-making at a symbolic level, Harder and Lysaker (2013), following Stern and colleagues (1998), propose that the procedural level of affective intersubjectivity is also severely disturbed in psychosis and needs to be addressed in psychotherapy, in order to restore the capacity to regulate affect during interpersonal exchange and to facilitate the process of meaning-making at a symbolic level.

The Attachment Model

Attachment theory has recently been applied to psychosis (Berry, Barrowclough, & Wearden, 2007; Harder, 2014; Liotti & Gumley, 2008; MacBeth, Gumley, Schwannauer, & Fisher, 2011; Read & Gumley, 2008). These theories typically hold that attachment status is an important mediating factor between childhood adversity and vulnerability to psychosis in later life. The attachment system is viewed as a developmental system construct organizing affect, cognition, and behavior in rela-tion to a caregiver (see Mikulincer & Shaver, Chapter 2, this volume, for a descrip-tion of attachment theory). As is well known, the organized forms of attachment in infancy or adulthood as measured by, respectively, the Strange Situation procedure (SSP; Ainsworth, Blehar, Waters, & Wall, 1970) or the Adult Attachment Interview (AAI; George, Kaplan, & Main, 1985), can be categorized as either secure or inse-cure, with insecure attachment being further divided into insecure ambivalent/pre-occupied or insecure avoidant/dismissing. Insecure/dismissing type of attachment is thought to emerge from experiences of consistent rejection from an attachment figure, when a need for comfort is present. This type of attachment is character- ized by deactivation or externalization of affects as the dominating affect regulation strategy. Disorganized forms of attachment, in turn, are conceptualized in terms of momentary or more profound breakdowns in the organized patterns of attachment and are, together with avoidant/dismissing attachment, of special interest in relation to psychosis. Infants characterized as disorganized/disoriented seem unable to use a consistent strategy toward the caregiver for downregulation of high arousal when experiencing a strong need for comfort. This pattern is thought to emerge from trau- matic experience, where an attachment figure is both a source of fear and comfort. Instead of a consistent attachment strategy the infant exhibits contradictory behav- ioral patterns of comfort-seeking mixed with avoidance, freezing, stereotypes, inter- ruptions, or other confused behaviors. These behaviors are interpreted as expressing "fear without solution." Fear plays a central role in disorganization because fear in relation to perceived danger is assumed to result in high levels of arousal of the attachment system. The perceived availability and responsibility of a caregiver are central to the infant's ability to downregulate this affective arousal. In adults, disor- ganization is identified at the representational level in the AAI as loss of coherence of thought in relation to loss or abuse (the category of "unresolved" state of mind) or, in more severe cases, throughout the interview (the "cannot classify" category). Disor- ganized attachment is thought to be produced by frightening or frightened parental behavior associated with severe aversive conditions in the caretaker–infant relation- ship, such as the caretaker's depression, mourning over loss, or trauma during the child's infancy, or the experience of loss or trauma by the child him- or herself (for a review, see Lyons-Ruth & Jacobvitz, 2008).

Severe forms of avoidant/dismissing and disorganized attachment, possibly in combination with other risk factors, have been hypothesized to be involved in several areas of disturbed development related to psychosis, such as negative symptoms, dis- turbed affect regulation, difficulties with interpersonal relationships, fragmentation of self-experience, and serious impairments in mentalizing/metacognition, as well as the specific psychotic symptoms of delusions and hallucinations.

Some forms of negative symptoms in schizophrenia such as blunted affect and emotional withdrawal might be expressions of deactivation of affect as part of a severely dismissing attachment pattern. Furthermore, the externalizing affect regula- tion strategy in dismissing attachment might be involved in development of positive psychotic symptoms such as hallucinations and delusions (Harder, 2014).

The high levels of anxiety and heightened reactivity to stress seen in psychosis are proposed to be part of disorganized attachment patterns where disturbed affect regulation strategies make the individual unable to down-regulate arousal related to fear and anxiety (Liotti & Gumley, 2008). These "fear without solution" experiences are further hypothesized to lead to a defensive dismissive attachment pattern in addi- tion to disorganization. Dismissive withdrawal defends the mind against interper- sonal encounters that may lead to these painful levels of arousal and disorganization (Liotti & Gumley, 2008). Activation of these "fear without solution" experiences may lead to dissociative processes, defined as disruptions in the usually integrated functions of consciousness, memory, identity, or perception of the environment, and fragmented "self with other" representations (Ogawa, Sroufe, Weinfield, Carlson, & Egeland, 1997). Dissociation has been empirically linked to the experience of trauma in general and with the later development of hallucinations in posttraumatic stress disorders (Moskowitz, Read, Farelly, Rudegeair, & Williams, 2009). Based on these findings, Moskowitz and colleagues (2009) proposed that several psychotic symptoms might have a traumatic origin and a dissociative nature. Furthermore, Liotti (1992) proposed that attachment organization might have a central role in the development of dissociative symptoms. Combining these ideas, Read and Gumley (2008) proposed a developmental model linking childhood trauma to psychosis. They argue that dissociative processes are better understood as part of disorganized attachment patterns than as a direct outcome of traumatic experiences. Furthermore, they propose that an interaction between disorganized attachment and other risk factors such as temperamental variables of schizotypy and proneness to dissociation might be necessary for childhood trauma to lead to psychosis and not to other forms of psychopathology.

A related area of interest is the disturbance in metacognitive or mentalizing capacities in psychosis. Based on the understanding that the attachment system is a developing, adaptive system that organizes affect, cognition, and behavior, Liotti and Gumley (2008) proposed that the metacognitive difficulties in psychosis could be understood as being associated with the affective problems and fragmentation of self that are related to disorganized attachment (as described above). Mentalizing and metacognitive functions refer to individuals' understanding of their own and others' behavior in terms of mental states, and the impact of mental states on one's cognition, affective state, and behavior. In addition, metacognition specifically includes the ability to make use of this understanding in dealing with interpersonal problems and distressing states of mind (the "mastery" dimension). These concepts overlap with the concepts of theory of mind and social cognition, but these notions are less focused on issues of affect regulation and affective reflectivity. The development of mentalizing capacities is thought to be fostered by secure attachment relationships, again emphasizing the potential role of attachment experiences in psychosis. Fonagy and Target (2006) have proposed that it is not the attachment style per se, but impairments in mentalizing capacities that are often observed in the context of attachment disruptions that render individuals vulnerable to development of psychopathology. The metacognitive difficulties seen in psychosis are thought to be at least partly rooted in such early disruptions of affective bonds and insecure or disorganized forms of attachment (Gumley, 2010). This represents an alternative hypothesis to the purely genetic hypothesis formulated by the theory of mind tradition (Frith, 1992). In this context, Gumley and Schwannauer (2006) have proposed an integrative cognitive interpersonal therapy model that is based on attachment theory concepts. It focuses on emotional recovery, self-coherence, and interpersonal functioning, and it uses an attachment approach to guide work in the therapeutic relationship. These psychodynamic principles are combined with cognitive interventions such as rational reasoning, structured sessions, and symptom-focused intervention. The compassion-focused approach to psychological treatment of psychosis integrates attention theory with cognitive and evolutionary psychology into its treatment model

(Gumley, Braehler, Laithwaite, MacBeth, & Gilbert, 2010). Furthermore, Lysaker and colleagues combining intersubjective and cognitive approaches, has developed a metacognitive reflection and insight therapy that is currently being tested (Van Donkersgoed et al., 2014).

Empirical Findings

Empirical research in schizophrenia and other kinds of psychosis is painting an increasingly complex picture of the possible causes that give rise to the conditions described as schizophrenia. In this section we review biological findings in relation to schizophrenia, as well as research concerning each of the psychodynamic views outlined above. We also review relevant outcome research in therapy models.

Biological Findings

The presence of genetic risk factors conferring vulnerability to schizophrenia is well established (Harrison & Weinberger, 2005), although most individuals diagnosed with schizophrenia do not have an affected relative (Gottesman, 1991). Several genetic (genes affecting neuron migration, synaptic pruning, and myelinization), intrauterine (pre- and perinatal exposure to viruses, complications at birth), and environmental (traumatic early life experiences, urbanization, cannabis abuse) risk factors have been identified (McGrath et al., 2004; Tienari et al., 2004; van Os, Krabbendam, Myin-Germeys, & Delespaul, 2005; Varese et al., 2012), but no single factor seems to be specific to schizophrenia. On the basis of the current evidence, schizophrenia and other psychoses are most likely the result of developmental pathways that are influenced by a complex interaction between multiple genetic and environmental risk factors whose crucial interactions are determined by nonlinear dynamics. Findings of morphometric changes in the brains of some patients diagnosed with schizophrenia, increased frequency of obstetric complications, and abnormal social, motor, and cognitive maturation during childhood have led to formulation of a neurodevelopmental hypothesis of schizophrenia. However, a direct causal link between these findings and abnormal brain development is lacking, and current evidence indicates a role for environmental factors in the development of schizophrenia. In addition, other psychiatric disorders may also have a neurodevelopmental component (Marenco & Weinberger, 2000).

Genetic and neurodevelopmental research (Hirsch, 2003; Kapur, 2003; Parnas, 1999) also suggests that changes at the molecular level (chromosomal deviations) influence the endophenotypic level (compromised ability to integrate perception, thought, and affect) and the transphenotypic level (basic symptoms and signs of disturbed experience of the self), which are thought to give rise to overt psychotic symptoms and disturbed reality testing on the phenomenological level. Although developmental psychopathology and psychodynamic approaches to psychopathology question the narrow biological focus and the linear causal view in these biological models, these biological findings and models challenge the emphasis of psychodynamic approaches on ego development, attachment, and the dynamics of the self in the development of psychosis.

Dynamic Models of Psychosis

The Dynamics of Drive, Drive Representation, and the Ego

A literature search identified only a few relevant systematic empirical studies of ego functions in psychosis. For instance, the ego-psychological assumption of disturbances in ego functions in psychosis was explored in depth by Bellak and colleagues (1973), who found that a group of individuals within the schizophrenia spectrum scored significantly lower on four factors: reality orientation, socialization, adaptive thinking, and integrative capacity. More recently, Scharfetter (2008) studied ego pathology in schizophrenia. Participants with a diagnosis of schizophrenia (N = 552) consistently reported the highest levels of pathology within the areas of identity, demarcation consistence/coherence, vitality, and activity (e.g., experiences of being controlled or manipulated by others or outside powers) compared with individuals with borderline personality disorder and depression. This indicates that a specific distribution of type and severity of ego disturbances may be present in schizophrenia. Empirical approaches to the study of self-experience in psychosis, integrating ego-psychological and phenomenological thinking, are emerging (Pérez-Álvarez, García-Montes, Vallina-Fernández, Perona-Garcelán, & Cuevas-Yust, 2011), but more research is definitely needed.

The Dynamics of Internal Object Relations

The Kleinian approach has used case studies only to empirically underpin the development of its theories, but studies from more integrative dynamic and other approaches have lent some support to some aspects of the Klein–Bion view regarding psychosis. Considerable empirical research, especially during the period from the 1970s to the 1990s, has established the validity of measures of object representations for describing and differentiating psychosis and other types of psychopathology (for a review, see Huprich & Greenberg, 2003). Early studies in this tradition have suggested that psychosis involves general boundary disruption (Blatt & Ritzler, 1974; Blatt & Wild, 1976), that is, a deficit in maintaining the distinction between self and other (Lerner, Sugarman, & Barbour, 1985) and diminished capacity to attribute autonomous identity to self and other (Harder, Greenwald, & Wechsler, 1984), congruent with object relational views. Furthermore, research also suggests that addressing and changing these difficulties during psychotherapy seem to be possible (Blatt, Ford, Berman, Cook, & Meyer, 1988). While confirming the presence of severe disturbances in object representation in psychosis, these studies are rooted more in Mahler's (1968) developmental phase model than in the "pure" Kleinian understanding of splitting and projective identification processes as the basis for development of psychotic functioning. Moreover, both the Kleinian and the Mahlerian developmental models have been criticized for being at odds with empirical infant research in several aspects (Stern, 1985).

At the same time, the hypothesis that splitting is a defense separating idealized from devaluated (part) objects has gathered initial support in two studies (Gerson, 1984; Glassman, 1986). More recent studies have also identified mental processes in psychosis that bear some resemblance to splitting. Trower and Chadwick (1995) and Melo, Taylor, and Bentall (2006), for instance, described two types of paranoia, "poor me" and "bad me," which can be interpreted as an expression of splitting into good and bad inner objects as proposed by Klein. In Kleinian theory, childhood adversity is seen as one factor in creating this split. This idea is supported by the finding of elevated levels of splitting in the form of "hostile–helpless" states of mind in disorganized attachment, as expressed in unintegrated alternating positive and negative evaluations of attachment figures in the AAI (Lyons-Ruth & Jacobvitz, 2008). "Hostile–helpless" states of mind were found to be strongly related to childhood trauma.

The Kleinian view of a process of excessive splitting in psychosis and the subsequent loss of self-coherence, self–other differentiation, and inner–outer boundaries gathers some empirical support if it is understood broadly as contained in the concept of dissociation (see below for a discussion of research on dissociation). Some support can be found for the projective aspect of the concept of projective identification, as projection and the cognitive concept of external attribution show some overlap. People showing paranoia have been found to make external-personal causal attributions for negative events, in contrast to normal individuals, who attribute such events to external-situational factors, and depressive individuals, whose attribution tends to be primarily internal (Melo et al., 2006).

The Interpersonal Approach and Social Risk Factors

The assumption in Sullivan's (1962) interpersonal approach of the importance of broader social factors during childhood for the development of psychosis is supported by several lines of research. Social childhood risk factors such as growing up in poverty, urban living, and belonging to an ethnic minority group, combined with unemployment, have been found to be linked to higher rates of psychosis (for a review, see Read & Gumley, 2008). The mechanisms behind these associations are not well understood. Poverty has been found to moderate the quality of the infant–parent relationship (Sroufe, Egeland, Carlson, & Collins, 2005); this indicates that at least some of the associations may be mediated by the family environment. It also suggests that the quality of family relationships and child care is, in itself, restricted or facilitated by the social context.

The impact of relationship with parents on the development of psychosis as assumed in object relational, interpersonal, and attachment approaches is supported by a number of studies. Family environment has been found to predict psychosis both in interaction with genetic risk (Tienari et al., 2004) and without such a risk (Goldstein, 1987). More severe adversity, such as loss of a parent, has also been found to be a risk factor for psychosis (Morgan et al., 2007). Other research has provided growing evidence for an association between childhood trauma, including sexual abuse, physical and emotional abuse and neglect, and the development of psychosis in later life (Varese et al., 2012).

Goldstein (1987) found that high levels of expressed emotion in the families of adolescents with lower levels of clinical disturbance predicted the likelihood of schizophrenia-spectrum disorders 15 years later. This finding lends some support to Sullivan's hypothesis that strong negative emotions could be transmitted from parents to infants and be involved in the development of psychosis. Together with a large amount of research showing that expressed emotion is an important risk factor for relapse, this study supports a more general hypothesis that unregulated or uncontained strong negative emotions are an important factor in eliciting psychotic symptoms—a hypothesis that is shared by most psychodynamic approaches. Furthermore, using a prospective momentary assessment design, one study demonstrated a specific link between negative emotions and the development of psychotic symptoms (Thewissen et al., 2011). These authors found that paranoid episodes were associated with high levels of negative emotions and that an increase in the level of anxiety predicted the onset of paranoid episodes. Depressive affectivity has been linked to relapse of psychosis (Birchwood, Iqbal, Chadwick, & Trower, 1993) and is common in psychosis. In a study on annihilation anxiety (Hurvich, 2003), Davidsen and Rosenbaum (2012) found that the level of annihilation anxiety was significantly higher in subjects at risk of psychosis than in healthy individuals, while the level in the at-risk group did not significantly differ from that of a group of patients with schizophrenia.

Attachment and Affect Regulation

Dismissing attachment is found to be the dominating attachment pattern in psychosis and more so in chronic (72%; Tyrell, Dozier, Teague, & Fallot, 1999) than in first-episode samples (62%; MacBeth et al., 2011). Unresolved/disorganized attachment styles are the second most common (29–44%). Dozier, Stovall-McClough, and Albus (2008) have argued that findings of disorganized attachment in psychosis, as measured by the AAI, should be interpreted with caution, as "lapses in monitoring of reasoning and discourse" are both a sign of thought disorder, which is a symptom of schizophrenia, and a sign of disorganized (unresolved) attachment status. MacBeth and colleagues (2011) found no association between attachment status and severity of symptoms, which indicates that attachment ratings may not be compromised by psychotic symptoms. A recent study found that degree of attachment security predicted recovery of negative symptoms (Gumley et al., 2014). However, further research is needed into the possible causal role of disorganized and avoidant forms of attachment in psychosis, as well as the more specific hypothesis of avoidant attachment as a defense against disorganized attachment (Liotti & Gumley, 2008)—a subject that remains unexplored.

The proposal that the disturbed affect regulation, also described as increased emotional stress reactivity, seen in psychosis is an expression of disorganized attachment has received indirect empirical support. A considerable body of research supports an attachment theory–based approach to the understanding of affect regulation in adults in general (Mikulincer & Shaver, 2008) and suggests that increased stress reactivity is a risk factor for development of psychosis (Myin-Germeys & van Os, 2007). It remains unknown to what degree this reactivity is an expression of a genetic vulnerability to psychosis, a result of childhood adversities possibly mediated by disorganized attachment, or a combination of both. Newborns differ in their reactivity and ability to adapt to external stimuli (Lester et al., 2004), but little is known about the neonatal affective reactivity status of people with psychosis. Furthermore, initial reactivity may be changed by healthy relationship experiences. This may, for example, partly explain why positive family conditions seem to protect against development of psychosis in genetically vulnerable individuals (Tienari et al., 2004). Childhood adversity alone has also been found to lead to increased stress reactivity. For example, Lardinois, Latester, Menglers, van Os, and Myin-Germeys (2011) found that a history of childhood trauma in patients with psychosis was associated with increased stress reactivity later in life. While this study did not assess attachment status, the findings indicate an underlying process of behavioral sensitization.

Dissociation and Psychotic Symptoms

The proposed role of dissociation in the development of psychotic symptoms is supported empirically in several ways. Dissociation has been identified in individuals diagnosed with schizophrenia, with studies suggesting a consistent association between dissociative experiences and acute symptoms of schizophrenia (Schäfer, Aderhold, Freyberger, & Spitzer, 2008). Patients show lower correlations between dissociation and schizophrenia symptoms in remission than in acute states. Hallucinations and delusions have been found to be strongly related to dissociation, whereas findings of negative symptoms are inconsistent (Schäfer et al., 2008). Furthermore, the Minnesota study found that both avoidant and disorganized patterns of attachment were strong predictors of later dissociative functioning (Carlson, 1998; Ogawa et al., 1997). This finding supports the assumption by Liotti (1992) of a central role of attachment organization in the development of dissociative symptoms.

The model proposed by Read and Gumley (2008), which links childhood trauma to psychosis mediated through disorganized attachment, rests on the above findings and on several additional empirical findings related specifically to childhood abuse and neglect. As noted, childhood abuse has consistently been linked to the development of disorganized attachment (Lyons-Ruth & Jacobvitz, 2008). Patients diagnosed with psychosis with a history of physical or sexual abuse during childhood reported significantly higher dissociation scores than patients without such experiences. The strongest correlation was found when emotional abuse and emotional and physical neglect were assessed in addition to childhood sexual abuse (Schäfer et al., 2008). Of particular interest, as pointed out by these researchers, is that childhood trauma and disorganized attachment are also associated with other forms of psychopathology. However, it remains to be explored in more detail how these factors may interact with other risk factors, for example, schizotypy, in the development of psychosis. Finally, only a subsample of individuals diagnosed with psychosis has experienced childhood trauma. This model therefore describes at best only one possible developmental pathway to psychosis, as pointed out by Liotti and Gumley (2008).

Mentalizing/Metacognition

There is robust evidence that theory of mind in patients with schizophrenia is compromised compared with nonclinical controls. Similarly, there is evidence of more profound theory of mind difficulties in individuals with more severe symptomatology, including disorganization, than in individuals with less severe symptomatology (Sprong, Scothorst, Vos, Hox, & van Engeland, 2007). Mentalizing has been studied in a small sample of patients with first-episode psychosis (MacBeth et al., 2011); in this study, the measure of mentalizing was reflective functioning assessed on the basis of the AAI. Individuals with secure attachment displayed significantly better mentalizing than individuals with an insecure dismissing classification. This observation supports the hypothesis of Liotti and Gumley (2008) that attachment status is involved in mentalizing deficits in psychosis. The attachment pattern is presumed to organize self-experience, affect, cognition, and behavior. This assumption is supported by Lysaker and colleagues (2011), who reported that metacognition in schizophrenia is related to displaying more adaptive coping in general, as well as better self-esteem and less social anxiety.

PSYCHODYNAMIC TREATMENT OF PSYCHOSIS

Only a few studies have investigated the effects of psychodynamic psychotherapy in psychosis, and most of these studies are several decades old, methodologically flawed, and report mixed results. An early study (May, 1968) found no significant effect of supportive psychotherapy compared with standard treatment and with medication alone. The supportive psychotherapy was performed by untrained therapists and over a variable time frame of between seven sessions and one year of therapy. In contrast, a study by Karon and Van den Bos (1981), which used insight-oriented techniques, found significant effects of psychodynamic psychotherapy compared with standard treatment. This study has been criticized for lacking control of medication and for applying different additional treatment conditions in the two comparison groups. Supportive weekly psychotherapy was compared with interpersonal insight-oriented intensive psychotherapy three times a week in a well-designed study (Gunderson et al., 1984). No standard treatment control group was included, as the aim was to compare the effects of an insight-oriented approach and a supportive approach. Contrary to expectations, the two treatment modalities turned out to be equally effective on most of the outcome measures. Only minor differences were found, with a shorter hospitalization time and better role performance (in terms of both family and work roles) for the supportive therapy group and better ego function and cognition for the insight-oriented therapy group. Furthermore, the therapists from both modalities were found to use both supportive and insight-oriented techniques, indicating that the therapies received by the two groups were less different than was intended. In another study (Harder, 2014; Rosenbaum et al., 2012), a psychotherapy approach that combined supportive and insight-oriented techniques, including Kleinian elements of containing and interpreting projective identificatory processes, reduced symptoms and improved social functioning significantly compared with a standard treatment at 2-year follow-up. This study also had methodological limitations, including its naturalistic design. Supportive communication-oriented psychodynamic group psychotherapy in addition to medication and social skills training has been found to increase improvement in factors and items related to emotional communication and anhedonia, as well as to increase free-time activities, and entry and reentry into the social field (Malm, 1982). Emerging therapy models that build on attachment models have not yet been tested empirically.

CLINICAL ILLUSTRATION

Camellia was age 20 when she had her first episode of psychosis, which was diagnosed as schizophrenia. She was referred to psychodynamic psychotherapy. She was a good-looking, smiling, and likeable person. In the months before seeking help, she had begun studies at a university but felt she was unable to cope. She developed symptoms—first anxiety related to trains and buses, then paranoid ideation and fears of being attacked by foreigners. All this distress culminated in an event with visual hallucinatory experiences of merging with an advertisement board above a metro station, feeling that she was falling down into the metro when the board was rolling to display a new advertisement. Following that experience, she felt depressed, lost her capacity to concentrate, and became unable to read books and to manage her life on her own. She dropped out of her studies and moved home to live with her father.

During her childhood, Camellia lived with both parents and an older sister. She links her actual problems to childhood experiences and her mother's abuse of alcohol during her childhood. Camellia remembers her mother's repeated, unpredictable shifts from being a caring mother to a drunken person who terrorized the family, including her father, who was nice and caring but unable to protect the two daughters from their mother's abuse and conflicts and from the violence between the parents. Camellia describes herself during childhood as unsuccessfully preoccupied with trying to take control at home and manage things. Her parents are now divorced.

Camellia's goal for the therapy is to get rid of her symptoms, to be able to start studying again, and to learn to know and understand herself better. She later describes herself as good at reading other's minds but out of contact with her own.

In the first sessions she is able to pay attention to the therapist only briefly, often losing contact, with periods of not listening or contributing. Although this might partly be due to sedation caused by her antipsychotic medication, it also seems to be related to distress that she experiences in new interpersonal relationships. She answers questions but does not raise topics of her own. She sometimes reacts by suddenly becoming very sleepy. Initially, she is sometimes unable to remain in the therapy session for more than 20 minutes because she is feeling too tense and starts experiencing hallucinations of the table in the room moving. Slowly, a more trusting therapeutic relationship develops.

In one session, she reports the following episode: Her former boyfriend phoned her late at night on his birthday. During their relationship, she was very dependent on him. She was so preoccupied with him and his needs that she completely lost contact with her own needs and boundaries. They had split up a year ago due to conflicts and frustrations, but it remained a very "unfinished business." On the phone, he asked her to come over for a glass of wine. She agreed, and though she did not want to stay overnight, she ended up staying over anyway because he asked her to. The next morning, she hurried home, her anxiety and paranoid ideation worsened, and she began to hallucinate again after a period free of hallucinations. She stayed at home in bed for the next few days, and the symptoms slowly diminished.

We will now illustrate possible foci and interventions based on the various dynamic approaches.

An ego-psychological supportive approach would assess Camellia's ego weaknesses in light of her difficulties with studying at the university and her interpersonal and social functioning. Interventions such as clarification of her problems and reactions would be applied, as would directive interventions aiming at helping her to find solutions to actual problems. Members of her family and/or social network could be included in sessions if suitable.

A Kleinian/object relational approach would understand the fear of attack from foreigners and her preoccupation with the former boyfriend's needs at the expense of her own as expressions of splitting and projective identification processes, both aggressive (toward foreigners) and idealized (toward the ex-boyfriend). These projections leave her self-fragmented and empty, and her capacity to think and act is impaired. The source of the unbearable affect that sparks these processes is thought to be inner conflicts. These inner conflicts need to be revealed by further exploring her inner mental life. Central to the therapy would be a focus on containing the fears and anxieties related to the paranoid-schizoid mode of experience and the projective identification processes taking place in the therapeutic relationship/transference. Here, her fears of foreigners would be reactivated and mixed with her habitual way of relating to her former boyfriend in her transference to the therapist. Interventions would aim at understanding the inner processes leading to these projective processes and helping her to acknowledge and contain the affects and related fantasies projected and, in that way, separate the inner fantasies from external reality and the self from others.

An interpersonal insight-oriented approach would understand her difficulties in the context of her actual task of finding her role in society in relation to success in education and romantic relationships. The problems relating to this task are thought to provoke "uncanny" emotions related to earlier dissociated "not-me" parts of her personality and cause acute disorganization, seen in her symptom formation and loss of the ability to manage her own life. In a collaborative approach, her fears and forgotten memories of former anxiety-provoking experiences may be seen as being possibly related to the frightening behavior of her parents. This insight would support the primary focus on reorganization of her disintegrated personality.

From an attachment perspective, a disorganized, hostile–helpless attachment pattern seems to be present, as seen in Camellia's relation to her former boyfriend and to the therapist. This could be understood as originating from the continuous and severe unpredictable availability of her parents and frightening experiences of abusive and violent behaviors at home during her childhood. Her symptom development and difficulties with managing her life would be understood in relation to heightened stress reactivity and disorganization of attachment in combination with other possible risk factors. A therapeutic approach would aim to promote the development of a more secure attachment relationship to the therapist. This approach might be combined with more focused interventions that aim to enhance affect-regulation and mentalizing capacities and facilitate the development of a more coherent self.

An intersubjective perspective would emphasize both verbal and nonverbal levels of interactions in the therapeutic relationship and focus on the co-creation of meaning.

These various approaches are, in our opinion, not mutually exclusive. In the Danish National Schizophrenia project, we combined the supportive approach from ego psychology with Kleinian techniques of containing and exploring inner object relations and mental states (Rosenbaum et al., 2012). In contrast to a classical Kleinian approach, our approach placed a stronger emphasis on the importance of actual interpersonal relationships and the struggle toward a normative development in relation to education, work, and family life, in line with the interpersonal approach.

Camellia's actual therapy was conducted from this integrative perspective, but with a stronger focus on nonverbal intersubjective processes, attachment, affect regulation, and mentalizing (Harder & Daniel, 2014). Her practical difficulties relating to finances, independent living, family, and work as well as options for medication, were addressed by a case manager and psychoeducational groups from a psychosis team independent of the psychotherapy. The medication she received initially helped to diminish her psychotic symptoms, but she suffered from severe side effects, and other types of medication did not decrease her symptoms. After about a year in treatment, she stopped taking medication altogether. During the first couple of years she suffered severely from social anxiety and anxiety attacks, and had repeated periods of depression and suicidal ideation as well as regular outbursts of psychotic experiences.

The therapy focused on understanding interpersonal encounters, such as the episode with her former boyfriend described in the case summary. Here the focus was on Camellia's lack of contact with her own feelings and needs when she was with others, her tendency to do what others wanted, and her inability to set boundaries or express any agency of her own. The therapy also explored how these experiences and difficulties were related to fluctuations in her various symptoms. For example, it became clear how much she ruminated, unable to solve or rid herself of frustrating experiences or fearful expectations, trying in her fantasy in an almost magical way to control what would happen next in relation to people she encountered. She slowly became increasingly able to express her feelings and needs more clearly in these encounters, both within and outside the therapy, to disentangle her needs from that of her friends or romantic partners, and to feel an emerging right to have needs of her own.

After almost 3 years (session 93) in therapy, Camellia stated how much better she felt in general:

"I can still remember how it felt like to be ill. . . . Also, before I got my diagnosis I felt so strange, but I was used to feeling like that and thought this is how I am normally. . . . Also after having been on medication, and getting off it again and then having been in therapy so much, I just feel totally different. . . . I am not so much within a bubble. . . . I felt always like everything, the world, was just too much. . . . I don't feel that way any more, generally. And I am much more full of energy. I was very physically, like, I didn't have that much energy and [was] unwell, in fact, as well, like physically, tired all the time and physically unwell. . . . Also more like, uhh, present now, I feel I am not like in my head. . . . Also very much those ruminations, I had those so often, also when I was a teenager. . . . And very much like, what we have been talking about, about things that got very big within me, I had to act or such, I was very much overwhelmed. I am not any more. . . . They [boyfriends] do not take up massively too much space anymore, I myself am still taking up space as well. . . . And this is very nice, that I am more able to keep track of myself, what I want, what I need."

On the supportive level, there was a focus on her daily living and wishes to resume her studies. Feeling that she was wasting her life, Camellia tried to start studying again after a year and a half in treatment, but she had to stop after a month. This worsened her feelings of depression and suicidality. In the year following this unsuccessful attempt to resume her studies, she became mentally able to prepare herself on a practical level for studying. She engaged in some work training and focused on establishing a daily rhythm, eating regularly, doing physical exercise, and so on. At the time of writing, she had recently started studying again and had just passed an exam for the first time in her four attempts to study—and with good marks. She is still in psychotherapy (almost 3 years in therapy) and is still in contact with her case manager.

The case presented here, as well as our previous research (Harder, 2014; Rosenbaum et al., 2012), indicates that psychodynamic psychotherapy/counseling can be an important adjunct to the case-management approach to treating psychosis. Other authors (Lehman & Steinwachs, 1998; Mueser & Berenbaum, 1990) have argued that psychodynamic psychotherapies may have harmful effects, insofar as they are too emotionally intensive and ignore more supportive, reality-focused aspects of treatment. Therapy based on supportive psychodynamic principles avoids such pitfalls. In a recent study (Rosenbaum et al., 2012), we did not observe any iatrogenic effects of psychodynamic psychotherapy. Psychodynamic psychotherapy offers a framework for mental recovery and development due to its therapeutic foci and its resemblance to an attachment relationship—that is, its continuity over time and the position of the therapist as a significant other. Thus, psychodynamic treatment may be an important addition to case management, with its main focus on social support, medication, and problem solving, and may integrate well with it.

CONCLUSIONS AND FUTURE DIRECTIONS

Psychodynamic Models of Psychosis

Psychodynamic models of psychosis have sought mainly to describe the role of affects, affect regulation, formation of thoughts and thinking, and object relations and interpersonal relationships in shaping the expressions of schizophrenic forms of psychosis—expressions that we delineated in the beginning of this chapter. All the models discussed in this chapter take a developmental approach to psychosis, whereby early developmental processes forming the basic structures of the personality lay the ground for the later development of psychosis, even if the models differ in their focus and understanding of specific disease processes.

Ego psychology focused on identifying and exploring ego disturbances, where two main causes were discussed—either an innate, neurodevelopmental deficit or a deficit based on dynamic processes related to drives and defenses against them. We noted a few empirical studies, one of which was recent (Pérez-Álvarez et al., 2011), which identified the presence of ego disturbances in psychosis. Within ego psychology and self psychology, a conceptual link has recently been established to trends in phenomenology, with emerging empirical approaches to the study of self-experience in psychosis. We consider this approach to be coherent with psychodynamic technique and understanding, and this line of research may well contribute to the empirical exploration of core elements in the development from at-risk states to psychosis as seen from a psychodynamic perspective. However, the phenomenological, descriptive approach needs to be integrated with investigations of the pathogenic processes involved in these disturbances in relation to both possible innate neurodevelopmental deficits and deficits related to ego disturbances. Turning to therapy, some empirical support was found for an ego-psychological supportive psychotherapy, but this conclusion is based on only a few studies with several methodological shortcomings.

The Kleinian approach focuses on assumed innate factors such as aggression, but it has been disputed whether and to what degree these factors reflect biological predispositions or result from frustrations. This underlines the importance of examining the interplay between genetics, neurobiology, mind, and social environment in future research. Furthermore, the Kleinian approach focuses on the importance and consequences of unbearable affect, splitting, and interpersonal projective identificatory processes in the development of psychosis. Empirical research has provided support for the presence of boundary disruptions and difficulties in maintaining self–other and inner–outer differentiation in psychosis. The developmental models that have inspired these studies, however, have been disputed by empirical infant research (Stern, 1985), and difficulties with defining and operationalizing the concept of object representations have been noted (Huprich & Greenberg, 2003). During the 1990s, research in attachment gradually became more common, which led to a decline in research on object representations. Attempts to integrate these two approaches (Blatt, Auerbach, & Levy, 1997) have not gained momentum. Despite these drawbacks, object relational thinking has proposed many concepts and disease mechanisms that have proved clinically useful. It is thus important to integrate new empirical knowledge into these models and to explore these concepts empirically and more systematically in individuals suffering from or at risk for psychosis. For instance, more research is needed on the potential role of excessive splitting and maladaptive projective identification, the process of attacks on linking, the relationship between unbearable affects and loss of symbolization, mechanisms of evacuation instead of symbolization, and psychotic and nonpsychotic parts of the personality.

Several of these concepts have been criticized for being far removed from clinical experience and thus difficult to explore empirically, but the empirical studies summarized here indicate that their systematic study is indeed possible.

Interpersonal theory and later developments focus on the contribution of interpersonal experiences to the development of psychopathology. The early interpersonal and intersubjective models focused exclusively on relational processes. Yet, contemporary models, including emerging models that build on attachment theory, embrace genetic and neurobiological considerations in their discussion of the cause of the heightened stress reactivity in psychosis. Similarly, these models acknowledge possible contributions from constitutional factors of schizotypy or dissociation proneness when seeking to explain why childhood adversities that are risk factors for several psychic disorders result in psychosis.

Very few studies have explored attachment in psychosis. The role of dismissive and disorganized attachment in psychosis needs further exploration. The proposed developmental pathway identifying childhood adversity, attachment disorganization, dissociative responses, and deficits in mentalizing, all of which are related to affective distress, needs further empirical research. Prospective longitudinal developmental research is difficult but necessary in order to explore the interplay between genes, neurobiology, mind, and social environment in the development of, for example, heightened stress reactivity and mentalizing deficits—how they are expressed at birth, how they change during infancy and childhood, and how they combine with other risk factors and differentiate into different psychiatric conditions.

Only a few studies, of varying quality, have explored the outcomes of psychotherapy that draws on relational models in psychosis, and only in a very broad sense. A recent study (Harder, Køster, Valbak, & Rosenbaum, 2014; Rosenbaum et al., 2012) found promising results. Yet, there remains a need for better designed psychotherapy process and outcome studies that build on well-defined models of psychotherapy focusing on well-described psychopathological and pathogenic processes.

Implications of Research Findings for Future Editions of ICD and DSM

Psychodynamic models do not support the idea of schizophrenia as a "nonaffective" psychosis. Rather, the term *schizophrenia* is used to describe more severe disturbances in the dimensions of self-coherence and organization of thinking, but the affective dimension and problems with affect regulation are seen as being involved in this disorganization rather than as independent and categorical aspects. This is at odds with the views expressed in ICD-10 (WHO, 1992) and DSM-IV, which feature purely descriptive diagnoses of categorically distinct types of psychosis and subtypes of schizophrenia. However, some changes toward a more dimensional approach characterize the recently published DSM-5 (APA, 2013), even though the categorical diagnosis of schizophrenia is maintained in DSM-5. Yet, the diagnostic criteria no longer include several distinct subtypes, acknowledging their lack of validity and lack of clinical utility. Furthermore, Section III (Emerging Measures and Models) in

DSM-5 now underlines the need for a more dimensional approach to mental disorders in future editions. Eight scales for dimensional assessments of psychosis are proposed, including five primary symptom domains of psychosis: delusions, hallucinations, disorganized speech, abnormal psychomotor behavior, and negative symptoms (restricted emotional expression or avolition). In addition, three more domains—impaired cognition, depression, and mania—are included because they are regarded as important for treatment planning.

Research has consistently shown that the existing categorical diagnoses of schizophrenia and schizoaffective disorders indeed have poor validity and need revision (van Os & Kapur, 2009). From a psychodynamic viewpoint, the important features of the schizophrenia type of psychosis lie in the fragmentation of self and the disorganization of thought. However, this is not to be understood as independent from affective and interpersonal difficulties—a viewpoint that has received growing empirical support, as outlined above, even if more research is needed. From this perspective, it would seem more appropriate to broaden the diagnosis of psychosis with dimensional ratings of symptomatology. The above eight dimensions would need to be supplemented with additional dimensions that are common in psychosis and important in treatment planning and outcome. We propose the addition of (1) affect regulation (stress reactivity), (2) self and other observing capacities (mentalizing), and (3) attachment (capacities for relatedness and intimacy). These dimensions have all been found to be important for treatment and outcome (Gumley, Taylor, Schwannauer, & MacBeth, 2014; Harder, 2006; Lysaker et al., 2011; Myin-Germeys & van Os, 2007). The present picture of the etiology of psychotic states does not permit a diagnosis to be made on the basis of knowledge of etiology, but we recommend that a checklist of the most important risk factors for psychosis be added to the diagnostic procedure in order to inform clinicians of possible pathways to psychosis in each individual case, which may be important for treatment.

Limitations

The psychodynamic understanding of psychosis has been controversial and in decline for decades, due to long-running polarized debates about the importance of genes versus environment, and biological treatment versus psychotherapy, that have emerged from simplistic linear etiological models of psychosis as either biological or psychosocial in nature. The psychodynamic models reviewed here have contributed to this polarization in the past, but today they are increasingly rooted in integrative views that take into account neuropsychological and genetic factors. More empirical research on psychodynamic models of psychosis and psychotherapy is needed, however. Some progress has already been made; for example, the role of social factors and trauma in the development of psychosis is now broadly acknowledged, and some psychodynamic ideas have been adopted by other theoretical approaches. Yet, there is still an urgent need for a considerable increase in research in order to turn around the negative mainstream attitude toward psychodynamic conceptualizations and treatment of psychosis.

REFERENCES

Ainsworth, M. D. S., Blehar, M. C., Waters, E., & Wall, S. (1978). *Patterns of attachment: A psychological study of the Strange Situation.* Hillsdale, NJ: Erlbaum.

American Psychiatric Association. (2013). *Diagnostic and statistical manual of mental disorders* (5th ed.). Arlington, VA: Author.

Bellak, L., Hurvich, M., & Gediman, H. K. (1973). *Ego functions in schizophrenics, neurotics, and normals.* New York: Wiley.

Berry, K., Barrowclough, C., & Wearden, H. (2007). A review of the role of adult attachment style in psychosis: Unexplored issues and questions for further research. *Clinical Psychological Review, 27*(4), 458–475.

Bion, W. R. (1967). *Second thoughts: Selected papers on psychoanalysis (Maresfield Library).* London: William Heinemann.

Birchwood, M., Iqbal, Z., Chadwick, P., & Trower, P. (2000). Cognitive approach to depression and suicidal thinking in psychosis: I. Ontogeny of post-psychotic depression. *British Journal of Psychiatry, 177,* 516–528.

Blatt, S. J., Auerbach, J. S., & Levy, K. N. (1997). Mental representations in personality Development, psychopathology and therapeutic process. *Review of Clinical Psychology, 1,* 351–374.

Blatt, S. J., Ford, R. Q., Berman, W., Cook, B., & Meyer, R. (1988). The assessment of change during the intensive treatment of borderline and schizophrenic young adults. *Psychoanalytic Psychology, 5,* 127–158.

Blatt, S. J., & Ritzler, B. A. (1974). Thought disorder and boundary disturbances in psychosis. *Journal of Consulting and Clinical Psychology, 42,* 370–381.

Blatt, S. J., & Wild, C. M. (1976). *Schizophrenia—a developmental analysis.* New York: Academic Press.

Carlson, E. A. (1998). A prospective longitudinal study of attachment disorganization/disorientation. *Child Development, 69,* 1107–1128.

Davidsen, K., & Rosenbaum, B. (2012). Fear of annihilation in subjects at risk of psychosis: A pilot study. *Psychosis: Psychological, Social and Integrative Approaches, 4,* 149–160.

Damasio, A. (2000). *The feeling of what happens: Body, emotion and the making of consciousness.* London: Heinemann.

Dimaggio, G., & Lysaker, P. H. (2010). *Metacognition and severe adult metal disorders.* London: Routledge.

Dozier, M., Stovall-McClough, K. C., & Albus, K. E. (2008). Attachment and psychopathology in adulthood. In J. Cassidy & P. R. Shaver (Eds.), *Handbook of attachment: Theory, research, and clinical applications* (2nd ed., pp. 718–744). New York: Guilford Press.

Edelman, G. M. (1989). *The remembered present: A biological theory of consciousness.* New York: Basic Books.

Edelman, G. M. (1992). *Bright air, brilliant fire: On the matter of the mind.* New York: Basic Books.

Federn, P. (1952). *Ego psychology and the psychoses.* London: Imago.

Fonagy, P., & Target, M. (2006). The mentalization-focused approach to self pathology. *Journal of Personality Disorders, 20,* 544–576.

Freud, S. (1955). Group psychology and the analysis of the ego. In J. Strachey (Ed. & Trans.), *The standard edition of the complete psychological works of Sigmund Freud* (Vol. 18, pp. 67–143). London: Hogarth Press. (Original work published 1921)

Freud, S. (1958). Psychoanalytic notes on an autobiographical account of a case of paranoia (dementia paranoids). In J. Strachey (Ed. & Trans.), *The standard edition of the complete psychological works of Sigmund Freud* (Vol. 12, pp. 3–82). London: Hogarth Press. (Original work published 1911)

Freud, S. (1961a). The loss of reality in neurosis and psychosis. In In J. Strachey (Ed. & Trans.), *The standard edition of the complete psychological works of Sigmund Freud* (Vol. 19, pp. 183–187). London: Hogarth Press. (Original work published 1924)

Freud, S. (1961b). *Neurosis and psychosis.* In In J. Strachey (Ed. & Trans.), *The standard edition of the complete psychological works of Sigmund Freud* (Vol. 19, pp. 149–158). London: Hogarth Press. (Original work published 1924)

Freud, S., & Abraham, K. (1965). *A Psycho-Analytic Dialogue. The Letters of Sigmund Freud and Karl Abraham, 1907–1926* (H. C. Abraham & E. L. Freud, Eds.). New York: Basic Books.

Frith, C. D. (1992). *The cognitive neuropsychology of schizophrenia.* Hove, UK: Erlbaum.

Fromm-Reichmann, F. (1950). *Psychoanalysis and psychotherapy.* Chicago: University of Chicago Press.

Frosch, J. (1983). *The psychotic process.* New York: International Universities Press.

George, C., Kaplan, N., & Main, M. (1985). *The Adult Attachment Interview.* Unpublished manuscript, Department of Psychology, University of California at Berkeley.

Gerson, M. (1984). Splitting: The development of a measure. *Journal of Clinical Psychology, 40,* 157–162.

Glassman, M. B. (1986). Splitting: Further contributions to the development of a measure. *Journal of Clinical Psychology, 42,* 895–904.

Goldstein, M. J. (1987). The UCLA High-Risk Project. *Schizophrenia Bulletin, 13,* 505–514.

Gottesman, I. I. (1991). *Schizophrenia genesis: The origins of madness.* New York: Freeman.

Gumley, A. (2010). The developmental roots of compromised mentalization in complex mental health disturbances of adulthood: An attachment-based conceptualization. In G. Dimaggio & P. H. Lysaker (Eds.), *Metacognition and severe adult mental disorders* (pp. 45–63). London: Routledge.

Gumley, A., & Schwannauer, M. (2006). *Staying well after psychosis. A cognitive interpersonal approach to recovery and relapse prevention.* Chichester, UK: Wiley.

Gumley, A. I., Braehler, C., Laithwaite, H., MacBeth, A., & Gilbert, P. (2010). A compassion focused model of recovery after psychosis. *International Journal of of Cognitive Therapy, 1,* 186–201.

Gumley, A. I., Schwannauer, M., MacBeth, A., Fisher, R., Clark, S., Rattrie, L., et al. (2014). Insight, duration of untreated psychosis and attachment in first-episode psychosis: Prospective study of psychiatric recovery over 12-months follow-up. *British Journal of Psychiatry, 205,* 60–67.

Gumley, A. I., Taylor, H. E. F., Schwannauer, M., & MacBeth, A. (2014). A systematic review of attachment and psychosis: Measurement, construct validity and outcomes. *Acta Psychiatrica Scandinavica, 129,* 257–274.

Gunderson, J. G., Frank, A. F., Katz, H. M., Vannicelli, M L., Frosch, J. P., & Knapp, P. H. (1984). Effects of psychotherapy in schizophrenia: II. Comparative outcome of two forms of treatment. *Schizophrenia Bulletin, 10,* 564–584.

Harder, D. W., Greenwald, D. F., & Wechsler, S. (1984). The Urist Rorschach mutuality of autonomy scale as an indicator of psychopathology. *Journal of Clinical Psychology, 40,* 1078–1083.

Harder, S. (2006). Self-image and outcome in first-episode psychosis. *Clinical Psychology and Psychotherapy, 13,* 285–296.

Harder, S. (2014). Attachment in schizophrenia: Implications for research, prevention, and treatment. *Schizophrenia Bulletin, 40,* 1189–1193.

Harder, S., & Daniel, S. (2014). The relationship between metacognitive profile, symptom development, therapeutic process and recovery in the treatment of a person experiencing first episode psychosis. In G. Dimaggio & M. Brüne (Eds.), *Social cognition and metacognition in schizophrenia: Pschopathology and treatment approaches* (pp. 261–264). London: Elsevier.

Harder, S., Køster, A., Valbak, K., & Rosenbaum, B. (2014). Long-term outcome in social functioning. Five-year follow-up of supportive psychodynamic psychotherapy in first-episode psychosis. *Psychiatry: Interpersonal and Biological Processes, 77,* 155–168.

Harder, S., & Lysaker, P. H. (2013). Narrative coherence and recovery of self-experience in integrative psychotherapy. In A. Gumley, A. Gillham, K. Taylor, & M. Schwannauer (Eds.), *Psychosis and emotion. The role of emotion in understanding psychosis, therapy and recovery* (pp. 56–67). London: Routledge.

Harrison, P. J., & Weinberger, D. R. (2005). Schizophrenia genes, gene expression, and neuropathology: on the matter of their convergence. *Molecular Psychiatry*, 10, 40–68.

Hirsch, S. R. (2003). *Schizophrenia*. Oxford, UK: Blackwell Publishing.

Huprich, S. K., & Greenberg, R. P. (2003). Advances in the assessment of object relations in the 1990s. *Clinical Psychological Review*, 23, 665–698.

Hurvich, M. (2003). The place of annihilation anxieties in psychoanalytic theory. *Journal of the American Psychoanalytic Association*, 51, 579–616.

Jackson, M. (2001). *Weathering the storms: Psychotherapy for psychosis*. London: Karnac Books.

Jackson, M., & Williams, P. (1994). *Unimaginable storms: A search for meaning in psychosis*. London: Karnac Books.

Kapur, S. (2003). Psychosis as a state of aberrant salience: A framework linking biology, phenomenology, and pharmacology in schizophrenia. *American Journal of Psychiatry*, 160, 13–23.

Karon, B. P., & Van den Bos, G. R. (1981). *Psychotherapy of schizophrenia: The treatment of choice*. New York: Jason Aronson.

Klein, M. (1946). Notes on some schizoid mechanisms. In *The writings of Melanie Klein* (Vol. 3, pp. 1–24). New York: Free Press.

Kohut, H. (1977). *The restoration of the self*. New York: International Universities Press.

Lardinois, M., Latester, T., Menglers, R., van Os, J., & Myin-Germeys, I. (2011). Childhood trauma and increased stress sensitivity in psychosis. *Acta Psychiatrica Scandinavica*, 123, 28–35.

Lehman, A., & Steinwachs, D. (1998). Translating research into practice: The Schizophrenia Patient Outcomes Research Team (PORT) treatment recommendations. *Schizophrenia Bulletin*, 24, 1–10.

Lerner, H., Sugarman, A., & Barbour, C. G. (1985). Patterns of ego boundary disturbance in neurotic, borderline and schizophrenic patients. *Psychoanalytic Psychology*, 2, 47–66.

Lester, B. M., Tronick, E. Z., LaGasse, L., Seifer, R., Bauer, C. R., Shankaran, S., et al. (2004). Summary statistics of neonatal intensive care unit network neurobehavioral scale scores from the maternal lifestyle study: A quasinormative sample. *Pediatrics*, 113, 668–675.

Liotti, G. (1992). Disorganized/disoriented attachment in the etiology of the dissociative disorders. *Dissociation*, 5, 196–204.

Liotti, G., & Gumley, A. (2008). An attachment perspective on schizophrenia: The role of disorganized attachment, dissociation and mentalization. In A. Moskowitz, Schäfer, I., & Doraty, J. M. (Eds.), *Psychosis, trauma and dissociation. Emerging perspectives on severe psychopathology* (pp. 117–135). Chichester, UK: Wiley.

Lyons-Ruth, K., & Jacobvitz, D. (2008). Attachment disorganization: Genetic factors, parenting contexts, and developmental transformation from infancy to adulthood. In J. Cassidy & P. R. Shaver (Eds.), *Handbook of attachment. Theory, research, and clinical applications* (pp. 666–697). New York: Guilford Press.

Lysaker, P. H., Erickson, M., Ringer, J., Buck, K. D., Semerari, A., Carcione, A., et al. (2011). Metacognition in schizophrenia: The relationship of mastery to coping, insight, self-esteem, social anxiety, and various facets of neurocognition. *British Journal of Clinical Psychology*, 50, 412–424.

MacBeth, A., Gumley, A., Schwannauer, M., & Fisher, R. (2011). Attachment states of mind, mentalization, and their correlates in a first-episode psychosis sample. *Psychology and Psychotherapy: Theory, Research and Practice*, 84, 42–57.

Mahler, M. S. (1968). *On human symbiosis and the vicissitudes of individuation*. New York: International Universities Press.

Malm, U. (1982). The influence of group therapy on schizophrenia. *Acta Psychiatrica Scandinavica*, 65(Suppl. 297), 1–65.

Marenco, S., & Weinberger, D. R. (2000). The neurodevelopmental hypothesis of schizophrenia: Following a trail of evidence from cradle to grave. *Development and Psychopathology*, 12, 501–527.

May, P. R. (1968). *Treatment of schizophrenia: A comparative study of five treatment methods.* New York: Science House.

McGrath, J., Saha, S., Welham, J., El Saardi, O., MacCauley, C., & Chant, D. (2004). A systematic review of the incidence of schizophrenia: The distribution of rates and the influence of sex, urbanicity, migrant status and methodology. *BMC Medicine, 2,* 1–22.

Melo, S. S., Taylor, J. L., & Bentall, R. P. (2006). "Poor me" versus "bad me" paranoia and the instability of persecutory ideation. *Psychology and Psychotherapy, Theory, Research and Practice, 79,* 271–287.

Meltzer, D. (1975). *Explorations in autism.* London: Clunie Press.

Mikulincer, M., & Shaver, P. R. (2008) Adult attachment and affect regulation. In J. Cassidy & P. R. Shaver (Eds.), *Handbook of attachment. Theory, research, and clinical applications* (pp. 503–531). New York: Guilford Press.

Morgan, C., Kirkbride, J., Leff, J., Craig, T., Hutchinson, G., McKenzie, K., et al. (2007). Parental separation, loss and psychosis in different ethnic groups: A case-control study. *Psychological Medicine, 37,* 495–503.

Moskowitz, A., Read, J., Farelly, S., Rudegeair, T., & Williams, O. (2009). Are psychotic symptoms traumatic in origin and dissociative in kind? In P. F. Dell & J. A. O'Neil (Eds.), *Dissociation and the dissociative disorders: DSM-V and beyond* (pp. 521–534). London: Routledge.

Mueser, K. T., & Berenbaum, H. (1990). Psychodynamic treatment of schizophrenia. Is there a future? *Psychological Medicine, 20,* 253–262.

Myin-Germeys, I., & van Os, J. (2007). Stress-reactivity in psychosis: Evidence for an affective pathway to psychosis. *Clinical Psychology Review 27,* 409–424.

Ogawa, J. R., Sroufe, L. A., Weinfield, N. S., Carlson, E. A., & Egeland, B. (1997). Development and the fragmentation of self: Longitudinal study of dissociative symptomatology in a nonclinical sample. *Development and Psychopathology, 9,* 855–879.

Ogden, T. (1980). On the nature of schizophrenic conflict. *International Journal of Psycho-Analysis, 61,* 513–533.

Parnas, J. (1999). From predisposition to psychosis: Progression of symptoms in schizophrenia. *Acta Psychiatrica Scandinavica. Supplementum, 395,* 2–29.

Pérez-Álvarez, M., García-Montes, J. M., Vallina-Fernández, O., Perona-Garcelán, S., & Cuevas-Yust, C. (2011). New life for schizophrenia psychotherapy in the light of phenomenology. *Clinical Psychology and Psychotherapy, 18,* 187–201.

Read, J., & Gumley, A. (2008). Can attachment theory help explain the relationship between childhood adversity and psychosis? *Attachment: New Directions in Psychotherapy and Relational Psychoanalysis, 2,* 1–35.

Read, J., van Os, J., Morrison, A. P., & Ross, C. A. (2005). Childhood trauma, psychosis and schizophrenia: A literature review with theoretical and clinical implications. *Acta Psychiatrica Scandinavica, 112,* 330–350.

Robbins, M. (2011). *The primordial mind in health and illness.* London: Routledge.

Rosenbaum, B. (2005). Psychosis and the structure of homosexuality: Understanding the pathogenesis of schizophrenic states of mind. *Scandinavian Psychoanalytic Review, 28,* 82–89.

Rosenbaum, B., Harder, S., Knudsen, P., Køster, A., Lajer, M., Lindhardt, A., et al. (2012). Supportive psychodynamic psychotherapy versus treatment as usual for first-episode psychosis: Two-year outcome. *Psychiatry, 75,* 331–341.

Rosenfeld, H. (1965). *Psychotic states.* London: Karnac Books.

Schäfer, I., Aderhold, V., Freyberger, H. J., & Spitzer, C. (2008). Dissociative symptoms in schizophrenia. In A. Moskowitz, I. Schäfer, & M. J. Dorahy (Eds.), *Psychosis, trauma and dissociation. Emerging perspectives on severe psychopathology* (pp. 151–165). Chichester, UK: Wiley-Blackwell.

Scharfetter, C. (2008). *Ego fragmentation in schizophrenia: A severe dissociation of self-experience.* In A. Moskowitz, I. Schäfer, & M. J. Dorahy (Eds.), *Psychosis, trauma and dissociation. Emerging perspectives on severe psychopathology* (pp. 51–64). Chichester, UK: Wiley-Blackwell.

Sprong, M., Scothorst, P., Vos, E., Hox, J., & van Engeland, H. (2007). Theory of mind in schizophrenia. *British Journal of Psychology, 191,* 5–13.

Sroufe, L. A., Egeland, B., Carlson, E. A., & Collins, W. A. (2005). *The development of the person: The Minnesota Study of Risk and Adaptation from Birth to Adulthood.* New York: Guilford Press.

Stern, D. N. (1985). *The interpersonal world of the infant.* New York: Basic Books.

Stern, D. N., Sander, L. W., Nahum, J. P., Harrison, A. M., Lyons-Ruth, K., Morgan, A. C., et al. (1998). Non-interpretive mechanisms in psychoanalytic therapy. The "something more" than interpretation. The Process of Change Study Group. *International Journal of Psychoanalysis, 79,* 903–921.

Stolorow, R. D., Brancroft, B., & Atwood, G. E. (1995). *Psychoanalytic treatment: An intersubjective approach.* Hillsdale, NJ: Analytic Press.

Sullivan, H. S. (1962). *Schizophrenia as a human process.* New York: Norton.

Thewissen, V., Bentall, R. P., Oorschot, M., à Campo, J., van Lierop, T., van Os, J., et al. (2011). Emotions, self-esteem, and paranoid episodes: An experience sampling study. *British Journal of Clinical Psychology, 50,* 178–195.

Tienari, P., Wynne, L. C., Sorri, A., Lahti, I., Laksy, K., Moring, J., et al. (2004). Genotype-environment interaction in schizophrenia-spectrum disorder. Long-term follow-up study of Finnish adoptees. *British Journal of Psychiatry, 184,* 216–222.

Trower, P., & Chadwick, P. (1995). Pathways to defense of the self: A theory of two types of paranoia. *Clinical Psychology: Science and Practice, 2,* 263–278.

Tyrell, C. L., Dozier, M., Tague, G. B., & Fallot, R. D. (1999). Effective treatment relationship for persons with serious psychiatric disorders: The importance of attachment states of mind. *Journal of Consulting and Clinical Psychology, 67,* 725–733.

Van Donkersgoed, R. J. M., De Jong, S., van der Gaag, M., Aleman, A., Lysker, P. H., Wunderink, L., et al. (2014). A manual-based individual therapy to improve metacognition in schizophrenia: Protocol of a multicenter RCT. *BMC Psychiatry, 14,* 27.

van Os, J., & Kapur, S. (2009). Schizophrenia. *Lancet, 374,* 635–645.

van Os, J., Krabbendam, L., Myin-Germeys, I., & Delespaul, P. (2005). The schizophrenia envirome. *Current Opinion in Psychiatry, 18,* 141–145.

Varese, F., Smeets, F., Drukker, M., Lieverse, R., Lataster, T., Viechtbauer, W., et al. (2012). Childhood adversities increase the risk of psychosis: A meta-analysis of patient-control, prospective and cross-sectional cohort studies. *Schizophrenia Bulletin, 38,* 661–671.

World Health Organization. (1992). *The ICD-10 classification of mental and behavioural disorders: Clinical descriptions and diagnostic guidelines.* Geneva, Switzerland: Author.

CHAPTER 14

Functional Somatic Disorders

Patrick Luyten, Manfred Beutel, and Golan Shahar

Many patients seen in clinical practice present with fatigue and pain-related complaints, either as a primary complaint or secondary to medical or psychiatric conditions (Fischhoff & Wessely, 2003). These complaints are often labeled as *psychosomatic* or *somatoform*, particularly in the psychoanalytic tradition. Both of these notions unduly emphasize the primacy of psychological factors or attributions in the causation of these disorders and are often based on obsolete models of the relationships between body and mind (Luyten & Van Houdenhove, 2013; Luyten, Van Houdenhove, Lemma, Target, & Fonagy, 2013). These labels also often meet with fierce resistance in patients—another reason to eschew their use (Dimsdale et al., 2013). Furthermore, these disorders are far from being "medically unexplained syndromes": Both biological and psychosocial factors have been implicated in the causation and pathophysiology of these disorders. DSM-5 has proposed the new diagnosis of somatic symptom disorder (SSD) (Dimsdale et al., 2013), which is an improvement on DSM-IV's somatoform disorder category. However, DSM-5 continues to emphasize disproportionate thoughts, feelings, and behaviors related to patients' symptoms in the definition of SSD. This means that the centrality of distorted cognition and affect is still emphasized, and it implies that SSD is a mental disorder—a view that is not empirically supported. In this chapter we prefer to use the notion of functional somatic symptoms or functional somatic disorders (FSDs), and the even more descriptive notion of persistent somatic complaints, as it is clear that, whatever their origin, these symptoms (1) involve (subtle) dysregulations of neurobiological systems and circuits involved in fatigue and pain processing and (2) become chronic in many patients, leading to high health care utilization and socioeconomic costs.

We first discuss the classification and prevalence of FSDs. We then go on to discuss the resurgence of interest in psychoanalytic approaches, as expressed in an

increasing emphasis on the importance of early adversity and life stress more generally in interaction with genetic vulnerability in these conditions. This resurgence of
interest has been paralleled by a renewed attention to interpersonal factors in the
causation and perpetuation of FSDs, including the roles of attachment, personality,
and social cognition or mentalizing. Congruent with these evolutions, we propose a
person–context interaction model of FSD rooted in contemporary attachment and
mentalizing approaches. We review evidence for this model that has accumulated
over the past two decades, and we discuss evidence for the efficacy and effectiveness
of psychodynamic treatments for FSDs. Finally, we outline the limitations of existing
research and suggest directions for future research.

CLASSIFICATION AND DIAGNOSIS

The group of FSDs comprises a wide variety of disorders and complaints, and each
medical subspecialty seems to have at least one specific FSD. These disorders include
but are not limited to chronic fatigue syndrome (CFS; infectious disease/internal
medicine); fibromyalgia (rheumatology); irritable bowel syndrome (IBS; gastroenterology); chronic pelvic pain (gynecology); noncardiac chest pain (cardiology); tension
headache (neurology); hyperventilation syndrome (respiratory medicine); multiple
chemical sensitivity (internal medicine); and chronic whiplash (emergency medicine)
(Fischhoff & Wessely, 2003; Wessely & White, 2004). Discussions concerning diagnosis and classification tend to center on two issues: (1) whether these disorders are
distinct entities ("splitters") or can best be seen as belonging to one functional somatic
syndrome ("lumpers"), and (2) whether they are purely biomedical diseases caused
by biological factors only, or whether they are influenced by both biological and psychological factors and the interaction between them. Both perspectives appear to be
unproductive and reflect ideological rather than scientific arguments.

Although these disorders differ substantially among themselves, there is also considerable evidence that different FSDs are not isolated disorders. Studies show high
comorbidity among these syndromes and high familial coaggregation (Aggarwal,
McBeth, Zakrzewska, Lunt, & Macfarlane, 2006; Anda et al., 2006), suggesting
that they are part of a spectrum of functional somatic syndromes (Ablin et al., 2012;
Creed et al., 2013; Lacourt, Houtveen, & van Doornen, 2013; Wessely & White,
2004). These disorders also show high comorbidity with emotional disorders such as
depression and anxiety (Arnold et al., 2006; Pae et al., 2008), leading to the assumption that they are also part of a spectrum of affective disorders (Hudson, Arnold,
Keck, Auchenbach, & Pope, 2004; Hudson et al., 2003; Hudson & Pope, 1996).

FSDs are highly prevalent. Estimates of the prevalence of CFS and fibromyalgia,
for instance, vary from 0.5 to 2.5% for CFS (Afari & Buchwald, 2003; Reeves et al.,
2007) and approximately 5% for fibromyalgia (Branco, 2008; Lawrence et al., 2008;
Spaeth, 2009). A more recent study reported a pooled prevalence of 11.2% for IBS
(Lovell & Ford, 2012). The prevalence of FSDs in the general population is estimated
to be 4%, and up to 9% of patients in tertiary care present with multiple FSDs (Bass
& May, 2002). The FSDs are diagnostic categories that are based on consensus.

Therefore, the true prevalence of these disorders is unknown, but their high medical, economic, and psychosocial costs have been clearly demonstrated (Afari & Buch-wald, 2003; Annemans, Le Lay, & Taeb, 2009; Annemans et al., 2008; Sicras et al., 2009; Spaeth, 2009).

Several psychosocial treatments have been developed and empirically evaluated with these disorders, typically showing improvements in core symptoms (Hauser, Bernardy, Arnold, Offenbacher, & Schiltenwolf, 2009; Malouff, Thorsteinsson, Rooke, Bhullar, & Schutte, 2008; National Institute for Health and Clinical Excel-lence, 2007; van Koulil et al., 2007). These treatments include cognitive-behavioral therapy (CBT), experiential and psychodynamic treatments, and several more body-oriented treatments such as graded exercise therapy. However, their efficacy is rel-atively limited in many patients, particularly in the long term. Furthermore, their effects are probably even more limited in the most severely affected patients, who are typically excluded from existing trials (which tend to focus on outpatients), although, as we explain later, a growing evidence base supports the relative effectiveness of intensive psychotherapy in patients with severe FSDs. Moreover, many of these treat-ments, including psychodynamic treatments, lag behind insights into the nature of these disorders, and thus there is ample room for improvement in the effectiveness of existing treatments (Luyten, Kempke, & Van Houdenhove, 2009; Van Houdenhove & Luyten, 2007, 2008).

The field is therefore witnessing a move toward broader and more integrative theoretical and intervention approaches, which has also led to a revival of psycho-analytic approaches. Three related developments are particularly relevant to the psy-chodynamic approach. First, optimism about the treatability of these patients has given way to a renewed awareness that many patients with FSDs feel severely mis-understood and stigmatized, particularly by proponents of psychosocial approaches, and are therefore hostile to such approaches. Indeed, patients with FSDs are often known as "difficult to treat" patients (Fischhoff & Wessevly, 2003). These hostile views are often reinforced by mental health professionals' use of unhelpful diagnostic labels, obsolete theories about the etiology of these disorders, a pessimistic prognosis (Rudich, Lerman, Gurevich, & Shahar, 2010; Rudich, Lerman, Gurevich, Weksler, & Shahar, 2008), and, last but not least, (perceived) negative responses by others (e.g., family, friends, colleagues), which further foster feelings of invalidation and embitterment (Blom et al., 2012; Kool, van Middendorp, Boeije, & Geenen, 2009). Not surprisingly, treatment of these patients is often associated with turbulent rela-tionships with health professionals. For instance, patients often cling to idealized specialists as a last resort, which often rapidly gives rise to their disappointment and reproach. This attitude, in turn, tends to induce contempt and rejection on the part of the professionals, which may even be demonstrated nonverbally based on mimi-cal interactions (Rasting, Brosig, & Beutel, 2005). These interaction patterns often impede the patient's response to treatment, particularly if the dynamics between patient and professional are not appropriately addressed (Luyten & Abbass, 2013).

Recently, we have argued that these features reflect problems with *epistemic trust* rooted in disruptions in attachment experiences (Fonagy, Luyten, & Allison, in press). Epistemic trust refers to the capacity to trust others as a source of knowledge about the world, which first develops in the context of relationships with attachment figures. Attachment disruptions are typically associated not only with problems trusting others on an emotional level, but also with problems with epistemic trust. These difficulties may range from difficulty trusting others as a source of knowledge about the world to more severe disruptions that manifest as the individual cycling between being overtrustful and complete epistemic distrust, expressed in *epistemic hypervigilance*. Epistemic distrust impedes an individual's capacity to form a therapeutic alliance and accept help more generally. It is particularly common among individuals with dismissive and disorganized attachment styles, which are highly prevalent in patients with FSDs (Waller & Scheidt, 2006). This may help to explain the distrustful attitude of some FSD patients toward (mental) health professionals.

Second, increasing numbers of studies suggest that early adversity and related personality/attachment issues play a role as predisposing and perpetuating factors in many patients with FSDs (Lumley, 2011; Luyten & Van Houdenhove, 2013).

Finally, this has also led to renewed interest in the role of interpersonal factors in FSDs. Patients with FSDs often tend to show high levels of emotional avoidance and distancing, rigidly adhering to somatic attributions, and relentlessly criticizing those who want to offer help. Alternatively, they may show high levels of catastrophizing, and claiming and clinging behavior, leading to push–pull cycles in interpersonal relationships—including their relationships with mental health professionals, who may as a result feel increasingly irritated, helpless, and angry (Luyten & Van Houdenhove, 2013; Maunder & Hunter, 2008).

Taken together, these findings call for a broader, developmental, person-centered, and transdiagnostic approach to the classification (and treatment) of FSDs that is at the heart of contemporary psychodynamic approaches (Luyten, Mayes, Target, & Fonagy, 2012; Westen, 1998). Rather than focusing on vulnerability to different types of FSD, psychodynamic approaches typically take a person-centered approach that attempts to map the developmental pathways of individuals who are vulnerable to developing FSD. Moreover, psychodynamic approaches also focus on the subjective experiences of individuals affected by FSD. In this chapter, we focus in particular on how FSDs are associated with a severe collapse of subjectivity, which often has dramatic negative effects on the course of the disorder and the patient's interpersonal relationships, leading to a vicious cycle characterized by increasing levels of stress, mood dysregulation, and unhelpful cognitions and behavior. The focus on the internal world, and particularly on the rooting of the embodied mind in interpersonal relationships, differentiates psychodynamic approaches from most other approaches in the field of behavioral medicine, which tend to focus on biological, cognitive-perceptual, and behavioral factors.

PSYCHODYNAMIC APPROACHES TO FSDs

Patients suffering from chronic fatigue and pain have played a key role in the development of psychoanalysis. Freud's typical patients included on the one hand people with a variety of symptoms and complaints ranging from paralyses and chronic pain symptoms to "unexplained" temporary blindness or deafness, and on the other hand patients suffering from profound fatigue and lethargy, a clinical picture we would now call chronic fatigue but was then known as neurasthenia (Beard, 1880; Freud, 1894/1962). Psychoanalysis can be said to have originated when Freud started listening to the stories—today we would say narratives—of these patients. These narratives, he argued, pointed the way to the underlying psychological conflicts and issues implicated in these disorders, although he never lost sight of the role of biological and social factors, such as heredity and lifestyle.

During Freud's lifetime, however, psychoanalysis paid relatively little attention to patients with chronic fatigue and pain-related conditions. The focus was on hysterical conversion, and other than a renewed interest in fatigue and pain in soldiers of World War I suffering from "shell shock," Freud's views on fatigue (neurasthenia) never gained much popularity (Hartocollis, 2002). It was not until the 1950s, mainly under the impetus of Alexander (1950), one of the founding fathers of psychosomatic medicine (Taylor, 1987), that psychoanalysis again became interested in FSDs. Alexander proposed the so-called *specificity hypothesis*, arguing that various "psychosomatic" conditions were associated with specific unconscious conflicts, leading to excessive and often chronic states of emotional arousal, which, in turn, were thought to have pathogenic effects on bodily systems and functions. However, again, Alexander's focus was not on chronic pain and fatigue conditions, but on what has become known as the "psychoanalytic seven": bronchial asthma, rheumatoid arthritis, ulcerative colitis, hypertension, neurodermatitis, hyperthyroidism, and duodenal ulcer.

These views quickly became discredited (Aronowitz & Spiro, 1988; Taylor, 1987). In addition, expectations concerning the efficacy of psychoanalysis did not materialize, and some commentators even suggested that psychoanalytic treatment for patients with functional somatic complaints was not only extremely difficult, but could even be harmful, leading to worsened symptoms (Krystal, 1982–1983; Sifneos, 1972). These views were mainly rooted in the notion that these patients were not amenable to psychoanalytic treatments because of what we would now term their limited mentalizing abilities (the capacity to interpret the self and others in terms of intentional mental states—feelings, wishes, desires, goals, and so on), expressed in so-called operational or mechanical thinking ("la pensée opératoire") and accompanying "blank relationships" ("relations blanches") characterized by a lack of affect and poverty of emotional inner life (Marty & de M'Uzan, 1963). Similarly, in the United States, Nemiah and Sifneos (1970) argued that these patients characteristically suffered from alexithymia, literally, "a lack of words for emotions" (Taylor & Bagby, 2013), expressed in (1) difficulties in identifying feelings and distinguishing them from bodily sensations and arousal, (2) difficulties in communicating about feelings, (3) poverty of inner life (feelings and fantasies), and (4) and an externally oriented cognitive style.

At the same time, evidence for the efficacy of more supportive and cognitive-behavioral treatments was rapidly increasing as part of the general growth in popularity of cognitive-behavioral approaches and the parallel decline in interest in psychoanalysis.

However, psychodynamic views have witnessed a revival in recent years. This chapter is part of our ongoing attempt to integrate contemporary findings concerning the nature of FSDs, and particularly findings concerning stress dysregulation in these disorders (Ablin et al., 2012; Heim et al., 2009; Tak & Rosmalen, 2010), within a psychodynamic approach to the conceptualization and treatment of these disorders rooted in attachment and mentalizing approaches. Central to our view are the high metabolic *and* interpersonal costs associated with the excessive use of so-called secondary attachment strategies—that is, stress or affect regulation strategies that involve hyperactivation or deactivation of the attachment system in response to stress, leading to further stress dysregulation and impairments in mentalizing. These impairments, in turn, give rise to (interpersonal) behaviors that perpetuate symptoms and complaints, leading to a typical pattern of stress dysregulation, high symptomatic distress, and interpersonal problems in patients with FSDs that also negatively influences their treatment seeking and response to treatment (see Figure 14.1).

A Contemporary Psychodynamic View of FSDs

The model that we have advanced assumes that FSDs result from negative vicious cycles of increasingly negative person–environment interactions, and distinguishes predisposing, precipitating, and perpetuating factors (see Figure 14.1) (Luyten & Van Houdenhove, 2013; Van Houdenhove & Luyten, 2009).

Predisposing Factors

Many studies have suggested that biological and environmental factors may predispose individuals to FSDs. Genetic polymorphisms, for instance, have been implicated in FSDs (Camilleri & Katzka, 2012; Landmark-Høyvik et al., 2010; Lee, Choi, Ji, & Song, 2012), although the evidence is not always clear. Other recent studies suggest

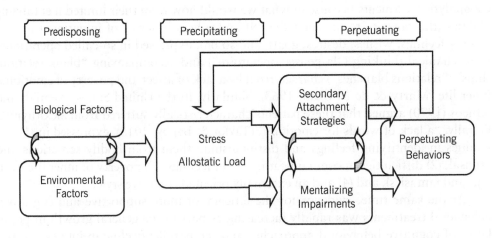

FIGURE 14.1. An attachment and mentalizing approach to FSDs.

a role for epigenetic modification of genes that are implicated in stress and affect regulation as a result of adverse circumstances in early and later life (Buskila, Sarzi-Puttini, & Ablin, 2007; Heim et al., 2009; Rajeevan et al., 2007), such as emotional abuse and neglect (Kempke et al., 2013). Indeed, recent meta-analyses and narrative reviews suggest that there are increased levels of early adversity at least in a substantial subgroup of patients with FSDs (Afari et al., 2014; Borsini, Hepgul, Mondelli, Chalder, & Pariante, 2013).

Precipitating Factors

Both psychological (e.g., problems related to work or relationships) (Aslakson, Vollmer-Conna, Reeves, & White, 2009) and biological (e.g., chronic infections or whiplash) factors have been identified as precipitating the onset of FSDs. In many patients, an accumulation of precipitating factors, often over an extended period of time, most probably disturbs allostasis, resulting in what has been termed a state of *allostatic load* (McEwen, 2007), a severe and often lasting disruption of the dynamic equilibrium that characterizes normal stress regulation. Studies suggest that the pathophysiology of this disruption involves important dysfunctions in the hypothalamic–pituitary–adrenal (HPA) axis, the main stress system in human beings (Heim et al., 2009; Powell, Liossi, Moss-Morris, & Schlotz, 2013; Tak & Rosmalen, 2010; Van Houdenhove, Luyten, & Kempke, 2013). These dysfunctions may lead to a cascade of negative effects such as abnormal inflammatory activity, with proinflammatory cytokines inducing feelings of lethargy, increased fatigability, loss of concentration, light fever, generalized hyperalgesia, hypersensitivity to stress (Dantzer, O'Connor, Freund, Johnson, & Kelley, 2008; Watkins & Maier, 2005), and, in interaction with negative affect, catastrophizing and sleep problems, and sensitization to pain (Ablin et al., 2012; Van Houdenhove & Luyten, 2008).

Perpetuating Factors

We believe it is crucial to realize that, regardless of the precise causes of the onset of FSDs, as the patient's arousal increases, and thus their difficulties in affect regulation worsen, their ability to reflect on what is happening progressively fades, congruent with studies showing that increasing arousal leads to deactivation of the capacity for controlled mentalizing (Luyten, Fonagy, Lowyck, & Vermote, 2012). As a result, there is an increasing reliance on so-called secondary attachment strategies (i.e., attachment deactivating and attachment hyperactivating strategies). These strategies in turn lead to further impairments in mentalizing, particularly *embodied mentalizing* (the capacity to see the body as the seat of emotions, wishes, and feelings, and the capacity to reflect on one's own bodily experiences and sensations and their relationships to intentional mental states in the self and others). Secondary attachment strategies and mentalizing impairments lead to an exacerbation of symptoms, further stress, and thus allostatic load (e.g., as a result of excessive catastrophizing and somatic attributions in a nonmentalizing mode) (see Figure 14.1), congruent with person–environment transactional models (Hammen, 2005; Luyten et al., 2011; Sha-har, 2006).

A Developmental Psychopathology Perspective on FSDs

In support of the model outlined above, burgeoning research suggests the existence of inherent relationships among attachment experiences, mentalization, and stress regulation throughout the lifespan. Research in animals as well as in humans strongly suggests that secure attachment experiences play a key role in the development of the stress system and of resilience when faced with adversity (Gunnar & Quevedo, 2007).

In securely attached individuals, stress typically leads to seeking proximity to attachment figures, either real or internalized, resulting in the downregulation of stress. Thus, normative stress regulation always involves the effective coregulation of stress in relation to attachment figures (Diamond, Stovall-McClough, Clarkin, & Levy, 2003; Luyten, Mayes, Fonagy, & van Houdenhove, 2014; Sbarra & Hazan, 2008). This process appears to be firmly rooted in neurobiology. The neuropeptide oxytocin, for instance, has been shown to play a key role both in fostering attachment and mentalizing, and in regulating stress (Fonagy & Luyten, 2009; Neumann, 2008). From a neurobiological perspective, activation of the attachment system leads to (1) the activation of a mesocorticolimbic, dopaminergic "reward" system (Insel & Young, 2001), (2) downregulation of neuroendocrine stress regulation systems (the HPA axis and sympathetic nervous system), and (3) activation of neural systems involved in mentalization, including the lateral prefrontal cortex, medial prefrontal cortex, lateral parietal cortex, medial parietal cortex, medial temporal lobe, and rostral anterior cingulate cortex (Fonagy & Luyten, 2009; Lieberman, 2007). High levels of mentalizing, particularly in high-stress situations, have been associated with resilience (Fonagy, Steele, Steele, Higgitt, & Target, 1994) through so-called broaden and build (Fredrickson, 2001) cycles of attachment security. These cycles reinforce feelings of secure attachment, agency, and stress and affect regulation ("build"), leading one to being "pulled into" more adaptive environments ("broaden") (Hauser, Allen, & Golden, 2006; Mikulincer & Shaver, 2007).

Secure attachment experiences, through their rewarding nature, reinforce affiliative behavior and mentalization, fostering the effective regulation of stress. In contrast, insecure attachment experiences (and early adversity in particular) have been associated with greater vulnerability to stress in both animals (Champagne & Curley, 2009; Neumann, 2008) and humans (Bakermans-Kranenburg, van IJzendoorn, Mesman, Alink, & Juffer, 2008; Gunnar & Quevedo, 2007). This vulnerability seems to be in large part mediated by dysfunctions in the HPA axis (Heim et al., 2009; Kempke et al., 2013; Van Houdenhove & Luyten, 2008).

Again, these claims are supported by ample empirical research. Until recently, studies concerning the role of early adversity in FSDs were still controversial owing to their many methodological limitations. Good evidence has now been presented to suggest that at least a subgroup of patients with FSDs are characterized by high levels of early adversity (particularly high levels of emotional abuse and neglect) (Afari et al., 2014; Borsini et al., 2013; Kempke et al., 2013) and insecure attachment (Luyten,

Van Houdenhove, Cosyns, & Van den Broeck, 2006; Maunder & Hunter, 2008; Waller & Scheidt, 2006). Typically, individuals characterized by insecure attachment histories rely excessively on so-called secondary attachment strategies in response to stress (Dozier & Kobak, 1992; Mikulincer & Shaver, 2007; Roisman et al., 2007).

Not all patients with FSDs, however, are characterized by a history of insecure attachment experiences, and even fewer patients with FSDs have a history of serious early adversity and/or premorbid mentalizing impairments. The overreliance on secondary attachment strategies and mentalizing impairments observed in many patients with FSDs may be a *consequence* rather than a *cause* of the disorder, or may be further *exacerbated* by the disorder, which has important implications for treatment. As noted, earlier psychoanalytic theories that argued for a close causal association between early adversity and problems with mentalizing in FSDs were clearly overspecified. They were mostly based on outdated assumptions concerning mind–body relationships, and they failed to account for biological findings in FSDs (Luyten, Mayes, et al., 2012; Luyten & Van Houdenhove, 2013). These views have rightfully been questioned.

Both clinical practice and research suggest that many patients with FSDs, in an attempt to cope with their illness, begin to rely excessively on *attachment deactivation* strategies, expressed in an often complete denial of attachment needs and assertion of their autonomy, independence, and strength (Cassidy & Kobak, 1988; Mikulincer & Shaver, 2007). Yet, underneath this appearance of autonomy and resilience is much vulnerability (Van Houdenhove & Luyten, 2008). As studies suggest, the use of attachment deactivation strategies is also often associated with high levels of self-critical perfectionism and related features such as persistence, overactivity, and so-called all-or-nothing behavior (Creed, 2007; Luyten et al., 2011). These represent a defensive attempt to affirm the self and soothe negative introjects, and there is now increasing evidence that these features are related to FSDs in a subset of patients (Luyten et al., 2011).

In the long term, these tendencies are associated with considerable interpersonal and metabolic costs. Attachment deactivating strategies (and high levels of self-critical perfectionism in particular) have been shown to lead to increasing isolation and loneliness (Mikulincer & Shaver, 2007), and the suppression of distress has been associated with increasing allostatic load, HPA axis dysregulation because of the "wear and tear" caused by prolonged stress (Hill-Soderlund et al., 2008; Miller, Chen, & Zhou, 2007; Wirtz, Siegrist, Rimmele, & Ehlert, 2008), and disturbed immune system functioning (Gouin et al., 2009). Furthermore, deactivating strategies progressively fail under increasing stress, as expressed in heightened feelings of stress and insecurity (Mikulincer, Dolev, & Shaver, 2004).

Particularly in patients with a history of serious early adversity and/or comorbid dependent and borderline features, *attachment hyperactivating strategies* tend to predominate. This is shown in anxious efforts to find support and relief, often through demanding, clinging, and claiming behaviors (Waller & Scheidt, 2006). These strategies are similarly associated with high interpersonal and metabolic costs. Demanding behavior tends to lead to frustration and resentment toward others, often confirming these individuals' worst fears that they are misunderstood and rejected by others. Their relationships with (mental) health professionals mimic this pattern. Thus, "broaden-and-build" cycles are inhibited. High levels of physiological stress and increased HPA axis activity (Diamond, Hicks, & Otter-Henderson, 2008; Gordon et al., 2008) further increase allostatic load. This leads to a vicious cycle because these patients tend to respond to increased stress and anxiety with even greater reliance on attachment hyperactivating strategies in an attempt to find relief, support, and understanding (Maunder & Hunter, 2008; Maunder, Lancee, Nolan, Hunter, & Tannenbaum, 2006).

Impairments in (Embodied) Mentalization in FSDs

The experience of symptoms and the resulting excessive use of secondary attachment strategies in patients with FSDs also has a negative effect on patients' mentalizing abilities, leading to the reemergence of so-called *nonmentalizing modes* (discussed later; see also Fonagy, 1998). This, in turn, leads to behaviors that further perpetuate the symptoms and exacerbate problems in interpersonal relationships (see Figure 14.1). As noted, mentalizing impairments are often the consequence of FSDs or are further exacerbated by the distress and interpersonal problems associated with FSDs. FSD symptoms can be seen as an "attack" from within on the capacity to reflect, particularly on the capacity to see the body as a "lived body" that one has ownership of and that is the seat of one's relationships with others. Driver (2005), for instance, has vividly described the "otherness of the illness" in patients with CFS, which leads to regressive fears and fantasies. Schattner, Shahar, and Abu-Shakra (2008), in turn, found that patients with a chronic illness typically treat their illness as an "internal object" that constantly threatens the patient and that needs to be negotiated with and soothed. Persistent somatic complaints increase stress, which further impairs and/ or exacerbates already-existing impairments in (embodied) mentalizing, congruent with studies showing an inverse relationship between stress and mentalizing capacity (Fonagy & Luyten, 2009; Luyten, Fonagy, et al., 2012).

Psychoanalytic approaches have long hypothesized the presence of mentalizing deficits in FSD patients. Earlier formulations emphasized high levels of alexithymia and problems with emotional awareness in these patients (Pedrosa Gil, Scheidt, Hoeger, & Nickel, 2008; Pedrosa Gil, Weigl, et al., 2008; Subic-Wrana, Beutel, Knebel, & Lane, 2010). However, studies suggest that only a minority of patients with FSD (in fibromyalgia, for instance, between 15 and 22%) are characterized by clinically elevated levels of alexithymia and lack of emotional awareness (Pedrosa Gil, Scheidt, et al., 2008; Pedrosa Gil, Weigl, et al., 2008; Waller & Scheidt, 2006). Moreover, these features are not specific to FSDs, but rather seem to reflect the effects of trauma and emotional neglect. Hence, although these patients are often seen in tertiary care, their premorbid deficits in mentalizing cannot be generalized to the total population of patients with FSDs. Neither should one underestimate the impact of FSDs (and negative responses by the environment) on mentalizing, even in these patients, as many of them have been caught up in vicious interpersonal cycles for many years, often compounded if they lose their employment and live on disability benefits.

The mentalization-based approach proposed in this chapter suggests that rather than considering patients with FSDs as "alexithymic" in general, their impairments in (embodied) mentalizing are often much more specific (i.e., associated with specific experiences and symptoms) and related to interpersonal situations and symptoms that involve high arousal or stress (Luyten, Van Houdenhove, Lemma, Target, & Fonagy, 2012). In fact, on one hand, both clinical experience and systematic research have shown that many of these patients exhibit, interchangeably, excessive mentalizing or so-called *hypermentalizing* (as expressed in apparently highly sophisticated narratives that lack any affective grounding in subjective experiences). On the other hand, they almost totally deny the importance of inner mental states. Rather than showing general impairments in emotional awareness, many of these patients are unable to link their emotional and bodily states (Oldershaw et al., 2011; Stonnington, Locke, Hsu, Ritenbaugh, & Lane, 2013; Subic-Wrana et al., 2010). Studies suggest that patients with FSDs are less likely to interpret physical sensations in terms of negative emotional states (Dendy, Cooper, & Sharpe, 2001) and are less interoceptively accurate, particularly in symptom-related contexts (Bogaerts et al., 2008, 2010). They also tend to have negative beliefs about their own emotions, particularly the expression of emotions (Hambrook et al., 2011), and tend to exhibit a strong need to control their own thoughts and feelings (Maher-Edwards, Fernie, Murphy, Nikcevic, & Spada, 2012; Rimes & Chalder, 2010), rather than showing "deficits" in processing emotions.

Nonmentalizing Modes of Experiencing Subjectivity and Perpetuating Factors

Context-specific impairments in (embodied) mentalizing lead to the reemergence of nonmentalizing modes that perpetuate symptoms and interpersonal problems (see Figure 14.1).

The first nonmentalizing mode that plays an important role in FSDs is the *psychic equivalence mode*. In this mode of experiencing subjectivity, patients equate inner and outer reality, leaving no room for alternative interpretations. In FSD patients, this is often associated with a lack of desire and/or an inability to explore inner mental states, which hampers treatment. This is particularly the case in patients who primarily use attachment deactivating strategies, which also may explain these patients' problems in accepting help and their difficulty in believing that professionals can be genuinely concerned about them. Psychic equivalence leads to equating psychological pain with physical pain, and emotional exhaustion with physical exhaustion. This may in part explain the high comorbidity between pain, fatigue, and depression (Hudson et al., 2004; Van Houdenhove & Luyten, 2008). It also fosters these patients' resistance to acknowledging the role of psychological factors ("I am exhausted, not angry or depressed"). They tend to experience psychological pain in terms of bodily pain: worries literally "depress" or "press down on" the patient and feel like a painful, heavy weight. Helplessness ensues, often in combination with catastrophizing ("I think there is something terribly wrong with me, so there *is* something terribly wrong with me [psychic equivalence], but no one notices me [feeling of invalidation]; I am beyond help [catastrophizing]").

Psychic equivalence also negatively influences their relationships: In this mode, thinking that others do not care *means* that others do not care. In situations where another person criticizes the patient, the patient feels this as an attack on the (bodily) integrity of the self. Research findings concerning the common neural circuits of psychological and physical pain are particularly relevant in this context. Rejection hurts (Eisenberger, Lieberman, & Williams, 2003), but in these patients often only the physical pain associated with rejection seems to be real ("I felt upset when my wife left me, but I can handle that, but it's these pains that are killing me"). In the psychic equivalence mode, the body begins to feel like an "alien self-part," "a thing that is out of control." As a result, patients are under constant pressure to externalize these alien self-parts in a defensive attempt to evacuate their pain and feelings of anxiety, helplessness, and depression, and to restore the coherence of the self. However, others are made to feel what the patient feels; this often has a destructive influence on the patient's relationships, including those with health professionals.

In the *teleological mode*, the patient recognizes mental states as driving behavior, but this recognition is limited to mental states that have clearly observable causes (i.e., observable behavior reflecting rational, goal-directed behavior and material causes). For many patients with FSDs, only rational, goal-directed behaviors and actions can be effective, hence their tendency to be excessively concerned with finding "objective proof" of their illness. If the patient is in the teleological mode, he or she may draw clinicians into endless discussions about the purported role of biological versus psychosocial factors in the etiology of their FSD.

This tendency to ruminate about the causes of their disorder often leads to what is called hypermentalization or "mentalization on the loose" in an extreme *pretend mode*. In this mode of thinking, the relationship between thoughts and feelings and reality is typically severed. Pretend-mode functioning may give rise to often extensive narratives that on first impression strike the clinician as sensible accounts of the patient's history and the factors contributing to his or her problems. Yet, upon closer consideration, these narratives are often overly analytical and cognitive, lacking any grounding in real affective experiences. They are often very repetitive, and the patient also typically lacks the ability to switch perspective. Attempts to encourage the patient to switch perspective are often met with fierce resistance ("What do you mean by considering what she might feel? We are talking about me").

These prementalizing modes perpetuate symptoms and interpersonal problems. Pretend-mode thinking is associated with often excessive worrying and rumination, expressed in symptoms such as excessive anxious concerns about one's health, sleeping problems, and sometimes anxiety attacks, further impairing stress regulation. Associated with this is the patient's tendency to mull over what he or she experiences as an unwillingness of others to take their illness seriously (Van Houdenhove & Luyten, 2008). Studies have shown that this unwillingness is related to these patients' feelings of invalidation, loneliness, and even embitterment (Kool et al., 2009). These feelings are further increased by psychic-equivalence thinking ("Nobody cares") and often given rise to a paranoid-like distrust in the medical profession ("They want to harm us"). Teleological thinking frequently leads to desperate attempts to find relief in surgery (e.g., the patient may have all his or her dental fillings replaced), experimental medical treatments, or alternative medicine. At the same time, many patients attempt to cope with their feelings of worthlessness by desperate attempts to prove the contrary, leading to overactivity (so-called boom-and-bust patterns), which results in extreme pain, exhaustion, and helplessness.

PSYCHODYNAMIC TREATMENT OF FSDs

The views expressed in this chapter have important implications for the psychodynamic treatment of patients with FSDs. It is often believed that psychoanalytic treatments are contraindicated in FSD patients because of these patients' alexithymic features. These features often seem to be the result rather than the cause of FSDs in many patients, or they may be exacerbated by FSDs. Thus, interventions that aim to recover the patient's capacity to mentalize, and to understand and communicate his or her feelings, can be expected to be effective.

In line with these assumptions, more structured psychodynamic treatments have been demonstrated to be efficacious in both randomized and nonrandomized trials in patients with FSDs. A meta-analysis by Abbass, Kisely, and Kroenke (2009) of 23 studies (13 randomized controlled trials and 10 case series with pre–post outcome assessments) showed significant effects on physical symptoms, psychiatric symptoms, and social adjustment, which were maintained at long-term follow-up. Importantly, this meta-analysis showed that brief dynamic treatment was associated with a 54% greater rate of retention in treatment compared to control conditions. This finding suggests that these interventions can address many of the interpersonal issues that frequently hamper treatment in these patients.

It is also important to note that even very brief treatments were associated with considerable improvement. Abbas, Campbell, Magee, and Tarzwell (2009), for instance, showed in patients with FSDs such as abdominal pain that an average of 3.8 sessions led to a reduction of 70% in the number of emergency department visits they made in the following year. Creed and colleagues (2003), in turn, reported evidence for the efficacy and cost-effectiveness of eight sessions of brief interpersonal dynamic therapy in patients with IBS. Although more research is needed, these studies suggest that brief dynamic treatments may be cost-effective in FSD, a finding that is in line with a recent meta-analysis of the cost-effectiveness of brief dynamic treatment more generally (Abbass & Katzman, 2013). These treatments also influence the neurobiological circuits involved in stress, affect regulation, and mentalizing (Abbass, Nowoweiski, Bernier, Tarzwell, & Beutel, 2014), congruent with the views advanced in this chapter.

Furthermore, a recent meta-analysis showed that longer-term multicomponent interventions—many of which are psychodynamic in orientation, such as the one described by Beutel, Michal, and Subic-Wrana (2008)—may be particularly effective in patients with severe FSDs (i.e., severe and often chronic complaints, often with substantial psychiatric comorbidity). These interventions improved symptoms and distress by fostering the patients' capacity to mentalize and engage in social interaction. Specifically, in 10 randomized controlled trials and six nonrandomized trials, with a total of 890 patients receiving psychotherapy and 548 receiving treatment as usual (TAU), multicomponent treatment was more effective than TAU for physical symptoms ($d = 0.80$ vs. 0.31, $p < .05$) and functional impairment ($d = 0.45$ vs. 0.15, $p < .01$), but not for psychological symptoms ($d = 0.75$ vs. 0.51, $p = .21$). These effects were maintained at long-term follow-up (Koelen et al., 2014), consistent with the notion that these treatments were associated with sustained changes in health functioning in these patients.

Whether these sustained changes are indeed related to changes in attachment, mentalizing, and affect regulation in patients with FSDs remains to be investigated. However, the theoretical model outlined in this chapter suggests that a focus on restoring patients' capacity for stress regulation by (1) addressing their typical attachment strategies in response to stress and (2) recovering their capacity for (embodied) mentalizing (Luyten & Van Houdenhove, 2013) may lead to sustained changes in person–environment exchanges, fostered by the "broaden and build" cycles (discussed earlier) associated with more secure attachment strategies and mentalizing. In fact, all effective treatments, regardless of their theoretical orientation, may achieve these changes in patients with FSDs (Luyten et al., 2013). Cognitive-behavioral interventions, for instance, typically challenge these patients' dysfunctional assumptions about their body and their self more generally, leading to changes in core assumptions about the self, and thus in mentalizing, likely followed by changes in attachment strategies. More intrapsychically oriented psychoanalytic approaches similarly aim to challenge the patient's core beliefs about the (embodied) self, the roots of such beliefs in the past, and their influence on the present. In these treatments, the therapeutic relationship is often used as a vehicle to understand typical patterns of thinking about the self and relating to others, as well as the relationship between them, and to link them to past experiences. Similarly, body-oriented work, such as graded exercise therapy, may lead to patients beginning to question their assumptions about mind–body relationships, with resulting changes in how they relate to the self and others. At the same time, however, this type of intervention may also reinforce these patients' exclusively somatic focus.

The effectiveness of treatments for patients with FSDs can most likely be enhanced by a greater focus on our growing insights into the nature of these disorders. On the basis of the views summarized in this chapter, treatments can be expected to be effective to the extent that they closely attend to (1) the patient's feelings of invalidation, (2) interpersonal issues and the use of secondary attachment strategies in particular, (3) the easy loss of (embodied) mentalizing and the reemergence of nonmentalizing modes, particularly when the patient is under conditions likely to cause high arousal, and (4) empowerment of the patient—that is, supporting the patient in applying new ways of thinking, feeling, and acting outside of the treatment setting, as patients often need considerable support to achieve this. It is important for clinicians to remain constantly aware of the potential iatrogenic nature of interventions for FSDs, given these patients' common use of secondary attachment strategies and/ or nonmentalizing modes as either a cause or a consequence of their symptoms. In our opinion, more insight-oriented psychodynamic treatments often tend to overestimate the mentalizing capacities of patients with FSDs. This runs the risk of strongly activating the patient's attachment system, resulting in the activation of secondary attachment strategies and severe impairments in mentalizing. Ultimately, this may lead to high rates of dropout and/or stormy transference and countertransference issues (e.g., idealization–denigration cycles, regressive dependency, sadomasochistic transferences) that are difficult to resolve even in long-term treatment (Luyten & Abbass, 2013).

These formulations are in line with the core tenets of more interpersonally oriented psychodynamic treatments for these patients, such as brief interpersonal psychotherapy (Guthrie et al., 1999; Sattel et al., 2012; Thomas, Else, Barbara, & Francis, 2009) and dynamic interpersonal therapy (DIT; Lemma, Target, & Fonagy, 2010). These treatments have a greater focus on the "here-and-now" than the "there-and-then" (see also Luyten, Mayes, Blatt, Target, & Fonagy, Chapter 1, this volume), related to their greater emphasis on current interpersonal issues and their relation to the presenting symptoms, and their focus on the process of reflecting on the connections between current interpersonal events and current symptoms. DIT in particular involves a stronger focus on the *process* of mentalizing than on the *content* of emotional issues, as a focus on content (e.g., the connection between presenting symptoms and interpersonal issues in the present or past) often surpasses these patients' mentalizing abilities, particularly in the early stages of treatment and/or in patients with chronic, multiple FSDs.

DIT for FSDs (DIT-FSD) consists of three phases. The first phase (sessions 1–4) focuses on engaging the patients, given the obvious problems many of these patients have in forming a treatment alliance, and on the collaborative formulation of a treatment focus. In this phase, acknowledgment of the patient's feelings of invalidation and his or her experiences of a lack of being understood (Kool et al., 2009) is central. This phase typically also includes a discussion of the anxieties activated by starting the therapy, which is often crucially important to prevent pseudoengagement and/or early treatment dropout.

Furthermore, in this phase, a discussion of unhelpful theories regarding the illness, and particularly of the high "costs" associated with insecure attachment strategies, is often indicated. This may lead to the formulation, through consensus rather than conflict, of a shared and acceptable illness theory that recognizes the complexity of the disorder (Salmon, 2007).

A final central aspect of the early phase of treatment is the joint formulation of what is called an Interpersonal Affective Focus (IPAF), which becomes the central focus of the treatment. The IPAF refers to a recurrent cognitive-affective relational or attachment pattern that is associated with the onset and perpetuation of functional somatic symptoms and interpersonal problems. It consists of a (nonconscious) representation of self-in-relation-to-others and the defensive function of this constellation. For instance, patients who typically use attachment deactivating strategies often depict the self as highly autonomous and self-reliant, and describe others as critical, ambivalent, and nonunderstanding. Affects that accompany this IPAF often include aggression, depression, and helplessness. However, this constellation typically defends against feelings of dependency and longing for approval and love. In patients who rely primarily on attachment hyperactivating strategies, the IPAF may consist of a representation of the self as caring and concerned about others (sometimes leading to compulsive caregiving), while others, by contrast, are described as indifferent and uncaring, which gives rise to feelings of helplessness and hopelessness. However, this constellation defends against feelings of frustration, resentment, and aggression toward others who are seen as unresponsive and uncaring.

The second phase of DIT-FSD (sessions 5–12) consists of working through the IPAF and consolidating treatment gains. The IPAF is used as a guide to explore the high allostatic and interpersonal costs of typical interpersonal patterns, with the aim of fostering the patient's capacities to reflect on the (bodily) self, others, and the self-in-relation-to-others. In most patients, this entails exploring impairments in embodied mentalizing, which may lead to reinvesting the body with positive affective meaning through decoupling bodily experiences from relational experiences. Experiencing the interpersonal world in terms of mental states, as is intended, in and of itself brings about relief from the physical stress that the collapse of mentalizing brings with it for these individuals. Furthermore, the intrinsic relationships among presenting symptoms (e.g., fatigue, pain), feelings (e.g., feeling misunderstood), and interpersonal relationships are explored. This entails both affect differentiation (e.g., recognizing that feeling "not good" may actually mean that one feels sad and rejected as well as depressed) and affect amplification (e.g., recognizing the influence of emotional states on the self), and linking both to interpersonal experiences (e.g., that one feels so tired because one feels rejected and misunderstood by others).

Affect differentiation and affect amplification foster a move from narrative incoherence and inconsistence with regard to both the past and the present toward a more consistent narrative about one's life history, present feelings, and relationships. This also opens up future possibilities to the patient to live his or her life differently. Indeed, the ability to regulate stress more effectively and relate to others better fosters "broaden-and-build" cycles. In addition to more basic mentalizing (e.g., affect recognition, differentiation, and amplification) and supportive (i.e., reassurance, support, and empathy) interventions, this phase uses more advanced expressive interventions (e.g., interpretations of interpersonal patterns, including the transference when appropriate) as well as directive techniques (e.g., encouraging new ways of relating).

The final phase of treatment (sessions 13–16) focuses on the end of the treatment and aims to transfer what the patient has "learned" in the course of treatment to the everyday context to prevent future relapses. This process is initiated by sharing a draft "goodbye" letter written by the therapist. The letter contains a summary of what the treatment has achieved and has *not* achieved. Its aim is to foster mentalizing with regard to what the patient has and has not gained from the treatment. DIT-FSD marks only the beginning of a change process, particularly as patients with FSDs often have a long history of illness. The goodbye letter is also a physical reminder of the treatment that patients can fall back upon in times of difficulty, for instance. It typically evokes strong reactions, as it is experienced as both supportive and challenging, and frequently leads to intensifying of the patient's fears about the end of treatment and issues related to the IPAF. This provides another opportunity to explore the links between symptoms, subjective responses, and interpersonal relationships. Hence, the aim of the final phase of DIT-FSD is to foster autonomy and resilience in the long run (empowering the patient). The use of directive techniques is quite pertinent in this phase of the treatment, as patients are actively encouraged to think about and try out new ways of thinking, feeling and relating to others and themselves. A substantial proportion of patients with FSDs are trapped in negative vicious cycles that are not easy to change. Consequently, in addition to FSD-DIT, psychiatric consultation and rehabilitation may be indicated, as well as couple/family treatment in some cases.

CONCLUSIONS AND FUTURE DIRECTIONS

Functional somatic symptoms or FSDs comprise a wide variety of highly prevalent disorders and complaints in each medical subspecialty, with high comorbidity. These disorders typically involve (subtle) dysregulations of neurobiological systems and circuits involved in fatigue and pain processing, which become chronic in many patients, leading to high health care utilization and socioeconomic costs. Recent empirical findings call for a broader, developmental, person-centered, and transdiagnostic approach to the classification (and treatment) of FSDs that is at the heart of contemporary psychodynamic approaches. From a developmental psychopathology perspective, we find that patients with FSDs have impairments in (embodied) mentalizing and nonmentalizing modes of experiencing subjectivity, which tend to perpetuate symptoms and interpersonal problems typically associated with FSDs.

Although psychodynamic approaches to FSDs are clearly experiencing a revival, much more research is needed. First, there is a need for large-scale prospective studies to tease out causality. These should entail a focus on the interpersonal sphere and link to the neurobiological circuits underpinning interpersonal issues at multiple levels of the stress response. Second, there is a need for more integrative approaches in which considerations concerning the psychodynamics of patients with FSDs play an important role. In response to these challenges, we have formulated a broad and integrative model that distinguishes between predisposing biological and environmental factors (e.g., childhood trauma, insecure attachment styles, impaired affect regulation), precipitating factors (e.g., stress, increased allostatic load), and perpetuating factors (overreliance on secondary attachment strategies and impaired mentalization). Third, treatment research should focus on changes in patient–environment interactions, starting from a focus on the patient's symptoms and improvements in mentalizing in the here-and-now. Thus, the field of treatment research should move beyond an almost exclusive emphasis on head-to-head trials to a focus on purported mechanisms of change, which may lead to the development of more integrative treatments. Furthermore, there is a need to identify predictors of treatment outcome that allow tailoring of treatments to individual patients. In line with our assumptions, some patients with FSDs, particularly those who are more reflective and have higher levels of epistemic trust, may respond well to brief and perhaps even Internet-based interventions. Other patients (e.g., those with substantial comorbidity and severe epistemic distrust) might require more intensive treatment programs. Finally, research on the cost-effectiveness and dissemination of effective treatments remains important, particularly in view of the high prevalence and socioeconomic costs associated with these disorders.

REFERENCES

Abbass, A., Campbell, S., Magee, K., & Tarzwell, R. (2009). Intensive short-term dynamic psychotherapy to reduce rates of emergency department return visits for patients with medically unexplained symptoms: Preliminary evidence from a pre–post intervention study. *Canadian Journal of Emergency Medicine, 11*, 529–534.

Abbass, A., & Katzman, J. W. (2013). The cost-effectiveness of intensive short-term dynamic psychotherapy. *Psychiatric Annals, 43*, 496–501.

Abbass, A., Kisely, S., & Kroenke, K. (2009). Short-term psychodynamic psychotherapy for somatic disorders. *Psychotherapy and Psychosomatics, 78*, 265–274.

Abbass, A., Nowoweiski, S. J., Bernier, D., Tarzwell, R., & Beutel, M. (2014). Review of psychodynamic psychotherapy neuroimaging studies. *Psychotherapy and Psychosomatics, 83*, 142–147.

Ablin, J. N., Buskila, D., Van Houdenhove, B., Luyten, P., Atzeni, F., & Sarzi-Puttini, P. (2012). Is fibromyalgia a discrete entity? *Autoimmunity Reviews, 11*, 585–588.

Afari, N., Ahumada, S. M., Wright, L. J., Mostoufi, S., Golnari, G., Reis, V., & Cuneo, J. G. (2014). Psychological trauma and functional somatic syndromes: A systematic review and meta-analysis. *Psychosomatic Medicine, 76*, 2–11.

Afari, N., & Buchwald, D. (2003). Chronic fatigue syndrome: A review. *American Journal of Psychiatry, 160*, 221–236.

Aggarwal, V. R., McBeth, J., Zakrzewska, J. M., Lunt, M., & Macfarlane, G. J. (2006). The epidemiology of chronic syndromes that are frequently unexplained: Do they have common associated factors? *International Journal of Epidemiology, 35*, 468–476.

Alexander, F. (1950). *Psychosomatic medicine, its principles and applications.* New York: Norton.

Anda, R., Felitti, V., Bremner, J., Walker, J., Whitfield, C., Perry, B., et al. (2006). The enduring effects of abuse and related adverse experiences in childhood. *European Archives of Psychiatry and Clinical Neuroscience, 256*, 174–186.

Annemans, L., Le Lay, K., & Taeb, C. (2009). Societal and patient burden of fibromyalgia syndrome. *Pharmacoeconomics, 27*, 547–559.

Annemans, L., Wessely, S., Spaepen, E., Caekelbergh, K., Caubere, J. P., Le Lay, K., et al. (2008). Health economic consequences related to the diagnosis of fibromyalgia syndrome. *Arthritis and Rheumatism, 58*, 895–902.

Arnold, L. M., Hudson, J. I., Keck, P. E., Auchenbach, M. B., Javaras, K. N., & Hess, E. V. (2006). Comorbidity of fibromyalgia and psychiatric disorders. *Journal of Clinical Psychiatry, 67*, 1219–1225.

Aronowitz, R., & Spiro, H. M. (1988). The rise and fall of the psychosomatic hypothesis in ulcerative colitis. *Journal of Clinical Gastroenterology, 10*, 298–305.

Aslakson, E., Vollmer–Conna, U., Reeves, W., & White, P. (2009). Replication of an empirical approach to delineate the heterogeneity of chronic unexplained fatigue. *Population Health Metrics, 7*, 17.

Bakermans-Kranenburg, M. J., van IJzendoorn, M. H., Mesman, J., Alink, L. R. A., & Juffer, F. (2008). Effects of an attachment-based intervention on daily cortisol moderated by dopamine receptor D4: A randomized control trial on 1- to 3-year-olds screened for externalizing behavior. *Development and Psychopathology, 20*, 805–820.

Bass, C., & May, S. (2002). Chronic multiple functional somatic symptoms. *British Medical Journal, 325*, 323–326.

Beard, G. M. (1880). *A practical treatise on nervous exhaustion.* New York: William Wood.

Beutel, M., Michal, M., & Subic-Wrana, C. (2008). Psychoanalytically-oriented inpatient psychotherapy of somatoform disorders. *Journal of the American Academy of Psychoanalysis and Dynamic Psychiatry, 36*, 125–142.

Blom, D., Thomaes, S., Kool, M. B., van Middendorp, H., Lumley, M. A., Bijlsma, J. W. J., et al. (2012). A combination of illness invalidation from the work environment and helplessness is associated with embitterment in patients with FM. *Rheumatology, 51*, 347–353.

Bogaerts, K., Millen, A., Li, W., De Peuter, S., Van Diest, I., Vlemincx, E., et al. (2008). High symptom reporters are less interoceptively accurate in a symptom-related context. *Journal of Psychosomatic Research, 65*, 417–424.

Bogaerts, K., Van Eylen, L., Li, W., Bresseleers, J., Van Diest, I., De Peuter, S., et al. (2010). Distorted symptom perception in patients with medically unexplained symptoms. *Journal of Abnormal Psychology, 119*, 226–234.

Borsini, A., Hepgul, N., Mondelli, V., Chalder, T., & Pariante, C. M. (2013). Childhood stressors in the development of fatigue syndromes: a review of the past 20 years of research. *Psychological Medicine, 7*, 1–15.

Branco, J. (2008). Milnacipran for the treatment of fibromyalgia syndrome: A European multicenter, double-blind, placebo-controlled trial. *European Neuropsychopharmacology, 18*, S574–S575.

Buskila, D., Sarzi-Puttini, P., & Ablin, J. N. (2007). The genetics of fibromyalgia syndrome. *Pharmacogenomics, 8*, 67–74.

Camilleri, M., & Katzka, D. A. (2012). Irritable bowel syndrome: Methods, mechanisms, and pathophysiology. Genetic epidemiology and pharmacogenetics in irritable bowel syndrome. *American Journal of Physiology. Gastrointestinal and Liver Physiology, 302*, G1075–G1084.

Cassidy, J., & Kobak, R. R. (1988). Avoidance and its relation to other defensive processes. In J. Belsky & T. Nezworski (Eds.), *Clinical implications of attachment* (pp. 300–323). London: Routledge.

Champagne, F. A., & Curley, J. P. (2009). Epigenetic mechanisms mediating the long-term effects of maternal care on development. *Neuroscience and Biobehavioral Reviews, 33*, 593–600.

Creed, F. (2007). Cognitive behavioural model of irritable bowel syndrome. *Gut, 56*, 1039–1041.

Creed, F., Fernandes, L., Guthrie, E., Palmer, S., Ratcliffe, J., Read, N., et al. (2003). The cost-effectiveness of psychotherapy and paroxetine for severe irritable bowel syndrome. *Gastroenterology, 124*, 303–317.

Creed, F. H., Tomenson, B., Chew-Graham, C., Macfarlane, G. J., Davies, I., Jackson, J., et al. (2013). Multiple somatic symptoms predict impaired health status in functional somatic syndromes. *International Journal of Behavioral Medicine, 20*, 194–205.

Dantzer, R., O'Connor, J. C., Freund, G. G., Johnson, R. W., & Kelley, K. W. (2008). From inflammation to sickness and depression: When the immune system subjugates the brain. *Nature Reviews. Neuroscience, 9*, 46–56.

Dendy, C., Cooper, M., & Sharpe, M. (2001). Interpretation of symptoms in chronic fatigue syndrome. *Behaviour Research and Therapy, 39*, 1369–1380.

Diamond, D., Stovall-McClough, C., Clarkin, J. F., & Levy, K. N. (2003). Patient–therapist attachment in the treatment of borderline personality disorder. *Bulletin of the Menninger Clinic, 67*, 227–259.

Diamond, L. M., Hicks, A. M., & Otter-Henderson, K. D. (2008). Every time you go away: Changes in affect, behavior, and physiology associated with travel-related separations from romantic partners. *Journal of Personality and Social Psychology, 95*, 385–403.

Dimsdale, J. E., Creed, F., Escobar, J., Sharpe, M., Wulsin, L., Barsky, A., et al. (2013). Somatic symptom disorder: An important change in DSM. *Journal of Psychosomatic Research, 75*, 223–228.

Dozier, M., & Kobak, R. (1992). Psychophysiology in attachment interviews: Converging evidence for deactivating strategies. *Child Development, 63*, 1473–1480.

Driver, C. (2005). An under-active or over-active internal world? *Journal of Analytical Psychology, 50,* 155–173.

Eisenberger, N. I., Lieberman, M. D., & Williams, K. D. (2003). Does rejection hurt?: An fMRI study of social exclusion. *Science, 302,* 290–292.

Fischhoff, B., & Wessely, S. (2003). Managing patients with inexplicable health problems. *British Medical Journal, 326,* 595–597.

Fonagy, P. (1998). An attachment theory approach to treatment of the difficult patient. *Bulletin of the Menninger Clinic, 62,* 147–169.

Fonagy, P., & Luyten, P. (2009). A developmental, mentalization-based approach to the understanding and treatment of borderline personality disorder. *Development and Psychopathology, 21,* 1355–1381.

Fonagy, P., Luyten, P., & Allison, E. (in press). Epistemic petrification and the restoration of epistemic trust: A new conceptualization of borderline personality disorder and its psychosocial treatment. *Journal of Personality Disorders.*

Fonagy, P., Steele, M., Steele, H., Higgitt, A., & Target, M. (1994). The theory and practice of resilience. *Journal of Child Psychology and Psychiatry and Allied Disciplines, 35,* 231–257.

Fredrickson, B. L. (2001). The role of positive emotions in positive psychology. The broaden-and-build theory of positive emotions. *American Psychologist, 56,* 218–226.

Freud, S. (1962). The neuro-psychoses of defence. In J. Strachey (Ed. & Trans.), *The standard edition of the complete psychological works of Sigmund Freud* (Vol. 3, pp. 43–61). London: Hogarth Press. (Original work published 1894)

Gordon, I., Zagoory-Sharon, O., Schneiderman, I., Leckman, J. F., Weller, A., & Feldman, R. (2008). Oxytocin and cortisol in romantically unattached young adults: Associations with bonding and psychological distress. *Psychophysiology, 45,* 349–352.

Gouin, J.-P., Glaser, R., Loving, T. J., Malarkey, W. B., Stowell, J., Houts, C., et al. (2009). Attachment avoidance predicts inflammatory responses to marital conflict. *Brain, Behavior, and Immunity, 23,* 898–904.

Gunnar, M., & Quevedo, K. (2007). The neurobiology of stress and development. *Annual Review of Psychology, 58,* 145–173.

Guthrie, E., Moorey, J., Margison, F., Barker, H., Palmer, S., McGrath, G., et al. (1999). Cost-effectiveness of brief psychodynamic-interpersonal therapy in high utilizers of psychiatric services. *Archives of General Psychiatry, 56,* 519–526.

Hambrook, D., Oldershaw, A., Rimes, K., Schmidt, U., Tchanturia, K., Treasure, J., et al. (2011). Emotional expression, self-silencing, and distress tolerance in anorexia nervosa and chronic fatigue syndrome. *British Journal of Clinical Psychology, 50,* 310–325.

Hammen, C. (2005). Stress and depression. *Annual Review of Clinical Psychology, 1,* 293–319.

Hartocollis, P. (2002). "Actual neurosis" and psychosomatic medicine: The vicissitudes of an enigmatic concept. *International Journal of Psychoanalysis, 83,* 1361–1373.

Hauser, S., Allen, J., & Golden, E. (2006). *Out of the woods: Tales of resilient teens.* Cambridge, MA: Harvard University Press.

Hauser, W., Bernardy, K., Arnold, B., Offenbacher, M., & Schiltenwolf, M. (2009). Efficacy of multicomponent treatment in fibromyalgia syndrome: A meta-analysis of randomized controlled clinical trials. *Arthritis and Rheumatism, 61,* 216–224.

Heim, C., Nater, U. M., Maloney, E., Boneva, R., Jones, J. F., & Reeves, W. C. (2009). Childhood trauma and risk for chronic fatigue syndrome: Association with neuroendocrine dysfunction. *Archives of General Psychiatry, 66,* 72–80.

Hill-Soderlund, A. L., Mills-Koonce, W. R., Propper, C., Calkins, S. D., Granger, D. A., Moore, G. A., et al. (2008). Parasympathetic and sympathetic responses to the strange situation in infants and mothers from avoidant and securely attached dyads. *Developmental Psychobiology, 50,* 361–376.

Hudson, J. I., Arnold, L. M., Keck, P. E., Jr., Auchenbach, M. B., & Pope, H. G., Jr. (2004). Family study of fibromyalgia and affective spectrum disorder. *Biological Psychiatry, 56,* 884–891.

Hudson, J. I., Mangweth, B., Pope, H. G., Jr, De Col, C., Hausmann, A., Gutweniger, S., et al.

(2003). Family study of affective spectrum disorder. *Archives of General Psychiatry, 60,* 170–177.

Hudson, J. I., & Pope, H. G., Jr. (1996). The relationship between fibromyalgia and major depressive disorder. *Rheumatic Diseases Clinics of North America, 22,* 285–303.

Insel, T., & Young, L. (2001). The neurobiology of attachment. *Nature Reviews. Neuroscience 2,* 129–136.

Kempke, S., Luyten, P., Claes, S. J., Van Wambeke, P., Bekaert, P., Goossens, L., et al. (2013). The prevalence and impact of early childhood trauma in chronic fatigue syndrome. *Journal of Psychiatric Research, 47,* 664–669.

Koelen, J. A., Houtveen, J. H., Abbass, A., Luyten, P., Eurelings-Bontekoe, E. H., Van Broeckhuysen-Kloth, S. A., et al. (2014). Effectiveness of psychotherapy for severe somatoform disorder: meta-analysis. *British Journal of Psychiatry, 204,* 12–19.

Kool, M. B., van Middendorp, H., Boeije, H. R., & Geenen, R. (2009). Understanding the lack of understanding: Invalidation from the perspective of the patient with fibromyalgia. *Arthritis Care and Research, 61,* 1650–1656.

Krystal, J. (1982–1983). Alexithymia and the effectiveness of psychoanalytic treatment. *International Journal of Psychoanalytic Psychotherapy, 9,* 353–378.

Lacourt, T., Houtveen, J., & van Doornen, L. (2013). "Functional somatic syndromes, one or many?"" An answer by cluster analysis. *Journal of Psychosomatic Research, 74,* 6–11.

Landmark-Høyvik, H., Reinertsen, K. V., Loge, J. H., Kristensen, V. N., Dumeaux, V., Fosså, S. D., et al. (2010). The genetics and epigenetics of fatigue. *PM&R, 2,* 456–465.

Lawrence, R. C., Felson, D. T., Helmick, C. G., Arnold, L. M., Choi, H., Deyo, R. A., et al. (2008). Estimates of the prevalence of arthritis and other rheumatic conditions in the United States: Part II. *Arthritis and Rheumatism, 58,* 26–35.

Lee, Y., Choi, S., Ji, J., & Song, G. (2012). Candidate gene studies of fibromyalgia: A systematic review and meta-analysis. *Rheumatology International, 32,* 417–426.

Lemma, A., Target, M., & Fonagy, P. (2010). The development of a brief psychodynamic protocol for depression: Dynamic interpersonal therapy (DIT). *Psychoanalytic Psychotherapy, 24,* 329–346.

Lieberman, M. D. (2007). Social cognitive neuroscience: A review of core processes. *Annual Review of Psychology, 58,* 259–289.

Lovell, R. M., & Ford, A. C. (2012). Global prevalence of and risk factors for irritable bowel syndrome: A meta-analysis. *Clinical Gastroenterology and Hepatology, 10,* 712–721.e714.

Lumley, M. A. (2011). Beyond cognitive-behavioral therapy for fibromyalgia: Addressing stress by emotional exposure, processing, and resolution. *Arthritis Research and Therapy, 13,* 136.

Luyten, P., & Abbass, A. (2013). What is the evidence for specific factors in the psychotherapeutic treatment of fibromyalgia?: Comment on "Is brief psychodynamic psychotherapy in primary fibromyalgia syndrome with concurrent depression an effective treatment? A randomized controlled trial." *General Hospital Psychiatry, 35,* 675–676.

Luyten, P., Fonagy, P., Lowyck, B., & Vermote, R. (2012). The assessment of mentalization. In A. Bateman & P. Fonagy (Eds.), *Handbook of mentalizing in mental health practice* (pp. 43–65). Washington, DC: American Psychiatric Association.

Luyten, P., Kempke, S., & Van Houdenhove, B. (2009). Treatment of chronic fatigue syndrome: Findings, principles and strategies. *Psychiatry Investigation, 5,* 209–212.

Luyten, P., Kempke, S., Van Wambeke, P., Claes, S. J., Blatt, S. J., & Van Houdenhove, B. (2011). Self-critical perfectionism, stress generation and stress sensitivity in patients with chronic fatigue syndrome: Relationship with severity of depression. *Psychiatry: Interpersonal and Biological Processes, 74,* 21–30.

Luyten, P., Mayes, L. C., Fonagy, P., & van Houdenhove, B. (2014). *The interpersonal regulation of stress: A developmental framework.* Manuscript submitted for publication.

Luyten, P., Mayes, L. C., Target, M., & Fonagy, P. (2012). Developmental research. In G. O. Gabbard, B. Litowitz, & P. Williams (Eds.), *Textbook of psychoanalysis* (2nd ed., pp. 423–442). Washington, DC: American Psychiatric Press.

Luyten, P., & Van Houdenhove, B. (2013). Common and specific factors in the psychotherapeutic treatment of patients suffering from chronic fatigue and pain disorders. *Journal of Psychotherapy Integration, 23,* 14–27.

Luyten, P., Van Houdenhove, B., Cosyns, N., & Van den Broeck, A. L. (2006). Are patients with chronic fatigue syndrome perfectionistic—or were they?: A case-control study. *Personality and Individual Differences, 40,* 1473–1483.

Luyten, P., Van Houdenhove, B., Lemma, A., Target, M., & Fonagy, P. (2012). An attachment and mentalization-based approach to functional somatic disorders. *Psychoanalytic Psychotherapy, 26,* 121–140.

Luyten, P., Van Houdenhove, B., Lemma, A., Target, M., & Fonagy, P. (2013). Vulnerability for functional somatic disorders: A contemporary psychodynamic approach. *Journal of Psychotherapy Integration, 23,* 14–27.

Maher-Edwards, L., Fernie, B. A., Murphy, G., Nikcevic, A. V., & Spada, M. M. (2012). Metacognitive factors in chronic fatigue syndrome. *Clinical Psychology and Psychotherapy, 19,* 552–557.

Malouff, J. M., Thorsteinsson, E. B., Rooke, S. E., Bhullar, N., & Schutte, N. S. (2008). Efficacy of cognitive behavioral therapy for chronic fatigue syndrome: A meta-analysis. *Clinical Psychology Review, 28,* 736–745.

Marty, P., & de M'Uzan, M. (1963). La pensée opératoire. *Revue Française de Psychanalyse, 27,* 1345–1356.

Maunder, R. G., & Hunter, J. J. (2008). Attachment relationships as determinants of physical health. *Journal of the American Academy of Psychoanalysis and Dynamic Psychiatry, 36,* 11–32.

Maunder, R. G., Lancee, W. J., Nolan, R. P., Hunter, J. J., & Tannenbaum, D. W. (2006). The relationship of attachment insecurity to subjective stress and autonomic function during standardized acute stress in healthy adults. *Journal of Psychosomatic Research, 60,* 283–290.

McEwen, B. S. (2007). Physiology and neurobiology of stress and adaptation: Central role of the brain. *Physiological Reviews, 87,* 873–904.

Mikulincer, M., Dolev, T., & Shaver, P. R. (2004). Attachment-related strategies during thought suppression: Ironic rebounds and vulnerable self-representations. *Journal of Personality and Social Psychology, 87,* 940–956.

Mikulincer, M., & Shaver, P. R. (2007). *Attachment in adulthood: Structure, dynamics and change.* New York: Guilford Press.

Miller, G. E., Chen, E. Y., & Zhou, E. S. (2007). If it goes up, must it come down?: Chronic stress and the hypothalamic-pituitary-adrenocortical axis in humans. *Psychological Bulletin, 133,* 25–45.

National Institute for Health and Clinical Excellence. (2007). Chronic fatigue syndrome/myalgic encephalomyelitis (or encephalopathy): Diagnosis and management of CFS/ME in adults and children. Clinical Guideline 53. London: National Institute for Health and Clinical Excellence. Available at *http://guidance.nice.org.uk/CG53.*

Nemiah, J. C., & Sifneos, P. E. (1970). Affect and fantasy in patients with psychosomatic disorders. In O. W. Hill (Ed.), *Modern trends in psychosomatic medicine* (Vol. 2, pp. 26–34). London: Butterworths.

Neumann, I. D. (2008). Brain oxytocin: A key regulator of emotional and social behaviours in both females and males. *Journal of Neuroendocrinology, 20,* 858–865.

Oldershaw, A., Hambrook, D., Rimes, K. A., Tchanturia, K., Treasure, J., Richards, S., et al. (2011). Emotion recognition and emotional theory of mind in chronic fatigue syndrome. *Psychology and Health, 26,* 989–1005.

Pae, C. U., Luyten, P., Marks, D. M., Han, C., Park, S. H., Patkar, A. A., et al. (2008). The relationship between fibromyalgia and major depressive disorder: A comprehensive review. *Current Medical Research and Opinion, 24,* 2359–2371.

Pedrosa Gil, F., Scheidt, C. E., Hoeger, D., & Nickel, M. (2008). Relationship between attachment style, parental bonding and alexithymia in adults with somatoform disorders. *International Journal of Psychiatry in Medicine, 38*, 437–451.

Pedrosa Gil, F., Weigl, M., Wessels, T., Irnich, D., Baumuller, E., & Winkelmann, A. (2008). Parental bonding and alexithymia in adults with fibromyalgia. *Psychosomatics, 49*, 115–122.

Powell, D. J. H., Liossi, C., Moss-Morris, R., & Schlotz, W. (2013). Unstimulated cortisol secretory activity in everyday life and its relationship with fatigue and chronic fatigue syndrome: A systematic review and subset meta-analysis. *Psychoneuroendocrinology, 38*, 2405–2422.

Rajeevan, M. S., Smith, A. K., Dimulescu, I., Unger, E. R., Vernon, S. D., Heim, C., et al. (2007). Glucocorticoid receptor polymorphisms and haplotypes associated with chronic fatigue syndrome. *Genes, Brain and Behavior, 6*, 167–176.

Rasting, M., Brosig, B., & Beutel, M. E. (2005). Alexithymic characteristics and patient-therapist interaction: A video analysis of facial affect display. *Psychopathology, 38*, 105–111.

Reeves, W., Jones, J., Maloney, E., Heim, C., Hoaglin, D., Boneva, R., et al. (2007). Prevalence of chronic fatigue syndrome in metropolitan, urban, and rural Georgia. *Population Health Metrics, 5*, 5.

Rimes, K. A., & Chalder, T. (2010). The Beliefs about Emotions Scale: Validity, reliability and sensitivity to change. *Journal of Psychosomatic Research, 68*, 285–292.

Roisman, G. I., Holland, A., Fortuna, K., Fraley, R. C., Clausell, E., & Clarke, A. (2007). The Adult Attachment Interview and self-reports of attachment style: An empirical rapprochement. *Journal of Personality and Social Psychology, 92*, 678–697.

Rudich, Z., Lerman, S. F., Gurevich, B., & Shahar, G. (2010). Pain specialists' evaluation of patient's prognosis during the first visit predicts subsequent depression and the affective dimension of pain. *Pain Medicine, 11*, 446–452.

Rudich, Z., Lerman, S. F., Gurevich, B., Weksler, N., & Shahar, G. (2008). Patients' self-criticism is a stronger predictor of physician's evaluation of prognosis than pain diagnosis or severity in chronic pain patients. *Journal of Pain, 9*, 210–216.

Salmon, P. (2007). Conflict, collusion or collaboration in consultations about medically unexplained symptoms: The need for a curriculum of medical explanation. *Patient Education and Counseling, 67*, 246–254.

Sattel, H., Lahmann, C., Gundel, H., Guthrie, E., Kruse, J., Noll-Hussong, M., et al. (2012). Brief psychodynamic interpersonal psychotherapy for patients with multisomatoform disorder: randomised controlled trial. *British Journal of Psychiatry, 200*, 60–67.

Sbarra, D. A., & Hazan, C. (2008). Coregulation, dysregulation, self-regulation: An integrative analysis and empirical agenda for understanding adult attachment, separation, loss, and recovery. *Personality and Social Psychology Review, 12*, 141–167.

Schattner, E., Shahar, G., & Abu-Shakra, M. (2008). "I used to dream of lupus as some sort of creature": Chronic illness as an internal object. *American Journal of Orthopsychiatry, 78*, 466–472.

Shahar, G. (2006). Clinical action: Introduction to the special section on the action perspective in clinical psychology. *Journal of Clinical Psychology, 62*, 1053–1064.

Sicras, A., Rejas, J., Navarro, R., Blanca, M., Morcillo, A., Larios, R., et al. (2009). Treating patients with fibromyalgia in primary care settings under routine medical practice: A claim database cost and burden of illness study. *Arthritis Research and Therapy, 11*, R54.

Sifneos, P. E. (1972). Is dynamic psychotherapy contraindicated for a large number of patients with psychosomatic diseases? *Psychotherapy and Psychosomatics, 21*, 133–136.

Spaeth, M. (2009). Epidemiology, costs, and the economic burden of fibromyalgia. *Arthritis Research and Therapy, 11*, 117.

Stonnington, C. M., Locke, D. E. C., Hsu, C.-H., Ritenbaugh, C., & Lane, R. D. (2013). Somatization is associated with deficits in affective Theory of Mind. *Journal of Psychosomatic Research, 74*, 479–485.

Subic-Wrana, C., Beutel, M. E., Knebel, A., & Lane, R. D. (2010). Theory of Mind and emotional awareness deficits in patients with somatoform disorders. *Psychosomatic Medicine, 72*, 404–411.

Tak, L. M., & Rosmalen, J. G. M. (2010). Dysfunction of the stress responsive systems as a risk factor for functional somatic syndromes. *Journal of Psychosomatic Research, 68*, 461–468.

Taylor, G. J. (1987). *Psychosomatic medicine and contemporary psychoanalysis.* Madison, CT: International Universities Press.

Taylor, G. J., & Bagby, R. M. (2013). Psychoanalysis and empirical research: The example of alexithymia. *Journal of the American Psychoanalytic Association, 61*, 99–133.

Thomas, H., Else, G., Barbara, T., & Francis, C. (2009). Psychodynamic interpersonal therapy and improvement in interpersonal difficulties in people with severe irritable bowel syndrome. *Pain, 145*, 196–203.

Van Houdenhove, B., & Luyten, P. (2007). Fibromaylgia and related syndromes characterized by stress intolerance and pain hypersensitivity: Do we need a new nosology? *Current Rheumatology Reviews, 3*, 304–308.

Van Houdenhove, B., & Luyten, P. (2008). Customizing treatment of chronic fatigue syndrome and fibromyalgia: the role of perpetuating factors. *Psychosomatics, 49*, 470–477.

Van Houdenhove, B., & Luyten, P. (2009). Central sensitivity syndromes: Stress system failure may explain the whole picture. *Seminars in Arthritis and Rheumatism, 39*, 218–219.

Van Houdenhove, B., Luyten, P., & Kempke, S. (2013). Chronic fatigue syndrome/fibromyalgia: A "stress-adaptation" model. *Fatigue: Biomedicine, Health and Behavior, 1*, 137–147.

van Koulil, S., Effting, M., Kraaimaat, F. W., van Lankveld, W., van Helmond, T., Cats, H., et al. (2007). Cognitive-behavioural therapies and exercise programmes for patients with fibromyalgia: State of the art and future directions. *Annals of the Rheumatic Diseases, 66*, 571–581.

Waller, E., & Scheidt, C. E. (2006). Somatoform disorders as disorders of affect regulation: A development perspective. *International Review of Psychiatry, 18*, 13–24.

Watkins, L. R., & Maier, S. F. (2005). Immune regulation of central nervous system functions: From sickness responses to pathological pain. *Journal of Internal Medicine, 257*, 139–155.

Wessely, S., & White, P. (2004). There is only one functional somatic syndrome. *British Journal of Psychiatry, 185*, 95–96.

Westen, D. (1998). The scientific legacy of Sigmund Freud: Toward a psychodynamically informed psychological science. *Psychological Bulletin, 124*, 333–371.

Wirtz, P. H., Siegrist, J., Rimmele, U., & Ehlert, U. (2008). Higher overcommitment to work is associated with lower norepinephrine secretion before and after acute psychosocial stress in men. *Psychoneuroendocrinology, 33*, 92–99.

CHAPTER 15

Personality Disorders

Kevin B. Meehan and Kenneth N. Levy

Generally, psychoanalytically or psychodynamically oriented clinicians find the classification system of personality disorders given in DSM-IV and DSM-5 (American Psychiatric Association [APA], 2000, 2013) to be of limited use in conceptualizing their patients. For that reason, there has been little interest in the DSM. Instead, psychodynamic clinicians have relied more on conceptualizations of character structure, but with little systematic basis for doing so consistently across patient groups. In fact, psychoanalytic explorations of personality disorders not only predate but also attempt to go beyond the symptom-and-sign approach of the DSM classification system (Blatt, 1995; Blatt & Levy, 1998; Kernberg, 1975; Levy & Blatt, 1999; Luyten & Blatt, 2011). With the introduction of the *Psychodynamic Diagnostic Manual* (PDM; PDM Task Force, 2006), and the DSM-5, psychoanalytic and psychodynamic clinicians are increasingly becoming interested in empirically evaluating psychodynamic constructs for underlying personality pathology and establishing a stronger evidence base for a classification system based on psychodynamic ideas (Fonagy & Target, 1998; Levy & Blatt, 1999; Shedler & Westen, 2004).

This chapter contributes to that dialogue by reviewing and evaluating current psychodynamic approaches to personality disorders (a more specific discussion of both dependent personality disorder and borderline personality disorder [BPD] will be covered in Bornstein, Chapter 16, and Clarkin, Fonagy, Levy, & Bateman, Chapter 17, this volume; see also Luyten & Blatt, Chapter 5, this volume). First, we review the current psychodynamic conceptualization of personality disorders. This review includes early efforts by Kernberg, Blatt, and others to think about personality pathology in a developmental/representational context, as well as more recent effort to systematize these models in the form of the PDM. Second, we discuss empirical research pertaining to this psychodynamic conceptualization. Specifically, we examine Shedler and Westen's work suggesting a prototype/dimensional model of personality pathology. Third, we provide a clinical vignette illustrating the disparity between a DSM-based and psychodynamic-based conceptualization of a patient with a personality disorder. Finally, we discuss the implications of the current state of psychodynamic models of personality disorders for future research and future editions of the DSM. We explore the extent to which a new classification system should incorporate dimensional and prototype-based approaches, as well as the limitations of a system that does not integrate the etiology, predicted course, and treatment implications of personality pathology.

PSYCHODYNAMIC APPROACHES TO PERSONALITY DISORDERS

Psychodynamic theories of personality disorders must first be understood in the context of the central role that personality as a construct has played in conceptualizing both healthy and pathological psychological processes. Psychodynamic theories emphasize that the individual's personality structure organizes his or her characteristic ways of thinking, feeling, behaving, and being in relationships (Kernberg & Caligor, 2005; McWilliams, 1994; PDM Task Force, 2006). Thus, the individual's personality has significant implications for his or her success or difficulty in being in the world, including the capacity "to love and to work" as Freud famously said (quoted by Erikson, 1950). Although other theoretical orientations have emphasized some aspects of personality (with an emphasis on "thinking" in the cognitive perspective, "behaving" in the behavioral perspective, and a relative deemphasis on "feeling" and "loving" in each), what sets psychodynamic theory apart is (1) consideration of not only each of these facets of personality but also the level of integration and differentiation among personality structures (Blatt, 1995; Kernberg, 1975), and (2) a central emphasis on the unconscious nature of personality processes, particularly the unconscious affective and motivational processes that have been overlooked in other theoretical approaches (Westen, 1998).[1] Thus, how our personality shapes the ways we think, feel, act, and relate to others often, though not exclusively, operates outside of our awareness, and at times causes conflicts (e.g., one may hold unconscious attitudes that conflict with one's conscious self-perception).

Personality interacts with all aspects of our experience of the world, including our experience of distress and psychological symptoms (Kernberg & Caligor, 2005; McWilliams, 1994; PDM Task Force, 2006). Although DSM-5 continues to distinguish between "symptom disorders" and "personality disorders," psychodynamic theories have long maintained that personality will significantly shape the experience and expression of symptoms of all kinds, including those of the "symptom disorders."

---

[1] Many "third-wave" CBT treatments place a much greater emphasis on affect than did earlier iterations of CBT, although they are primarily focused on the capacity to accept and tolerate negative affect states. Psychodynamic approaches are unique in emphasizing unconscious affective and motivational processes. A notable exception can be seen in recent developments in the social-cognitive approach, which has increasingly focused on unconscious affective and motivational processes, though often with little credit to its psychodynamic origins (see Hassin, Uleman, & Bargh, 2005).

Thus, for example, the experience and expression of panic attacks will differ as a function of the individual's underlying personality organization (Powers & Westen, 2009). Underlying personality pathology may also have prescriptive implication for treating panic attacks (Milrod, Leon, Barber, Markowitz, & Graf, 2007). Thus, conceptualizing the influence of personality on the experience and expression of all symptomatology is a central tenet of psychodynamic theory.

Personality disorders involve chronic, long-standing patterns of responding to distress, which are often limited in variability and rigidly applied regardless of appropriateness to context (PDM Task Force, 2006). Because such personality patterns tend to enact the very experiences the patient is trying to avoid, these patterns come to define the patient's experience (Wachtel, 1997). Thus, in personality disorders, the ways in which the individual thinks, feels, acts, and relates directly restrict his or her capacity to love and work, pursue goals, and enjoy intimate relationships.

Psychodynamic theories conceptualize personality along a continuum, from a healthy personality to severe personality pathology (Kernberg, 1975; Kernberg & Caligor, 2005; McWilliams, 1994; PDM Task Force, 2006). In a healthy personality, the individual's characteristic styles of thinking, feeling, and acting allow a flexible response to stressors with a range of adaptive defenses and coping strategies. Healthy personality functioning also allows the individual to establish stable, mutual, and intimate relationships with others. Higher-level personality pathology may negatively affect functioning, but this may be limited to a particular area of conflict, allowing adaptive functioning in other facets of the individual's life. For example, people with higher-functioning narcissistic pathology may be socially adept and successful enough to function in social and occupational environments and receive some degree of the sought admiration, although they may struggle with deeper intimacy. In contrast, the impact of severe personality pathology on functioning will likely be pervasive across all contexts. For example, individuals with the most severe narcissistic pathology, malignant narcissism, are likely to display antisocial and paranoid features, as well as take pleasure in their aggression and sadism toward others, which would significantly inhibit most aspects of functioning (Kernberg, 1975).

Psychodynamic Models of Personality Pathology

Ego psychology (A. Freud, 1936; Hartmann, 1939) has influenced psychodynamic models of personality pathology through its emphasis on psychological resources (i.e., ego functions and defenses) at an individual's disposal for adapting to internal and external demands. Personality pathology is viewed as the result of the habitual use of maladaptive defense mechanisms, with corresponding problems in functioning such as impulsive behavior, poor affect control, and an impaired capacity for accurate self-reflection. Mature defense mechanisms, such as humor or sublimation, may address the conflict with little interference in (or possible improvement in) the individual's functioning or feeling state. Neurotic defense mechanisms, such as repression or reaction formation, may address the conflict at the cost of circumscribed psychological symptoms, such as anxiety or impaired functioning, as in compulsive behaviors. The most primitive defenses, such as splitting or projective identification, characterize the rigid and distortion-prone psychological structures found in personality disorders. Primitive defenses are likely to provide only the most immediate (and likely inadequate) decrease in anxiety, or they may successfully reduce anxiety at the expense of successful adaptation to life.

The self psychology model, developed by Kohut (1971, 1977), views personality pathology as resulting from a deficit in the structure of the self, without emphasis on conflict among structures within the psyche (Ornstein, 1998). Self psychology focuses on the cohesiveness and vitality versus weakness and fragmentation of the self, and on the role that external relationships play in helping to maintain the cohesion of the self. It posits that primary infantile narcissism, or love of self, is disturbed in the course of development by inadequacies in caretaking. In an effort to safeguard a primitive experience of perfection, the infant places the sense of perfection both in an image of a "grandiose self" and in an "idealized parent imago," which are considered the archaic but healthy nuclei of the "bipolar self" that is the normal product of the evolution of these two nuclei. In the development of the bipolar self, the grandiose self evolves into self-assertive ambitions and involves self-esteem regulation, goal-directedness, and the capacity to enjoy physical and mental activities. The idealized parental imago becomes the individual's internalized values and ideals that function as self-soothing, self-calming, affect-containing structures that maintain internal psychological balance.

Problems in either of these evolutions lead to personality pathology. Inadequate development of the grandiose self results in low self-esteem, lack of motivation, anhedonia, and malaise. Inadequate development of the idealized parental imago results in difficulty regulating tension and the many behaviors that can attempt to achieve this function (e.g., addictions, promiscuity), and a sense of emptiness, depression, and chronic despair. The individual responds to these deficits in psychic structure by developing defensive structures that attempt to fill that gap and lead to the manifest personality pathology.

Object relations models (Bion, 1962; Kernberg, 1975; Kernberg & Caligor, 2005; Klein, 1957) have had the most direct influence on current dynamic conceptualizations of personality pathology (e.g., the PDM). According to such models, in normal psychological development representations of self in relation to others become increasingly more differentiated and integrated. The infant's experience, initially organized around moments of pain ("I am uncomfortable and in need of someone to care for me") and pleasure ("I am now being soothed by someone and feel loved"), become increasingly differentiated and integrated representations of self and other. These mature representations allow for the realistic blending of good and bad, such that positive and negative qualities can be integrated into a complex, multifaceted representation of an individual. Such integrated representations allow for the tolerance of ambivalence, difference, and contradiction in oneself and others.

For Kernberg (1975; Kernberg & Caligor, 2005), the degree of differentiation and integration of these representations of self and other, along with their affective valence, constitutes personality organization. The level of organization of the personality is thought to differ as a function of the nature of the psychological structures that organize the individual's experience and behavior. In a normal personality organization, the individual has an integrated model of self and others, allowing for stability and consistency within his or her identity and in the perception of others, as well as a capacity for becoming intimate with others while maintaining one's sense of self. For example, such an individual would be able to tolerate hateful feelings in the context of a loving relationship without internal conflict or a sense of discontinuity in the perception of the other. Focusing on the degree of identity consolidation versus identity pathology (or "diffusion"), patients are classified according to their capacity to establish and maintain realistic, stable and meaningful experiences of self and significant others and to contextualize their day-to-day experience.

In this context, Kernberg (1975; Kernberg & Caligor, 2005) distinguishes between three levels of personality organization: neurotic, borderline, and psychotic. In the borderline level of organization, the lack of integration in representations of self and other leads to the use of primitive defense mechanisms (e.g., splitting, projective identification, dissociation), identity diffusion (inconsistent view of self and others), and unstable reality testing (inconsistent differentiation between internal and external experience). The high end of the borderline level of organization is thought to include the histrionic, dependent, avoidant, and narcissistic personality disorders as well as the sadomasochistic personality disorder. The low end of the borderline level of organization includes the paranoid, schizoid, schizotypal, borderline, malignant narcissistic and antisocial personality disorders as well as the hypochondriacal and hypomanic personality disorders. In the neurotic level of organization, the more integrated representations of self and other allow for the use of more mature defense mechanisms (e.g., repression, reaction formation) and stable reality testing, with more isolated areas of conflict repressed from the individual's conscious experience. The neurotic level of organization includes the obsessive–compulsive, hysterical, and depressive-masochistic personality disorders. Finally, in contrast to the fluctuations in reality testing seen in the borderline organization, the psychotic level of organization is characterized by chronic breaks in reality testing.

Relatedness and Self-Definitional Dimensions of Personality Pathology

Blatt and colleagues (Blatt, 1995; Blatt & Shichman, 1983) conceptualized personality development as involving two fundamental parallel developmental lines—(1) an *anaclitic* or relatedness line that involves the development of the capacity to establish increasingly mature and mutually satisfying interpersonal relationships, and (2) an *introjective* or self-definitional line that involves the development of a consolidated, realistic, essentially positive, differentiated, and integrated self-identity (see also Luyten & Blatt, Chapter 5, this volume). These two developmental lines normally evolve throughout life in a reciprocal or dialectic transaction. An increasingly differentiated, integrated, and mature sense of self is contingent on establishing satisfying interpersonal relationships, and, conversely, the continued development of increasingly mature and satisfying interpersonal relationships is contingent on developing a more mature self-concept and identity. In normal personality development, these two developmental processes evolve in an interactive, reciprocally balanced, mutually facilitating fashion from birth to senescence.

Blatt (1995) and colleagues (e.g., Blatt & Levy, 1998; Blatt & Shichman, 1983; Levy & Blatt, 1999) conceptualize various forms of psychopathology as an overemphasis and exaggeration of one of these developmental lines (relatedness or self-definition) at the expense of the development of the other line. This overemphasis defines two distinctly different configurations of psychopathology, each containing several types of disordered behavior that range from relatively severe to relatively mild. Anaclitic psychopathologies are those disorders in which patients are preoccupied mainly with issues of relatedness, and who use primarily avoidant defenses (e.g., withdrawal, denial, repression) to cope with psychological conflict and stress. Anaclitic disorders involve a primary preoccupation with interpersonal relations and issues of trust, caring, intimacy, and sexuality, ranging developmentally from more to less disturbed, and include nonparanoid-undifferentiated schizophrenia, BPD, infantile (or dependent) character disorder, anaclitic depression, and hysterical disorders.

In contrast, introjective psychopathology includes disorders in which the patients are primarily concerned with establishing and maintaining a viable sense of self, with issues ranging from a basic sense of separateness, through concerns about autonomy and control, to more complex and internalized issues of self-worth. These patients use primarily counteractive defenses (projection, rationalization, intellectualization, doing and undoing, reaction formation, overcompensation) to cope with conflict and stress. Introjective patients are more ideational and concerned with establishing, protecting, and maintaining a viable self-concept than they are with the quality of their interpersonal relations and with achieving feelings of trust, warmth, and affection. Issues of anger and aggression, directed toward the self or others, are usually central to their difficulties. Introjective disorders, ranging developmentally from more to less severely disturbed, include paranoid schizophrenia; overideational borderline, paranoia, and obsessive–compulsive personality disorders; introjective (guilt-ridden) depression; and phallic narcissism.

Attachment-Based Models of Personality Pathology

From its inception, Bowlby conceptualized attachment theory in both normal and psychopathological development. He (1973) believed that attachment difficulties increase vulnerability to psychopathology and can help identify the specific types of difficulties that arise. Bowlby contended that internal working models of attachment help explain "the many forms of emotional distress and personality disturbances, including anxiety, anger, depression, and emotional detachment, to which unwilling separations and loss give rise" (Bowlby, 1977, p. 201). Bowlby (1977) held that childhood attachment underlies the "later capacity to make affectional bonds as well as a whole range of adult dysfunctions," including "marital problems and trouble with children as well as . . . neurotic symptoms and personality disorders" (p. 206).

Bowlby postulated that insecure attachment lies at the center of disordered personality traits, and he actually tied the overt expression of felt insecurity to specific characterological disorders. For instance, he connected anxious ambivalent attachment to "a tendency to make excessive demands on others and to be anxious and clingy when they are not met, such as is present in dependent and hysterical personalities," and avoidant attachment to "a blockage in the capacity to make deep relationships, such as is present in affectionless and psychopathic personalities" (Bowlby, 1973, p. 14). Avoidant attachment, Bowlby (1973) postulated, results from the individual constantly being rebuffed in his or her appraisals for comfort or protection, and the individual "may later be diagnosed as narcissistic" (p. 124). Thus, Bowlby proposed that early attachment experiences not only have effects that tend to persist across the lifespan but are among the major determinates of personality organization and pathology.

Levy and Blatt (1999), integrating Blatt's (1995) cognitive-developmental psychoanalytic theory with attachment theory, proposed that within each attachment pattern, there may exist more and less adaptive forms of dismissing and preoccupied attachment. These developmental levels are based on the degree of differentiation and integration of representational or working models that underlie attachment patterns. In terms of personality disorders, Levy and Blatt noted that several personality disorders (i.e., histrionic, dependent, borderline) appear to be focused in different ways, and possibly at different developmental levels, on issues of interpersonal relatedness. They proposed that preoccupied attachment would run along a relatedness continuum from nonpersonality-disordered individuals, who value attachment, intimacy, and closeness; to the gregarious, who may exaggerate relatedness; to those with a hysterical style, who not only exaggerate closeness and overly value others but may defend against ideas inconsistent with their desires; to more histrionic individuals, who are overly dependent and easily show anger in attachment relationships; to those with BPD. In contrast, another set of personality disorders (i.e., avoidant, paranoid, obsessive–compulsive, narcissistic) appear to express a preoccupation with establishing, preserving, and maintaining a sense of self, possibly in different ways and at different developmental levels. Levy and Blatt proposed that avoidant attachment would run along a self-definitional continuum from nonpersonality-disordered individuals, who are striving for personal development, to those who are more obsessive; to those with avoidant personality disorder; to those with narcissistic personality disorder (NPD); and finally, at the lowest developmental levels, to those with BPD and antisocial personality disorder.

Levy and Blatt (1999) note that this integration allows us to observe that the two primary types of insecure attachment, avoidant and anxious-preoccupied, can occur at several developmental levels. Differences in the content and structure of mental representations (or internal working models) distinguish more and less adaptive forms of avoidant and anxious-preoccupied attachment, thereby bringing a fuller developmental perspective to the study of attachment patterns. Different patterns of attachment involve not only differences in the content of internal working models but also differences in the structure of those models (e.g., the degree of differentiation and integration). It may be the structure of these models, more so than the content, that results in different capacities and potentials for adaptation. Research has supported the notion that within specific attachment styles, internal working models may vary in the degree of differentiation, integration, and internalization (Levy, Blatt, & Shaver, 1998).

More recently, Peter Fonagy, Mary Target, and colleagues have developed a psychodynamic developmental theory about impairments in the emergence of the agentive self in relation to personality disorders, stressing the importance of the capacity to mentalize, that is, the ability to conceive of mental states as explanations of behavior in oneself and in others (Fonagy, Gergely, Jurist, & Target, 2002; Fonagy, Gergely, & Target, 2007). This model, rooted in attachment theory, goes beyond Bowlby's claims concerning the evolutionary advantages of a system that regulates proximity seeking to the protective caregiver by arguing that the capacity for mentalizing has provided humans with a major evolutionary advantage in terms of the capacity for social intelligence and meaning-making (Bateman & Fonagy, 2003).

This capacity is assumed to develop primarily within the context of secure attachment relationships, with attachment figures promoting the understanding of internal mental states (e.g., emotions, thoughts, wishes), which contributes in turn to the development and consolidation of the self, effortful control, and affect regulation more generally. In contrast, attachment disruptions typically lead to impairments in the capacity for mentalizing, resulting in a disorganized self structure and poor affect, stress regulation, and attentional control systems. This may even completely inhibit mentalizing as a defensive attempt to avoid thinking about the abuser's potentially malevolent and dangerous states of mind. Specifically in attachment contexts, when arousal is high, there is a constant pressure for externalization of this persecutory part of the self, which explains many of the key features of patients with severe personality pathology, including persistent projective identification, self-harm, and parasuicidal behavior. Considerable empirical support for this model has accumulated (Fonagy et al., 2007; Fonagy & Luyten, 2009), and a range of empirically supported treatment and intervention strategies have been developed based on these views (Allen, Fonagy, & Bateman, 2008). Research has also begun to explore the underlying neural circuits of mentalizing as well as neuroendocrine processes underlying relationships among mentalizing, attachment, and affect regulation (Fonagy & Luyten, 2009; Fonagy et al., 2010; Luyten, Fonagy, Lowyck, & Vermote, 2012) (see also Clarkin et al., Chapter 17, this volume).

The PDM: An Integrative Approach to Personality Pathology

The PDM (PDM Task Force, 2006) has integrated many of the aforementioned theories in its approach to classifying personality disorders. First, it explicitly states that patients with personality disorders should be characterized according to level of severity. Following Kernberg (1975), the PDM describes a continuum from neurotic to more severely disturbed personality pathology. Second, in contrast to the DSM-5's description of manifest signs and symptoms, the PDM specifies other aspects of mental functioning to be considered when diagnosing personality disorders, including quality of cognitive capacities (regulation, attention, learning), affect (experience, expression, communication), relationships (depth, range, consistency), internal representations (differentiation, integration, self-regard, morality, self-reflection), and defenses (range, flexibility). Third, the PDM outlines prototypes of personality disorders, moving away from the observable trait approach of the DSM toward typologies of patients characterized by patterns of thinking, feeling, behaving, and relating to others.

Although the prototypes of personality disordered patients in the PDM share some overlap with the DSM categories, there are notable differences. The selection of prototypes is based on a body of clinical literature (McWilliams, 1994) and research findings (Westen & Shedler, 2000), although some key divergences from the research literature are discussed here. The PDM highlights six personality disorders that are not in the DSM-5 system: depressive, sadistic/sadomasochistic, masochistic/self-defeating, dissociative, somatizing, and anxious personality disorders. The first few of these additions resemble categories that are relegated to the DSM's "criteria sets and axes provided for further study" (i.e., depressive and passive-aggressive personality disorders). In fact, significant empirical support exists for depressive personality disorder as a valid construct that can be reliably measured, although challenges remain in discriminating it from similar disorders, most notably dysthymia and other personality disorders with predominantly internalizing symptoms (Bradley, Shedler & Westen, 2006; Huprich, 2009). Passive-aggressive personality disorder has similarly evidenced strong reliability and validity data. Although it has been criticized as better representing a pathological behavior found in multiple personality disorders, recent research has shown it to be a distinct construct (Bradley et al., 2006; Hopwood et al., 2009). However, there is significantly less evidence for sadistic/sadomasochistic or masochistic/self-defeating personality disorders as conceptualized in the PDM, which are better conceptualized as subtypes of other personality disorders (Bradley et al., 2006). Sadistic personality disorder was found to be better represented as a subtype of antisocial personality disorder, whereas self-defeating personality disorder was found to be better represented by borderline and dependent personality disorders. Thus, despite having a rich tradition in the clinical literature, the empirical literature is less supportive of the inclusion of sadistic/sadomasochistic and masochistic/self-defeating personality disorders.

A number of the other personality disorder additions in the PDM (dissociative, somatizing, and anxious personality disorders) are conceptualized by the DSM as "symptom disorders" with little consideration for the influence of personality pathology (i.e., dissociative identity disorder, somatization disorder, generalized anxiety disorder). With regard to these "symptom disorders" in the DSM, it is notable that the differential diagnoses for generalized anxiety disorder and somatization disorder do not list personality disorders as diagnoses to be considered, and they receive a cursory mention in the differential diagnosis for dissociative identity disorder. This stands in contrast to research on Axis I and Axis II comorbidity, which has found the Cluster C personality disorders to be strongly associated with anxiety and somatoform disorders (Tyrer, Gunderson, Lyons, & Tohen, 1997), and BPD to be distinguished from other personality disorders by high rates of comorbid anxiety and somatoform disorders (Zanarini et al., 1998). In contrast, the PDM conceptualizes the symptom presentation of these disorders (anxiety, somatization, dissociation) as the manifestation of disturbances in the individual's underlying personality organization. However, despite strong empirical support for the co-occurrence of personality pathology with anxiety and somatoform disorders, suggesting a central role of personality organization in these pathologies, to date no empirical support has been presented for somatizing and anxious personality disorders as distinct diagnostic constructs that can be reliably measured.

The PDM also omits two categories in the DSM system: schizotypal personality disorder and BPD. Schizotypal personality disorder as described in the DSM-5 is considered a problematic category for many reasons. From a diagnostic perspective, research has demonstrated that the observable features of schizoid and schizotypal personality disorders overlap considerably and tend to load together in factor-analytic models, making it quite difficult to distinguish them in the DSM system (Huprich, Schmitt, Richard, Chelminski, & Zimmerman, 2010; Shedler & Westen, 2004). From a biological perspective, research indicates that patients with schizotypal personality disorder share more commonalities with patients with schizophrenia, in terms of genetic basis as well as structural and functional brain abnormalities, than with patients with other personality disorders (Parnas, Licht, & Bovet, 2005). This finding has led some authors to suggest that clinicians should evaluate the trait of schizotypy independently from personality pathology (Shedler & Westen, 2004). Furthermore, in the PDM system, consistent with Kernberg's model (Kernberg, 1975; Kernberg & Caligor, 2005), borderline personality is conceptualized as a level of organization within which many of the aforementioned disorders will fall (i.e., sadistic and sadomasochistic personality disorders) rather than a specific prototype with characteristic features. However, there is considerable support for BPD as a distinct diagnostic construct, albeit a heterogeneous one in which patients may vary in important ways in terms of their symptom picture and prognosis and yet each meet criteria for the disorder (Clarkin, 1998; Johansen, Karterud, Pedersen, Gude, & Falkum, 2004). As is discussed in more detail later, while some research has supported the notion of borderline personality as a superordinate structure encompassing subgroups, specifically an emotionally dysregulated group and a histrionic-impulsive group, borderline cannot be implicated as organizationally encompassing all personality disorders (Shedler & Westen, 2004; Westen & Shedler, 2007).

In contrast to the DSM-5's (APA, 2013) description of manifest signs and symptoms, the PDM characterizes each disorder in terms of prototypical internal representations of self and others, predominant defenses, central affects, and possible temperamental contributions. As is noted below, proposed revisions for future editions of DSM, included in Section III of DSM-5, consider the inclusion of evaluating higher-order personality trait domains (i.e., negative affectivity, detachment, antagonism, disinhibition, and psychoticism) as well as evaluating levels of both self and interpersonal functioning. This balance of internal dimensions and external manifestations is essential for case conceptualization, as there are often disparities between these aspects of functioning in patients with personality disorders—a level of nuance that is often lost in the DSM-5 system. For example, the manifest presentation of schizoid personality disorder is an apparent indifference to the interpersonal world, and the DSM-5 criteria reflect such behaviors (i.e., has no desire for friendships or sexual relationships, chooses solitary activities, is indifferent to praise/criticism, is emotionally detached). However, the PDM characterizes the internal experience of an individual with schizoid personality disorder as highly vigilant of and intolerably pained by difficulty engaging the social world, which is defended against by an apparent indifference toward relationships. Such individuals often long for intimacy and yet have intense fears of the implications of such closeness; therefore, withdrawal becomes a safe but unsatisfying method of coping with this fear. Thus, the DSM-IV captures only the defensive manifestation, rather than the internal experience of individuals with this disorder—a difference that has significant implications for treatment.

EMPIRICAL FINDINGS

Research on Personality Disorder Prototypes

From an empirical standpoint, the most influential contributor to the PDM's personality disorder sets has been Shedler and Westen's work on empirically derived prototypes of personality disorders (Shedler & Westen, 2004; Westen & Shedler, 2007). Using a Q-sort method called the Shedler–Westen Assessment Procedure, large samples of clinicians characterized their own patients as well as prototypical patients on a wide range of personality descriptors, and the results were used to create empirically derived diagnostic factors. Although their work is influenced by core principles of psychodynamic case conceptualization (experience-near descriptors of mental life, focus on both internal experience and external behaviors), their personality descriptors are atheoretical, and clinician-based prototypes have been consistent across both dynamic and nondynamic therapists.

Shedler and Westen's empirically derived prototypes for personality disorders share some overlap with the DSM categories, but notable differences were found. With regard to the Cluster A disorders, as previously discussed, the observable features of schizoid and schizotypal (and to a lesser extend paranoid) personality disorders overlap considerably, making them difficult to distinguish empirically (Shedler & Westen, 2004). The empirically derived prototypes also include a greater emphasis on the internal experience of these disorders. For example, their description of paranoid personality disorder goes beyond the overt suspiciousness emphasized in the DSM to include an inner experience of anger, victimization, and hypersensitivity to slights. Furthermore, their description of schizoid personality disorder goes beyond interpersonal avoidance to describe an inner experience of fear of embarrassment and humiliation.

With regard to the Cluster B disorders, their prototype of antisocial personality disorder differs from the DSM criteria in important ways. In contrast to the focus in the DSM on criminality and other asocial behaviors, their prototype more closely resembles psychopathy as originally described by Cleckley (1976), with an emphasis instead on internal dimensions such as lack of empathy, remorse, and concern for consequences. In terms of narcissistic personality disorder (NPD), they found that the DSM captured most of the important features as seen in clinical practice. However, narcissistic patients as described by clinicians were characterized as more controlling and competitive, more likely to get into power struggles, and more externalizing of blame than DSM-5 suggests.

Not surprisingly, BPD as characterized by the DSM was found to have significant limitations in terms of its correspondence to clinician ratings. Shedler and Westen (2004) identified prominent symptoms of the disorder not adequately represented in the DSM, including feeling intense emotional pain, dysphoria, rage, inadequacy, helplessness, anxiety, and victimization. Furthermore, they identified distinctions among symptoms that distinguish BPD from other disorders (Bradley et al., 2006). For example, although negative affect (i.e., dysphoria) is characteristic of BPD, it does not distinguish it from other disorders (e.g., dysthymia). In contrast, they note that emotional dysregulation is not only characteristic but also distinctive of BPD. Lastly, they note that not all symptoms of BPD emerge in all contexts (e.g., cutting) and therefore may be distinctive but unstable. Another limitation of the diagnosis concerns the fact that borderline and histrionic personality disorders share many key features (fear of abandonment, dependency, provocative behaviors), leading to difficulty distinguishing between the two (Blagov & Westen, 2008; Shedler & Westen, 2004). They instead found support for a hierarchical structure, with borderline as a superordinate structure encompassing an emotionally dysregulated group and a histrionic-impulsive group (Westen & Shedler, 2007). (See Luyten & Blatt, Chapter 5, and Clarkin et al., Chapter 17, this volume, for a discussion of other limitations of the BPD diagnosis.)

Similarly, with regard to the Cluster C disorders, avoidant and dependent personality disorders were found to share many key features, leading to some difficulty distinguishing between the two (Shedler & Westen, 2004). However, unlike the overlap between the borderline and histrionic disorders, the core features shared between the avoidant and dependent disorders are not included in the DSM-5 criteria but are revealed in their respective prototypes. Shedler and Westen found that patients with avoidant and dependent personality disorders share a depressive core (i.e., "tends to feel inadequate, inferior, a failure," "helpless, powerless," and "will be rejected/ abandoned") from which different coping strategies arise: excessively avoiding and needing people, respectively. While these manifest behaviors appear at odds, the fact that they share such high comorbidity suggests that clinicians recognize and make diagnostic decisions based on this core similarity, even though it is not represented in the DSM. Lastly, in terms of obsessive–compulsive personality disorder, the DSM was found to capture most of the important features as seen in clinical practice, although the empirically derived prototype described a somewhat healthier patient than the DSM would suggest.

As mentioned earlier, Shedler and Westen (2004) evaluated a hierarchical structure for these empirically derived prototypes for personality disorders and identified three superordinate categories: internalizing, externalizing, and borderline. The internalizing category encompasses the depressive, anxious, dependent, and schizoid groups. The externalizing category encompasses the psychopathic, narcissistic, and paranoid groups. The borderline category encompasses an emotionally dysregulated group and a histrionic-impulsive group.

These empirically derived prototypes for personality disorders have a number of advantages over the DSM's categorical system. A study by Westen, Shedler, and Bradley (2006) found that using a prototype approach to diagnosis led to significant decreases in comorbidity, improved clinical utility, and no loss of validity in predicting external measures of functioning. Furthermore, they found that the inclusion of a prototype considering aspects of personality health accounted for additional variance in predicting external measures of functioning. Thus, consideration of personality strengths and adaptive personality features can strengthen assessment of personality disorders.

Research on Subtypes within Personality Disorders

One of the major controversies regarding the DSM-5 personality disorders concerns whether or not they represent distinct diagnostic entities. The controversy has been most clearly seen in the diagnosis of NPD, which has been the focus of controversy since its introduction in DSM-III. Studies have generally confirmed the validity of some of the overt characteristics of NPD as defined in DSM-IV (and thus also in DSM-5), such as grandiosity, grandiose fantasy, desire for uniqueness, need for admiring attention, and arrogant, haughty behavior (Morey, 1988; Ronningstam & Gunderson, 1990; Westen, 1990). However, theoretical and empirical work has suggested that NPD is not a homogeneous disorder, and subtypes likely exist within this group. Several prominent theories and a few empirical studies are summarized below.

Kernberg (1975) classified narcissism along a dimension of severity from normal to pathological and distinguished between three levels of pathological narcissism—high, middle-, and low-functioning groups. At the highest functioning level, patients are able to achieve the admiration necessary to gratify their grandiose needs. These patients may function successfully during their lifetime but are susceptible to breakdowns with advancing age as their grandiose desires go unfulfilled. At the middle level, patients present with a grandiose sense of self and have little interest in true intimacy. At the lowest level, patients present with comorbid borderline personality traits. These patients' sense of self is generally more diffuse and less stable; they frequently vacillate between pathological grandiosity and suicidality. Finally, Kernberg also identified an NPD subtype known as malignant narcissism. These patients are characterized by the typical NPD; however, they also display antisocial behavior, tend toward paranoid features, and take pleasure in their aggression and sadism toward others. Malignant narcissists are at high risk for suicide, despite the absence of depression, given that suicide for these patients represents sadistic control over others, a dismissal of a denigrated world, or a display of mastery over death. Despite the richness of Kernberg's descriptions, we could find no direct research on malignant narcissism. It will be important to differentiate malignant narcissism from NPD proper (as well as from antisocial, paranoid, and borderline personality disorders) and to show that patients meeting Kernberg's criteria for malignant narcissism are at risk for the kind of difficulties that Kernberg described clinically.

Other subtype distinctions in the expression of NPD have been noted. Kohut and Wolf (1978) described three subtypes based on interpersonal relationships. "Merger-hungry" individuals must continually attach and define themselves through others; "contact-shunning" individuals avoid social contact because of fear that their behaviors will not be admired or accepted; and "mirror-hungry" individuals tend to display themselves in front of others. Millon (1998) conceptualized NPD as a prototype and distinguished among the several variations, or subtypes, in which the basic personality style may manifest itself. These subtypes represent configurations of a dominant personality style (e.g., NPD) and traits of other personality styles. For example, in addition to meeting criteria for NPD, Millon's "amorous" subtype would show elevations in histrionic traits, his "unprincipled" subtype would show elevations in antisocial traits, and his "compensatory" subtype would show elevations in avoidant and/ or passive-aggressive traits. To date, little research has been performed to establish the reliability or validity of Kohut and Wolf's or Millon's distinctions.

The DSM criteria for NPD were derived mainly from the theoretical and clinical work of Kernberg, Kohut, and Millon, with little empirical input. Since DSM-III, the criteria for NPD have transitioned from a mixed polythetic/monothetic set of criteria to an entirely polythetic set. The interpersonal criteria, which originally included four parts (entitlement, interpersonal exploitativeness, alternating between extremes of overidealization and devaluation of self and others, lack of empathy), were reduced to three parts through elimination of alternating between extremes of overidealization and devaluation of self and others. The criterion that included grandiosity and uniqueness was split into two separate criteria, and a criterion about preoccupation with feelings of envy was added.

Several theorists and researchers have noted that the DSM criteria for NPD, following the conceptual approaches of Kernberg and Millon, have emphasized a more overt form of narcissism. More recently, Cooper (1981), Akhtar and Thomson (1982), Gabbard (1989), and Wink (1991) suggested that there are two subtypes of NPD: an overt form, also referred to as grandiose, oblivious, willful, exhibitionist, thick-skinned, or phallic; and a covert form, also referred to as vulnerable, hypersensitive, closet, or thin-skinned (Bateman, 1998; Britton, 2000; Gabbard, 1989; Masterson, 1981; Rosenfeld, 1987). The grandiose type is characterized by attention seeking, entitlement, arrogance, and little observable anxiety. These individuals can be socially charming despite being oblivious of others' needs, interpersonally exploitative, and envious. In contrast, the vulnerable type is hypersensitive to others' evaluations, inhibited, manifestly distressed, and outwardly modest. Gabbard described these individuals as shy and "quietly grandiose," with an "extreme sensitivity to slight" that "leads to an assiduous avoidance of the spotlight" (p. 527). Both types are extraordinarily self-absorbed and harbor unrealistically grandiose expectations of themselves. This grandiose–vulnerable distinction has been empirically supported in a number of studies using factor analyses and correlational methods (Dickinson & Pincus, 2003; Hendin & Cheek, 1997; Hibbard & Bunce, 1995; Rathvon & Holmstrom, 1996; Rose, 2002; Wink, 1992).

Using cluster analysis, DiGiuseppe, Robin, Szeszko, and Primavera (1995) reported three clusters of narcissistic patients in an outpatient setting. They named these clusters the *True Narcissist*, the *Compensating Narcissist*, and the *Detached Narcissist*. Patients in all three clusters exhibited self-centeredness and entitlement. However, patients in the True and Detached clusters reported experiencing little emotional distress; in contrast, patients in the Compensating cluster reported high levels of emotional vulnerability. The True and Detached clusters were similar, except that the Detached cluster was characterized by extreme interpersonal avoidance.

Using Q-factor analysis for all patients meeting criteria for NPD, Russ, Shedler, Bradley, and Westen (2008) also found three subtypes: grandiose/malignant, fragile, and high-functioning/exhibitionistic. Grandiose narcissists were described as angry, interpersonally manipulative, and lacking empathy and remorse; the grandiosity was not defensive or compensatory. Fragile narcissists demonstrated grandiosity under threat (defensive grandiosity) and experienced feelings of inadequacy and anxiety, indicating that they vacillate between superiority and inferiority. High-functioning narcissists were grandiose, competitive, attention-seeking, and sexually provocative; they tended to show adaptive functioning and utilize their narcissistic traits to succeed.

Overall, theory and empirical evidence suggest that NPD is a heterogeneous diagnosis that likely contains different subtypes not reflected in the current DSM system. While the problem of heterogeneity of diagnosis is most evident in NPD, it is not limited to this disorder (see Clarkin et al., Chapter 17, this volume, on BPD for further elaboration).

PSYCHODYNAMIC TREATMENT OF PERSONALITY DISORDERS

A meta-analysis by Perry, Banon, and Ianni (1999) suggested that psychotherapy is an effective treatment for personality disorders and may be associated with up to a sevenfold faster rate of recovery in comparison with the natural history of disorders. A more recent meta-analysis examined the effectiveness of psychodynamic therapy and cognitive-behavioral therapy (CBT) in the treatment of personality disorders (Leichsenring & Leibing, 2003; see also Leichsenring, Kruse, & Rabung, Chapter 23, this volume). The study found that psychodynamic therapy yielded a large overall effect size of 1.46, with effect sizes of 1.08 for self-report measures and 1.79 for observer-rated measures. This contrasted with CBT, for which the corresponding values were somewhat lower (i.e., 1.00, 1.20, and 0.87, respectively). Furthermore, it was found that the longer the treatment, the greater the effect size. However, these studies are difficult to interpret because the studies differ, even within the same therapy group, in terms of therapy content, patient diagnosis, length of treatments, outcome assessments, and other variables.

Few controlled studies exist on treatment outcomes for specific personality disorders. To date, there have been no controlled or uncontrolled outcome studies for histrionic, dependent, schizotypal, schizoid, narcissistic, passive-aggressive, or paranoid personality disorders. Most studies have focused on BPD, supporting the efficacy of specific psychodynamic psychotherapies for this condition (see Clarkin et al., Chapter 17, and Leichsenring et al., Chapter 23, this volume, for a review of these studies). In addition, a number of studies have used samples that included Cluster C patients or a mixture of personality disorders with primarily Cluster C patients (Abbass, Sheldon, Gyra, & Kalpin, 2008; Diguer et al., 1993; Hellerstein et al., 1998; Karterud et al., 1992; Monsen, Odland, & Eilertsen, 1995; Rosenthal, Muran, Pinsker, Hellerstein, & Winston, 1999; Turkat, 1990; Winston et al., 1991, 1994). Although these studies generally show improvement in treated patients, particularly with the brief psychodynamic treatments, they are difficult to interpret in terms of specific personality disorders because they do not denote specific diagnostic cohorts.

Svartberg, Stiles, and Seltzer (2004) reported findings from a randomized controlled trial examining the treatment of Cluster C personality disorders. They compared a short-term psychodynamic treatment with CBT and found a significant main effect for reduction in symptomatology for the psychodynamic group but not the CBT group (although there were no between-group differences). Hardy and colleagues (1995) reported the outcome for a subsample of patients with Cluster C personality disorders who had participated in a larger study comparing interpersonal-psychodynamic psychotherapy with cognitive therapy for major depression. Findings indicated that Cluster C patients continued to show more severe symptomatology than non-Cluster C patients if they received dynamic therapy, but not if they received cognitive therapy. In a comparative outcome study, Muran, Safran, Samstag, and Winston (2005) found brief relational therapy, short-term dynamic therapy, and CBT all to be effective in reducing symptomatology (with no significant between-group differences) in a sample of mixed personality disorder patients with primarily Cluster C features. Abbass and colleagues (2008) found that intensive short-term dynamic therapy, in comparison to a delayed-treatment control group, was associated with significant improvements in symptomatic and interpersonal functioning in a sample of mixed personality disorder patients with primarily borderline, avoidant, and obsessive–compulsive personality disorder diagnoses. Patients evidenced an 83% reduction of personality disorder diagnoses at 2-year follow-up.

Numerous uncontrolled outcome studies also suggest promising treatment approaches for personality disorders (for a review, see Fonagy, Roth, & Higgitt, 2005). For example, in an open trial, Barber, Morse, Krakauer, Chittams, and Crits-Cristoph (1997), found that a supportive-expressive psychodynamic psychotherapy was effective for treating both obsessive–compulsive and avoidant personality disorders. At the end of one year of treatment, 85% of obsessive–compulsive and over 60% of avoidant personality disorder patients no longer met criteria for the disorders.

Finally, preliminary research suggests that Axis I patients with comorbid personality pathology may be more likely to benefit from psychodynamic therapy than those without such comorbidity. For example, Milrod and colleagues (2007) found that the presence of comorbid Cluster C personality diagnosis in patients with panic disorder moderated treatment outcome, with superior improvement in panic-focused psychodynamic psychotherapy. Thus, the presence of personality pathology may act as a prescriptive indicator for psychodynamic treatments. This finding reinforces the importance of clinicians attending to personality pathology when planning treatment for patients with Axis I disorders.

CLINICAL ILLUSTRATION

The following vignette is a clinical illustration of the value of a psychodynamic framework for diagnosing personality disorders, using the example of NPD. As discussed earlier in this chapter, DSM-5 presents a number of limitations to the diagnosis of NPD, most notably increased emphasis on overtly haughty and arrogant behaviors, and decreased emphasis on the pattern of alternating between idealization and devaluation of self and others. As a result, many personality-disordered patients who struggle with narcissistic issues do not meet the criteria for NPD, and yet narcissistic dynamics have significant implications for the assessment and treatment of these individuals.

Jennifer is a single, 32-year-old woman who is underemployed for her level of education and intelligence. She was administered a structured interview for personality disorders by an independent evaluator prior to the beginning of treatment. She met the criteria for BPD, endorsing unstable relationships, impulsivity, affective instability, anger, identity disturbance, and emptiness. In contrast, she did not meet the full criteria for any symptoms of NPD, although she was found to have subclinical features of a grandiose sense of self-importance, fantasies of success and power, and belief in oneself as special or unique.

In her initial presentation, Jennifer came across as somewhat entitled, but not haughty or arrogantly so, and the primary expression of this entitlement was a resentment of others in a superior position whom she felt did not deserve that status. Although she did not act superior to others or express the feeling that she should receive special treatment, there was a feeling of envy toward others for their superior standing as well as contempt for their not deserving their status. Similarly, she did not express a global grandiose sense of self-importance or achievement—in specific contexts, such as work, she thought she could do a given task better than the "idiot" above her, but not better than people in general. Jennifer did not act in interpersonally exploitative ways but, rather, she was very sensitive to perceived exploitativeness from others. Similarly, she never appeared to be overtly lacking in empathy, but she was quite sensitive to the unempathic behaviors of others, and would react with anger and resentment at these perceived behaviors from others.

Thus, the three main domains of NPD in the DSM-5 criteria (entitlement, interpersonal exploitativeness, and lack of empathy) are not overt in Jennifer's behavior but, rather, covertly expressed through a fear of being victim to such behaviors from others. In terms of NPD symptoms no longer included in DSM-5, one of Jennifer's most notable features concerns extremes of overidealization and devaluation of self and others. This aspect was evident in her self-perception (i.e., "I am right because I know how life works, but my life is a mess so apparently I know nothing") and her perception of others (i.e., "the therapist's opinion has enormous weight because he is a professional, but has no weight because he appears incompetent"). Jennifer also displays many of the features described by Russ and colleagues (2008) in their narcissistic prototype but not found in DSM (i.e., controlling, competitive, power struggles). She was noted to exert a high level of control in her relationships, including with her therapist, motivated by fear that she would be made too vulnerable if others took control, which often led to power struggles in her relationships.

In conclusion, this vignette demonstrates how a patient may not meet DSM-5 criteria for NPD and yet narcissistic dynamics may dominate within sessions and in external life.

CONCLUSIONS AND FUTURE DIRECTIONS

Proposals for modifying personality disorder diagnosis in the fifth edition of the DSM for a time suggested a radical restructuring of the way in which these disorders are diagnosed, but due to a lack of research support for such changes the DSM-5 has retained the categories of the DSM-IV. Although such radical changes will likely require further research before being adopted in future editions of the DSM, a consideration of the advantages and disadvantages of the proposed changes from the Personality Disorders Workgroup is warranted. During the open-comment phase of DSM-5's development, a system was offered that involved evaluating a limited number of personality disorder types (i.e., antisocial, avoidant, borderline, narcissistic, obsessive–compulsive, and schizotypal) dimensionally; evaluating higher-order personality trait domains (i.e., negative affectivity, detachment, antagonism, disinhibition, and psychoticism) as well as lower-order trait facets for each trait domain; evaluating levels of both self and interpersonal functioning; and evaluating failures in adaptive functioning (APA, 2013). Taken together, this system was intended to provide a multidimensional profile of personality types and traits, pathology, and level of functioning.

Including a prototype approach to the classification of personality pathology in future editions of the DSM has many advantages. Many authors have noted that in such an approach the most prototypical behavioral qualities of a disorder form the center of a diagnostic category, while less descriptive behaviors form the periphery (Livesley & Jackson, 1986; Westen, 1997). This approach allows clinicians to distinguish between essential and nonessential symptoms, which a categorical system cannot do (Shedler & Westen, 2007). Ideally, this method of classification would reduce overlap between personality disorder criteria and lead to more precise diagnoses.

Furthermore, the evaluation of self and interpersonal functioning bears some resemblance to the structural models of Blatt and Kernberg (Luyten & Blatt, 2011). Impairments in self-functioning would be indicated by problems related to identity and self-direction; this is consistent with Blatt's (1995) *introjective* or self-definitional line of development, as well as the central role of identity cohesion/diffusion in Kernberg's (1975) model. Impairments in interpersonal functioning would be indicated by problems in the capacity for empathy and intimacy; this is consistent with Blatt's *anaclitic* or relatedness line of development, as well as the central place of the identity role of love, intimacy, and healthy sexual relations in Kernberg's model.

However, a number of experts in the field of personality disorders (Shedler et al., 2010) have expressed concern about an approach that blends prototype and trait-based dimensional ratings. Clinicians tend not to think of their patients along trait-based dimensions, nor do they tend to draw from multiple conceptually unrelated models to identify dimensions of personality pathology. A blended system calls to mind the axiom "A camel is a horse designed by committee" (D. Westen, quoted in Holden, 2010) in that it is "an unwieldy conglomeration of disparate models that cannot happily coexist and raises the likelihood that many clinicians will not have the patience and persistence to make use of it in their practices" (Shedler et al., 2010, p. 1026).

Future editions of the DSM would benefit from moving beyond overt descriptions of signs and symptoms to include multiple domains of functioning—affect, behavior, cognitions, and quality of relatedness. Such an approach should include not just deficits in these domains of functioning, but also the presence of internal resources that might buffer against the impact of symptoms, for example, the capacity for intimacy (Shedler & Westen, 2007). Diagnosis needs to account for not only overt behaviors but also inner experience (Shedler & Westen, 2004). Thus the patient's total life circumstances need to be taken into account in diagnosing personality disorders (Kernberg & Caligor, 2005).

Future editions of the DSM would also benefit from increased consideration of levels of pathology within personality disorders (Kernberg, 1975). Personality disorder diagnosis needs to be placed in the context of etiology, predicted course, and treatment implications. Finally, the assessment of personality pathology cannot remain segregated from the assessment of "symptom disorders." Rather, there needs to be an appreciation of how they interact, and often the dichotomy between these groups of disorders may be a false one.

REFERENCES

Abbass, A., Sheldon, A., Gyra, J., & Kalpin, A. (2008). Intensive short-term dynamic psychotherapy for DSM IV personality disorders. A randomized controlled trial. *Journal of Nervous and Mental Disease, 196,* 1–6.

Akhtar, S., & Thomson, J. A. (1982). Overview: Narcissistic personality disorder. *American Journal of Psychiatry, 139,* 12–20.

Allen, J., Fonagy, P., & Bateman, A. (2008). *Mentalizing in clinical practice.* Washington, DC: American Psychiatric Press.

American Psychiatric Association. (2000). *Diagnostic and statistical manual of mental disorders* (4th ed., text rev.). Washington, DC: Author.

American Psychiatric Association. (2013). *Diagnostic and statistical manual of mental disorders* (5th ed.). Arlington, VA: Author.

Barber, J. P., Morse, J. Q., Krakauer, I. D., Chittams, J., & Crits-Christoph, K. (1997). Change in obsessive–compulsive and avoidant personality disorders following time-limited supportive-expressive therapy. *Psychotherapy, 34,* 133–143.

Bateman, A. W. (1998). Thick- and thin-skinned organizations and enactment in borderline and narcissistic disorders. *International Journal of Psychoanalysis, 79,* 13–25.

Bateman, A. W., & Fonagy, P. (2003). The development of an attachment-based treatment program for borderline personality disorder. *Bulletin of the Menninger Clinic, 67,* 187–211.

Bion, W. R. (1962). A theory of thinking. *International Journal of Psycho-Analysis, 43,* 306–310.

Blagov, P., & Westen, D. (2008). Questioning the coherence of histrionic personality disorder: Borderline and hysterical personality subtypes in adults and adolescents. *Journal of Nervous and Mental Disease, 196,* 785–797.

Blatt, S. J. (1995). Representational structures in psychopathology. In D. Cicchetti & S. L. Toth (Eds.), *Emotion, cognition, and representation. Rochester Symposium on Developmental Psychopathology* (Vol. 6, pp. 1–33). Rochester, NY: University of Rochester Press.

Blatt, S. J., & Levy, K. N. (1998). A psychodynamic approach to the diagnosis of psychopathology. In J. W. Barron (Ed.), *Making diagnosis meaningful: Enhancing evaluation and treatment of psychological disorders* (pp. 73–109). Washington, DC: American Psychological Association Books.

Blatt, S. J., & Shichman, S. (1983). Two primary considerations of psychopathology. *Psychoanalysis and Contemporary Thought, 6,* 187–254.

Bowlby, J. (1973). *Attachment and loss: Vol. 2. Separation.* New York: Basic Books.

Bowlby, J. (1977). The making and breaking of affectional bonds: I. Etiology and psychopathology in the light of attachment theory. *British Journal of Psychiatry, 130,* 201–210.

Bradley, R., Shedler, J., & Westen, D. (2006). Is the appendix a useful appendage?: An empirical examination of depressive, passive-aggressive (negativistic), sadistic, and self-defeating personality disorders. *Journal of Personality Disorders, 20,* 524–540.

Britton, R. (2000). Hyper-sensitivity and hyper-objectivity in narcissistic disorders. *Fort Da: The Journal of the Northern California Society for Psychoanalytic Psychology, 6,* 18–23.

Clarkin, J. F. (1998). Research findings on the personality disorders. *In Session: Psychotherapy in Practice, 4,* 91–102.

Cleckley, H. (1976). *The mask of sanity* (5th ed.). St Louis, MO: Mosby.

Cooper, A. (1981). Narcissism. In S. Arieri, H. Keith, & H. Brodie (Eds.), *American Handbook of Psychiatry* (Vol. 4, pp. 297–316). New York: Basic Books.

Dickinson, K. A., & Pincus, A. L. (2003). Interpersonal analysis of grandiose and vulnerable narcissism. *Journal of Personality Disorders, 17,* 188–207.

DiGiuseppe, R., Robin, M., Szeszko, P. R., & Primavera, L. H. (1995). Cluster analyses of narcissistic personality disorders on the MCMI-II. *Journal of Personality Disorders, 9,* 304–317.

Diguer, L., Luborsky, L., Luborsky, E., McLellan, A., Woody, G., & Alexander, L. (1993). Psychological health-sickness (PHS) as a predictor of outcomes in dynamic and other psychotherapies. *Journal of Consulting and Clinical Psychology, 61,* 542–548.

Erikson, E. H. (1950). *Childhood and society.* New York: Norton.

Fonagy, P., Gergely, G., Jurist, E., & Target, M. (2002). *Affect regulation, mentalization and the development of the self.* New York: Other Press.

Fonagy, P., Gergely, G., & Target, M. (2007). The parent–infant dyad and the construction of the subjective self. *Journal of Child Psychology and Psychiatry, 48,* 288–328.

Fonagy, P., & Luyten, P. (2009). A developmental, mentalization-based approach to the understanding and treatment of borderline personality disorder. *Development and Psychopathology, 21,* 1355–1381.

Fonagy, P., Luyten, P., Bateman, A., Gergely, G., Strathearn, L., Target, M., et al. (2010). Attachment and personality pathology. In J. F. Clarkin, P. Fonagy, & G. O. Gabbard (Eds.), *Psychodynamic psychotherapy for personality disorders. A clinical handbook* (pp. 37–87). Washington, DC: American Psychiatric Publishing.

Fonagy, P., Roth, A., & Higgitt, A. (2005). The outcome of psychodynamic psychotherapy for psychological disorders. *Clinical Neuroscience Research, 4,* 367–377.

Fonagy, P., & Target, M. (1998). Mentalization and the changing aims of child psychoanalysis. *Psychoanalytic Dialogues, 8,* 87–114.

Freud, A. (1936). *The ego and the mechanisms of defense.* London: Hogarth Press.

Gabbard, G. (1989). Two subtypes of narcissistic personality disorder. *Bulletin of the Menninger Clinic, 53,* 527–532.

Hardy, G., Barkham, M., Shapiro, D., Stiles, W., Rees, A., & Reynolds, S. (1995). Impact of Cluster C personality disorders on outcomes of contrasting brief psychotherapies for depression. *Journal of Consulting and Clinical Psychology, 63,* 997–1004.

Hartmann, H. (1939) *Ego-psychology and adaptation.* New York: International Universities Press.

Hassin, R., Uleman, J., & Bargh, J. (2005). *The new unconscious.* New York: Oxford University Press.

Hellerstein, D. J., Rosenthal, R. N., Pinsker, H., Samstag, L. W., Muran, J. C., & Winston, A. (1998). A randomized prospective study comparing supportive and dynamic therapies. Outcome and alliance. *Journal of Psychotherapy Practice and Research, 7,* 261–271.

Hendin, H. M., & Cheek, J. M. (1997). Assessing hypersensitive narcissism: A reexamination of Murray's narcissism scale. *Journal of Research in Personality, 31,* 588–599.

Hibbard, S., & Bunce, S. C. (1995, August). *Two paradoxes of narcissism.* Paper presented at the annual meeting of the American Psychological Association, New York.

Holden, C. (2010). APA seeks to overhaul personality disorder diagnoses. *Science, 327,* 1314.

Hopwood, C., Morey, L., Markowitz, J., Pinto, A., Skodol, A., Gunderson, J., et al. (2009). The construct validity of passive–aggressive personality disorder. *Psychiatry: Interpersonal and Biological Processes, 72(3),* 256–267.

Huprich, S. K. (2009). What should become of depressive personality disorder in DSM-V? *Harvard Review of Psychiatry, 17,* 41–59.

Huprich, S. K., Schmitt, T. A., Richard, D. C., Chelminski, I., & Zimmerman, M. A. (2010). Comparing factor analytic models of the DSM-IV personality disorders. *Personality Disorders: Theory, Research, and Treatment, 1,* 22–37.

Johansen, M., Karterud, S., Pedersen, G., Gude, T., & Falkum, E. (2004). An investigation of the prototype validity of the borderline DSM-IV construct. *Acta Psychiatrica Scandinavica, 109,* 289–298.

Karterud, S., Vaglum, S., Friis, S., Irion, T., Johns, S., & Vaglum, P. (1992). Day hospital therapeutic community treatment for patients with personality disorders: An empirical evaluation of the containment function. *Journal of Nervous and Mental Disease, 180,* 238–243.

Kernberg, O. F. (1975). *Borderline conditions and pathological narcissism.* New Haven, CT: Yale University Press.

Kernberg, O. F., & Caligor, E. (2005). A psychoanalytic theory of personality disorders. In M. F. Lenzenweger & J. F. Clarkin (Eds.), *Major theories of personality disorder* (2nd ed., pp. 114–156). New York: Guilford Press.

Klein, M. (1957). *Envy and gratitude: A study of unconscious sources.* New York: Basic Books.

Kohut, H. (1971). *The analysis of the self.* New York: International Universities Press.

Kohut, H. (1977). *The restoration of the self.* New York: International Universities Press.

Kohut, H., & Wolf, E. S. (1978). The disorders of the self and their treatment: An outline. *International Journal of Psychoanalysis, 59,* 413–425.

Leichsenring, F., & Leibing, E. (2003). The effectiveness of psychodynamic therapy and cognitive behavior therapy in the treatment of personality disorders: A meta-analysis. *American Journal of Psychiatry, 160,* 1223–1232.

Levy, K., & Blatt, S. (1999). Attachment theory and psychoanalysis: Further differentiation within insecure attachment patterns. *Psychoanalytic Inquiry, 19,* 541–575.

Levy, K. N., Blatt, S. J., & Shaver, P. R. (1998). Attachment styles and parental representations. *Journal of Personality and Social Psychology, 74,* 407–419.

Livesley, W., & Jackson, D. (1986). The internal consistency and factorial structure of behaviors judged to be associated with DSM-III personality disorders. *American Journal of Psychiatry, 143,* 1473–1474.

Luyten, P., & Blatt, S. J. (2011). Integrating theory-driven and empirically-derived models of personality development and psychopathology: A proposal for DSM V. *Clinical Psychology Review, 31,* 52–68.

Luyten, P., Fonagy, P., Lowyck, B., & Vermote, R. (2012). The assessment of mentalization. In A. Bateman & P. Fonagy (Eds.), *Handbook of mentalizing in mental health practice* (pp. 43–65). Washington, DC: American Psychiatric Association.

Masterson, J. F. (1981). *The narcissistic and borderline disorders.* New York: Brunner/Mazel.

McWilliams, N. (1994). *Psychoanalytic diagnosis.* New York: Guilford Press.

Millon, T. (1998). DSM narcissistic personality disorder: Historical reflections and future directions. In E. F. Ronningstam (Ed.), *Disorders of narcissism: Diagnostic, clinical, and empirical implications* (pp. 75–101). Washington, DC: American Psychiatric Press.

Milrod, B., Leon, A. C., Barber, J. P., Markowitz, J. C., & Graf, E. (2007). Do comorbid personality disorders moderate psychotherapy response in panic disorder?: A preliminary empirical evaluation of the APA Practice Guideline. *Journal of Clinical Psychiatry, 68,* 885–891.

Monsen, J. T., Odland, T., & Eilertsen, D. E. (1995). Personality disorders: Changes and stability after intensive psychotherapy focusing on affect consciousness. *Psychotherapy Research, 5,* 33–48.

Morey, L. C. (1988). The categorical representation of personality disorder: A cluster analysis of DSM-III–R personality features. *Journal of Abnormal Psychology, 97,* 314–321.

Muran, J. C., Safran, J. D., Samstag, L. W., & Winston, A. (2005). Evaluating an alliance-focused treatment for personality disorders. *Psychotherapy: Theory, Research, Practice, Training, 42*, 532–545.

Ornstein, P. H. (1998). Psychoanalysis of patients with primary self-disorder. In E. F. Ronningstam (Ed.), *Disorders of narcissism: Diagnostic, clinical, and empirical implications* (pp. 147–169). New York: American Psychiatric Press.

Parnas, J., Licht, D., & Bovet, P. (2005). Cluster A personality disorders: A review. In M. Maj, H. Akiskal, J. E. Mezzich, & A. Okasha (Eds.), *Personality disorders* (pp. 1–74). New York: Wiley.

PDM Task Force. (2006). *Psychodynamic diagnostic manual.* Silver Spring, MD: Alliance of Psychoanalytic Organizations.

Perry, J. C., Banon, E., & Ianni, F. (1999). Effectiveness of psychotherapy for personality disorders. *American Journal of Psychiatry, 156*, 1312–1321.

Powers, A., & Westen, D. (2009). Personality subtypes in patients with panic disorder. *Comprehensive Psychiatry, 50*, 164–172.

Rathvon, N., & Holstrom, R. W. (1996). An MMPI-2 portrait of narcissism. *Journal of Personality Assessment, 66*, 1–19.

Ronningstam, E., & Gunderson, J. (1990). Identifying criteria for narcissistic personality disorder. *American Journal of Psychiatry, 147*, 918–922.

Rose, P. (2002). The happy and unhappy faces of narcissism. *Personality and Individual Differences, 33*, 379–392.

Rosenfeld, H. A. (1987). *Impasse and interpretation: Therapeutic and anti-therapeutic factors in the psychoanalytic treatment of psychotic, borderline, and neurotic patients.* London: Tavistock and the Institute of Psycho-Analysis.

Rosenthal, R. N., Muran, J. C., Pinsker, H., Hellerstein, D., & Winston, A. (1999). Interpersonal change in brief supportive psychotherapy. *Journal of Psychotherapy Practice and Research, 8*, 55–63.

Russ, E., Shedler, J., Bradley, R., & Westen, D. (2008). Refining the construct of narcissistic personality disorder: Diagnostic criteria and subtypes. *American Journal of Psychiatry, 165*, 1473–1481.

Shedler, J., Beck, A., Fonagy, P., Gabbard, G. O., Gunderson, J., Kernberg, O., et al. (2010). Personality disorders in DSM-5. *American Journal of Psychiatry, 167*, 1026–1028.

Shedler, J., & Westen, D. (2004). Refining personality disorder diagnoses: Integrating science and practice. *American Journal of Psychiatry, 161*, 1–16.

Shedler, J., & Westen, D. (2007). The Shedler–Westen Assessment Procedure (SWAP): Making personality diagnosis clinically meaningful. *Journal of Personality Assessment, 81*, 41–55.

Svartberg, M., Stiles, T., & Seltzer, M. (2004). Randomized, controlled trial of the effectiveness of short-term dynamic psychotherapy and cognitive therapy for Cluster C personality disorders. *American Journal of Psychiatry, 161*, 810–817.

Turkat, I. (1990). *The personality disorders: A psychological approach to clinical management.* Elmsford, NY: Pergamon Press.

Tyrer, P., Gunderson, J., Lyons, M., & Tohen, M. (1997). Extent of comorbidity between mental state and personality disorders. *Journal of Personality Disorders, 11*, 242–259.

Wachtel, P. L. (1997). *Psychoanalysis, behavior therapy, and the relational world.* Washington, DC: American Psychological Association.

Westen, D. (1990). The relations among narcissism, egocentrism, self-concept, and self-esteem: Experimental, clinical and theoretical considerations. *Psychoanalysis and Contemporary Thought, 13*, 183–239.

Westen, D. (1997). Divergences between clinical and research methods for assessing personality disorders: Implications for research and the evolution of Axis II. *American Journal of Psychiatry, 154*, 895–903.

Westen, D. (1998). The scientific legacy of Sigmund Freud: Toward a psychodynamically informed psychological science. *Psychological Bulletin, 124*, 333–371.

Westen, D., & Shedler, J. (2000). A prototype matching approach to diagnosing personality disorders: Toward DSM-V. *Journal of Personality Disorders, 14*, 109–126.

Westen, D., & Shedler, J. (2007). Personality diagnosis with the Shedler–Westen assessment procedure (SWAP): Integrating clinical and statistical measurement and prediction. *Journal of Abnormal Psychology, 116*, 810–822.

Westen, D., Shedler, J., & Bradley, R. (2006). A prototype approach to personality disorder diagnosis. *American Journal of Psychiatry, 163*, 846–856.

Wink, P. (1991). Two faces of narcissism. *Journal of Personality and Social Psychology, 61*, 590–597.

Wink, P. (1992). Three narcissism scales for the California Q-Set. *Journal of Personality Assessment, 58*, 51–66.

Winston, A., Laikin, M., Pollack, J., Samstag, L., McCullough, L., & Muran, J. C. (1994). Short-term psychotherapy of personality disorders. *American Journal of Psychiatry, 151*, 190–194.

Winston, A., Pollack, J., McCullough, L., Flegenheimer, W., Kestenbaum, R., & Trujillo M. (1991). Brief psychotherapy of personality disorders. *Journal of Nervous and Mental Disorders, 179*, 188–193.

Zanarini, M. C., Frankenburg, F. R., Dubo, E. D., Sickel, A. E., Trikha, A., Levin, A., et al. (1998). Axis I Comorbidity of Borderline Personality Disorder. *American Journal of Psychiatry, 155*, 1733–1739.

CHAPTER 16

Dependent Personality Disorder

Robert F. Bornstein

This chapter reviews psychodynamic research on trait dependency and dependent personality disorder (DPD), to point the way toward a more psychodynamically informed, empirically based conceptualization of pathological dependency. I begin by discussing classification and diagnosis, theoretical perspectives on dependency and DPD, and then review empirical research in this area. Following an overview of psychodynamic treatment and a brief case vignette illustrating how psychodynamic principles may be useful in clinical work with dependent patients, I suggest possible directions for continued refinement in our conceptualization of problematic dependency.

CLASSIFICATION AND DIAGNOSIS

Although Kraepelin (1913), Schneider (1923), and others (e.g., Abraham, 1927) provided early descriptions of patients with pathological dependency, formal diagnostic criteria for DPD were not developed until the publication of the first edition of the *Diagnostic and Statistical Manual of Mental Disorders* (DSM-I; American Psychiatric Association [APA], 1952). In DSM-I, DPD was conceptualized as a passive–dependent subtype of the passive–aggressive personality, with passive–dependent patients characterized by "helplessness, indecisiveness, and a tendency to cling to others as a dependent child to a supporting parent" (APA, 1952, p. 37). The evolution of DPD across successive revisions of the DSM has been characterized by a gradual "depsychoanalyzing" of the diagnostic criteria: By the time DSM-III (APA, 1980) was published all reference to psychodynamic processes had been excised from the description of DPD, and subsequent editions of the manual have maintained this atheoretical perspective (see Bornstein, 2006, for a discussion of the declining influence of psychodynamic concepts in the DSM conceptualization of personality disorders more generally).

As is true of several other forms of personality pathology (e.g., narcissism, avoidance, obsessiveness), there is considerable conceptual and empirical overlap between the more pathological manifestations of dependency (i.e., DPD) and normally distributed interpersonal dependency (sometimes called *trait dependency*) as found in the broader population (see Bornstein, 2005b, 2012). As a result, research on interpersonal dependency in clinical and nonclinical samples has helped inform contemporary conceptualizations of DPD (Bornstein, 1998, 2007a), and research on the etiology and dynamics of DPD has helped shape researchers' understanding of trait dependency (Overholser, 1996; Pincus & Gurtman, 1995). Although it is important to be cautious when generalizing from nonclinical participants to clinical populations, studies confirm that high levels of interpersonal dependency are associated with elevated levels of DPD symptoms and increased likelihood of a diagnosis of DPD in a variety of groups, including psychiatric inpatients, outpatients, college students, and adults in the community (Hirschfeld, Klerman, Clayton, & Keller, 1983; Johnson & Bornstein, 1992; Loas et al., 2002). As Skodol and colleagues (2011) noted, studies of trait dependency and DPD have yielded such consistent results that "current measures of DPD and trait dependency are virtually interchangeable" (p. 152).

Psychodynamic research reviewed in this chapter on interpersonal dependency and DPD has noteworthy implications for assessment, classification, and diagnosis. Detailed discussions of assessment-related issues are provided by Bornstein (2002, 2009), Cogswell (2008), and McGrath (2008). In the following sections I discuss the implications of the interactionist model and research presented in this chapter evaluating this model (see also Figure 16.1) for (1) extant DPD diagnostic criteria, (2) DPD as conceptualized in the *Psychodynamic Diagnostic Manual* (PDM; Alliance of Psychoanalytic Organizations [APO], 2006), and (3) DPD in DSM-5 (APA, 2013) and beyond.

Burdened by History: DPD in DSM

As Bornstein (1997) noted, the DSM criteria for DPD have been problematic in a number of respects: They overemphasize the passive, submissive elements of problematic dependency, and they ignore the fact that certain dependent people may behave assertively—sometimes downright aggressively—when important relationships are threatened. The implicit equating of dependency with passivity stems primarily from the initial DSM-I (APA, 1952) conceptualization of DPD as a form of "passive dependency," a subtext that has carried through successive revisions of the DSM. The more active manifestations of dependency have been documented in both laboratory (Bornstein, Masling, & Poynton, 1987; Bornstein, Riggs, Hill, & Calabrese, 1996) and field studies (Mongrain et al., 1998), as discussed in more detail below. Moreover, research confirms that dependent men are at increased risk for perpetrating domestic violence (Bornstein, 2006) and dependent women are at increased risk for perpetrating child abuse (Bornstein, 2002).

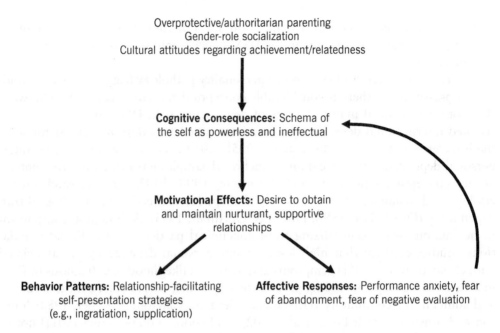

FIGURE 16.1. An interactionist model of interpersonal dependency and DPD. As this figure shows, dependent personality traits reflect the interplay of cognitive, motivational, emotional, and behavioral features, which stem in part from early learning and socialization experiences within and outside the family. Overprotective and authoritarian parenting, alone or in combination, play a key role in the development of a dependent personality because both lead to the construction of a "helpless self-concept," which is the core element of a dependent personality style. As the feedback loop in the right portion of the figure shows, dependency-related affective responses reinforce the dependent person's perception of the self as powerless and ineffectual: When a dependency-related affective response (e.g., fear of abandonment by a valued other) occurs, the helpless self-concept is primed (i.e., brought into working memory), and dependency-related responding increases.

In addition, the DSM DPD criteria ignore the cognitive elements of DPD: There is no allusion to the dependent patient's helpless self-concept anywhere in the essential feature or diagnostic criteria, or any mention of dependency-related beliefs or thought patterns. This omission not only ignores a central dynamic element of dysfunctional dependency (see Figure 16.1), but prevents clinicians and clinical researchers from making accurate predictions regarding situational variations in dependent responding, because these variations are rooted in the dependent patient's beliefs regarding interpersonal risks and opportunities in various contexts and settings.

A Psychodynamic Shift: DPD in the PDM

In most respects the PDM DPD criteria (APO, 2006) are stronger than those in DSM-IV (APA, 1994) and DSM 5 (APA, 2013). The PDM conceptualizes DPD on a continuum; makes explicit the fact that pathological dependency varies in severity from neurotic to borderline level; describes key intra- and interpersonal dynamics of dependency; specifies the early developmental antecedents of dependent personality traits; discusses the impact of culture on the experience and expression of dependent attitudes and urges; and notes that high levels of dependency may include adaptive as well as maladaptive features. It is ironic (to say the least) that the PDM diagnostic criteria for DPD are far more closely linked to empirical research on dependency and DPD than are the DSM-5 DPD criteria, despite the fact that DSM-5 is ostensibly an empirically based system, and psychodynamic models of personality and psychopathology have been criticized vociferously for being inattentive to empirical research.

In addition to describing the ways in which dependency impacts the patient's self-concept and interpersonal relationships, the PDM (APO, 2006, pp. 51–52) lists six specific correlates of DPD, as it does for each syndrome on the Personality Patterns and Disorders (P) Axis. These six correlates are:

1. Contributing constitutional-maturational patterns (placidity and sociophilia).
2. Central tension/preoccupation (keeping/losing relationships).
3. Central affects (pleasure when securely attached; sadness and fear when alone).
4. Characteristic pathogenic belief about the self (I am inadequate, needy, and impotent).
5. Characteristic pathogenic belief about others (Others are powerful and I need their care).
6. Central ways of defending (regression, reversal, and avoidance).

These putative correlates require additional investigation and empirical validation, but they represent a fruitful avenue for refining the psychodynamic perspective on dependency and DPD.

Looking Ahead: DPD in DSM-5 and Beyond

Without question, the delineation of heuristic, clinically useful criteria for DPD in future versions of the DSM requires that these criteria include a developmental perspective and make explicit the impact of parenting, culture, and gender role in the etiology and dynamics of DPD. These criteria must also be dimensional rather than categorical, recognizing that problematic dependency is best conceptualized as existing on a continuum of severity ranging from mild through moderate to severe, with no fixed threshold distinguishing normal from pathological dependency.

The DSM-5 Personality and Personality Disorders workgroup proposed that DPD be eliminated as a formal diagnostic category in future versions of the manual and described in terms of three trait domains: submissiveness, anxiousness, and separation insecurity (Skodol et al., 2011). As Bornstein (2011, 2012) noted, this decision is inconsistent with a plethora of empirical studies that have demonstrated that DPD fulfills all the criteria outlined by Kendler, Kupfer, Narrow, Phillips, and Fawcett (2009) for the inclusion of extant syndromes in future versions of the DSM. A thorough discussion of the evidence bearing on this issue is beyond the scope of this chapter (however, see Bornstein, 2011, for an extensive review). Scrutiny of the available evidence confirms that DPD meets the criteria of Kendler and colleagues for distinctiveness and diagnostic stability, as well as antecedent, concurrent, and predictive validity. In addition, studies have demonstrated the clinical utility of DPD in predicting risk for psychological and physical illness, health care utilization, functional impairment, perpetration of domestic violence and child abuse, and risk for parasuicidal and suicidal behavior (Bornstein, 2011, 2012).

Questions regarding the inclusion of DPD as a distinct category aside, the DSM-5 description of DPD as reflecting underlying submissiveness is problematic in and of itself. Converging evidence from studies of interpersonal dependency and DPD confirms that dependency is indeed associated with anxiousness and separation insecurity (Livesley, Schroeder, & Jackson, 1990; Pincus, 2005). However, evidence indicates that dependent people may be submissive in certain contexts (e.g., when they believe that passivity and compliance will strengthen ties to potential caregivers), but they are quite assertive in others (e.g., when important relationships are threatened). If DPD is described in trait terms in future editions of DSM, a different set of traits will be needed.

PSYCHODYNAMIC APPROACHES TO DPD

Contemporary psychodynamic conceptualizations of interpersonal dependency and DPD reflect the influence of four theoretical perspectives that unfolded over time, some originating within the psychoanalytic canon and others outside it, each model building upon one or more earlier frameworks.

Classical Psychoanalysis

In classical psychoanalytic theory, dependency is inextricably linked to events of the infantile, oral stage—the first few months of life. In Freud's (1905/1953) drive model, frustration or overgratification during the oral stage was presumed to result in oral fixation and in the development of an oral dependent personality type characterized by continued preoccupation during adulthood with the events and developmental challenges of the oral phase (i.e., preoccupation with food and oral activities, feelings of helplessness and vulnerability, and a passive, dependent stance in interpersonal relations). As Freud (1908/1959, p. 167) noted in describing the dual nature of oral fixation, "one very often meets with a type of character in which certain traits are very strongly marked while at the same time one's attention is arrested by the behavior of these persons in regard to certain bodily functions."

At least three noteworthy hypotheses emerge from the classical psychoanalytic conceptualization of dependency. First, this model contends that dependent personality traits in adulthood may be traced to frustration or overgratification during breastfeeding and weaning. However, this hypothesis has been repeatedly disconfirmed in observational studies of infant–mother dyads and in retrospective interview-based studies (e.g., Heinstein, 1963). Second, the classical psychoanalytic model predicts that individuals who show high levels of interpersonal dependency in adulthood will also show a preoccupation with oral activities (e.g., overeating, alcohol use, tobacco use). Although results in this domain have been mixed, in general research does not support the existence of a robust dependency–orality link (see Black, Goldstein, & Mason, 1992).

Third—and perhaps most important with respect to contemporary conceptual-izations of interpersonal dependency and DPD—the classical psychoanalytic model predicts that dependent persons will show varying degrees of insight regarding their underlying dependent strivings and the impact of these strivings on their behavior. Research has consistently confirmed this hypothesis: Some dependent people are clearly cognizant of their dependent thoughts and feelings, scoring high on question-naire and interview measures of interpersonal dependency and DPD, including those measures with high face validity (e.g., Hirschfeld et al.'s [1977] Interpersonal Depen-dency Inventory [IDI]). Other people score high on measures of implicit dependency (e.g., Masling, Rabie, & Blondheim's [1967] Rorschach Oral Dependency [ROD] scale), but low on various self-report dependency scales (see Bornstein, 2002, for an overview of studies in this area).

Object Relations Theory

Beginning in the 1920s, the focus of psychodynamic metapsychology shifted from Freud's (1905/1953) drive-based framework to a more person-centered approach that came to be known as object relations theory (see Greenberg & Mitchell, 1983). Within this framework—and associated interpersonal perspectives—personality dynamics are conceptualized in terms of (1) internalized mental representations of self and significant figures (identified as *introjects* by psychoanalytic theorists, and as *person schemas* by cognitive theorists), and (2) self–other interactions, both real and imag-ined, which represent templates, or "blueprints," that shape subsequent interpersonal relationships. These internalized templates are sometimes conceptualized as *internal working models* or *scripts*. As Galatzer-Levy and Cohler (1993) noted, the reconcep-tualization of psychoanalytic concepts in relational terms introduced a fundamentally new paradigm for conceptualizing continuity and change in personality development and dynamics, with personality stability now seen as stemming from stability in the core features of key object representations, including self-representation. Conversely, personality change is presumed to occur in part because internalized representations of self and other people evolve in response to changing life circumstances.

As object relations models of dependency gained influence, psychodynamic researchers began to investigate links between dependency and insecure attachment (e.g., Collins & Read, 1990). Although there are some noteworthy convergences between dependency-related behaviors and those associated with insecure attach-ment, there are some noteworthy differences as well (Bornstein, 2005b; Heiss, Ber-man, & Sperling, 1996). Most important, scores on measures of trait dependency and DPD tend to be modestly related to scores on indices of insecure attachment in adults, with correlations typically in the $r = .30–.40$ range (Bornstein, Ng, Gallagher, Kloss, & Regier, 2005; Pincus & Wilson, 2001).

As a result, researchers have devoted greater attention to delineating object relations models than attachment-focused models of dependency (cf., Heiss et al., 1996). In recent years, Blatt's (1974, 1991) theoretical framework has been the most influential perspective in this area. Integrating psychodynamic principles with research on social and cognitive development, Blatt and colleagues (e.g., Blatt & Homann, 1992) argued that dependent personality traits stem in part from a mental representation of the self as weak and ineffectual, along with parental introjects that are both conceptually immature and poorly internalized. Consequently, these introjects are experienced as unavailable or even absent, leading to failures in evocative constancy that leave the dependent person feeling depleted, isolated, and helpless, and at increased risk for anaclitic depression, especially following interpersonal conflict or loss.

Social Learning and Culture

The object relations perspective helped psychodynamic theorists recognize the ways in which early interpersonal relationships shape dependent attitudes and behaviors that were exhibited years—even decades—later. A natural outgrowth of this view was the recognition that key social influences on the development of dependent personality traits transcend the child–parent relationship and include other relationships as well. Beginning in the 1960s, social learning theorists delineated the ways that the child's interactions with siblings, peers, and adults (e.g., teachers) help shape the child's attitudes regarding dependent urges and feelings (e.g., Bandura & Walters, 1963).

Social learning theory provides a useful framework for conceptualizing how social reinforcement and observational learning contribute to the development of dependent personality traits. It also provides a ready explanation for the well-established finding that—at least in Western societies—women typically report higher levels of interpersonal dependency and DPD symptoms than men do when questionnaire or interview measures are used. In most Western cultures, boys are discouraged more strongly than girls from expressing (or even acknowledging privately) dependent thoughts and feelings, and studies confirm that in clinical settings women are about 40% more likely than men to receive a diagnosis of DPD (Bornstein, 2005a). Meta-analytic findings indicate that on questionnaire measures of trait dependency women obtain scores that are approximately 0.2 standard deviations higher than those of men (Bornstein, 1995).

Individualistic societies (e.g., the United States, Great Britain) tend to value autonomy and independence more strongly than more sociocentric cultures (e.g., Japan, India) do, although some studies suggest that traditional sociocentric socialization patterns are becoming more individualistic as sociocentric cultures assimilate Western norms and values (Yamaguchi, 2004). As a result of these contrasting cultural norms and expectations, gender differences in dependency and DPD are generally smaller in sociocentric cultures than in more individualistic cultures (Bhogle, 1978; Gupta & Mattoo, 2012), and adults in sociocentric cultures—women and men alike—report higher levels of interpersonal dependency on questionnaires and in interviews than adults raised in more individualistic cultures (Chen, Nettles, & Chen, 2009; Yasunaga, 1985).

An Interactionist Perspective

Combining key elements of the object relations perspective with concepts and findings from the social learning and cultural frameworks, Bornstein (1993, 1996, 2005a) delineated an interactionist model of interpersonal dependency and DPD. The interactionist model conceptualizes dependency in terms of four primary components: (1) *cognitive* (a perception of oneself as vulnerable and weak); (2) *motivational* (a desire to strengthen ties to potential protectors and caregivers); (3) *affective* (fear of abandonment, fear of negative evaluation by figures of authority); and (4) *behavioral* (relationship-facilitating self-presentation strategies aimed at precluding rejection and abandonment).

Key elements of the interactionist model are summarized in Figure 16.1, which illustrates how the dependent person's "helpless self-schema" results from overprotective or authoritarian parenting (both of which teach children that they are fragile and weak, and must look to others for protection and support), along with the effects of gender-role socialization and cultural attitudes regarding achievement and relatedness. More than two dozen empirical studies have documented the links between overprotective or authoritarian parenting and the subsequent development of dependency in offspring; these include both retrospective interview- and questionnaire-based studies and prospective observational studies, and involve participants from an array of backgrounds, including participants raised in the United States, Great Britain, India, Germany, Italy, Japan, and the Netherlands (see Bornstein, 1992, 1993, 2005a, for reviews).

As Figure 16.1 shows, the presence of a helpless self-schema in and of itself helps create dependency-related motivations: Individuals who perceive themselves as helpless, vulnerable, and weak are inclined to look to others for nurturance, guidance, and support. These motives in turn lead to dependency-related behaviors and affective responses. As the feedback loop in Figure 16.1 shows, when a dependency-related affective response (e.g., fear of abandonment) occurs, the helpless self-concept is primed—brought into working memory—resulting in an increase in the dependent person's perception of himself or herself as powerless and ineffectual.

Implicit in the interactionist model is recognition that dependency-related passivity is not invariably a reflexive, automatic, "mindless" response, but can also be a deliberate, goal-directed self-presentation strategy used by the dependent person to strengthen ties to others and meet various intra- and interpersonal needs. Moreover, the interactionist model argues that dependent individuals are not limited to passivity and compliance in interpersonal relations, but can—and do—use more active social influence strategies as well. Some of these strategies are maladaptive and self-destructive (e.g., when a borderline patient with strong underlying dependency needs engages in parasuicide to preclude abandonment by a valued other; Bornstein et al., 2010), but others are potentially adaptive and foster healthy functioning (e.g., when a dependent medical patient adheres conscientiously to a treatment regimen to please the physician; Greenberg & Fisher, 1977). Thus, in addition to elucidating situational variations in dependency-related responding, the interactionist model distinguishes unhealthy (maladaptive) expressions of dependency from healthy (adaptive) dependency (see Bornstein & Languirand, 2003, for a detailed discussion of this issue).

EMPIRICAL FINDINGS

Research on dependency and DPD has addressed a broad spectrum of issues (e.g., social support, sensitivity to interpersonal conflict, risk for illness; see Bornstein, 2012, for a review). Four issues central to a psychodynamic conceptualization of interpersonal dependency and DPD have been examined in particular detail: (1) the role of the dependent person's self-representation in the intra- and interpersonal dynamics of dependency; (2) situational variations in dependency-related responding; (3) the varying maladaptive and adaptive expressions of underlying dependency needs; and (4) the contrasting dynamics of unconscious (or implicit) and conscious dependency strivings.

The Helpless Self-Concept and Interpersonal Dependency

In one of the first studies to examine this issue directly, Bornstein, Leone, and Galley (1988) obtained open-ended descriptions of the self from college students who had been divided into dependent and nondependent groups using the ROD scale of Masling and colleagues (1967). When these open-ended responses were scored using Blatt, Chevron, Quinlan, and Wein's (1981) method for rating structural and qualitative aspects of descriptions of significant figures, patterns emerged that were consistent with object relations models of interpersonal dependency: Relative to dependent participants, nondependent participants in the sample of Bornstein and colleagues (1988) described themselves as ineffectual, insecure, anxious, and weak. In addition, the self-descriptions of dependent participants were at a more primitive conceptual level (i.e., less developmentally mature) than those of nondependent participants.

Researchers have assessed the impact of subliminally priming the dependent person's helpless self-concept on dependency-related responding and found that priming the helpless self-concept decreases lexical decision latency—the amount of time it takes to judge whether a series of letters is actually a word—for dependency-related words such as *timid, helpless, vulnerable,* and *weak* (but not for control words such as *table, book, lamp,* and *chair*). These patterns confirm that dependency-related concepts are chronically activated and easily accessible in dependent people's associative networks (Bornstein et al., 2005). Moreover, because these priming effects were obtained in dependent—but not nondependent—participants, it appears that chronic activation of dependency-related concepts is specific to individuals with high levels of dependency. Studies have shown that the presence of a dependent self-schema shapes social perceptions and behaviors as well (Mongrain, Vettese, Shuster, & Kendal, 1998).

Situational Variations in Dependency-Related Responding

A central tenet of the interactionist model is that intraindividual variability in dependency-related responding is largely a function of the dependent person's perceptions of interpersonal risks and opportunities. Initial support for this view was obtained by Bornstein, Masling, and Poynton (1987). In this study, same-sex pairs of college students, each consisting of one dependent and one nondependent person, were asked to debate an issue on which they had previously disagreed. In line with previous findings regarding dependency and yielding, it was expected that dependent participants would change their initial opinion, but the opposite occurred: In 70% of dyads the nondependent participant yielded to the opinion of the dependent participant. Postexperiment interviews revealed that a majority of dependent participants chose not to yield because they hoped to impress the experimenter. In other words, when forced to choose between impressing a figure of authority by holding their ground or accommodating a peer by yielding, the dependent participants opted to impress the authority figure.

These findings provided strong evidence that in certain situations dependency-related passivity represents a self-presentation strategy aimed at strengthening ties with those most able to provide help and support. In a follow-up experiment in which the presence (versus absence) of an authority figure was varied systematically across dyads (Bornstein, Riggs, Hill, & Calabrese, 1996), these initial results were confirmed: Dependent students competed aggressively with another student on a mock creativity task when told that a professor would be evaluating their performance at the end of the experiment, but acquiesced passively (and performed relatively poorly) when told that only the undergraduate experimenter would have access to their data.

More recently, Bornstein (2007b) found that dependent college students are more motivated than nondependent students to meet with a professor whom they believe can offer future help and support—but only if the professor represents a potential protector and caregiver. In an initial experiment, Bornstein (2007b) found that dependent students were willing to wait an average of 12 minutes to receive positive test feedback from the professor (versus approximately 6 minutes for nondependent students). A follow-up experiment showed that the professor's potential to offer future help was key in motivating dependent students' willingness to wait: When told that the professor providing test feedback would soon be leaving the university (and therefore would be unavailable in the future), dependent–nondependent differences disappeared completely. In this condition, dependent and nondependent students both averaged 6 minutes of waiting time (Bornstein, 2007b, Experiment 2).

Unhealthy and Healthy Dependency

Two issues are germane in this context. First, consistent with Bornstein's (1996, 2005) interactionist perspective, certain dependency-related behaviors (e.g., help-seeking) may be maladaptive in certain situations but adaptive in others. Thus, studies have shown that the dependent person's tendency to look to other people for help and support leads to conflicts with friends, romantic partners, and coworkers (Overholser,

1996) and may lead dependent patients to overuse health and mental health services (O'Neill & Bornstein, 2001). On the other hand, this same dependency-related help-seeking causes dependent women to delay less long than nondependent women in seeking medical help following the onset of a serious medical symptom (e.g., a possible lump in the breast; see Greenberg & Fisher, 1977), and leads dependent college students to seek advice from professors and academic advisors more readily than non-dependent college students, ultimately resulting in higher grade point averages even when scholastic aptitude is controlled for statistically (Bornstein & Kennedy, 1994).

Beyond these situational variations in the expression of dependent strivings, there are individual differences in the degree to which people express dependency needs in adaptive versus maladaptive ways. Using Bornstein and Languirand's (2003) Relationship Profile Test (RPT), a 30-item self-report scale that yields separate scores for Destructive Overdependence (DO) and Healthy Dependency (HD), researchers have found that healthy dependent individuals show better adjustment than dysfunctionally overdependent individuals in a wide variety of areas (e.g., with respect to defense style, affect regulation, self-concept, physical health, risk for depression and anxiety disorders, and overall life satisfaction; see Porcerelli, Bornstein, Markova, & Huprich, 2009). RPT, DO, and HD scores are stable for periods of at least 3 years in young adults (Bornstein & Huprich, 2006), attesting to their trait-like qualities. These findings not only confirm that there are distinct maladaptive and adaptive expressions of dependency, but also suggest that clinical work with dependent patients need not focus exclusively on reducing underlying and expressed dependency, but might instead aim toward replacing maladaptive expressions of dependency with more adaptive expressions of dependency (Bornstein, 2005a, 2007a).

Contrasting Dynamics of Unconscious and Conscious Dependency Strivings

Examining links between various indices of dependency and different categories of personality pathology, Bornstein (1998) demonstrated that individuals with DPD traits and symptoms scored high on both self-report and implicit measures of interpersonal dependency, whereas individuals with histrionic personality disorder traits and symptoms obtained high implicit—but low self-report—dependency scores (see Bornstein, 1998, for a discussion of the implications of these findings for the dynamics of dependent and histrionic personality disorders). Subsequent studies have also found that contrasting patterns of implicit and self-report dependency scores are associated with differential patterns of personality and personality pathology (Cogswell, 2008).

Approaching this issue from a slightly different perspective, Bornstein (2002) utilized findings from research on the cognitive and neurological underpinnings of implicit and explicit memory, combining these findings with psychoanalytic principles to develop the *process dissociation approach* to personality and personality disorder assessment. The process dissociation strategy involves identifying naturally occurring influences on test scores, then deliberately manipulating these influences to illuminate underlying response processes. Thus, Bornstein, Rossner, Hill, and Stepanian (1994) administered the IDI (Hirschfeld et al., 1977) and ROD scale (Masling et al., 1967) to a mixed-sex sample of adults under three conditions. One-third of participants completed the two measures under a *negative set* condition and were told that the study was part of a research program examining the negative aspects of dependent personality traits. One-third of participants completed the measures under a *positive set* condition and were told that the study was part of a research program examining the positive, adaptive aspects of dependency. The remaining participants completed the two measures under standard conditions, wherein no mention was made of the purpose of either scale or the fact that they assess dependency.

Bornstein and colleagues (1994) found that, relative to the baseline (control) condition, participants' IDI scores increased significantly in the positive set condition and decreased significantly in the negative set condition; ROD scores were unaffected by the instructional set. These patterns reflect the contrasting processes that occur as participants complete the IDI (introspection, retrospection, and deliberate self-presentation) and the ROD scale (focus on stimulus rather than self followed by attribution of meaning to ambiguous inkblots). In a follow-up investigation, Bornstein, Bowers, and Bonner (1996) examined the impact of induced mood state on IDI and ROD scores, asking participants to write essays regarding traumatic events, joyful events, or neutral events to induce a corresponding mood immediately prior to testing. As expected, induction of a negative mood prior to testing led to a significant increase in ROD—but not IDI—scores (see Bornstein, 2002, and Cogswell, 2008, for descriptions of these and other process dissociation studies involving self-report and implicit dependency scales).

PSYCHODYNAMIC TREATMENT OF DPD

A fair amount of writing has been done on psychodynamic treatment of dependent patients (e.g., Abramson, Cloud, Keese, & Keese, 1994; Coen, 1992; Colgan, 1987; Kantor, 1992; van Sweden, 1995), but there is a paucity of research testing these concepts empirically. Among the few noteworthy empirical contributions in this area are those of Blatt (1992) and Blatt and Ford (1994), who found that dependent psychotherapy patients tend to show more positive results in psychoanalytic therapy than classical psychoanalysis, presumably because pychoanalytic therapy affords more interaction and interpersonal contact between patient and therapist (Blatt, 1992). They also found that positive therapeutic effects in dependent patients are manifested most strongly in improvements in object relations and interpersonal functioning (Blatt & Ford, 1994).

The interactionist model suggests that effective clinical work with dependent patients should emphasize three goals: (1) helping patients gain insight into their underlying dependency needs and the way these needs are manifest in various contexts and settings; (2) altering the dependent patient's helpless self-concept to increase self-efficacy and diminish dependency-related urges and affective responses; and (3) helping the patient find ways to express dependency needs that foster adaptation rather than impairing intra- and interpersonal functioning. For most patients, this means moving beyond superficial awareness of how their dependency needs have affected past and present relationships to a more nuanced understanding of how these relationships have influenced (and, in some instances, helped propagate) their dependency-related feelings, motives, and fears (see Bruch, Rivet, Heimberg, Hunt, & McIntosh, 1999).

Bornstein (2005a, 2007a) outlined therapeutic strategies aimed at meeting these goals. Central to this approach is examination of core conflictual relationship themes (CCRTs; Luborsky & Crits-Christoph, 1990) to elucidate the impact of the patient's dependency on others, and using transference interpretation to illuminate distorted perceptions of authority figures and the self-defeating emotional patterns that ensue. The basic elements of CCRT in therapeutic work with dependent patients can be divided into four domains, described in the following sections.

The Underlying Context: A Supportive–Expressive Frame

Luborsky and Crits-Christoph (1990) combine psychoanalytic interpretation with a milieu specifically designed to enhance the therapeutic alliance. The first task is to build a collaborative working relationship through empathic communication on the part of the therapist. This supportive "holding environment" may have curative value in and of itself, especially for dependent patients (see Blatt, 1992; Bornstein, 2007a), but it also helps minimize anxiety and defensiveness, especially in patients with limited insight into their underlying dependency needs (Crits-Christoph & Barber, 1991).

Insight through Analysis of CCRTs

CCRTs are derived from patient narratives that center on relationship episodes— memorable, meaningful interactions with other people. As patterns emerge in a patient's relationship episodes, these are analyzed in three areas: (1) the patient's wishes, intentions, and fears, (2) the response of the other person, and (3) the patient's reaction to the other person's response. By exploring consistencies in CCRTs across different relationships, the patient's dominant needs and defenses are made explicit, and the trait-like aspects of dependency become clear. By examining inconsistencies in CCRTs between different relationships, the contextual specificity of a patient's behavior can be understood.

Obstacles to Progress: Ambivalence in the Therapeutic Alliance

As the dependent patient becomes increasingly attached to the therapist, anxiety regarding abandonment increases and behaviors designed to minimize the possibility of relationship disruption begin to dominate (Kantor, 1992). Dependency-related resistance is not limited to the patient, however; it can also originate in the therapist (see Ryder & Parry-Jones, 1982). The therapist may fear that the patient's dependency will become increasingly intense over time (the "fantasy of insatiability") and that the patient's dependency will make termination impossible, so treatment can never end (the "fantasy of permanence"). If not managed properly, the patient's and therapist's fears may feed on each other: The patient becomes increasingly anxious about the risks of autonomy, and the therapist becomes increasingly anxious about the negative impact of the patient's dependency.

The Emotional Undercurrent: Transference and Countertransference

One way to prevent dependency-related fears from undermining treatment is to explore the patient's transference reaction and the therapist's countertransference response. As noted, common transference patterns in dependent patients include idealization, possessiveness, and projective identification. Common therapist responses to these transference reactions include frustration at the patient's insatiable neediness; hidden hostility (often accompanied by passive–aggressive acting out); overindulgence (ostensibly to protect the "fragile" patient); and pleasurable feelings of power and omnipotence (which can, on occasion, lead to exploitation or abuse).

CLINICAL ILLUSTRATION

Melissa was a 25-year-old outpatient who sought treatment for bulimia and the debilitating depression that often accompanied her binge–purge episodes. She received diagnoses of bulimia nervosa and major depressive disorder on DSM-IV-TR Axis I; on DSM-IV-TR Axis II she was diagnosed with DPD and borderline personality disorder. Although she did not meet formal DSM criteria, Melissa habitually used alcohol and sedatives to modulate her negative affect.

Melissa lived at home and had highly conflicted relationships with her parents and older sister. She functioned quite well at work, however, where she was an office manager in a small company, and she consistently received positive evaluations from her supervisor. Exploration of Melissa's presenting complaint and background during initial treatment sessions revealed a surprising duality: Although her relationships with family members were characterized by extreme dependency interspersed with emotional outbursts and regression, her relationships with coworkers were far healthier and more stable. It soon became clear that although Melissa was highly dependent and labile at home, at work she was confident, competent, and controlled. Although her lability and self-destructive behavior were such that she formally met DSM-5 criteria for a diagnosis of BPD, Melissa's ability to modulate affect effectively in certain contexts suggested that underlying dependency—not borderline pathology—played a more central role in her difficulties (see Bornstein et al., 2010, for a detailed discussion of the links between dependency and BPD symptomatology).

Because Melissa was aware of her dysfunctionally dependent family relationships, therapy initially focused on exploration of Melissa's work relationships, deconstructing her work-related CCRTs to better understand her healthy interaction patterns and the responses evoked by these patterns in colleagues and coworkers. As Melissa gained an understanding of the social influence strategies she used most effectively at work, we were able to contrast these patterns with those that occurred within the family, and understand the wishes and fears that impelled Melissa's volatile relationships with family members. Therapy moved to examining the responses—both gratifying and frustrating—elicited by Melissa's adaptive and dysfunctional behaviors, and her characteristic ways of responding when her dependency needs were unmet.

As therapy progressed, the focus shifted to exploration of the therapeutic relationship, including transference patterns and associated emotional responses. Melissa exhibited a positively toned idealizing transference throughout treatment, perceiving the therapist as "the only person who really gets me." As she became increasingly comfortable exploring her transference, we were able to connect her idealized view of the therapist with her idealized view of her supervisor at work, and the way in which her overvaluation of figures of authority (especially male figures of authority) provided an avenue through which she was able to get her dependency needs met in a reasonably healthy way.

Treatment ended after approximately 6 months, with mutually agreed-upon termination. At this time, Melissa had made some progress in moderating her bulimic episodes and substance use. Her family relationships remained conflicted, and when therapy ended she was in the process of obtaining her own apartment and making plans to live on her own for the first time.

CONCLUSIONS AND FUTURE DIRECTIONS

Although initially conceptualized in terms of problematic early parent–child relationships and "oral fixation," pathological dependency is increasingly viewed as stemming from a perception of the self as weak, coupled with a belief that others are comparatively competent and confident. As a result, the dependent person becomes preoccupied with obtaining and maintaining relationships with potential caregivers. Studies support the notion that a "helpless self-concept" plays a key role in the intra- and interpersonal dynamics of dependency, and that dependent individuals exhibit an array of relationship-facilitating self-presentation strategies—some passive, some active—designed to preclude rejection and abandonment by valued others. Certain dependency-related behaviors (e.g., frequent help-seeking) lead to difficulties in social, sexual, and professional relationships, but others (e.g., sensitivity to subtle interpersonal cues) may actually foster adaptation and functioning.

Because dependency is associated with adaptive as well as maladaptive consequences, psychotherapy with dependent patients may include interventions that enable patients to express underlying dependency needs in more adaptive ways. Such interventions are particularly important when the manifestations of dependency are associated with increased risk for self-harm or harm to others. As noted, research confirms that highly dependent men are at increased risk for perpetrating domestic violence when they believe that a close relationship is in jeopardy; that dependent women are at increased risk for perpetrating child abuse when affectively overwhelmed; and that dependent psychiatric patients—women and men alike—are at increased risk for suicide. Thus, continued research on the psychodynamics of DPD is important, not only because dependency has implications for a broad array of issues in clinical psychology, but also because increased understanding of interpersonal dependency can enhance therapeutic efficacy and improve patient functioning.

REFERENCES

Abraham, K. (1927). The influence of oral erotism on character formation. In C. A. D. Bryan & A. Strachey (Eds.), *Selected papers on psycho-analysis* (pp. 393–406). London: Hogarth Press.

Abramson, P. R., Cloud, M. Y., Keese, N., & Keese, R. (1994). How much is too much? Dependency in a psychotherapeutic relationship. *American Journal of Psychotherapy, 48,* 294–301.

Alliance of Psychoanalytic Organizations. (2006). *Psychodynamic diagnostic manual.* Silver Spring, MD: Author.

American Psychiatric Association. (1952). *Diagnostic and statistical manual of mental disorders.* Washington, DC: Author.

American Psychiatric Association. (1980). *Diagnostic and statistical manual of mental disorders* (3rd ed.). Washington, DC: Author.

American Psychiatric Association. (1994). *Diagnostic and statistical manual of mental disorders* (4th ed.). Washington, DC: Author.

American Psychiatric Association. (2013). *Diagnostic and Statistical Manual of Mental Disorders* (5th ed.). Arlington, VA: Author.

Bandura, A., & Walters, R. H. (1963). *Social learning and personality development.* New York: Holt, Rinehart, & Winston.

Bhogle, S. (1978). Child rearing practices among three cultures. *Psychological Studies, 28,* 92–95.

Black, D. W., Goldstein, R. B., & Mason, E. E. (1992). Prevalence of mental disorder in 88 morbidly obese bariatric clinic patients. *American Journal of Psychiatry, 149,* 227–234.

Blatt, S. J. (1974). Levels of object representation in anaclitic and introjective depression. *Psychoanalytic Study of the Child, 29,* 107–157.

Blatt, S. J. (1991). A cognitive morphology of psychopathology. *Journal of Nervous and Mental Disease, 179,* 449–458.

Blatt, S. J. (1992). The differential effect of psychotherapy and psychoanalysis with anaclitic and introjective patients. *Journal of the American Psychoanalytic Association, 40,* 691–724.

Blatt, S. J., Chevron, E. S., Quinlan, D. M., & Wein, S. J. (1981). *The assessment of qualitative and structural dimensions of object representations.* Unpublished manual, Yale University School of Medicine.

Blatt, S. J., & Ford, R. Q. (1994). *Therapeutic change: An object relations perspective.* New York: Plenum Press.

Blatt, S. J., & Homann, E. (1992). Parent–child interaction in the etiology of dependent and self-critical depression. *Clinical Psychology Review, 12,* 47–91.

Bornstein, R. F. (1992). The dependent personality: Developmental, social, and clinical perspectives. *Psychological Bulletin, 112,* 3–23.

Bornstein, R. F. (1993). *The dependent personality.* New York: Guilford Press.

Bornstein, R. F. (1995). Sex differences in objective and projective dependency tests: A meta-analytic review. *Assessment, 2,* 319–331.

Bornstein, R. F. (1996). Beyond orality: Toward an object relations/interactionist receonceptualization of the etiology and dynamics of dependency. *Psychoanalytic Psychology, 13,* 177–203.

Bornstein, R. F. (1997). Dependent personality disorder in the DSM-IV and beyond. *Clinical Psychology: Science and Practice, 4,* 175–187.

Bornstein, R. F. (1998). Implicit and self-attributed dependency needs in dependent and histrionic personality disorders. *Journal of Personality Assessment, 71,* 1–14.

Bornstein, R. F. (2002). A process dissociation approach to objective-projective test score interrelationships. *Journal of Personality Assessment, 78,* 47–68.

Bornstein, R. F. (2005a). *The dependent patient: A practitioner's guide.* Washington, DC: APA Books.

Bornstein, R. F. (2005b). Interpersonal dependency in child abuse perpetrators and victims: A meta-analytic review. *Journal of Psychopathology and Behavioral Assessment, 27,* 67–76.

Bornstein, R. F. (2006). The complex relationship between dependency and abuse: Converging psychological factors and social forces. *American Psychologist, 61,* 595–606.

Bornstein, R. F. (2007a). Dependent personality disorder: Effective time-limited therapy. *Current Psychiatry, 6,* 37–45.

Bornstein, R. F. (2007b). Self-schema priming and desire for test performance feedback: Further evaluation of a cognitive/interactionist model of interpersonal dependency. *Self and Identity, 5,* 110–126.

Bornstein, R. F. (2009). Heisenberg, Kandinsky, and the heteromethod convergence problem: Lessons from within and beyond psychology. *Journal of Personality Assessment, 91,* 1–8.

Bornstein, R. F. (2011). Reconceptualizing personality pathology in DSM-5: Limitations in evidence for eliminating dependent personality disorder and other DSM-IV syndromes. *Journal of Personality Disorders, 25,* 237–250.

Bornstein, R. F. (2012). From dysfunction to adaptation: An interactionist model of dependency. *Annual Review of Clinical Psychology, 8,* 291–316.

Bornstein, R. F., Becker-Matero, N., Winarick, D. J., & Reichman, A. E. (2010). Interpersonal dependency in borderline personality disorder: Clinical context and empirical evidence. *Journal of Personality Disorders, 24,* 109–127.

Bornstein, R. F., Bowers, K. S., & Bonner, S. (1996). Effects of induced mood states on objective and projective dependency scores. *Journal of Personality Assessment, 67,* 324–340.

Bornstein, R. F., & Huprich, S. K. (2006). Construct validity of the Relationship Profile Test: Three-year retest reliability and links with core personality traits, object relations, and interpersonal problems. *Journal of Personality Assessment, 86,* 162–171.

Bornstein, R. F., & Kennedy, T. D. (1994). Interpersonal dependency and academic performance. *Journal of Personality Disorders, 8,* 240–248.

Bornstein, R. F., & Languirand, M. A. (2003). *Healthy dependency.* New York: Newmarket Press.

Bornstein, R. F., Leone, D. R., & Galley, D. J. (1988). Rorschach measures of oral dependence and the internalized self-representation in normal college students. *Journal of Personality Assessment, 52,* 648–657.

Bornstein, R. F., Masling, J. M., & Poynton, F. G. (1987). Orality as a factor in interpersonal yielding. *Psychoanalytic Psychology, 4,* 161–170.

Bornstein, R. F., Ng, H. M., Gallagher, H. A., Kloss, D. M., & Regier, N. G. (2005). Contrasting effects of self-schema priming on lexical decisions and Interpersonal Stroop Task performance: Evidence for a cognitive/interactionist model of interpersonal dependency. *Journal of Personality, 73,* 731–761.

Bornstein, R. F., Riggs, J. M., Hill, E. L., & Calabrese, C. (1996). Activity, passivity, self-denigration, and self-promotion: Toward an interactionist model of interpersonal dependency. *Journal of Personality, 64,* 637–673.

Bornstein, R. F., Rossner, S. C., Hill, E. L., & Stepanian, M. L. (1994). Face validity and fakability of objective and projective measures of dependency. *Journal of Personality Assessment, 63,* 363–386.

Bruch, M. A., Rivet, K. M., Heimberg, R. G., Hunt, A., & McIntosh, B. (1999). Shyness and sociotropy: Additive and interactive relations in predicting interpersonal concerns. *Journal of Personality, 67,* 373–406.

Chen, Y., Nettles, M. E., & Chen, S. W. (2009). Rethinking dependent personality disorder: Comparing different human relatedness in cultural contexts. *Journal of Nervous and Mental Disease, 193,* 793–800.

Coen, S. J. (1992). *The misuse of persons: Analyzing pathological dependency.* Hillsdale, NJ: Analytic Press.

Cogswell, A. (2008). Explicitly rejecting an implicit dichotomy: Integrating two approaches to assessing dependency. *Journal of Personality Assessment, 90,* 26–35.

Colgan, P. (1987). Treatment of dependency disorders in men: Toward a balance of identity and intimacy. *Journal of Chemical Dependency Treatment, 1*, 205–227.

Collins, N. L., & Read, S. J. (1990). Adult attachment, working models, and relationship quality in dating couples. *Journal of Personality and Social Psychology, 58*, 644–663.

Crits-Christoph, P., & Barber, J. P. (1991). *Handbook of short-term dynamic psychotherapy.* New York: Basic Books.

Freud, S. (1953). Three essays on the theory of sexuality. In J. Strachey (Ed. & Trans.), *The standard edition of the complete psychological works of Sigmund Freud* (Vol. 7, pp. 125–248). London: Hogarth Press. (Original work published 1905)

Freud, S. (1959). Character and anal erotism. In J. Strachey (Ed. & Trans.), *The standard edition of the complete psychological works of Sigmund Freud* (Vol. 9, pp. 167–176). London: Hogarth Press. (Original work published 1908)

Galatzer-Levy, R. M., & Cohler, B. J. (1993). *The essential other: A developmental psychology of the self.* New York: Basic Books.

Greenberg, J. R., & Mitchell, S. J. (1983). *Object relations in psychoanalytic theory.* Cambridge, MA: Harvard University Press.

Greenberg, R. P., & Fisher, S. (1977). The relationship between willingness to adopt the sick role and attitudes toward women. *Journal of Chronic Disease, 30*, 29–37.

Gupta, S., & Mattoo, S. K. (2012). Personality disorders: Prevalence and demography at a psychiatric outpatient clinic in northern India. *International Journal of Social Psychiatry, 58*, 146–152.

Heinstein, M. I. (1963). Behavioral correlates of breast-bottle regimes under varying parent–infant relationships. *Monographs of the Society for Research in Child Development, 28*, 1–61.

Heiss, G. E., Berman, W. H., & Sperling, M. B. (1996). Five scales in search of a construct: Exploring continued attachment to parents in college students. *Journal of Personality Assessment, 67*, 102–115.

Hirschfeld, R. M. A., Klerman, G. L., Clayton, P. J., & Keller, M. B. (1983). Personality and depression: Empirical findings. *Archives of General Psychiatry, 40*, 993–998.

Hirschfeld, R. M. A., Klerman, G. L., Gough, H. G., Barrett, J., Korchin, S. J., & Chodoff, P. (1977). A measure of interpersonal dependency. *Journal of Personality Assessment, 41*, 610–618.

Johnson, J. G., & Bornstein, R. F. (1992). Utility of the Personality Diagnostic Questionnaire–Revised in a nonclinical population. *Journal of Personality Disorders, 6*, 450–457.

Kantor, M. (1992). *Diagnosis and treatment of the personality disorders.* St. Louis, MO: Ishiyaku EuroAmerica.

Kendler, K., Kupfer, D., Narrow, W., Phillips, K., & Fawcett, J. (2009). *Guidelines for making changes to DSM-V.* Unpublished manuscript, American Psychiatric Association, Washington, DC.

Kraepelin, E. (1913). *Psychiatrie: Ein lehrbuch.* Leipzig, Germany: Barth.

Livesley, W. J., Schroeder, M. L., & Jackson, D. N. (1990). Dependent personality disorder and attachment problems. *Journal of Personality Disorders, 4*, 131–140.

Loas, G., Corcos, M., Perez-Diaz, F., Verrier, A., Guelfi, J. D., Halfon, O., et al. (2002). Criterion validity of the Interpersonal Dependency Inventory: A preliminary study of 621 addictive subjects. *European Psychiatry, 17*, 477–478.

Luborsky, L., & Crits-Christoph, P. (1990). *Understanding transference: The Core Conflictual Relationship Theme method.* New York: Basic Books.

Masling, J. M., Rabie, L., & Blondheim, S. H. (1967). Obesity, level of aspiration, and Rorschach and TAT measures of oral dependence. *Journal of Consulting Psychology, 31*, 233–239.

McGrath, R. E. (2008). The Rorschach in the context of performance-based personality assessment. *Journal of Personality Assessment, 90*, 465–475.

Mongrain, M., Vettese, L. C., Shuster, B., & Kendal, N. (1998). Perceptual biases, affect, and behaviour in the relationships of dependents and self-critics. *Journal of Personality and Social Psychology, 75*, 230–241.

O'Neill, R. M., & Bornstein, R. F. (2001). The dependent patient in a psychiatric inpatient setting: Relationship of interpersonal dependency to consultation and medication frequencies. *Journal of Clinical Psychology, 57,* 289–298.

Overholser, J. C. (1996). The dependent personality and interpersonal problems. *Journal of Nervous and Mental Disease, 184,* 8–16.

Pincus, A. L. (2005). A contemporary integrative interpersonal theory of personality disorders. In M. F. Lenzenweger & J. F. Clarkin (Eds.), *Major theories of personality disorder* (2nd ed., pp. 282–331). New York: Guilford Press.

Pincus, A. L., & Gurtman, M. B. (1995). The three faces of interpersonal dependency: Structural analysis of self-report dependency measures. *Journal of Personality and Social Psychology, 69,* 744–758.

Pincus, A. L., & Wilson, K. R. (2001). Interpersonal variability in dependent personality. *Journal of Personality, 69,* 223–251.

Porcerelli, J. H., Bornstein, R. F., Markova, T., & Huprich, S. K. (2009). Physical health correlates of pathological and healthy dependency in urban women. *Journal of Nervous and Mental Disease, 197,* 761–765.

Ryder, R. D., & Parry-Jones, W. L. (1982). Fear of dependence and its value in working with adolescents. *Journal of Adolescence, 5,* 71–81.

Schneider, K. (1923). *Die psychopathischen Persönlichkeiten.* Vienna, Austria: Deuticke.

Skodol, A. E., Bender, D. S., Morey, L. C., Clark, L. A., Oldham, J. M., Alarcon, R. D., et al. (2011). Personality disorder types proposed for DSM-5. *Journal of Personality Disorders, 25,* 136–169.

van Sweden, R. C. (1995). *Regression to dependence.* Northvale, NJ: Jason Aronson.

Yamaguchi, S. (2004). Further clarifications of the concept of *amae* in relation to dependence and detachment. *Human Development, 47,* 28–33.

Yasunaga, S. (1985). The effects of dependency and strategy patterns on modeling. *Japanese Journal of Psychology, 55,* 374–377.

CHAPTER 17

Borderline Personality Disorder

John F. Clarkin, Peter Fonagy, Kenneth N. Levy,
and Anthony Bateman

Borderline personality disorder (BPD) is a chronic, serious disorder involving suicidal and self-destructive behavior, affective liability and dysregulation, intense interpersonal conflict, and incoherent internal representations of self and others. The mean prevalence for any personality disorder across contemporary epidemiological studies is 11.39% (Lenzenweger, 2008), and in the National Comorbidity Survey Replication (Kessler et al., 2004) BPD had a general population prevalence of 14%. Because of the severity of the pathology and the disruptions in interpersonal relations, these patients are both difficult to treat and high service utilizers (Bender et al., 2001).

There has been an intense interest in and explosion of information on borderline pathology. This chapter addresses the conception of borderline pathology in terms of the developmental aspects of the pathology, and the current functioning of adult patients that would be manifest both in their daily lives and in the treatment situation. We review the phenomenology, personality structure, and biological underpinnings of BPD in order to demonstrate how this growing body of information must influence the progressive adaptations of the existing psychotherapeutic treatments to the pathology. To accomplish this, one must go beyond a mere phenomenological description of the pathology to a developmental model that captures the dynamic interaction of the individual's temperament with environmental factors. This interaction results in adult functioning with the stigmata of borderline pathology—that is, attention difficulties, affect dysregulation, and problems in mentalization.

CLASSIFICATION AND DIAGNOSIS

History of the Borderline Construct

The American psychoanalyst Adolf Stern (1938) was the first to coin the term *borderline*, referring to a group of patients who appeared neurotic during the evaluation phase of treatment but who would "regress" into mild transient psychotic episodes during treatment. These patients were thought to be "on the borderline" between neurotic and psychotic functioning, hence the notion of borderline personality disorder. Other writers used the concept of preschizophrenic personality structure (Rapaport, Gill, & Schafer, 1945–1946), borderline states (Knight, 1953), and psychotic characters (Frosch, 1964). Borderline personality (Rangell, 1955; Robbins, 1956) grew out of clinical treatment experience with patients who were severely disturbed and multisymptomatic. Knight (1953), for instance, described the ego weakness that led to severe regression in the transference and the need for modification of psychotherapeutic approaches. Kernberg (1975) described these patients as having a specific and stable pathological ego structure differing from that in neurotic patients and those in the psychotic range, and termed the group as having borderline personality organization. These patients were seen as having symptoms typical of those with neurotic and character disorder, but experiencing transient psychotic episodes when under severe stress or under the influence of alcohol or drugs. When in classical analytic treatment, these patients were prone to develop loss of reality testing and delusional ideas restricted to the transference. Using concepts of defensive splitting from Fairbairn (1940/1952, 1944), Klein (1946), and Jacobson (1954, 1964), Kernberg (1975, 1984) described these patients both in terms of descriptive pathology and, most importantly, at the level of structural organization involving lack of anxiety tolerance, poor impulse control, and lack of developed sublimatory channels (ego weakness), tendency to shift toward primary process thinking, reliance on primitive defenses such as splitting, and pathological internalized object relations.

While Kernberg (1975, 1984) was describing these patients in terms of descriptive pathology and structural characteristics, others such as Grinker, Werble, and Drye (1968) and Gunderson and Kolb (1978) were using a purely descriptive approach to identify patients with intense affect, particularly anger and depression, and to indicate subgroups of these patients. Many of the descriptive characteristics of these patients were utilized to formulate the diagnosis of BPD for the first time in the diagnostic system (DSM-III; American Psychiatric Association [APA], 1980).

The Complex Phenomenology of Borderline Pathology

The group of patients currently captured by the DSM-5 BPD criteria (APA, 2013) is extremely heterogeneous. The dismantling of this heterogeneity is a major task facing the field at this time. Various statistical procedures have been used to resolve phenotypic heterogeneity in borderline pathology. Factor-analytic studies of the DSM-III (Becker, McGlashan, & Grilo, 2006; Clarkin, Hull, & Hurt, 1993; Rosenberg & Miller, 1989; Sanislow, Grilo, & McGlashan, 2000) and DSM-IV criteria (Benazzi,

2006; Blais, Hilsenroth, & Castlebury, 1997; Fossati et al., 1999; Johansen, Karterud, Pedersen, Gude, & Falkum, 2004; Taylor & Reeves, 2007) have resulted in two to four factors, depending on the sample and instruments utilized, including affective instability, identity problems, disturbed relationships, and impulsivity. A confirmatory factor analysis of BPD features (Sanislow et al., 2002) was consistent with a one-factor model or a three-factor model involving affective disturbance, identity disturbance, and impulse dyscontrol. Q-factor analysis results in groups of similar individuals rather than in grouping factors across individuals. Utilizing information from practicing clinicians, Bradley, Zittel Conklin, and Westen (2005) found four subtypes of adolescent borderline females: high-functioning internalizing, histrionic, depressive internalizing, and angry externalizing.

Since neither factor- nor cluster-analytic procedures are well suited to the classification problem of BPD heterogeneity, we (Lenzenweger, Clarkin, Yeomans, Kernberg, & Levy, 2008) have used finite mixture modeling guided by an object relations theory of the pathology (Kernberg, 1984; Kernberg & Caligor, 2005) to parse the heterogeneous BPD pathology. This identified three groups of borderline patients: (1) a nonparanoid and nonaggressive group, (2) a paranoid and moderately aggressive group, and (3) a nonparanoid, aggressive/antisocial group. These three groups thus vary in terms of paranoid, antisocial, and aggressive features. Refinement of the BPD phenotype is necessary to facilitate research at multiple levels of analysis (i.e., endophenotypic, neurobiological, genomic, and intervention).

Major Domains of BPD Pathology

Despite the heterogeneity of BPD, there is consensus about the major domains of BPD pathology. First, impulsivity is one of the defining criteria of BPD and is thought to be most characteristic of the condition (Henry et al., 2001; Koenigsberg et al., 2002; Links, Heslegrave, & van Reekum, 1999; Sanislow et al., 2002). However, the construct of impulsivity can include near-neighbor and overlapping constructs of sensation-seeking, risk-taking, lack of planning, inability to delay gratification, insensitivity to consequences of action, and alteration in the perception of time (Coffey, Schumacher, Baschnagel, Hawk, & Holloman, 2011; McCloskey et al., 2009). It has been pointed out (Coffey et al., 2011) that not only do BPD and substance abuse frequently co-occur, but impulsivity is a core feature of both disorders and may be a causal link in the co-occurrence.

Second, negative affects, such as irritability, anger, anxiety, and depression, are characteristic of a number of disorders, but BPD is uniquely marked by affective instability that is reactive to environmental stimuli in a transient and fluctuating course (Henry et al., 2001; Koenigsberg et al., 2002). Affective instability and the lack of constraint or the ability to modulate affect is most probably related to self-destructive and suicidal behavior, impulsivity, fluctuating and extreme representations of self and others, and interpersonal conflict. Borderline patients have particular difficulty processing negative stimuli efficiently and effectively (Silbersweig et al., 2007). Borderline patients rely on reflexive, automatically responding networks, whereas healthy controls use networks with access to higher-level conscious cortical processing (Koenigsberg, Siever, et al., 2009). Furthermore, borderline patients are deficient in the ability to reduce negative affect by reappraisal (Koenigsberg, Fan, et al., 2009). This finding is quite important to borderline pathology and has potential treatment implications, as in normal individuals affect regulation by reappraisal in contrast to suppression is associated with greater positive emotion, reduced negative emotion, and better interpersonal functioning (Gross & John, 2003). As is explained further later, both transference-focused psychotherapy (TFP) and mentalization-based treatment (MBT) encourage reappraisal, especially in the interpersonal perception of self and others, by the use of clarification, interpretation, and mentalizing.

Third, a core feature of BPD is severe disruptions in interpersonal behavior (APA, 2000; Clarkin, Widiger, Frances, Hurt, & Gilmore, 1983; Gunderson, 2007; Kehrer & Linehan, 1996) that endure even after other symptoms have declined (Skodol et al., 2002). The intense negative states that borderline patients experience are often stimulated by aspects of interpersonal relations such as rejection (Herpertz, 1995; Stiglmayr et al., 2005; Stiglmayr, Shapiro, Stieglitz, Limberger, & Bohus, 2001) and interpersonal events (Jovev & Jackson, 2006). In an event-contingent recording procedure study (Russell, Moskowitz, Zuroff, Sookman, & Paris, 2007), borderline patients experienced more unpleasant affect, were less dominant and more submissive, and more quarrelsome in their interpersonal behavior than were controls. They also showed greater variability in the use of these behaviors. In contrast to patients with other personality disorders and other psychiatric disorders without personality disorder, borderline patients showed more disagreements, confusion, hostility, emptiness, and ambivalence in their social interactions (Stepp, Pilkonis, Yaggi, Morse, & Feske, 2009).

These findings are consistent with the clinical hypothesis that borderline patients lack a stable sense of self to help guide them smoothly and efficiently through various interpersonal situations (Kernberg, 1984). Indeed, information-processing biases may be linked to internal beliefs, assumptions, and working models of self and others, which, in turn, guide interpersonal behavior. Beliefs about the social world, such as that one is powerless and vulnerable in the face of a malevolent social environment (Beck & Freeman, 1990), may bias appraisal of the environment. Borderline individuals selectively remember negative information (Korfine & Hooley, 2000), and they have an enhanced awareness of others' emotions (Fertuck et al., 2009; Lynch et al., 2006).

Course and Outcome

With the advantage of diagnostic criteria that can be reliably assessed at one point in time, the groundwork was laid for investigating the stability or change in these criteria over time. This has been examined in a number of prospective studies (Clark, 2007; Grilo, McGlashan, & Skodol, 2000; Sanislow et al., 2009). The very definition of personality disorder adopted in the DSMs assumed stability, but the overall picture that has emerged in five major studies suggests a more complicated picture.

The Children in the Community study (Johnson et al., 2000) found a steady and significant decline of personality disorder traits from age 14 to 22. The Collaborative Longitudinal Personality Disorders Study (CLPS) prospective study of four personality disorders reported significant diagnostic change over two years (Grilo et al., 2004; Shea et al., 2002), with only 44% of the patients meeting criteria every month during year 1. Remission rates ranged from 20 to 40% by year 2. In a study of depressed outpatients over a 10-year period, Durbin and Klein (2006) found a significant decline in personality disorder diagnoses. A longitudinal study of patients with BPD (Zanarini, Frankenburg, Hennen, Reich, & Silk, 2005) also reported significant decline in personality pathology as measured by the diagnostic criteria. In a longitudinal study of personality disorders among college students, Lenzenweger, Johnson, and Willett (2004) found significant decreases in the mean number of criteria at each year of follow-up.

In summary, these studies of adults with BPD across time indicate change at the symptom or criteria level, but stability in work and social dysfunction. Some view this optimistically as the amelioration of the disorder; another view is that the symptoms do not capture the structure of the personality, which is more stable without concerted intervention. It is not surprising that the field of personality disorders will face some of the same challenges that have beguiled the field of personality, notably, issues of stability and change. The variety of personality functioning between situations and across time has brought into question the intuitive sense that people's personalities do not change. In a current view of both stability and change, one must consider the interaction between specific environmental circumstances and challenges, and the adaptive behaviors driven by internal structures such as cognitive-affective units that transcend situations (Mischel, 2004).

Most relevant to the present chapter is the course of the symptom state (e.g., symptom criteria in DSM) over time, the underlying structure of the personality, and the timing of psychotherapeutic intervention. It has become clear that the symptom pattern of BPD changes with time, so that the focus of intervention depends in part on the individual patient's age and course of illness. In addition, the severity of the symptom pattern varies between individuals.

PSYCHODYNAMIC APPROACHES TO BPD

Development of Borderline Pathology

The development of BPD is usually linked to early adversity in the psychoanalytic literature (e.g., Terr, 1991). This is hardly surprising given that patients diagnosed with BPD tend to report severe adverse events in early childhood (e.g., Zanarini et al., 2002) and do so more frequently than patients with other personality disorder diagnoses (e.g., Yen et al., 2002). However, attempts to identify specific links between the presence of early adversity and specific changes in psychopathology in the course of adult life have, by and large, been unsuccessful (e.g., Paris, 2007).

Increasingly, authors have been looking toward interactional models that incorporate biological vulnerability with psychosocial risk such as early neglect and abuse, and pinning their hopes on emergent studies of gene–environment interactions (e.g.,

Wagner, Baskaya, Dahmen, Lieb, & Tadic, 2010; Wagner, Baskaya, Lieb, Dahmen, & Tadic, 2009). Modern psychodynamic views should go back to classical psychoanalysis (e.g., Freud, 1896, 1905; Freud & Breuer, 1893), which saw genetic factors in combination with adverse childhood experiences as the cause of both biological (neurobiological structures and dysfunctions) and psychosocial (neuroticism, interpersonal, and self-structure deficits) anomalies. It is the interaction of these two factors that accounts for the components of psychopathology that we recognize—in Freud's case hysteria, and in ours, BPD (see above).

As John Oldham (2009) has helpfully delineated, borderline psychopathology is most likely at least partially but complexly "hard-wired," whereby a biological endophenotype of the disorder (perhaps characterized by impulsive aggression and emotion dysregulation) disrupts early relationships that normally might have the function of facilitating the development of behavioral and affect regulation, thus aggravating further the biological vulnerability with which the young child constitutionally presents. It is the combination of biological propensity, for example, overanticipation of an overreaction to criticism or rejection, which compromises the attachment relationships that could, under normal circumstances, compensate for such subjective states. Emerging from this combination of suboptimal biology and environment are the unstable interpersonal relationships, characterized by excessive intensity, profound distortions, deep anxieties, and unfathomable psychic pain.

Accumulating evidence is indeed consistent with a model that sees abnormal interpersonal relationships in BPD as a consequence of a combination of early attachment insecurity linked to psychosocial deprivation and biological vulnerability. The disorganization of the attachment system in patients with BPD is manifest in the combination of two attachment styles, characterized by strongly negative views of the self but, interestingly, simultaneously *fearful* and *preoccupied* in their perception of others, indicating holding, side by side, both positive and negative views of them (Choi-Kain, Fitzmaurice, Zanarini, Laverdiere, & Gunderson, 2009). But attachment anxiety interacts with constitution, as evidence is overwhelming in relation to the genetic determination of BPD (Bornovalova, Hicks, Iacono, & McGue, 2009; Distel et al., 2008; Kendler et al., 2008; Torgersen et al., 2000, 2008; White, Gunderson, Zanarini, & Hudson, 2003; Zanarini, Barison, Frankenburg, Reich, & Hudson, 2009). There may be further epigenetic evidence of the complexity of gene × environment interactions. A recent study hinted at the role of environmental influence in the penetration of the *5-HTTLPR* polymorphism. It seems that, in line with the environmental vulnerability of those with the "s" allele, attachment disorganization (unresolved loss and trauma scores) is elevated for those with the "s" allele only in cases with lower levels of methylation (van IJzendoorn, Caspers, Bakermans-Kranenburg, Beach, & Philibert, 2010). Clearly, this literature will yield further exciting developments, and there may indeed be genetically determined serotonergic anomalies that genetically underpin the kind of aggressive impulsive symptoms that Kernberg (1967) placed at the center of his psychoanalytic theoretical model. The molecular nature of this association remains currently unclear, but adequate consideration being given to triggering psychosocial relational environment factors seems key to a proper understanding of the biological narrative (Wagner et al., 2010).

The Environmental Perspective

Within a psychodynamic model, it is inconceivable that a proper understanding of borderline pathology can be arrived at without thought to the nature of early object relationships. For a start, an immediate implication of a genetic model of BPD is that the parents of these individuals would be likely themselves to manifest BPD traits or even frank BPD, which would profoundly affect their caregiving. The implication goes beyond mere gene–environment correlations (Plomin & McGuffin, 2003) and suggests quite specific developmental paths for social inheritance. For example, children of mothers with BPD show deficits in emotion regulation and distorted self–other representations, as well as later problems in psychosocial functioning (Hobson, Patrick, Crandell, Garcia-Perez, & Lee, 2005; Hobson et al., 2009). It would be surprising, given the difficulties these patients have in affective communication and relatedness in their moment-to-moment interactions with others, if their children were spared from the impact of shortcomings that directly interfere with the caregiving function (Bowlby, 1988; Sroufe, Egeland, Carlson, & Collins, 2005). Young children of mothers with BPD manifest disorganized attachment (Hobson et al., 2005) associated with disrupted affective communication and fearful and disoriented responses in the mothers (Hobson et al., 2009). A fearful pattern of attachment persists in these children until adolescence: they show an inability to make close friends and to feel socially accepted (Herr, Hammen, & Brennan, 2008). In completing story stems in middle childhood, the children of mothers with BPD show increased fear of abandonment, fantasy-proneness, and role reversal (Macfie & Swan, 2009). Jane Macfie, for instance, reported that a girl aged 5, whose mother had BPD, completed a story about a birthday party using family dolls, a table, and a cake thus: "The girl tells how the family open presents and eat cake. She then adds: *And then Mom takes off her clothes and gets drunk*" (Macfie, 2009, p. 69).

The social environment of infancy is critical because the infant acquires a sense of self through interaction with the object (Fairbairn, 1952a, 1952b). Early attachment experiences will be robust predictors of later BPD pathology because it is in the attachment context that the infant comes to understand his own emotional states, acquires the capacity for affect regulation, and discovers himself as a psychological entity through marked mirroring interaction (Fonagy, Gergely, Jurist, & Target, 2002; Fonagy, Gergely, & Target, 2007). The evidence that links harsh treatment in early life with later BPD goes beyond patient recollections; it has been largely confirmed by numerous prospective studies (Carlson, Egeland, & Sroufe, 2009; Crawford, Cohen, Chen, Anglin, & Ehrensaft, 2009; Johnson, Cohen, Chen, Kasen, & Brook, 2006). A particularly impressive study following up several hundred abused and neglected children and matched controls into adulthood reported a 2.5-fold increase in the prevalence of BPD associated with abuse and neglect (Widom, Czaja, & Paris, 2009). Interestingly, in this prospective investigation, early neglect appeared to be the most potent risk factor for both genders, whereas physical abuse represented a risk only for men. Sexual abuse, which has been highlighted by retrospective studies as potentially causal of BPD, appeared not to increase the risk of BPD for either gender. In general, findings highlight the pernicious impact of early neglect, depriving children of the opportunity to use interpersonal interaction with the caregiver to acquire knowledge and control over their subjective worlds.

Micro-analytic studies of parent–infant interaction have contributed to understanding of the way the genetic predisposition of the child may interact with suboptimal parenting environments to increase the risks of attachment disorganization (Beebe et al., 2010) and BPD symptoms (Lyons-Ruth & Jacobvitz, 2008). In Lyons-Ruth's (2008) longitudinal study, disrupted maternal communication and maltreatment were found to be independent predictors of BPD symptoms at age 18. An unusual longitudinal study (Crawford et al., 2009) examined the trajectory of BPD symptoms over time. The authors found deprivation of early parenting influence (early separation) to be predictive of BPD symptoms in adolescence and early adulthood, and the slower developmental decline of symptom severity over this period. Importantly, temperament (presumably genetically determined) was a partial mediator between early development and later symptoms. We may speculate that those with a difficult temperament are on the whole somewhat more likely to be abandoned by parents who are themselves more impulsive and less able to feel emotional commitment toward their child (gene–environment correlation). But those with this type of environmental deprivation will miss out on the self-organizing influence of early parenting and will be more likely to experience these events in a more exaggerated manner, turning on themselves in relation to deprivation, blaming themselves for the separation, and ending up feeling unworthy of love and attention.

The same bidirectional process is brought into relief by perhaps the most exquisite study of the emergence of borderline symptoms in young adulthood. Carlson and colleagues (2009) reported weak but significant correlations between borderline symptoms at 28 years of age and indicators of a suboptimal early environment (maltreatment, maternal hostility, attachment disorganization, family stress) in the first 3–4 years of life. These symptoms culminated in a range of social-cognitive anomalies that were evident by 12 years of age: attentional disturbance, emotional instability, and relational disturbance. A path-analytic approach offered strong evidence that disturbances in self-representation in early adolescence mediated the link between the disorganization of early attachment relationships and personality disorder. A narrative projective task administered at age 12 yielded more intrusive violence related to the self, more unresolved feelings of guilt and fear, and more self-associated bizarre imagery in individuals with borderline symptoms 16 years later. Early adversity was strongly associated with these inauspicious anomalies. A combined indicator of early adversity predicted such effects both directly and via the disorganization of the attachment system. Carlson and colleagues conclude that "representations and related mentalizing processes are viewed as carriers of experience" (p. 1328) that link early attachment to later psychopathology.

The Diathesis–Stress Model of BPD

A bidirectional model between social influence and genetic vulnerability is by no means new in accounts of BPD (Crowell et al., 2005; Fonagy, 1998; Gunderson & Lyons-Ruth, 2008; Paris, 2005; Zanarini & Frankenburg, 2007). The emergent findings of behavioral genetic studies confirm that, in addition to gene–environment correlation (the genetically predictable increase in environmental adversity), there is also gene–environment interaction supportive of a diathesis–stress model of BPD (e.g., Distel et al., 2010, 2011). For example, it has been shown that the absolute contribution of genetic factors to predicting variation in BPD features in twins or siblings depends on the number of life events they have been exposed to. The proportion of variance accounted for by genetic contribution declines linearly with exposure to social adversity and decreases from 46 to 36% when those exposed to no life events are contrasted with those who report six or more life events (Distel et al., 2010).

To properly test the diathesis–stress model of BPD etiology, we need to test for the interaction between inherited risk and adverse early experience. This requires a prospective longitudinal design that monitors family liability, early adversity, and subsequently emerging symptoms of BPD. A recent report (Belsky et al., 2012) provided important information pertinent to this issue. The study of a nationally representative birth cohort of over 11,000 pairs of UK twins, followed from birth to age 12, assessed BPD symptomatology in terms of both a continuous and a dichotomous indicator of borderline status. Extreme scores on borderline symptoms were predicted by poor theory of mind scores at age 5 as well as by low IQ. Early behavioral and affective indicators from age 5 included maternal and teacher ratings of impulsivity, maternal rating of internalizing problems, and externalizing problems perceived by both teacher and mother. Maltreatment was only weakly associated with BPD symptoms overall. When genetic vulnerability (operationalized as *any* family history of psychological illness) was used as a moderator, maltreatment became a highly significant predictor of membership of the borderline group. The relative risk of BPD was only about twofold for those with an experience of maltreatment who carried no genetic risk through a family history of mental disorder. However, among those with a positive family history of psychiatric illness (as an indication of genetic vulnerability), experience of early maltreatment increased the risk of borderline group membership by a factor of 13. Forty-two percent of those with a positive family history of psychiatric illness and an observed record of maltreatment were in the borderline group, compared with only 7% of those with similar maltreatment experiences but no family history of psychiatric illness, and 3% in either genetic risk group with no maltreatment experience. Dimensional indicators of borderline personality provided the same pattern of results. For example, maternal negative expressed emotion about the child recorded when the child was 5 years of age was twice as strongly associated with borderline personality characteristics among those with genetic vulnerability/ family history than among those without.

Thus, the overwhelming weight of evidence favors an interactional route to the causation of BPD. Constitutional factors, such as anxious or aggressive temperament, and environmental factors, such as parental neglect and trauma, both have a role in causation, but they also exert influence in relation to each other. Genes may mark vulnerability to environmental influence, and environment triggers genetic propensities. Constitutional disadvantage most likely translates to a greater sensitivity to negative environmental perturbations but may also include within it an increase in the likelihood of benefiting from positive environmental influence. Negative events may overwhelm an individual's capacity to assimilate environmental influence and to accommodate its unchangeable aspects. By contrast, positive events may serve to strengthen these individuals, making them more likely to benefit from favorable experiences such as good, high-quality psychosocial therapy. Individuals without a constitutional load may be more "resilient" to adversities and are less likely to develop BPD under the same degree of stress. However, the same constitutional factors that serve to protect them may also make them less accessible to the potential benefits of therapy, if disorder has occurred.

A Dynamic Biopsychosocial Model for BPD

We can construct a relatively coherent biopsychosocial model from the developmental evidence that is currently available, which contains within it elements of the dynamic model of the mind that all psychologies with psychoanalytic origins share. We have suggested (see Fonagy & Bateman, 2008; Fonagy, Luyten, & Strathearn, 2011) that three capacities (affect regulation, attention control, and mentalization) may represent the developmental domains where genes and environment interact and generate the vulnerability in self-structure that ultimately creates the risk for BPD. Each of these capacities has been shown to be susceptible to environmental adversity, to be genetically conditioned, and to be flawed to some degree in BPD. Furthermore, there is neural imaging evidence implicating brain regions known to mediate these capacities (see summary by Leichsenring, Leibing, Kruse, New, & Leweke, 2011). In general, findings support a conceptualization of BPD as involving deficits in mentalizing, including problems in inferring others' mental states and in being emotionally accurately attuned to oneself and others. How does this come about in the course of the development of an individual? In summary, we believe that genetic and early attachment environmental influences act together to create vulnerability for the development of BPD via three convergent mechanisms: poor affect regulation, poor control of attention, and fragile interpersonal understanding. These processes converge substantially to disrupt the effective management of emotionally charged interpersonal relationships—in other words, to render the person's attachment system vulnerable to disorganization when encountering additional trauma and stress.

We speculate that the activating or provoking risk factors of BPD probably include not just those relatively dramatic experiences documented by epidemiological studies (e.g., emotional abuse or trauma, as reviewed above) but, more subtly, the presence of nonmentalizing social systems where the impact on the child is from a lack of protection rather than from explicit adversity or assault. The increased prevalence of BPD over recent decades (see Grant et al., 2008; Lenzenweger, 2008; Torgersen, Kringlen, & Cramer, 2001) cannot be accounted for by dramatic variations in the gene pool or the increased prevalence of trauma. Rather, more subtle changes in social structure are likely to be responsible—namely, the "disappearance" of social structures that serve as personal support systems for holding and maintaining individuals whose development leaves them in a social environment demanding individuation, struggling with issues of subjectivity, of self and other, of thoughts and feelings, and of internal and external experience. We view the impact of these provoking experiences as serving to create a hyperreactive attachment system where vulnerability to interpersonal stress and the experience of rejection become the hallmark of BPD phenomenology. The abnormalities of the functioning of the attachment system in BPD have recently been well documented (Levy, Beeney, & Temes, 2011; Levy, Beeney, Wasserman, & Clarkin, 2010; Levy, Ellison, Scott, & Bernecker, 2011; Scott, Levy, & Pincus, 2009).

The overactivation of attachment in BPD is the primary trigger for two of the key mechanisms that serve to move patients with BPD from a state of vulnerability to a state where symptoms become manifest. First, the adverse emotional experiences they encounter in their daily life trigger distress and fear, leading to an intensification of attachment needs. However, seeking and achieving (psychological or physical) proximity to an attachment figure does not meet these needs. Instead, individuals with the disorganized attachment system we are describing experience a further intensification of adverse emotional experiences because of the traumatic association that attachment feelings can bring with them.

Second, the arousal-sensitive social-cognitive (i.e., mentalizing) deficits noted above come to play a central role in this context. Numerous biases of social cognition emerge at these times. We have highlighted four biases that strike us as particularly central to the phenomenology of the disorder (Fonagy & Luyten, 2009). First, the mentalizing profile of the prototypical BPD patient is biased against explicit, controlled, conscious, reflective mentalizing in favor of implicit, automatic, nonconscious, intuitive, and impressionistic thinking about mental states. Second, these individuals are focused on external visible cues for internal states, and more complex inferences required to access internal states are not accessible to them.

Third, their thinking about mental states prioritizes affect, or at least the logic that we normally use to infer emotional states (Baron-Cohen, Golan, Chakrabarti, & Belmonte, 2008). In inferring affect, we all start from our own state of feeling and assume that someone else who has the same emotional state has experiences that correspond to ours. This process is most obvious in its absence, for example, in individuals with antisocial personality disorder (Bateman & Fonagy, 2008). The domination of social cognition by emotionally rooted thinking should be contrasted with mentalizing focused on cognitions. In these instances, the tendency is to separate one's own beliefs and thoughts from the beliefs of others. It is the collapse of this distinction in BPD that is particularly pernicious when the individual comes to *believe* something simply because they *feel* it to be the case—what we have called "psychic equivalence."

Fourth, we have described how the self–other distinction can collapse because the inhibition of imitative experience (the "chameleon effect" of experiencing something as funny because others laugh or as boring because others yawn) can blur this distinction (Fonagy et al., 2011). Patients with BPD feel vulnerable in interpersonal interchanges because they cannot adequately inhibit the alternative state of mind that is imposed on them through social contagion. We see their apparent determination to manipulate and control the minds of others as a defensive reaction protecting the integrity of the self within an attachment context. Without such "excessive control," they might feel excessively vulnerable to losing their sense of separateness and their individuality.

The imbalance in mentalizing between implicit and explicit, cognitive and affective, internal and external, and focus on the self versus the other, generates three prementalistic modes of subjective functioning we have described in some detail in the context of other psychoanalytic constructs (Fonagy, Gergely, & Target, 2008). The tendency for what has been called concrete thinking (i.e., to give the same weight and importance to an internal experience as one does to an external experience) or *psychic equivalence* follows from the kinds of self:affective-state propositions that dominate emotional thinking ("I think it, therefore it is true"). We have also described a complementary state of pretend thinking in which internal states are referred to without appropriate linkage to reality. The lack of reflective, conscious thinking about thoughts and the resulting impressionistic bias based on appearance rather than reflection provides a basis for excessive mentalizing or *hypermentalizing*, a meaningless ruminatory exploration of internal states never linked with reality. Notably, this hypermentalizing bias is an early indication of borderline personality features in adolescents (Sharp et al., 2011) and leads to the emotion dysregulation that is the hallmark of BPD. Most disturbing for those working with BPD, finally, is the *teleological nature* of prementalistic thought. Judging mental states solely on the basis of observable outcomes reveals the bias toward external, visible cues and nonreflective impulsive thought.

PSYCHODYNAMIC TREATMENT OF BPD

A number of complex day hospital and outpatient treatment packages have been found to be efficacious in treating borderline personality. These include dialectical behavior therapy (DBT) (Linehan, Armstrong, Suarez, Allmon, & Heard, 1991; Linehan et al., 2006), MBT (Bateman & Fonagy, 1999, 2009), schema-focused psychotherapy (Giesen-Bloo et al., 2006), TFP (Clarkin, Levy, Lenzenweger, & Kernberg, 2007; Doering et al., 2010; Levy, Clarkin, et al., 2006; Levy, Meehan, et al., 2006), a specific form of CBT (Davidson et al., 2006), and Systems Training for Emotional Predictability and Problem Solving (STEPPS) (Blum et al., 2008). Additionally, a number of treatments are promising as they have shown effectiveness in pre-post or quasi-experimental approaches (Brown, Newman, Charlesworth, Crits-Christoph, & Beck, 2004; Stevenson & Meares, 1992).

Until recent years, there was a great deal of pessimism about the possibility of change in the severe pathology of patients with BPD, but there is now optimism that various approaches to treatment are effective for a large and significant proportion of patients, at least in the reduction of symptoms, in the short term, and compared with treatment as usual (TAU).

The results of these efficacy studies suggest several important evidence-based principles. First, BPD is a treatable disorder. Second, because BPD is a chronic disorder, it may require ongoing or long-term treatment. Many of the treatments for it are conceptualized as a multiyear process. Third, therapists have a range of options across a number of orientations available to them, and it is premature to foreclose on any one of the available options that have been tested. Although there have been few direct comparisons, no credible evidence has been presented that any one treatment is significantly better than any other as a function of effect sizes or comparisons with bona fide alternative treatments. A recent meta-analysis examining treatment studies of DBT found that DBT had only a small to moderate effect in comparison to TAU and no discernible effect in comparison with alternative treatments such as TFP, psychodynamic therapy, or comprehensive validation therapy (Kliem, Kroger, & Kosfelder, 2010). Unpublished meta-analytic data from one of the authors' laboratories has found no differences between any treatments in terms of within- or between-group effect sizes (Levy, Ellison, Temes, & Khalsa, 2013). Most importantly, commonalities across these treatments suggest a number of important guidelines for clinicians, such as providing a structured, coherent treatment, being in supervision, paying particular attention to the treatment frame and therapeutic relationship, and avoiding enactments, collusions, and iatrogenic behaviors.

Next, we review two treatments, each developed by the authors of this chapter (MBT: Fonagy & Bateman; TFP: Clarkin & Levy) and their colleagues. We use these reviews of the treatments to synthesize information from them and to signal future developments. In this process, we identify overlapping and common elements of the treatments, and unique elements of each, that may have a role in future treatment development (see also Table 17.1).

TFP: Essential Characteristics

TFP was developed with an object relations theoretical conception of borderline pathology, based not only on the specific criteria of DSM-III and its successors, but more broadly on the concept of borderline personality organization, with major structural deficits in representations of self and others, and the use of primitive defenses such as splitting. The treatment is focused on the patient's present life rather than the past, and the goals of treatment are to reduce harmful action and to develop a therapeutic relationship with the patient in which the patient can gradually reflect on his or her active and reactive perceptions of self and others, including within the relationship with the therapist and within relationships with important others in the patient's current life circumstances. Techniques of clarification, confrontation, and interpretation in the here and now are utilized in order to expand the patient's awareness of conceptions of self and others, especially in "hot," conflictful situations in which affect dysregulation is paramount. The aim of the sequence of clarification, confrontation, and interpretation is to provide a context in which the patient does not simply continue his or her incoherent, contradictory sense of self and others, but can begin to reflect rather than react and to reappraise dominant themes of self–other situations.

MBT: Essential Characteristics

MBT is essentially a therapy that places mentalizing at the center of the therapeutic process. It is primarily defined not by a cluster of specific and related techniques, but more by the process that is stimulated in therapy. At the core of MBT is the argument

TABLE 17.1. Comparison of the features of TFP and MBT

	TFP	MBT
Treatment format	Individual	Individual and group
Treatment structure	Treatment contract Focus on the present rather than the past	Engagement through mentalizing assessment process and psychoeducation Identification of problems and formulation Focus on current function in external world and individual and group therapy context
Goals and strategies	Containment of destructive action Clarification of dominant object relations dyads. Observing and interpreting patient's relations with therapist and with others	Stabilize social function and manage destructive behaviors Focus on mind of patient Identification of nonmentalizing states of mind Formation of attachment relationship
Treatment targets and their relative priorities	Obstacles to transference exploration, such as suicidal threats, threatened treatment dropout, dishonesty Overt transference manifestations Nontransferential affect-laden material	Maintaining mentalizing mind in context of attachment process Identification of pathway to dysregulating affect states Mentalizing the patient–therapist relationship
Treatment techniques	Clarification Confrontation Interpretation	Clarification Exploration Challenge Affect focus Mentalizing the relationship
Therapeutic stance	Technical neutrality	Not-knowing

that the therapy works through the therapist, establishing an enduring attachment relationship with the patient while continuously stimulating a mentalizing process in the patient. Its aim is to develop a therapeutic process in which the mind of the patient becomes the focus of treatment. The objective is for patients to find out more about how they think and feel about themselves and others, how those thoughts and feelings influence their behavior, and how distortions in understanding themselves and others lead to maladaptive actions, albeit intended to maintain stability and manage incomprehensible feelings. It is not the therapist's job to tell patients how they feel, what they think, or how they should behave—or to explain the underlying conscious or unconscious reasons for their difficulties to them. On the contrary, we believe that any therapeutic approach that moves toward *knowing* how patients are, how they should behave and think, and why they are as they are, is likely to be harmful. Therapists must ensure that they hold to an approach that focuses on the mind of their patient as the patient experiences him- or herself and others at any given moment. We have endeavored to capture the spirit of this approach in the phrase "the mentalizing stance," that is, a stance of inquisitiveness, curiosity, open-mindedness, and—ironically—not-knowing. This requires a modesty and authenticity on the part of the MBT therapist.

The basic aim of the treatment is to reestablish mentalizing when it is lost and to maintain mentalizing when it is present. Therapists are expected to focus on the patient's subjective sense of self. To do so they need to (1) identify and work with the patient's mentalizing capacities, (2) represent internal states in themselves and in their patient, (3) focus on these internal states, and (4) sustain this in the face of constant challenges by the patient over a significant period of time. In order to achieve this level of focus, mentalizing techniques will need to be offered in the context of an attachment relationship, consistently applied over time, and used to reinforce the therapist's capacity to retain mental closeness with the patient.

Synthesis of TFP and MBT

The technique of interpretation has long been conceptualized as a chief mechanism of change in psychoanalytic treatments and as a distinguishing feature of dynamically oriented therapies. As the concept of transference has been elaborated and become more central in psychoanalytic theorizing, the interpretation of transference has also become more central. However, the concept of transference interpretation and its use has become controversial (Frances & Perry, 1983; Gabbard et al., 1994), particularly with patients with BPD (Gabbard et al., 1994; Gunderson & Sabo, 1993; Paris, 2002; Wheelis & Gunderson, 1998). Some clinical theorists have suggested that negative reactions to transference interpretations might lead to frequent dropout (Gunderson & Sabo, 1993). Gabbard and colleagues (1994) contend that although transference interpretations are potentially high-yield interventions, they are high-risk.

Early data on transference interpretations were mixed but at least partially supported this view. A number of studies have found that transference interpretations are related to poor psychotherapy outcome (Connolly et al., 1999; Høglend, 1996; Ogrodniczuk, Piper, Joyce, & McCallum, 1999; Piper, Azim, Joyce, & McCallum, 1991; Piper, Joyce, McCallum, & Azim, 1993). Piper and colleagues (Ogrodniczuk et al., 1999; Piper et al., 1991; Piper, Joyce, et al., 1993) found an inverse relationship between the frequency and proportion of transference interpretations and both therapeutic alliance and outcome of therapy. Høglend (1996) found that transference interpretations were related to less favorable outcome at both 2-year and 4-year follow-up. Patients appeared to respond more defensively, often asked for more advice, missed sessions, and tended to increase their habitual maladaptive interpersonal responses when these patterns were interpreted in the transference. Henry, Strupp, Schach, and Gaston (1994) found that patients often perceive transference interpretations as hostile.

Other research, however, has demonstrated the importance of the accuracy and the competent delivery of an interpretation as well as the correspondence of the interpretation to the therapist's treatment plan for predicting outcome (Crits-Christoph, Barber, & Kurcias, 1993; Crits-Christoph, Cooper, & Luborsky, 1988; Gabbard et al., 1994; Piper, McCallum, Azim, & Joyce, 1993; Silberschatz, Fretter, & Curtis, 1986). Gabbard and colleagues (1994) found that transference interpretations tended to have greater impact—both positive and negative—than other types of therapeutic interventions on the development of the therapeutic alliance. They suggest that transference interpretations may result in substantial improvement in the patient's ability to collaborate.

Both MBT and TFP utilize interpretation as a process that must be titrated to the momentary condition of the patient. The goal of this process is not necessarily "insight" but rather the patient's growing awareness that his or her understanding of others may at times be distorted and subject to his or her own internal biases and emotional state at that particular point in time.

Two misconceptions relevant to thinking about interpretation in MBT and TFP are (1) that MBT eschews transference interpretations and (2) that TFP is for highly intelligent patients because the therapist provides complex descriptions of the patient's internal experience and behavior that would be beyond the ability of less intelligent patients to process and integrate, particularly in moments of high arousal. With regard to the first of these misconceptions, as Bateman and Fonagy (2007) point out, in MBT, therapists work in the transference in a similar way to TFP. This requires attending to and tracking the transference as well as being aware of it when formulating interventions, including extratransferential and nontransferential interventions. The goal is the "creation of alternative perspectives within an interpersonal context fraught with emotion" (Bateman & Fonagy, 2007, p. 680). What is avoided in MBT is the use of complex descriptions of mental states and behavior that transcend the patient's ability to process while in states of high arousal. Additionally, MBT eschews what Bateman and Fonagy call "the 'expert stance' potentially implied by reinterpreting the patient's behavior to provide insights within a model of the mind alternative to that which the patient (at least initially) holds" (p. 680). In a Vygotskian sense, Bateman and Fonagy are concerned about interventions that are outside the patient's "zone of proximal development" and not about the use of transference interpretations per se.

With regard to the second misconception, experimental studies (e.g., randomized controlled trials) as well as pre–post and quasi-experimental trials have clearly shown, in contrast to the early correlational data from the work of Piper, Høglend, and others (Connolly et al., 1999; Høglend, 1996; Piper et al., 1991; Piper, Joyce, et al., 1993), that TFP is appropriate for a full range of individuals with BPD and not just those with strong intellectual capacity. In the various trials of TFP (Clarkin et al., 2001, 2007; Doering et al., 2010; Levy, Meehan, et al., 2006), participants were not selected or excluded on the basis of intelligence and represented the full range of intellectual functioning. Patients in these trials were highly disturbed, with high levels of comorbidity, trauma, suicidality, and low levels of reflective function (i.e., mentalization). The treatment was well tolerated (e.g., low dropout, no adverse events) and as effective as any other available empirically supported treatments (e.g., DBT) on standard outcome measures. Importantly, those in TFP compared with other treatments (e.g, DBT and supportive psychotherapy) showed statistically and clinically significant changes in mentalization as assessed through the Reflective Functioning Scale

(Levy, Meehan, et al., 2006). Moreover, in subsequent analyses, those with severely impaired reflective functioning were the patients who benefited the most from TFP in terms of dropout. Thus, contrary to clinical hypotheses, patients with severely impaired reflective functioning tend to stay in treatment and do well. An evidence-based principle, which awaits replication, may be that TFP is the treatment of choice for those with severely impaired reflective functioning (at least in comparison to DBT and supportive psychotherapy).

Recent findings from Høglend's First Experimental Study of Transference (Høglend et al., 2006, 2008, 2011; Johansson et al., 2010) are consistent with the appropriateness of transference interpretations for severely impaired patients. In contrast to Høglend's earlier correlational studies (Høglend, 1996), in this experimental randomized controlled trial, Høglend and colleagues (2008) found that although overall there was no difference in outcome between a transference interpretation treatment and a no transference interpretation treatment, there was a significant difference between treatment groups for patients with low quality of object relations (characterized by high levels of personality disorders). For those patients, the transference interpretation treatment was superior.

The cautious approach to transference interpretation in MBT underlines a further aspect of treatment, namely, the level of training required to deliver a treatment effectively without iatrogenic effects. Dynamic therapies have often been criticized for their complexity and difficulty to implement well without a long period of training. MBT was developed as a research-based treatment to be implemented by generic mental health professionals, and this may account for its perhaps overcautious approach. MBT is concerned to avoid the possible harmful effects of overzealous and clumsy transference interpretation delivered without the balancing aspects described by Kernberg. In other words, transference interpretation is a complex technique that is not easily learned and may specifically risk harm in patients with BPD if used inappropriately. In recent trials of MBT, the therapists have been practitioners with no specialist psychotherapy training, and MBT has minimal training and supervision demands because it uses a common-sense view of the mind, incorporates generic ideas from different models of psychotherapy, blending them into a healthy ecumenism relevant to borderline personality disorder, and in the trials had to meet realistic service and training patterns. Three days' basic training is provided, and supervision is offered in the workplace as practitioners see patients for treatment. Current results suggest that reasonable outcomes may be achievable within this framework of mental health services without lengthy specialist training. This supports the general utility of MBT.

CONCLUSIONS AND FUTURE DIRECTIONS

Given empirical findings suggesting that a number of treatment programs result in significant reductions in borderline symptoms and that these are maintained over time, the interesting question is raised of how this is so. An obvious first answer is that the treatments, while using different models of pathology, utilize a number of common treatment elements that account for the majority of variance in outcome, such as a clear framework for the treatment, relatively long duration, attention to the dynamics of the relationship between therapist and patient, focus on emotion and impulse regulation, and a conception of the stages of change expected in the treatment (e.g., stabilization, reduction of emotion dysregulation, understanding how past experiences are manifest in current patterns of interpersonal behavior, and reorganization of interpersonal relations (Bradley, Conklin, & Westen, 2007; Levy, 2008). In addition to the use of overlapping strategies and techniques, these various outcome studies have found that although there are mean effects that are significant, many patients do not change and continue to be impaired. In fact, in most randomized controlled trials only about 50% of patients achieve moderate levels of improvement (e.g., Global Assessment of Functioning scores above 60), while the other 50% tends to continue to be functionally impaired (Levy, 2008). Also, the borderline diagnosis identifies a very heterogeneous group of individuals who vary in terms of their severity of dysfunction and unique combination of dysfunctional domains within BPD symptomatology and in combination with other comorbid diagnoses (see Lenzenweger et al., 2008).

Furthermore, findings from the McLean Study of Adult Development and CLPS, consistent with the classic follow-up studies by Stone, Hurt, and Stone (1987) and McGlashan (1986), suggest that there are symptomatic changes in the expression of BPD over time. Specifically, these studies found that as patients with BPD age, they become less impulsive and have less chaotic relationships, but they remain identity disturbed. It is believed that the decrease in impulsivity is related to age (McGlashan, 1986; Stone et al., 1987), whereas the less chaotic relationship functioning is a result of isolating oneself from relationships that would otherwise evoke or provoke affect dysregulation.

Thus, it is likely that further treatment development must not only utilize strategies and techniques from the various treatment packages, but also target subgroups of patients with different levels of severity in different stages of the pathology over the lifespan (see Howe, Reiss, & Yuh, 2002).

Given the complex nature of the pathology, not one but a number of effective measures are likely involved (Gabbard & Horowitz, 2009) in positive change. A generic view of treatment would require therapeutic functions of containment, support, structure, involvement, and validation (Gunderson, 2001), all of which are approached in the various empirically supported treatments.

The goal of treatment is to assist the patient in developing the internal controls that allow impulse containment and affective discharge regulation in the context of cooperative and fulfilling relationships with others. The prior review of the literature suggests the normal way in which these internal controls are developed and matured, and treatment must be designed to assist in furthering these abilities in borderline patients who have not had the environmental supports to develop these mechanisms. We propose that treatment must provide (1) a setting in which the patient is motivated for change in a relationship with a therapist that provides a secure base in which to use his or her usual ways of relating to others that are not effective, and (2) treatment focus on the way in which the patient mentalizes his or her relationships with the therapist and with others.

However, the following questions remain: Are there important subgroups of borderline patients who might differentially respond to the various treatments? Do the treatment effects endure over time? It is in the intersection of treatment approaches and mechanisms of change that the nature of the borderline pathology is paramount. Therefore, future research should focus on (1) subgroups of patients; (2) attention to the role of personality functioning and underlying neurobiological processes in predicting treatment outcome; (3) a focus on critical processes in the treatment, such as (a) the focus and process of assessment, (b) structuring the treatment, (c) motivating the patient for change, (d) activating a relationship (attachment) between the patient and therapist, (e) the therapeutic stance that the therapist takes, (f) understanding the relationship between patient and therapist (mentalizing, managing therapeutic ruptures), and (g) the hierarchy of treatment targets (Clarkin, Livesley, & Dimaggio, in press); and (4) mechanism of change.

As this review indicates, there is emerging information regarding borderline pathology linking the major aspects of the phenomenology of the disorder to both theories of personality and its dysfunctions, and neurobiological and genetic elements. The combination of information from these systemic levels of organization gives impetus to the next round of treatment development in the field. Future treatment outcome studies should capture the heterogeneity of the disorder, possibly through measurement of risk factors, protective factors, and mechanisms of change hypothesized by the treatments under investigation. Patients do not start treatment during the same phase of the illness or at the same level of symptom and dysfunctional severity. Treatment should be focused on the assessment–appraisal–response modes of the patient, especially in the interpersonal sphere. Treatments may need to be phased, with a sequence of targets progressing from containment of impulsive, destructive behavior to appraisal and reevaluation of habitual ways of perceiving self and interactions with others.

REFERENCES

American Psychiatric Association. (1980). *Diagnostic and statistical manual of mental disorders* (3rd ed.). Washington, DC: Author.

American Psychiatric Association. (2000). *Diagnostic and statistical manual of mental disorders* (4th, text rev. ed.). Washington, DC: Author.

American Psychiatric Association. (2013). *Diagnostic and statistical manual of mental disorders* (5th ed.). Arlington, VA: Author.

Baron-Cohen, S., Golan, O., Chakrabarti, B., & Belmonte, M. K. (2008). Social cognition and autism spectrum conditions. In C. Sharp, P. Fonagy, & I. Goodyer (Eds.), *Social cognition and developmental psychopathology*. Oxford, UK: Oxford University Press.

Bateman, A., & Fonagy, P. (1999). Effectiveness of partial hospitalization in the treatment of borderline personality disorder: A randomized controlled trial. *American Journal of Psychiatry, 156,* 1563–1569.

Bateman, A., & Fonagy, P. (2007). The use of transference in dynamic psychotherapy [Letter]. *American Journal of Psychiatry, 164,* 680.

Bateman, A., & Fonagy, P. (2008). Comorbid antisocial and borderline personality disorders: Mentalization-based treatment. *Journal of Clinical Psychology, 64,* 181–194.

Bateman, A., & Fonagy, P. (2009). Randomized controlled trial of outpatient mentalization-based treatment versus structured clinical management for borderline personality disorder. *American Journal of Psychiatry, 166,* 1355–1364.

Beck, A. T., & Freeman, A. (1990). *Cognitive therapy of personality disorders.* Guilford Press.

Becker, D. F., McGlashan, T. H., & Grilo, C. M. (2006). Exploratory factor analysis of borderline personality disorder criteria in hospitalized adolescents. *Comprehensive Psychiatry, 47,* 99–105.

Beebe, B., Jaffe, J., Markese, S., Buck, K., Chen, H., Cohen, P., et al. (2010). The origins of 12-month attachment: A microanalysis of 4-month mother–infant interaction. *Attachment and Human Development, 12,* 3–141.

Belsky, D. W., Caspi, A., Arseneault, L., Bleidorn, W., Fonagy, P., Goodman, M., et al. (2012). Etiological features of borderline personality related characteristics in a birth cohort of 12-year-old children. *Development and Psychopathology, 24,* 251–265.

Benazzi, F. (2006). Borderline personality-bipolar spectrum relationship. *Progress in Neuro-Psychopharmacology and Biological Psychiatry, 30,* 68–74.

Bender, D. S., Dolan, R. T., Skodol, A. E., Sanislow, C. A., Dyck, I. R., McGlashan, T. H., et al. (2001). Treatment utilization by patients with personality disorders. *American Journal of Psychiatry, 158,* 295–302.

Blais, M. A., Hilsenroth, M. J., & Castlebury, F. D. (1997). Content validity of the DSM-IV borderline and narcissistic personality disorder criteria sets. *Comprehensive Psychiatry, 38,* 31–37.

Blum, N., St John, D., Pfohl, B., Stuart, S., McCormick, B., Allen, J., et al. (2008). Systems Training for Emotional Predictability and Problem Solving (STEPPS) for outpatients with borderline personality disorder: A randomized controlled trial and 1-year follow-up. *American Journal of Psychiatry, 165,* 468–478.

Bornovalova, M. A., Hicks, B. M., Iacono, W. G., & McGue, M. (2009). Stability, change, and heritability of borderline personality disorder traits from adolescence to adulthood: A longitudinal twin study. *Development and Psychopathology, 21,* 1335–1353.

Bowlby, J. (1988). *A secure base: Clinical applications of attachment theory.* London: Routledge.

Bradley, R., Conklin, C. Z., & Westen, D. (2007). Borderline personality disorder. In W. O'Donohue, K. A. Fowler, & K. A. Lillenfeld (Eds.), *Personality disorders: Toward the DSM-V* (pp. 167–202). Thousand Oaks, CA: Sage.

Bradley, R., Zittel Conklin, C., & Westen, D. (2005). The borderline personality diagnosis in adolescents: gender differences and subtypes. *Journal of Child Psychology and Psychiatry, 46,* 1006–1019.

Brown, G. K., Newman, C. F., Charlesworth, S. E., Crits-Christoph, P., & Beck, A. T. (2004). An open clinical trial of cognitive therapy for borderline personality disorder. *Journal of Personality Disorders, 18,* 257–271.

Carlson, E. A., Egeland, B., & Sroufe, L. A. (2009). A prospective investigation of the development of borderline personality symptoms. *Development and Psychopathology, 21,* 1311–1334.

Choi-Kain, L. W., Fitzmaurice, G. M., Zanarini, M. C., Laverdiere, O., & Gunderson, J. G. (2009). The relationship between self-reported attachment styles, interpersonal dysfunction, and borderline personality disorder. *Journal of Nervous and Mental Disease, 197,* 816–821.

Clark, L. A. (2007). Assessment and diagnosis of personality disorder: Perennial issues and an emerging reconceptualization. *Annual Review of Psychology, 58,* 227–257.

Clarkin, J. F., Livesley, W. J., & Dimaggio, G. (in press). A final review of integrated treatment for personality disorders. In J. Livesley, G. DiMaggio, & J. F. Clarkin (Eds.), *Integrated modular treatment for personality disorder.* New York: Guilford Press.

Clarkin, J. F., Foelsch, P. A., Levy, K. N., Hull, J. W., Delaney, J. C., & Kernberg, O. F. (2001). The development of a psychodynamic treatment for patients with borderline personality disorder: A preliminary study of behavioral change. *Journal of Personality Disorders, 15,* 487–495.

Clarkin, J. F., Hull, J. W., & Hurt, S. W. (1993). Factor Structure of Borderline Personality-Disorder Criteria. *Journal of Personality Disorders, 7*, 137–143.

Clarkin, J. F., Levy, K. N., Lenzenweger, M. F., & Kernberg, O. F. (2007). Evaluating three treatments for borderline personality disorder: A multiwave study. *American Journal of Psychiatry, 164*, 922–928.

Clarkin, J. F., Widiger, T. A., Frances, A., Hurt, S. W., & Gilmore, M. (1983). Prototypic typology and the borderline personality disorder. *Journal of Abnormal Psychology, 92*, 263–275.

Coffey, S. F., Schumacher, J. A., Baschnagel, J. S., Hawk, L. W., & Holloman, G. (2011). Impulsivity and risk-taking in borderline personality disorder with and without substance use disorders. *Personality Disorders: Theory, Research, and Treatment, 2*, 128–141.

Connolly, M. B., Crits-Christoph, P., Shappell, S., Barber, J. P., Luborsky, L., & Shaffer, C. (1999). Relation of transference interpretations to outcome in the early sessions of brief supportive-expressive psychotherapy. *Psychotherapy Research, 9*, 485–495.

Crawford, T. N., Cohen, P. R., Chen, H., Anglin, D. M., & Ehrensaft, M. (2009). Early maternal separation and the trajectory of borderline personality disorder symptoms. *Development and Psychopathology, 21*, 1013–1030.

Crits-Christoph, P., Barber, J. P., & Kurcias, J. S. (1993). The accuracy of therapists' interpretations and the development of the therapeutic alliance. *Psychotherapy Research, 3*, 25–35.

Crits-Christoph, P., Cooper, A., & Luborsky, L. (1988). The accuracy of therapists' interpretations and the outcome of dynamic psychotherapy. *Journal of Consulting and Clinical Psychology, 56*, 490–495.

Crowell, S. E., Beauchaine, T. P., McCauley, E., Smith, C. J., Stevens, A. L., & Sylvers, P. (2005). Psychological, autonomic, and serotonergic correlates of parasuicide among adolescent girls. *Development and Psychopathology, 17*, 1105–1127.

Davidson, K., Norrie, J., Tyrer, P., Gumley, A., Tata, P., Murray, H., et al. (2006). The effectiveness of cognitive behavior therapy for borderline personality disorder: Results from the Borderline Personality Disorder Study of Cognitive Therapy (BOSCOT) trial. *Journal of Personality Disorders, 20*, 450–465.

Distel, M. A., Middeldorp, C. M., Trull, T. J., Derom, C. A., Willemsen, G., & Boomsma, D. I. (2011). Life events and borderline personality features: The influence of gene–environment interaction and gene-environment correlation. *Psychological Medicine, 41*, 849–860.

Distel, M. A., Trull, T. J., Derom, C. A., Thiery, E. W., Grimmer, M. A., Martin, N. G., et al. (2008). Heritability of borderline personality disorder features is similar across three countries. *Psychological Medicine, 38*, 1219–1229.

Distel, M. A., Willemsen, G., Ligthart, L., Derom, C. A., Martin, N. G., Neale, M. C., et al. (2010). Genetic covariance structure of the four main features of borderline personality disorder. *Journal of Personality Disorders, 24*, 427–444.

Doering, S., Horz, S., Rentrop, M., Fischer-Kern, M., Schuster, P., Benecke, C., et al. (2010). Transference-focused psychotherapy v. treatment by community psychotherapists for borderline personality disorder: Randomised controlled trial. *British Journal of Psychiatry, 196*, 389–395.

Durbin, C. E., & Klein, D. N. (2006). Ten-year stability of personality disorders among outpatients with mood disorders. *Journal of Abnormal Psychology, 115*, 75–84.

Fairbairn, W. R. D. (1952). Schizoid factors in the personality. In *An object-relations theory of the personality* (pp. 3–28). New York: Basic Books. (Original work published 1940)

Fairbairn, W. R. D. (1944). Endopsychic structure considered in terms of object-relationships. *International Journal of Psychoanalysis, 25*, 70–93.

Fairbairn, W. R. D. (1952a). *An object-relations theory of the personality.* New York: Basic Books.

Fairbairn, W. R. D. (1952b). *Psychoanalytic studies of the personality.* London: Tavistock.

Fertuck, E. A., Jekal, A., Song, I., Wyman, B., Morris, M. C., Wilson, S. T., et al. (2009). Enhanced "Reading the Mind in the Eyes" in borderline personality disorder compared to healthy controls. *Psychological Medicine, 39*, 1979–1988.

Fonagy, P. (1998). An attachment theory approach to treatment of the difficult patient. *Bulletin of the Menninger Clinic, 62,* 147–169.

Fonagy, P., & Bateman, A. (2008). The development of borderline personality disorder: A mentalizing model. *Journal of Personality Disorders, 22,* 4–21.

Fonagy, P., Gergely, G., Jurist, E., & Target, M. (2002). *Affect regulation, mentalization and the development of the self.* New York: Other Press.

Fonagy, P., Gergely, G., & Target, M. (2007). The parent–infant dyad and the construction of the subjective self. *Journal of Child Psychology and Psychiatry, 48,* 288–328.

Fonagy, P., Gergely, G., & Target, M. (2008). Psychoanalytic constructs and attachment theory and research. In J. Cassidy & P. R. Shaver (Eds.), *Handbook of attachment: Theory, research, and clinical applications* (2nd ed., pp. 783–810). New York: Guilford Press.

Fonagy, P., & Luyten, P. (2009). A developmental, mentalization-based approach to the understanding and treatment of borderline personality disorder. *Development and Psychopathology, 21,* 1355–1381.

Fonagy, P., Luyten, P., & Strathearn, L. (2011). Borderline personality disorder, mentalization, and the neurobiology of attachment. *Infant Mental Health Journal, 32,* 47–69.

Fossati, A., Maffei, C., Bagnato, M., Donati, D., Namia, C., & Novella, L. (1999). Latent structure analysis of DSM-IV borderline personality disorder criteria. *Comprehensive Psychiatry, 40,* 72–79.

Frances, A., & Perry, S. (1983). Transference interpretations in focal therapy. *American Journal of Psychiatry, 140,* 405–409.

Freud, S. (1896). Heredity and the aetiology of the neuroses. In J. Strachey (Ed.), *The standard edition of the complete psychological works of Sigmund Freud* (Vol. 3, p. 141–156). London: Hogarth Press.

Freud, S. (1905). Fragment of an analysis of a case of hysteria. In J. Strachey (Ed.), *The standard edition of the complete psychological works of Sigmund Freud* (Vol. 7, pp. 7–122). London: Hogarth Press.

Freud, S., & Breuer, J. (1893). On the physical mechanism of hysterical phenomena: Preliminary communication. In J. Strachey (Ed.), *The standard edition of the complete psychological works of Sigmund Freud* (Vol. 3, pp. 25). London: Hogarth Press.

Frosch, J. (1964). The psychotic character: Clinical psychiatric considerations. *Psychiatric Quarterly, 38,* 81–96.

Gabbard, G. O., & Horowitz, M. J. (2009). Insight, transference interpretation, and therapeutic change in the dynamic psychotherapy of borderline personality disorder. *American Journal of Psychiatry, 166,* 517–521.

Gabbard, G. O., Horwitz, L., Allen, J. G., Frieswyk, S., Newsom, G., Colson, D. B., et al. (1994). Transference interpretation in the psychotherapy of borderline patients: A high-risk, high-gain phenomenon. *Harvard Review of Psychiatry, 2,* 59–69.

Giesen-Bloo, J., van Dyck, R., Spinhoven, P., van Tilburg, W., Dirksen, C., van Asselt, T., et al. (2006). Outpatient psychotherapy for borderline personality disorder: Randomized trial of schema-focused therapy vs transference-focused psychotherapy. *Archives of General Psychiatry, 63,* 649–658.

Grant, B. F., Chou, S. P., Goldstein, R. B., Huang, B., Stinson, F. S., Saha, T. D., et al. (2008). Prevalence, correlates, disability, and comorbidity of DSM-IV borderline personality disorder: Results from the Wave 2 National Epidemiologic Survey on Alcohol and Related Conditions. *Journal of Clinical Psychiatry, 69,* 533–545.

Grilo, C. M., McGlashan, T. H., & Skodol, A. E. (2000). Stability and course of personality disorders: The need to consider comorbidities and continuities between axis I psychiatric disorders and axis II personality disorders. *Psychiatric Quarterly, 71,* 291–307.

Grilo, C. M., Sanislow, C. A., Gunderson, J. G., Pagano, M. E., Yen, S., Zanarini, M. C., et al, T. H. (2004). Two-year stability and change of schizotypal, borderline, avoidant, and obsessive–compulsive personality disorders. *Journal of Consulting and Clinical Psychology., 72,* 767–775.

Grinker, R., Werble, B., & Drye, R. C. (1968). *The borderline syndrome: A behavioral study of ego functions.* New York: Basic Books.

Gross, J. J., & John, O. P. (2003). Individual differences in two emotion regulation processes: Implications for affect, relationships, and well-being. *Journal of Personality and Social Psychology, 85*, 348–362.

Gunderson, J., & Sabo, A. (1993). The phenomenal and conceptual interface between borderline personality disorder and PTSD. *American Journal of Psychiatry, 150*, 19–27.

Gunderson, J. G. (2001). *Borderline personality disorder: A clinical guide.* Washington, DC: American Psychiatric Publishing.

Gunderson, J. G. (2007). Disturbed relationships as a phenotype for borderline personality disorder. *American Journal of Psychiatry, 164*, 1637–1640.

Gunderson, J. G., & Kolb, J. E. (1978). Discriminating features of borderline patients. *American Journal of Psychiatry, 135*, 792–796.

Gunderson, J. G., & Lyons-Ruth, K. (2008). BPD's interpersonal hypersensitivity phenotype: A gene–environment-developmental model. *Journal of Personality Disorders, 22*, 22–41.

Henry, C., Mitropoulou, V., New, A. S., Koenigsberg, H. W., Silverman, J., & Siever, L. J. (2001). Affective instability and impulsivity in borderline personality and bipolar II disorders: Similarities and differences. *Journal of Psychiatric Research, 35*, 307–312.

Henry, W. P., Strupp, H. H., Schach, T. E., & Gaston, L. (1994). Psychodynamic approaches. In A. E. Bergin & S. L. Garfield (Eds.), *Handbook of psychotherapy and behavior change* (4th ed., pp. 467–508). New York: Wiley.

Herpertz, S. (1995). Self-injurious behaviour. Psychopathological and nosological characteristics in subtypes of self-injurers. *Acta Psychiatrica Scandincavica, 91*, 57–68.

Herr, N. R., Hammen, C., & Brennan, P. A. (2008). Maternal borderline personality disorder symptoms and adolescent psychosocial functioning. *Journal of Personality Disorders, 22*, 451–465.

Hobson, R. P., Patrick, M., Crandell, L., Garcia-Perez, R., & Lee, A. (2005). Personal relatedness and attachment in infants of mothers with borderline personality disorder. *Development and Psychopathology, 17*, 329–347.

Hobson, R. P., Patrick, M. P., Hobson, J. A., Crandell, L., Bronfman, E., & Lyons-Ruth, K. (2009). How mothers with borderline personality disorder relate to their year-old infants. *British Journal of Psychiatry, 195*, 325–330.

Høglend, P. (1996). Analysis of transference in patients with personality disorders. *Journal of Personality Disorders, 10*, 122–131.

Høglend, P., Amlo, S., Marble, A., Bogwald, K. P., Sorbye, O., Sjaastad, M. C., et al. (2006). Analysis of the patient–therapist relationship in dynamic psychotherapy: An experimental study of transference interpretations. *American Journal of Psychiatry, 163*, 1739–1746.

Høglend, P., Bogwald, K. P., Amlo, S., Marble, A., Ulberg, R., Sjaastad, M. C., et al. (2008). Transference interpretations in dynamic psychotherapy: Do they really yield sustained effects? *American Journal of Psychiatry, 165*, 763–771.

Høglend, P., Hersoug, A. G., Bogwald, K. P., Amlo, S., Marble, A., Sorbye, O., et al. (2011). Effects of transference work in the context of therapeutic alliance and quality of object relations. *Journal of Consulting and Clinical Psychology, 79*, 697–706.

Howe, G. W., Reiss, D., & Yuh, J. (2002). Can prevention trials test theories of etiology? *Developmental Psychopathology, 14*, 673–694.

Jacobson, E. (1954). On psychotic identifications. *International Journal of Psycho-Analysis, 35*, 102–108.

Jacobson, E. (1964). *The self and the object world.* New York: International Universities Press.

Johansen, M., Karterud, S., Pedersen, G., Gude, T., & Falkum, E. (2004). An investigation of the prototype validity of the borderline DSM-IV construct. *Acta Psychiatrica Scandincavica, 109*, 289–298.

Johansson, P., Hoglend, P., Ulberg, R., Amlo, S., Marble, A., Bogwald, K. P., et al. (2010). The mediating role of insight for long-term improvements in psychodynamic therapy. *Journal of Consulting and Clinical Psychology, 78,* 438–448.

Johnson, J. G., Cohen, P., Chen, H., Kasen, S., & Brook, J. S. (2006). Parenting behaviors associated with risk for offspring personality disorder during adulthood. *Archives of General Psychiatry, 63,* 579–587.

Johnson, J. G., Cohen, P., Kasen, S., Skodol, A. E., Hamagami, F., & Brook, J. S. (2000). Age-related change in personality disorder trait levels between early adolescence and adulthood: A community-based longitudinal investigation. *Acta Psychiatrica Scandincavica, 102,* 265–275.

Jovev, M., & Jackson, H. J. (2006). The relationship of borderline personality disorder, life events and functioning in an Australian psychiatric sample. *Journal of Personality Disorders, 20,* 205–217.

Kehrer, C. A., & Linehan, M. M. (1996). Interpersonal and emotional problem solving skills and parasuicide among women with borderline personality disorder. *Journal of Personality Disorders, 10,* 153–163.

Kendler, K. S., Aggen, S. H., Czajkowski, N., Roysamb, E., Tambs, K., Torgersen, S., et al. (2008). The structure of genetic and environmental risk factors for DSM-IV personality disorders: A multivariate twin study. *Archives of General Psychiatry, 65,* 1438–1446.

Kernberg, O. (1967). Borderline personality organization. *Journal of the American Psychoanalytic Association, 15,* 641–685.

Kernberg, O. F. (1975). *Borderline conditions and pathological narcissism.* New York: Jason Aronson.

Kernberg, O. F. (1984). *Severe personality disorders: Psychotherapeutic strategies.* New Haven, CT: Yale University Press.

Kernberg, O. F., & Caligor, E. (2005). A psychoanalytic theory of personality disorders. In M. F. Lenzenweger & J. F. Clarkin (Eds.), *Major theories of personality disorder* (2nd ed., pp. 114–156). New York: Guilford Press.

Kessler, R. C., Berglund, P., Chiu, W. T., Demler, O., Heeringa, S., Hiripi, E., et al. (2004). The US National Comorbidity Survey Replication (NCS-R): Design and field procedures. *International Journal of Methods in Psychiatric Research, 13,* 69–92.

Klein, M. (1946). Notes on some schizoid mechanisms. In M. Klein, P. Heimann, S. Isaacs, & J. Riviere (Eds.), *Developments in psychoanalysis* (pp. 292–320). London: Hogarth Press.

Kliem, S., Kroger, C., & Kosfelder, J. (2010). Dialectical behavior therapy for borderline personality disorder: A meta-analysis using mixed-effects modeling. *Journal of Consulting and Clinical Psychology, 78,* 936–951.

Knight, R. P. (1953). Borderline states. *Bulletin of the Menninger Clinic, 17,* 1–12.

Koenigsberg, H. W., Fan, J., Ochsner, K. N., Liu, X., Guise, K. G., Pizzarello, S., et al. (2009). Neural correlates of the use of psychological distancing to regulate responses to negative social cues: A study of patients with borderline personality disorder. *Biological Psychiatry, 66,* 854–863.

Koenigsberg, H. W., Harvey, P. D., Mitropoulou, V., Schmeidler, J., New, A. S., Goodman, M., et al. (2002). Characterizing affective instability in borderline personality disorder. *American Journal of Psychiatry, 159,* 784–788.

Koenigsberg, H. W., Siever, L. J., Lee, H., Pizzarello, S., New, A. S., Goodman, M., et al. (2009). Neural correlates of emotion processing in borderline personality disorder. *Psychiatry Research, 172,* 192–199.

Korfine, L., & Hooley, J. M. (2000). Directed forgetting of emotional stimuli in borderline personality disorder. *Journal of Abnormal Psychology, 109,* 214–221.

Leichsenring, F., Leibing, E., Kruse, J., New, A. S., & Leweke, F. (2011). Borderline personality disorder. *Lancet, 377,* 74–84.

Lenzenweger, M. F. (2008). Epidemiology of personality disorders. *Psychiatric Clinics of North America, 31,* 395–403.

Lenzenweger, M. F., Clarkin, J. F., Yeomans, F. E., Kernberg, O. F., & Levy, K. N. (2008). Refining the borderline personality disorder phenotype through finite mixture modeling: implications for classification. *Journal of Personality Disorders, 22*, 313–331.

Lenzenweger, M. F., Johnson, M. D., & Willett, J. B. (2004). Individual growth curve analysis illuminates stability and change in personality disorder features: The longitudinal study of personality disorders. *Archives of General Psychiatry, 61*, 1015–1024.

Levy, K. N. (2008). Psychotherapies and lasting change. *American Journal of Psychiatry, 165*, 556–559.

Levy, K. N., Beeney, J. E., & Temes, C. M. (2011). Attachment and its vicissitudes in borderline personality disorder. *Current Psychiatry Reports, 13*, 50–59.

Levy, K. N., Beeney, J. E., Wasserman, R. H., & Clarkin, J. F. (2010). Conflict begets conflict: Executive control, mental state vacillations, and the therapeutic alliance in treatment of borderline personality disorder. *Psychotherapy Research, 20*, 413–422.

Levy, K. N., Clarkin, J. F., Yeomans, F. E., Scott, L. N., Wasserman, R. H., & Kernberg, O. F. (2006). The mechanisms of change in the treatment of borderline personality disorder with transference focused psychotherapy. *Journal of Clinical Psychology, 62*, 481–501.

Levy, K. N., Ellison, W., Temes, C. M., & Khalsa, S. (2013). *The outcome of psychotherapy for borderline personality disorder: A meta-analysis.* Paper presented at the annual conference of the North American Society for the Study of Personality Disorders, Boston.

Levy, K. N., Ellison, W. D., Scott, L. N., & Bernecker, S. L. (2011). Attachment style. *Journal of Clinical Psychology, 67*, 193–203.

Levy, K. N., Meehan, K. B., Kelly, K. M., Reynoso, J. S., Weber, M., Clarkin, J. F., et al. (2006). Change in attachment patterns and reflective function in a randomized control trial of transference-focused psychotherapy for borderline personality disorder. *Journal of Consulting and Clinical Psychology, 74*, 1027–1040.

Linehan, M. M., Armstrong, H. E., Suarez, A., Allmon, D., & Heard, H. L. (1991). Cognitive-behavioral treatment of chronically parasuicidal borderline patients. *Archives of General Psychiatry, 48*, 1060–1064.

Linehan, M. M., Comtois, K. A., Murray, A. M., Brown, M. Z., Gallop, R. J., Heard, H. L., et al. (2006). Two-year randomized controlled trial and follow-up of dialectical behavior therapy vs therapy by experts for suicidal behaviors and borderline personality disorder. *Archives of General Psychiatry, 63*, 757–766.

Links, P. S., Heslegrave, R., & van Reekum, R. (1999). Impulsivity: Core aspect of borderline persoanlity disorder. *Journal of Personality Disorders, 13*, 1–9.

Lynch, T. R., Rosenthal, M. Z., Kosson, D. S., Cheavens, J. S., Lejuez, C. W., & Blair, R. J. (2006). Heightened sensitivity to facial expressions of emotion in borderline personality disorder. *Emotion, 6*, 647–655.

Lyons-Ruth, K. (2008). Contributions of the mother–infant relationship to dissociative, borderline, and conduct symptoms in young adulthood. *Infant Mental Health Journal, 29*, 203–218.

Lyons-Ruth, K., & Jacobvitz, D. (2008). Attachment disorganization: Genetic factors, parenting contexts, and developmental transformation from infancy to adulthood. In J. Cassidy & P. R. Shaver (Eds.), *Handbook of attachment: Theory, research, and clinical applications* (2nd ed., pp. 666–697). New York: Guilford Press.

Macfie, J. (2009). Development in children and adolescents whose mothers have borderline personality disorder. *Child Development Perspectives, 3*, 66.

Macfie, J., & Swan, S. A. (2009). Representations of the caregiver–child relationship and of the self, and emotion regulation in the narratives of young children whose mothers have borderline personality disorder. *Development and Psychopathology, 21*, 993–1011.

McCloskey, M. S., New, A. S., Siever, L. J., Goodman, M., Koenigsberg, H. W., Flory, J. D., et al. (2009). Evaluation of behavioral impulsivity and aggression tasks as endophenotypes for borderline personality disorder. *Journal of Psychiatric Research, 43*, 1036–1048.

McGlashan, T. H. (1986). The Chestnut Lodge follow-up study. III. Long-term outcome of borderline personalities. *Archives of General Psychiatry, 43*, 20–30.

Mischel, W. (2004). Toward an integrative science of the person. *Annual Review of Psychology, 55*, 1–22.

Ogrodniczuk, J. S., Piper, W. E., Joyce, A. S., & McCallum, M. (1999). Transference interpretations in short-term dynamic psychotherapy. *Journal of Nervous and Mental Disease, 187*, 571–578.

Oldham, J. M. (2009). Borderline personality disorder comes of age. *American Journal of Psychiatry, 166*, 509–511.

Paris, J. (2002). Commentary on the American Psychiatric Association guidelines for the treatment of borderline personality disorder: evidence-based psychiatry and the quality of evidence. *Journal of Personality Disorders, 16*, 130–134.

Paris, J. (2005). The development of impulsivity and suicidality in borderline personality disorder. *Development and Psychopathology, 17*, 1091–1104.

Paris, J. (2007). The nature of borderline personality disorder: Multiple dimensions, multiple symptoms, but one category. *Journal of Personality Disorders, 21*, 457–473.

Piper, W. E., Azim, H. F., Joyce, A. S., & McCallum, M. (1991). Transference interpretations, therapeutic alliance, and outcome in short-term individual psychotherapy. *Archives of General Psychiatry, 48*, 946–953.

Piper, W. E., Joyce, A. S., McCallum, M., & Azim, H. F. A. (1993). Concentration and correspondence of transference interpretation in short-term psychotherapy. *Journal of Consulting and Clinical Psychology, 61*, 586–610.

Piper, W. E., McCallum, M., Azim, H. F., & Joyce, A. S. (1993). Understanding the relationship between transference interpretation and outcome in the context of other variables. *American Journal of Psychotherapy, 47*, 479–493.

Plomin, R., & McGuffin, P. (2003). Psychopathology in the postgenomic era. *Annual Review of Psychology, 54*, 205–228.

Rangell, L. (1955). The borderline case. *Journal of the American Psychoanalytic Association, 3*, 285–298.

Rapaport, D., Gill, M. M., & Schafer, R. (1945–1946). *Diagnostic psychological testing* (2 vols.). Chicago: Year Book.

Robbins, L. L. (1956). Panel report: The borderline case. *Journal of the American Psychoanalytic Association, 4*, 550–563.

Rosenberg, P. H., & Miller, G. A. (1989). Comparing borderline definitions: DSM-III borderline and schizotypal personality disorders. *Journal of Abnormal Psychology, 98*, 161–169.

Russell, J. J., Moskowitz, D. S., Zuroff, D. C., Sookman, D., & Paris, J. (2007). Stability and variability of affective experience and interpersonal behavior in borderline personality disorder. *Journal of Abnormal Psychology, 116*, 578–588.

Sanislow, C. A., Grilo, C. M., & McGlashan, T. H. (2000). Factor analysis of the DSM-III-R borderline personality disorder criteria in psychiatric inpatients. *American Journal of Psychiatry, 157*, 1629–1633.

Sanislow, C. A., Grilo, C. M., Morey, L. C., Bender, D. S., Skodol, A. E., Gunderson, J. G., et al. (2002). Confirmatory factor analysis of DSM-IV criteria for borderline personality disorder: Findings from the Collaborative Longitudinal Personality Disorders Study. *American Journal of Psychiatry, 159*, 284–290.

Sanislow, C. A., Little, T. D., Ansell, E. B., Grilo, C. M., Daversa, M., Markowitz, J. C., et al. (2009). Ten-year stability and latent structure of the DSM-IV schizotypal, borderline, avoidant, and obsessive-compulsive personality disorders. *Journal of Abnormal Psychology, 118*, 507–519.

Scott, L. N., Levy, K. N., & Pincus, A. L. (2009). Adult attachment, personality traits, and borderline personality disorder features in young adults. *Journal of Personality Disorders, 23*, 258–280.

Sharp, C., Pane, H., Ha, C., Venta, A., Patel, A. B., Sturek, J., et al. (2011). Theory of mind and emotion regulation difficulties in adolescents with borderline traits. *Journal of the American Academy of Child and Adolescent Psychiatry, 50*, 563–573.

Shea, M. T., Stout, R., Gunderson, J., Morey, L. C., Grilo, C. M., McGlashan, T., et al. (2002). Short-term diagnostic stability of schizotypal, borderline, avoidant, and obsessive–compulsive personality disorders. *American Journal of Psychiatry, 159,* 2036–2041.

Silberschatz, G., Fretter, P. B., & Curtis, J. T. (1986). How do interpretations influence the process of psychotherapy? *Journal of Consulting and Clinical Psychology, 54,* 646–652.

Silbersweig, D., Clarkin, J. F., Goldstein, M., Kernberg, O. F., Tuescher, O., Levy, K. N., et al. (2007). Failure of frontolimbic inhibitory function in the context of negative emotion in borderline personality disorder. *American Journal of Psychiatry, 164,* 1832–1841.

Skodol, A. E., Siever, L. J., Livesley, W. J., Gunderson, J. G., Pfohl, B., & Widiger, T. A. (2002). The borderline diagnosis: II. Biology, genetics, and clinical course. *Biological Psychiatry, 51,* 951–963.

Sroufe, L. A., Egeland, B., Carlson, E. A., & Collins, W. A. (2005). *The development of the person: The Minnesota Study of Risk and Adaptation from Birth to Adulthood.* New York: Guilford Press.

Stepp, S. D., Pilkonis, P. A., Yaggi, K. E., Morse, J. Q., & Feske, U. (2009). Interpersonal and emotional experiences of social interactions in borderline personality disorder. *Journal of Nervous and Mental Disease, 197,* 484–491.

Stern, A. (1938). Psychoanalytic investigation and therapy in borderline group of neuroses. *Psychoanalytic Quarterly, 7,* 467–489.

Stevenson, J., & Meares, R. (1992). An outcome study of psychotherapy for patients with borderline personality disorder. *American Journal of Psychiatry, 149,* 358–362.

Stiglmayr, C. E., Grathwol, T., Linehan, M. M., Ihorst, G., Fahrenberg, J., & Bohus, M. (2005). Aversive tension in patients with borderline personality disorder: A computer-based controlled field study. *Acta Psychiatrica Scandinavica, 111,* 372–379.

Stiglmayr, C. E., Shapiro, D. A., Stieglitz, R. D., Limberger, M. F., & Bohus, M. (2001). Experience of aversive tension and dissociation in female patients with borderline personality disorder: A controlled study. *Journal of Psychiatric Research, 35,* 111–118.

Stone, M. H., Hurt, S. W., & Stone, D. K. (1987). The PI 500: Long-term follow-up of borderline inpatients meeting DSM-III criteria: I. Global outcome. *Journal of Personality Disorders, 1,* 291–298.

Taylor, J., & Reeves, M. (2007). Structure of borderline personality disorder symptoms in a nonclinical sample. *Journal of Clinial Psychology, 63,* 805–816.

Terr, L. C. (1991). Childhood traumas: An outline and overview. *American Journal of Psychiatry, 148,* 10–20.

Torgersen, S., Czajkowski, N., Jacobson, K., Reichborn-Kjennerud, T., Roysamb, E., Neale, M. C., et al. (2008). Dimensional representations of DSM-IV cluster B personality disorders in a population-based sample of Norwegian twins: A multivariate study. *Psychological Medicine, 38,* 1617–1625.

Torgersen, S., Kringlen, E., & Cramer, V. (2001). The prevalence of personality disorders in a community sample. *Archives of General Psychiatry, 58,* 590–596.

Torgersen, S., Lygren, S., Oien, P. A., Skre, I., Onstad, S., Edvardsen, J., et al. (2000). A twin study of personality disorders. *Comprehensive Psychiatry, 41,* 416–425.

van IJzendoorn, M. H., Caspers, K., Bakermans-Kranenburg, M. J., Beach, S. R., & Philibert, R. (2010). Methylation matters: Interaction between methylation density and serotonin transporter genotype predicts unresolved loss or trauma. *Biological Psychiatry, 68,* 405–407.

Wagner, S., Baskaya, O., Dahmen, N., Lieb, K., & Tadic, A. (2010). Modulatory role of the brain-derived neurotrophic factor Val66Met polymorphism on the effects of serious life events on impulsive aggression in borderline personality disorder. *Genes, Brain and Behavior, 9,* 97–102.

Wagner, S., Baskaya, O., Lieb, K., Dahmen, N., & Tadic, A. (2009). The 5-HTTLPR polymorphism modulates the association of serious life events (SLE) and impulsivity in patients with borderline personality disorder. *Journal of Psychiatric Research, 43,* 1067–1072.

Wheelis, J., & Gunderson, J. G. (1998). A little cream and sugar: Psychotherapy with a borderline patient. *American Journal of Psychiatry, 155*, 114–122.

White, C. N., Gunderson, J. G., Zanarini, M. C., & Hudson, J. I. (2003). Family studies of borderline personality disorder: A review. *Harvard Review of Psychiatry, 11*, 8–19.

Widom, C. S., Czaja, S. J., & Paris, J. (2009). A prospective investigation of borderline personality disorder in abused and neglected children followed up into adulthood. *Journal of Personality Disorders, 23*, 433–446.

Yen, S., Shea, M. T., Battle, C. L., Johnson, D. M., Zlotnick, C., Dolan-Sewell, R., et al. (2002). Traumatic exposure and posttraumatic stress disorder in borderline, schizotypal, avoidant, and obsessive–compulsive personality disorders: Findings from the Collaborative Longitudinal Personality Disorders Study. *Journal of Nervous and Mental Disease, 190*, 510–518.

Zanarini, M. C., Barison, L. K., Frankenburg, F. R., Reich, D. B., & Hudson, J. I. (2009). Family history study of the familial coaggregation of borderline personality disorder with axis I and nonborderline dramatic cluster axis II disorders. *Journal of Personality Disorders, 23*, 357–369.

Zanarini, M. C., & Frankenburg, F. R. (2007). The essential nature of borderline psychopathology. *Journal of Personality Disorders, 21*, 518–535.

Zanarini, M. C., Frankenburg, F. R., Hennen, J., Reich, D. B., & Silk, K. R. (2005). The McLean Study of Adult Development (MSAD): Overview and implications of the first six years of prospective follow-up. *Journal of Personality Disorders, 19*, 505–523.

Zanarini, M. C., Yong, L., Frankenburg, F. R., Hennen, J., Reich, D. B., Marino, M. F., et al. (2002). Severity of reported childhood sexual abuse and its relationship to severity of borderline psychopathology and psychosocial impairment among borderline inpatients. *Journal of Nervous and Mental Disease, 190*, 381–387.

PART III

PSYCHOPATHOLOGY IN CHILDHOOD AND ADOLESCENCE

CHAPTER 18

Child–Parent Psychotherapy in the Treatment of Infants and Young Children with Internalizing Disorders

Maria S. St. John and Alicia F. Lieberman

The patient herself . . . christened this novel kind of treatment the "talking cure."
—FREUD (1910/1957, p. 13)

What emerged, then, was a form of "psychotherapy in the kitchen," so to speak, which will strike you as both familiar in its methods and unfamiliar in its setting. The method, a variant of psychoanalytic psychotherapy, made use of transference, the repetition of the past in the present, and interpretation. Equally important, the method included continuous developmental observations of the baby and a tactful, non-didactic education of the mother in the recognition of her baby's needs and signals.
—FRAIBERG, ADELSON, AND SHAPIRO (1987, p. 108)

Infants fascinate. They capture the attention of individuals and groups, children and adults, laypeople, artists, and professionals alike. This alluring quality makes sense from an evolutionary perspective because the human species begins life in a state of such utter physical immaturity that survival depends on the infant's capacity to elicit and sustain attention. To the mature members of the species, an infant may represent many things, including a link between the past, the present, and the future. But, as understandable and critical for ensuring care as the infant's allure may be, this power to fascinate can also be problematic. Imagination and emotion are stirred so readily by the evocative specter of infancy that perceiving infants with developmental accuracy and individual specificity is an elusive—although essential—endeavor.

In the early decades of psychoanalysis, infancy was theorized rather than studied; it was conceptual territory serving as fodder for theory-building. In time, psychoanalytic practitioners with expertise in infant development and pediatric care demonstrated how infants might not only further psychoanalytic understanding of the human condition but, in certain instances, benefit directly from psychoanalytically informed intervention. The intersecting streams of scholarship and practice in such fields as pediatrics, attachment research, developmental psychopathology, and infant psychiatry have in recent decades moved understanding of the experiences, capacities and vulnerabilities of infants, toddlers, and preschoolers forward by leaps and bounds. At present, families of struggling infants and small children may access a diverse, multidisciplinary field of infant mental health service providers that includes early intervention specialists, early care and education experts, and mental health professionals representing a broad range of disciplines and theoretical allegiances.

This chapter describes child–parent psychotherapy (CPP), an evidence-based psychodynamic approach to the treatment of social-emotional disorders and behavioral difficulties in infancy and early childhood. We discuss the application of this approach to children with a range of difficulties, with special emphasis on internalizing disorders and the ways that stress and trauma often complicate the clinical picture presented by small children (for externalizing disorders, see Hill & Sharp, Chapter 19, this volume). A clinical example illustrates how this treatment approach helped restore a vulnerable toddler to a more promising developmental trajectory.

CLASSIFICATION AND DIAGNOSIS

The idea that an infant, toddler, or preschooler may exhibit a mental health disorder is difficult for many to countenance, but very small children can behave in ways that exasperate their caregivers to the point that the highest rates of child maltreatment and fatalities as the result of physical abuse occur in the first five years of life (U.S. Department of Health and Human Services, 2007), and preschoolers are expelled from childcare and preschool at a rate three times higher than children in the K–12 age range (Gilliam, 2005). The majority of these children are experienced by their caregivers as too difficult to manage as the result of externalizing behaviors such as disruptive or aggressive acts. Equally worrisome, though less often noticed, are the counterparts to those who "act out": children who exhibit symptoms of internalizing disorders such as anxiety and depression, many of whom may not draw the attention of adults and, as a result, may not receive the intervention they need (Tandon, Cardeli, & Luby, 2009). Other young children present with such a mixture of symptoms and behavioral challenges that categorizing them as showing either internalizing or externalizing disorders would not do justice to the complexity of the clinical problems or to the subjective experience of the child or the caregivers. Research consistently shows significant correlations between children's internalizing and externalizing scores in assessment instruments, supporting the long-standing clinical consensus that aggression and defiance are often the external manifestation of deep-rooted anxieties (Silverman, Lieberman, & Pekarsky, 1997).

Rene Spitz is well known for initially alerting the world to the lethal danger posed by depression in infants as young as 12–18 months old (Spitz, 1946). Many subsequent investigators have observed in infants, toddlers, and preschoolers the depressive symptoms initially described by Spitz (Emde, Polak, & Spitz, 1965; Harmon, Wagonfeld, & Emde, 1982; Tandon et al., 2009). In spite of this cumulative evidence, there is still a pervasive tendency to deny the presence of depression in young children. The mother of a listless, withdrawn, and underresponsive 11-month-old whose beloved full-time nanny had left her position precipitously asked the infant–parent psychotherapist in disbelief, "You mean babies can get depressed?" There were several impediments to this generally psychologically minded woman's ability to recognize her daughter's depression, including her own competitiveness with the nanny and jealous guarding of the maternal role, which led her to minimize the nanny's emotional importance to the child. Her question suggested, however, a more basic and quite common reluctance to imagine that a child as young as her daughter was vulnerable to experiencing the emotional chasm and libidinal vacuum that we refer to as depression in older children and adults. A further complicating matter in many instances is the fact that depression in infants and small children does not always appear as clearly as it did for this little girl. Behavioral symptoms such as difficulties with state and body systems regulation, irritability, and attentional difficulties can signal depression in small children as surely as the more familiar symptoms such as vegetative retardation and anhedonia with which this child presented.

Recognition of symptoms of anxiety in infants and young children can likewise be challenging. In their review of the literature, Tandon and colleagues (2009) cite studies documenting a range of DSM-IV anxiety disorders in preschool-aged children, including generalized anxiety disorder, separation anxiety disorder, obsessive–compulsive disorder and posttraumatic stress disorder (PTSD). Although they are sometimes apparent as worry or fear, anxiety and traumatic stress responses in infants and small children more often present as exaggerated startle response and dysregulation of affect states, sleep, toileting, feeding, and biological rhythms; restlessness/irritability; difficulty concentrating and cooperating; emotional restriction or numbing; hypervigilance; restricted or noncreative play; and/or clingy, whiny, demanding, and/or controlling behavior. Behavioral difficulties can range from freezing, emotional constriction, and social withdrawal to impulsivity, recklessness, and counterphobic acting out.

PTSD in particular defies neat categorization as either an internalizing or an externalizing disorder. Falling under the general heading of the anxiety disorders, PTSD is often considered to be an internalizing disorder, yet many of the signs exhibited by toddlers and preschoolers suffering from PTSD—such as fighting, biting, and reckless behavior—are more immediately recognizable as externalizing behaviors. Even very young infants can exhibit symptoms of PTSD following traumatic experiences. As an illustration, the parents of a prematurely born infant who spent many weeks in the neonatal intensive care unit (NICU) and underwent regular, painful medical procedures reported the following remarkable story. At 2 months postdischarge, when the now healthy infant seemed well settled into home life, the parents realized that every week on Wednesday morning they were awakened by their baby crying at a pitch and intensity that they did not hear from the infant at any other time, and they found soothing him uncharacteristically difficult. The parents realized that Wednesday morning was trash day, and the beeping sound of the garbage trucks resembled the sounds of the NICU equipment. This traumatic trigger awakened the baby from his sleep on a weekly basis with typical traumatic stress responses of reexperiencing and hyperarousal.

Infants, toddlers, and preschoolers are thus vulnerable to a range of difficulties that may defy the traditional internalizing/externalizing dichotomy and may not be readily identifiable to nonspecialists as social-emotional disorders. Difficulties exhibited during early childhood "are commonly regarded as transient despite growing evidence to the contrary" (Tandon et al., 2009, p. 596). A study by Egger and Angold (2004) showed that 60% of parents with preschoolers with anxiety thought their children needed help, but only 10% reported having been referred for evaluation or treatment. The impact of untreated early difficulties may become increasingly severe, chronic, and complex over time, resulting in even young children showing co-occurring psychiatric diagnoses as the result of cumulative adversities and traumatic stressors and the relational strains they create in the child–caregiver relationship.

Considerable empirical effort has been directed at identifying specific pathogenic factors leading to psychopathology in infants and small children (Zeanah & Zeanah, 2009). Increasing new evidence suggests that child outcomes may be determined less by *which* risk factors a child is exposed to than by *how many* (Trentacosta et al., 2008). In their study of the developmental trajectories of externalizing and internalizing behaviors in physically abused children, for example, Lansford and colleagues (2006) examined several specific vulnerability and protective factors as potentially exacerbating or mitigating the adverse effects of physical abuse. They found, in tracing the arc of symptomatic behavior over time in these abused children, that protective factors were related to less acute trajectories of internalizing and externalizing problems, while vulnerability factors were related to higher levels of internalizing and externalizing problems, but an additive or main-effect perspective was more predictive of child outcome than examining discrete factors in isolation.

The nature of the child–caregiver relationship is among the most powerful moderating factors influencing the child's developmental course and emotional health (Zeanah & Zeanah, 2009). The healthy development and emotional well-being of young children is tied to the quality of caregiving they receive, which in turn is influenced by the overall level of stress experienced by the caregivers as well as by broader environmental factors (National Research Council & Institute of Medicine, 2000). In a study of families with toddlers who were affected by Hurricane Katrina, for example, cumulative family stress (characterized by financial strain and community violence) was linked with parental depression, which in turn was related to poorer parenting efficacy and more internalizing and externalizing problems in the toddlers (Scaramella, Sohr-Preston, Callahan, & Mirabile, 2008). The quality of the child's attachment to the caregiver also influences the child's resilience in the face of psychosocial stressors. A longitudinal study of 78 children exposed to traumatic events, for example, showed that disorganized attachment status at 12 months of age predicted higher PTSD symptoms at school age (specifically, avoidance and reexperiencing symptom clusters) than nondisorganized attachment (MacDonald et al., 2008).

The following sections explore the implications of these findings for mental health intervention with children in the birth-to-5 age range, with specific focus on the contributions made by a psychoanalytic perspective to the development and dissemination of CPP as an evidence-based approach to treatment.

PSYCHODYNAMIC APPROACHES TO INFANT AND EARLY CHILDHOOD MENTAL HEALTH

As Zeanah and Zeanah (2009) describe it, the field of infant mental health stands in the early 21st century "as a broad-based, multidisciplinary, and international effort to enhance the social and emotional well-being of young children and which includes the efforts of clinicians, researchers, and policymakers" (p. 5). Infant mental health professionals examine and address the factors contributing to positive versus adverse outcomes for infants, toddlers, and preschoolers, and their caregivers, from a range of disciplinary perspectives. Interventions exist along a continuum that encompasses promotion, prevention, early intervention, and treatment of mental health difficulties in the birth-to-5 age range (Zeanah & Zeanah, 2009). Among this array of approaches, how does one delineate which of them should be designated as psychodynamic?

Elucidating the scope and impact of psychoanalytic perspectives on early mental health interventions is challenging because there has been a widespread adaptation in clinical practice of concepts and therapeutic strategies that originated in psychoanalysis. As Jonathan Shedler (2010) has suggested, many elements of nonpsychodynamic evidence-based models of intervention may in fact be effective in part because skilled therapists practicing within these models actually incorporate interventions that are core to psychoanalytic practice and were described long ago by Freud and other early psychoanalytic writers. Such widely borrowed practices include a focus on affect and the expression of emotion; the exploration of attempts to avoid distressing thoughts and feelings; discussion of past experiences as a way of understanding the origins of current difficulties; and an emphasis on interpersonal relations. Additional key concepts derived from psychodynamic perspectives are highlighted below as nodal organizing constructs within the field of infant mental health (see also Luyten, Mayes, Blatt, Target, & Fonagy, Chapter 1, and Malberg & Mayes, Chapter 3, this volume).

"There's No Such Thing as an Infant"

When the psychoanalyst and pediatrician D. W. Winnicott (1975, p. xxxvii) made this assertion, he added, "Whenever one finds an infant one finds maternal care, and without maternal care there would be no infant." This single-minded focus on maternal care gradually expanded in optimal infant mental health practice to include the range of primary caregivers who make up the infant's caregiving network, and it is now widely acknowledged within the field that young children should not be assessed or treated without taking the caregiving relational matrix fully and actively into consideration. For example, the *Diagnostic Classification of Mental Health and Developmental Disorders of Infancy and Early Childhood—Revised* (DC:0–3R), a diagnostic system designed to redress the paucity of representation in the DSM system of disorders afflicting infants and toddlers, stipulates that infants cannot be ethically assessed or diagnosed without considering the child's functioning in the context of all significant caregiving relationships and environments (Zero to Three, 2005). Similarly, the administration protocol for the Bailey Scales of Infant Development includes instructions for the inclusion of the caregiver in the assessment process and suggests that this may well occur not in a clinic or testing facility but in a naturalistic setting such as a child's home (Bayley, 2006). In keeping with key tenets of diversity-informed infant mental health practice (St. John, Thomas, & Noroña, 2012), professionals are reminded to "honor diverse family structures." This means in part "[recognizing and striving] to counter the historical bias toward idealizing (and conversely blaming) biological mothers as primary caregivers while overlooking the critical childrearing contributions of other parents and caregivers including fathers, second mothers, foster parents, kin and felt family, early care and educational providers, and others" (p. 15). A comprehensive understanding of a child's functioning must extend beyond a consideration of the critical contributions of parents to an appreciation of the important influence of siblings and extended family, professional caregivers, and all the networks of relationships in which infants and families are embedded (Zeanah & Zeanah, 2009).

"There's No Such Thing as a Parent"

This extension of Winnicott's assertion indicates that parents are defined at least in part in relation to their baby. Parenthood is a malleable category, culturally constructed in important ways and inhabited differently by different individuals within and across cultures. Historically and geographically, specific expectations define who may be recognized as parent to a particular infant or child, and most industrialized societies reserve the right to rescind parental status should an individual be deemed unfit. Divergences may exist at times between who the child treats as his or her psychological parent and who society and/or the law recognizes as the child's parent. At the level of the individual and the family, particular babies carry particular meanings and elicit particular responses from caregivers depending on, for instance, the circumstances surrounding the pregnancy and childbirth; the baby's gender, birth order, health, temperament, and physical appearance; and the parents' ecological context and systems of support. For example, the parent of several children may have a very different psychological experience of parenthood in relation to each of his or her children and may act according to this individualized experience, thus in fact *being* a different parent to each child. A parent is co-created by the baby and the social world that recognizes that adult as parent to that baby, and these complex psychological processes are acknowledged, studied, and addressed in a range of ways within the field of infant mental health. An important outgrowth of this set of psychodynamic understandings of parenthood is the ethical mandate within the field of infant mental health to be guided by the family's own self-definition rather than importing or imposing a ready-made idea of who a child's parent may be or who comprises the family. As the National Research Council and Institute of Medicine state, "We use the term 'parenting' to capture the focused and differentiated relationship that the young child has with the adult (or adults) who is (are) most emotionally invested in and consistently available to him or her. . . . *Who* fills this role is far less important than the quality of the relationship he or she establishes with the child" (2000, p. 226).

Culture Matters

As with a great deal of psychological theory, psychoanalysis has been (rightly) criticized for its historical blind spots regarding the psychological significance of ethnicity, race and culture, and gender and sexual orientation. Nevertheless, psychoanalysis offers an interpretive framework that makes it impossible to disregard the powerful influence of culture on identity development, endogamous and exogamous group mapping, interpersonal relationships, and broader social systems of meaning. In recent decades, extensive cross-disciplinary psychoanalytic writing has addressed the psychodynamics of race as well as racism (e.g., Abel, Christian, & Moglen, 1997; Johnson, 1998; Lane, 1998; Seshadri-Crooks, 2000; Walton, 2001). The field of infant mental health has embraced an awareness of the importance of culture to infant/family experience, and culturally attuned service delivery has been adopted as a criterion for best practice within the field (Banerjee Brown, 2007; Maschinot, 2008).

A Baby Is a Subject (Coming-into-Being) with Agency

Freud asserted that, far from being a simple, passive creature devoid of ideas about the world or designs on it, the infant is in fact a complex, active being who strives from the first moments after birth to make sense of and influence the environment. Infant development research, partly spurred by psychoanalytically trained infancy researchers such as Daniel Stern (1995) and Beatrice Beebe (Beebe & Lachmann, 1994, 1998), has substantiated Freud's theories by demonstrating the amazing capacity of the newborn to seek out, take in, and respond to information, and organize him- or herself in relation to the caregiving environment. The field of infant mental health embraces this recognition of the personhood of the infant and seeks to protect and promote the possibility of the infant's full participation in social life in ways that are meaningful within a particular family, culture, and society.

Parental Deprivation Damages Infants and Young Children

Spitz (1946) demonstrated the critical importance of loving, individualized caregiving relationships by studying the devastation wrought by their absence for institutionalized infants even in the presence of adequate nourishment and physical care. The term *maternal deprivation* is commonly used, although loving caregiving is not gender-specific (Pruett, 1997). Young children are affected psychologically by separation from important caregivers, and, although expectable amounts of separation from the primary caregiver are growth-promoting while the infant is learning to navigate culturally and developmentally, prolonged separations may cause psychological harm requiring psychological healing—perhaps aided by intervention (Bowlby, 1969, 1973; Winnicott, 1971).

Some Infants/Families Are Haunted by "Ghosts in the Nursery"

This assertion by the social worker and psychoanalyst Selma Fraiberg (1987) has been credited with giving birth to the field of infant mental health (Stern, 1995). Fraiberg's galvanizing insight was that deeply entrenched, unresolved conflicts from the parent's past can be reenacted in the present parent–infant relationship, creating impediments to the parent's ability to perceive or respond to the infant as an individual by converting the baby into a transference object and leading the parent to "repeat the tragedy of his childhood with his baby in terrible and exacting detail" (Fraiberg, 1987, p. 101). The intergenerational repetition of problematic patterns of relating could, without intervention, repeat itself across many generations. Although the effort to interrupt such pathogenic cycles calls for specialized treatment and specific training, the field of infant mental health as a whole is informed by the acknowledgment of the power of intergenerational transmissions and by the awareness that service providers intervene at this consequential crossroad across a range of areas of expertise.

The basic psychodynamic principles described above constitute organizing axes within the multidisciplinary field of infant and early-childhood mental health. In the next section we describe CPP as a treatment approach that borrows from different theoretical orientations and clinical practices but is firmly rooted in the psychoanalytic model of infant mental health treatment pioneered by Selma Fraiberg (1980).

CPP: A PSYCHODYNAMIC TREATMENT APPROACH

The origins of CPP are traced to infant–parent psychotherapy, a relationship-based psychodynamic intervention developed by Selma Fraiberg and colleagues first at the University of Michigan, Ann Arbor, and then at the University of California, San Francisco (Fraiberg, 1980; Lieberman, Silverman, & Pawl, 2000; St. John & Pawl, 2000). Designed in response to the needs of a clinical population of parents and infants who also face dire economic and social hardship, CPP aims at improving the quality of the infant–parent relationship as a means of securing optimal developmental outcomes for the child. Its core components consist of psychodynamic psychotherapy, concrete assistance with challenges of daily life, and nondidactic developmental guidance, all offered in a single, integrated approach. An important adaptation of infant–parent psychotherapy was prompted by the understanding of pregnancy as a critical period for intervention to prevent the newborn baby's engulfment in maternal ambivalence, marital difficulties, or unresolved parental conflicts (Lieberman, 1983; Lieberman & Blos, 1980).

Three extensions of this approach have been developed in recent decades: trauma-focused relationship-based intervention (Lieberman & Van Horn, 2005, 2008), mental health consultation to early childhood settings (Johnston & Brinamen, 2006), and perinatal CPP to prepare expectant mothers traumatized by domestic violence and other stressors for the transition to parenthood (Lieberman, Diaz, & Van Horn, 2010). Clinicians across the United States and around the globe practice in the Fraiberg tradition (Weatherston, 2002). The terms *toddler–parent psychotherapy* (Lieberman, 1992; Toth, Rogosch, Manly, & Cicchetti, 2006) and *preschool–parent psychotherapy* (Toth, Maughan, Manly, Spagnola, & Cicchetti, 2002) have been coined to describe relational CPP at specific developmental stages of the child. The overarching term *child–parent psychotherapy* has been proposed as an umbrella term that encompasses relationship-based intervention in the Fraiberg tradition of psychoanalytically informed joint sessions of children in the birth-to-5 age range together with their parent(s) (Lieberman, Ghosh Ippen, & Marans, 2008; Lieberman & Van Horn, 2008), as well as perinatal CPP with expectant mothers (Lieberman et al., 2010).

Infants, toddlers, and preschoolers enter treatment with a wide range of presenting problems that include internalizing disorders, externalizing disorders, and symptom presentations that defy neat categorization as one or the other. In addition, infants and small children may be referred for treatment when a parent's mental health problems endanger the child's safety or healthy development. (This situation may be most familiar in the case of postpartum depression, in which a woman's capacity to provide the intensity of emotionally attuned care required by a newborn is severely compromised.) Alternatively, families may be referred because the parent–child relationship is imperiled as a result of a life event that has strained or ruptured it, such as domestic violence, bereavement, or the child's premature birth or congenital birth defect. CPP is grounded in the idea that whatever the difficulty, a small child's best chance at recovery and sustained healthy development rests with interventions that support and enhance the quality, adaptive functioning, and level of satisfaction in the parent–child relationship. When presented with a description of CPP, one young mother who found her active, curious, locomoting 8-month-old infuriatingly difficult to manage stated excitedly, "I get it. It's like couples therapy for me and my baby. That's just what we need!"

A central premise of CPP is that ordinary parent–child relationships are characterized by a set of relationship competencies that, in tandem with the maturational processes, provide mutual pleasure and promote healthy life-course development for children and parents. These competencies may be compromised or undeveloped due to myriad intrapsychic or environmental deficits. Intervention is aimed at building or restoring absent or impaired parent–child relationship competencies, and symptom reduction follows from this effort (St. John, 2015).

In addition, as noted above, CPP recognizes and responds to environmental threats to child and family well-being and frequently involves home visiting and clinical efforts that might be described as "advocacy" or "case management." CPP avoids such compartmentalized conceptualization of clinical efforts, instead viewing home visiting, advocacy, and concrete assistance when clinically indicated as inextricable from insight-oriented intervention. Lieberman and Harris (2007) have described the historical development and philosophical underpinnings of this component of CPP:

> An integral component of the [child]–parent psychotherapist's work is the mandate of attempting to ameliorate environmental stresses through active intervention with the social systems impinging on the parent and the child. Practical interventions, including

crisis management and assistance with problems of living, are implemented in tandem with insight-oriented clinical strategies. The [child]–parent psychotherapist integrates a sense of social justice into the therapeutic work. . . . In creating what she called "psychoanalysis in the kitchen," Fraiberg (1980) implicitly blended psychoanalysis with the ecological theory developed by Bronfenbrenner (1979, 1986), which urged an examination of individual functioning in the context of the family, neighborhood, and broader society. (p. 223)

This multidirectional focus of CPP—on the intrapsychic worlds of the child and the parent, the intersubjective field between them, and the broader environment in which they are nested (or through the cracks of which they are falling, as the case may be)—enables the therapist to synthesize diagnostic impressions of both parent and child together with an assessment of the quality of the relationship between them and the external forces impacting these, and to pinpoint critical targets of intervention. This approach brings together Stern's (1995) concept of representational "ports of entry" with Emde, Everhart, and Wise's (2004) "leverage" framework, where intervention strategies are guided by an analysis of perceived "best opportunities for engaging therapeutic or preventative change in a relationship that is embedded in a network of other relationships" (p. 278).

Informed by such an ecological analysis, the full range of psychodynamic interventions might come into play in any CPP treatment, as well as insights borrowed from other theoretical orientations. CPP flexibly incorporates techniques derived from social learning and cognitive-behavioral approaches, but these are offered in the context of a psychodynamic clinical framework, in keeping with Fraiberg's original approach of incorporating concrete assistance and other traditionally extrapsychoanalytic techniques into relationship-based treatment guided by fundamental principles of psychoanalysis, including the inevitability of ambivalence, conflict, and defense; consistent attention to unconscious processes; and belief in the healing power of symbolization. Here, we give brief and specific examples of six central therapeutic techniques of CPP. The common thread linking these techniques is the effort to *translate the child's experience to the parent and the parent's experience to the child*, so that bridges of understanding can be built between two subjectivities that are alienated or simply unaware of each other.

Addressing Two Generations of Infants Simultaneously

Perhaps the hallmark of psychodynamic child–parent interventions, this technique involves making a statement about an internal experience or relational template that is hypothesized to be true about both the present-day child and the parent-as-child long ago. It aims to interrupt the repetition of the past in the present whereby the parent's unresolved conflicts are being replayed at the child's expense. It is proffered in a generalized way because this approach may bypass parental defenses such as identification with the aggressor/disidentification from the victim. The therapist might say, for example, "A little girl needs her mother and gets frightened when she feels all alone." The therapist in this instance is attempting to interrupt an intergenerational pattern of parental abandonment by increasing the parent's capacity for empathy with a lonely child—both the parent-as-child and the present-day child. The hypothesis is that if the therapist can make the historic specter of the lonely little child less abhorrent to the parent, the parent will be better able to empathize with the present-day child, and that this shift can begin to occur outside of the parent's conscious awareness. This technique may be used with parents who are likely to defensively reject more direct interpretations.

Ghosts-in-the-Nursery Interpretations

Another classic CPP technique, the ghost-in-the-nursery intervention (Fraiberg 1980) is based on the same premise as the first, but the formulation is stated explicitly to the parent. The therapist might say, for example, "I think that when he cries and cries and nothing seems to help it makes you feel as helpless as when you were very little and your father yelled at you and blamed you even though you tried your hardest to please him and cooperate." As with the first intervention, the therapist is attempting to expand the parent's capacity for empathy both with the self and with the child, but in this instance the hope is to draw the parent's attention to the links between the present and the past. These direct links between the parent's unresolved emotional experiences from the past and current conflicts between parent and child are made when solid groundwork and a sturdy therapeutic alliance are present that will help the parent tolerate the pain that may be involved in bringing a defensively fended-off idea or affect to conscious awareness.

Interpretation-in-Action

Any psychotherapy with a small child involves a lot of action, and CPP is no exception. Interpretation-in-action (Renschler, 2009) engages nonverbal modes of symbolization as a means of communicating the therapist's understanding of the parent–child dynamics. A graphic example (Renschler, 2009) involves a therapist walking into a home visit with a father who had been routinely demeaned and undermined by his own father and who was now repeating these dynamics both with his son and with the therapist. On this particular day, the therapist found the father surrounded by parts of a stroller he was unsuccessfully attempting to assemble. The therapist sensed that this father's sense of incompetence was at risk of being confirmed yet again, but the therapist also knew that addressing this state of mind directly would be met with defensive denial and hostility. The therapist's interpretation-in-action took the form of asking the father if he would like a hand and then assisting with the project of constructing the stroller while painstakingly avoiding taking the lead. A verbal version of this interpretation might have been something like, "Your father would have made you feel incompetent at a moment like this as a way of making himself feel powerful when what you really would have wanted would be to work side-by-side with him." In this instance, the fragile ego of the father would likely have felt tantalized, exposed, abandoned, and humiliated by such a statement. *Doing* it (collaboratively joining him in the effort) seemed much more potent—and humane—than *saying* it (pointing out his desire for this).

Maintaining Inclusive Interaction

As described by St. John and Pawl (2000), this psychodynamic technique, inclusive interaction, stems from the recognition that all children, including preverbal infants, have a desire and the capacity to enter into "conversations" with their caregivers about matters of importance to them, and that ultimately it is what parents and children communicate to and understand from *each other*—not to and from therapists— that matters the most in healing relational disturbances. The technique involves a mode of listening and responding on the part of the therapist that takes the communications of child and parent(s) into constant consideration simultaneously and is directed at enhancing the capacity of each to register and respond to the communications of the other. Three levels of inclusive interaction intervention have been identified (Pawl & St. John, 1998). In the first level, the therapist conceptualizes whatever is occurring in the therapeutic encounter as representing something having to do with the parent–child relationship (e.g., the therapist interprets a mother's cold reception of her and the toddler's sour look as signals that parent and child were struggling in their relationship prior to her arrival at this home visit). The second level involves the therapist finding a way to communicate this understanding to the parent and child (e.g., "Looks like the two of you are having a rough time together!"). The third level entails involving the parent and child in the process of making meaning of their relational experience (e.g., "Did the two of you have different ideas of how to spend your time this morning?" or "Did something happen between you that left you both unhappy?").

Speaking for and to the Baby

As the examples above suggest, maintaining inclusive interaction frequently entails articulating the infant's imagined experience. For example, a therapist might say to a parent about a persistently crying baby, "The bottle doesn't seem to be soothing him. How frustrating! I wonder what else he might be telling us he wants with those cries?" In other instances, the therapist will speak directly *to* the baby in the presence of the parent. This is done, even with preverbal infants, in all seriousness. It is not that a preverbal infant is expected to comprehend the content of the communication in linguistic terms, of course. But even preverbal infants orient themselves to human interaction and appear to register when they are being addressed in a purposeful and affectful manner. And, beyond that, it does appear that the content of the interpretation—whether or not the therapist "gets it" —makes a difference. Thus, the therapist might say to the crying baby, "Your mother is trying to feed you but it seems it is not milk that you want. Are you crying because things have been so topsy-turvy in your family? Maybe you are having a hard time because your mother is so upset inside herself." Such an intervention may be effective in part as an interpretation for the benefit of the mother, but it has been regularly observed that infants as well as young children respond immediately and enduringly to well-timed interpretations expressed to them directly, regardless of the immediate effect on the parent (Norman, 2001, 2004; Salomonsson, 2010).

Creating a Trauma Narrative

Developing an account of stressful or traumatic experiences that has shared meaning between parent and child is an essential ingredient of healing from a significant disruption, loss, or trauma (Lieberman & Van Horn, 2008). Historically, infant–parent psychotherapy relied on the psychoanalytic practices of free association and free play, and therapists waited for the parent or the child to initiate discussion of a traumatic event such as physical abuse, exposure to domestic violence, or a death in the family. The rationale was that patients bring up clinically charged material when they are psychologically ready to work with it. In CPP, the influence of trauma theory, research, and clinical practice has led to a change in this practice when the therapist knows that a traumatic event has occurred. Child–parent therapists now initiate conversations about known traumatic events because failure to do so confirms and reinforces avoidance, which is one of the fundamental traumatic stress responses. When the child–parent psychotherapist, in the context of a "good enough" therapeutic alliance and using a judicious sense of timing, forthrightly addresses the painful (perhaps shattering) things that have happened to a parent and child, the clinician models a way of giving words to the unspeakable that helps to interrupt the pattern of phobic avoidance, shame-drenched silence, or worried expectation that the therapist's silence on the topic conveys a message of "Don't ask, don't tell" that confirms the child's and the parent's fears that what happened is too terrible to disclose. An example involves a 30-month-old who witnessed the battering of his mother by his father, who subsequently left the family. After carefully planning with the mother during preliminary individual meetings how to address this issue in the joint parent–child sessions, the therapist said to the child in the first joint session, "Your mommy told me that you saw your dad hitting her, and then he left, and now you hit and you bite and you can't sleep because you are so sad and scared." The toddler responded by going to the doll house and putting the mother and father dolls on the same bed. The therapist responded, with much feeling, "You miss your daddy. You want him to come back." This scene became the starting point for the course of treatment, which focused on the child's and mother's range of positive and negative feelings toward their often loving, intermittently abusive father and husband.

EMPIRICAL FINDINGS

There is rapidly growing evidence of empirical support for the efficacy of many psychodynamic intervention modalities aimed at treating childhood mental health difficulties, including evidence-based psychodynamic, relationship-focused, and/or attachment-based interventions geared specifically toward addressing difficulties arising in the first few years of life (see Buysse & Wesley, 2006; Midgley, 2009). The effective treatment of PTSD with psychoanalytic treatment approaches is specifically documented (Lieberman et al., 2008). A recent comparison of mother–infant psychoanalysis (Salomonsson, 2010) with nonpsychoanalytic mother–child interaction approaches for mother–infant dyads within the child protection services in Sweden showed differential improvement for dyads treated with the psychoanalytic modality.

The efficacy of CPP is supported by several randomized studies with samples varying in child age, referring problems, and ethnic and socioeconomic backgrounds in two separate university settings. The samples include maltreated infants in the child protection system (Cicchetti, Rogosh, & Toth, 2006), anxiously attached toddlers of low-income, recently immigrated, and often undocumented Latina mothers (Lieberman, Weston, & Pawl, 1991), toddlers of middle-class depressed mothers (Cicchetti, Rogosh, & Toth, 2006), maltreated preschoolers in the child welfare system (Toth et al., 2002), and preschoolers who witnessed domestic violence against the mother in addition to other violence-related traumatic stressors (Lieberman, Ghosh Ippen, & Van Horn, 2006; Lieberman, Van Horn, & Ghosh Ippen, 2005). Outcome findings include reductions in child and maternal psychiatric symptoms; more positive child attributions of parents, themselves, and relationships; improvement in the quality of the child–mother relationship and measures of security of attachment; and improvements in child cognitive functioning. In the United States, the Substance Abuse and Mental Health Services Administration National Registry of Evidence-based Programs and Practices (NREPP) recognizes CPP as an evidence-based treatment.

CLINICAL ILLUSTRATION

The following case illustrates the application of CPP with a parent–child dyad in the grip of a painful pattern of intergenerational repetition of neglect and maltreatment.

Referral and Presenting Problems

The dyad, comprising 18-month-old Dante and his 20-year-old mother, Brenda, were referred for CPP by Child Protective Services (CPS) in an effort to support them in the reunification process after Dante was removed from his mother's care and placed in foster care following an incident when she took him to the emergency room with a cut on his face. Brenda reported that Dante had injured himself when he fell while in her sister's care. During their investigation, emergency response child protection workers encountered a chaotic and high-conflict extended family situation and were unable to determine what had actually occurred, but the court found sufficient grounds to take jurisdiction based on the fact that Dante had clearly not been well enough protected from harm. The child welfare worker was committed to supporting reunification because she recognized that Dante was attached to his mother, who, in turn, expressed remorse at not having kept him out of harm's way and showed a passionate desire to "get him back." Weekly CPP sessions were undertaken by a child–parent therapist intern, occurring first in a supervised visiting room at the child welfare department and then in Brenda's home. Dante was returned to his mother's care four months into the treatment, and his CPS case was closed 2 months later, with CPP continuing for an additional 10 months beyond the reunification to further consolidate gains made in treatment.

Assessment, Diagnosis, and Case Formulation

At 18 months, Dante showed many symptoms of internalizing disorders, both depressive and anxious. He met the criteria for PTSD according to the DC:0-3R. He had experienced at least one known traumatic event resulting in an injury; frequently awoke from sleep crying and disoriented (suggesting that he suffered from nightmares); was withdrawn socially; tended to stare out into space in situations in which he was exposed to interpersonal conflict; and exhibited a restricted range of affect and little pleasure in most activities or interactions. He also showed co-occurring symptoms of depression and anxiety, and it seemed certain that many of his symptoms preceded the discrete traumatic event (the cut to his face). His play skills and interests were quite limited and characteristic of a younger child, and his vocabulary was limited to very few words. The symptom that Dante's mother found most distressing did not fall neatly into any single diagnostic category: Dante was preoccupied with food and unable to focus on anything else if food was present. He stuffed the food he was offered into his mouth in a frenzied way, held food in his mouth for long periods, insisted on keeping food in his pockets, stroller, and crib, and became distraught when food was taken from him. Brenda found these behaviors inexplicable and repulsive, and tended to berate him or ignore him in response.

Brenda met the criteria for a DSM-IV diagnosis of dysthymic disorder. She also had several symptoms of posttraumatic stress, including hypervigilance and emotional numbing. Brenda had spent several years in foster care herself—first between 4 and 5 years of age when she was removed due to neglect during a period when her mother was heavily engaged in substance abuse, and then again as an adolescent after being sexually abused by her mother's boyfriend. She became pregnant with Dante almost immediately after aging out of foster care and moving out of the group home where she had resided for the prior 3 years. Her sexual encounter with Dante's father had been an isolated event. She did not have an ongoing relationship with him, and he was in no way involved in Dante's rearing. Brenda now lived with a boyfriend, Joe, who had lost custody of two children due to physical abuse. As conditions for reunification, CPS stipulated that Joe needed to complete a 36-week anger management class and that both Brenda and Joe should participate in CPP as long as Brenda resided with Joe. Joe originally consented but soon discontinued attending both services, so the treatment constellation for CPP consisted of the mother–child dyad.

We hypothesized that Brenda was repeating in her relationship with Dante aspects of her own childhood experiences of abandonment and abuse. We speculated that she was enacting a pattern of identification with the aggressor/disidentification from the victim in part as an unconscious expression of loyalty to her mother, whom she professed not to care for. The clinical formulation included several related hypotheses, including the following propositions: (1) Brenda held a deep conviction that attachments constituted liabilities; (2) she was perpetuating a vacuum of emotional deprivation as a result of early experiences of emotional starvation that led her to feel that numbness was preferable to experiencing feelings; (3) the prospect of dependence was terrifying to her given how alone, unprotected, and unnurtured she had been as a dependant child; and (4) her ability to distinguish safety from danger was impaired as a result of her sexual abuse by a father figure and other traumatic experiences she had suffered.

With respect to Dante, we hypothesized that he had been exposed to chronic emotional neglect and chaotic caregiving, that his preoccupation with food was an expression of emotional starvation, and that food served both sensory and emotional soothing functions for him. In a vicious circle, his constant evocation of hunger and need (his gorging) led his mother to feel overwhelmed by the confrontation with her own deprivation and to distance herself from him in an effort at self-protection and perhaps to protect him from her defensive rage and desire to punish him. We understood that the events leading to his face injury, the medical treatment, and the extended sudden separation from his mother were traumatic events superimposed on a backdrop of prior emotional/relational/developmental difficulties, and were exacerbated by parental deprivation introduced by the removal from his mother and caregiving network. The racial and cultural components of the situation served to complicate the clinical picture further because Dante and Brenda were African American while the child welfare worker, the foster mother, and the child–parent therapist were all white, raising the likelihood that Brenda perceived these representatives of the dominant culture as menacing authorities who behaved in accordance with a historical pattern of hostile disregard for and active undermining of black family ties.

Treatment

In keeping with the core infant mental health principle that culture matters, the therapist and her supervisor (M. St. J.) recognized that establishing a productive therapeutic alliance depended on the therapist's ability to address the potential meanings for Brenda of the racial and cultural differences between them in the context of group and personal history, given Brenda's own foster care placement. Initially defensive and wary, Brenda seemed more open to the treatment following an initial conversation in which the therapist raised the question of how Brenda imagined Dante might experience being in a white foster home, and how the two of them were holding up with the array of white workers they were both contending with. While issues of race and culture were addressed at many points throughout the treatment, it was deemed unlikely that the therapeutic relationship would have been effective if these early transference-focused conversations had not taken place.

Within the first months of treatment, Brenda had to reckon with Joe's failure to follow through with the CPS requirements, which meant that he was impeding her ability to progress toward reunification with Dante. A stalemate was constellated for Brenda where her relationships with Joe and with Dante were in direct competition because the authorities in charge of reunification deemed Joe to be unsafe for Dante. This conundrum led the treatment directly into the issues of intergenerational repetition and Brenda's identification with, unconscious loyalty to, and unmourned love/loss of love of, her mother. The therapist used multiple CPP intervention techniques to work with these issues, including addressing two generations simultaneously ("It is harsh when a woman has to choose between her baby and her man") and ghosts-in-the-nursery interpretations ("I think it must have felt so horrible and scary to you when your mother chose her boyfriend over you. Maybe at some point you decided it was safer to be like her than to be somebody who gets hurt by her."). As these issues were addressed, important parent–child relational ground was gained because the more Brenda could consciously remember and experience her own past and present feelings, the more she could recognize and respond to these feelings as they arose in her relationship with Dante.

Dante proved a felicitous partner in this process because he responded readily and in clearly legible ways to his mother's increased capacities for attunement and empathy. The therapist made direct speaking-to-the-baby interpretations such as "Dante, you will not need to hold onto that cookie when you feel your mother is holding you and will not let you go again." She also made speaking-for-the-baby interpretations to Brenda (e.g., "I think Dante is using food to fill up a hole in his heart that can really only be filled by your love and closeness"). Dante's gorging and hoarding symptoms abated as Brenda became better able to recognize and respond to his emotional needs and to nurture/nourish him accordingly. This in turn was easier for her when the food-related symptoms that she had found repulsive began to decrease. Dante was gradually able to rely on his mother's body, voice, and interactions for both soothing and stimulation, and his repertoire of speech and play expanded as he relinquished his reliance on food for self-organization.

Brenda was eventually able to recognize Joe's dangerousness as she revisited her childhood exposure to sexual and physical violence in the context of the therapeutic relationship, which served as a safe holding environment where she could feel and express the pain that had so long been warded off. She ultimately decided to leave Joe in order to move forward in the reunification process and the child welfare worker assisted her in securing subsidized housing. Dante was placed with her full time at this point (4 months into treatment), but a spike in conflict between Dante and Brenda ensued immediately. The therapist arrived at a home visit during this period to find both of them sullen and exhausted, and Brenda reported that they had been engaging in struggles over nearly every logistic issue that had to be navigated. The therapist used a range of techniques of intervention, including maintaining inclusive interaction, speaking for and to the child, interpretation-in-action, and ghosts-in-the-nursery interpretations to address the issues she saw as salient.

The therapist hypothesized that the mother–child conflicts following reunification had erupted in part because the negative side of Brenda's ambivalence about parenting had been repressed during the time leading up to reunification, as she organized herself around the goal to "get Dante back" and admitted into consciousness only her wish to be with him. Now that the externalized struggle with CPS was over, Brenda was back in the throes of her internal conflict, and the parts of her that wished to be rid of Dante were holding sway. The therapist conveyed to Brenda her psychoanalytically informed assumption of parental ambivalence as a universal experience, and the mother seemed relieved by the therapist's empathic acceptance of what she had seen as evidence that she was an inherently "bad mother."

It may seem surprising that the therapist pursued all these conversations in the presence of the now 22-month-old Dante. A core principle of CPP holds that infants and small children are, at one level of consciousness or another, exquisitely sensitive to the suffering and struggles of their important caregivers, and that they process what they perceive through the filter of cognitive and emotional capacities that are in formation. In keeping with the developmentally expectable egocentrism of early childhood, for example, small children are quite prone to holding the conviction that they themselves have brought about events that are in fact entirely beyond their control.

Grounded in this set of convictions about the complex nature of early-childhood experience, the therapist assumed that Dante registered his mother's wish to be rid of him, and she sought to help him as well as his mother make sense of this perception. She said, "Dante, your mom is mad at herself because she didn't take good enough care of you before and that is why you had to go away to Mary's house where you would be safe. Your mom wasn't ready to keep you safe then, but she worked very hard to make sure the two of you could be together again and be safe now. Today she's a little confused and scared. She thinks that just because she is tired and grumpy and sometimes needs to be alone and rest that she is messing everything up again. But she is wrong. All mothers need to be alone sometimes, and that doesn't mean that they are bad mothers or their little boys are bad boys. You are both learning to be together in your new house, and you will keep learning every day." Both Dante and Brenda listened with rapt attention to the therapist's words, which served as the germ of the trauma narrative that the three of them elaborated further in the weeks and months that followed.

The development of the trauma narrative did not entail establishing a definitive account of all of the injuries and ruptures Dante and Brenda had suffered. The question of how Dante's face had been cut, for example, was never answered (although it was addressed straightforwardly with him), and many parts of Brenda's painful childhood remained inaccessible to her as conscious memory. But many things that had seemed unspeakable were brought into symbolization through the CPP. Brenda was able, for example, to avow her own failures in the care of Dante prior to his removal by CPS. She echoed the therapist's words regarding her abandonment of Dante, saying to him sadly (and bravely) on one occasion, "I handed you off, little man"—a powerful statement of agency that contrasted with her prior defensive stance that the system "took [her] baby away," a position that had left Dante all alone with the reality of his early emotional abandonment.

Dante, as his symbolic repertoire expanded in the context of the emotional holding he now experienced more often than not, played out themes of hunger and nurture, separation and reunion, danger and safety, with increased degrees of nuance and sophistication. With the therapist's help, Brenda embraced the idea that Dante's play was a form of communication and she learned to join him in it. When Brenda complained that she was bored of Dante's wanting her to feed the pretend food to the dinosaur again and again session after session, the therapist suggested that he might be patiently trying to tell them something that they had not yet understood. Brenda replied, "But we've been over and over it. I know he used to stuff himself because he was starved for love, but that doesn't happen anymore." The therapist suggested that perhaps Brenda needed to find a way to show Dante "in his own language" what she understood. Brenda narrowed her eyes and thought about this for a moment, and then in a beautiful application of her newfound capacities said to Dante, "That one's a meat-eating dinosaur. Forget that fake cake. Feed him somma' this!" and she held out her arm. Delighted, Dante had the dinosaur devour his mother, who was proud of this proof of her new literacy. The dinosaur tasted the therapist too, but it returned to feast on the mother. This joint act of symbolization represented the heart of the reparative work of CPP—the "talking/playing/doing cure" in the parent–child matrix.

CONCLUSIONS AND FUTURE DIRECTIONS

Newborns tend to take their families by storm, and development during the first few years of life unfolds with unparalleled force and rapidity. Experiences during these years are powerfully influential with respect to children's senses of themselves, expectations of others, and hopes for what promise the world might hold. Parents' experiences of these years are likewise consequential, as parental identity, though powerfully influenced by imported identifications and fantasies, is forged in the crucible of parent–child interactions. The stage is set during infancy and early childhood for who a parent and child will be to each other and how they will move through the world together. Rewarding relational experiences during these years can lead to cooperative partnerships that enable families to creatively manage adversity encountered down the road, whereas relational deprivations and injuries in the early years may drain and disable parent–child relationships in lasting ways, lending power to the inevitable external challenges that life brings.

CPP can benefit any family seeking to establish a new equilibrium that includes the new member of the family or struggling to manage the ordinary yet monumental challenges of early development and parenting. It is indicated when parental mental health difficulties are likely to impede parental functioning; when an infant, toddler, or small child is already symptomatic or seems to be at risk of developing emotional/relational difficulties; and when an infant–family suffers a significant loss or trauma, the effects of which might be lasting without developmentally attuned and relationship-focused working through. In our view, because of the formative influence of caregiving relationships and the family environment on small children's development, individual treatment of small children is to be considered only as an approach of last resort. We do practice CPP-informed individual play therapy with small children when dyadic or triadic intervention is impossible, such as when a child is orphaned, a parent is hospitalized or incarcerated, or an adult's parental rights have been severed and a child is awaiting adoption. Even in such instances, however, we rely on intensive collateral contact with foster parents, child welfare workers, and so on, to ensure that the work of the treatment considers and influences the caregiving environment. Whereas older children who are fully constituted as individuals can make good use of individual treatment, infants, toddlers, and preschoolers are in the process of differentiating themselves from their environments and consolidating senses of themselves using their caregiving relationships as the primary building blocks. Treatment at this age is most effective when it takes place in the parent–child matrix.

In a similar vein, we would caution those who treat adults who happen to have babies to be attentive to signs of struggle in the parent–child relationship and to consider referral for collateral CPP as indicated. While children may benefit to some degree from the long-term gains of their parents' individual treatment, opportunities may be lost for immediate improvements in the quality of the parent–child relationship that could ease the struggle in the short run and reroute the relationship so that it constitutes primarily a source of pleasure rather than strife for both parties, thus reducing the chances of overdetermined intergenerational repetitions of problematic patterns of relating. The power of the maturational processes, the potency of intergenerational resonance, and the passionate intensity of infant–parent interaction belong to infants and parents; CPP can support families in harnessing these forces in the service of relational healing, child and parent growth and well-being, and family self-determination.

While a psychodynamic approach has proven effective in decreasing symptoms and enhancing quality of attachment, cognitive performance, and sense of self in young children with a range of emotional problems that include internalizing disorders, additional research is needed to ascertain whether specific CPP modalities have a greater mutative impact in generating positive outcomes. Studies that compare psychodynamic intervention with other treatment modalities while controlling for treatment dose need to be conducted to address this question. The existing follow-up studies have been conducted at 6 and 12 months, and there is no information on whether the improvements persist for longer periods of time. Longer-term longitudinal studies are needed to address this important question.

ACKNOWLEDGMENT

We thank Robin Silverman, PhD, JD, for her contributions to the conceptualization of this chapter.

REFERENCES

Abel, E., Christian, B., & Moglen, H. (1997). *Female subjects in black and white: Race, psychoanalysis, feminism.* Berkeley: University of California Press.

Banerjee Brown, L. (2007). *Circles in the nursery: Practicing multicultural family therapy.* Washington, DC: Zero to Three Press.

Bayley, N. (2006). *Bayley scales of infant and toddler development* (3rd ed.). San Antonio, TX: Harcourt Assessment.

Beebe, B., & Lachmann, F. M. (1988). The contribution of mother–infant mutual influence to the origins of self- and object representations. *Psychoanalytic Psychology, 5,* 305–337.

Beebe, B., & Lachmann, F. M. (1994). Representation and internalization in infancy: Three principles of salience. *Psychoanalytic Psychology, 11,* 127–165.

Bowlby, J. (1969). *Attachment and loss: Vol. 1. Attachment.* London: Hogarth Press.

Bowlby, J. (1973). *Attachment and loss: Vol. 2. Separation: Anxiety and anger.* London: Hogarth Press.

Bronfenbrenner, U. (1979). *The ecology of human development: Experiments by nature and design.* Cambridge, MA: Harvard University Press.

Bronfenbrenner, U. (1986). Ecology of the family as a context for human development: Research perspectives. *Developmental Psychology, 22,* 723–742.

Buysse, V., & Wesley, P. W. (2006). *Evidence-based practice in the early childhood field.* Washington, DC: Zero to Three Press.

Cicchetti, D., Rogosch, F. A., & Toth, S. L. (2006). Fostering secure attachment in infants in maltreating families through preventive interventions. *Development and Psychopathology, 18,* 623–649.

Egger, H. L., & Angold, A. (2006). Common emotional and behavioral disorders in preschool children: Presentation, nosology, and epidemiology. *Journal of Child Psychology and Psychiatry and Allied Disciplines, 47,* 313–337.

Emde, R. N., Everhart, K. D., & Wise, B. K. (2004) Therapeutic relationships in infant mental health and the concept of leverage. In A. J. Sameroff, S. C. McDonough, & K. L. Rosenblum (Eds.), *Treating parent–infant relationship problems: Strategies for intervention* (pp. 267–292). New York: Guilford Press.

Emde, R. N., Polak, P. R., & Spitz, R. A. (1965). Anaclitic depression in an infant raised in an institution. *Journal of the American Academy of Child Psychiatry, 4,* 545–553.

Fraiberg, S. (1980). *Clinical studies in infant mental health: The first year of life.* New York: Basic Books.

Fraiberg, S., Adelson, E., & Shapiro, V. (1987). Ghosts in the nursery: A psychoanalytic approach to the problems of impaired infant–mother relationships. In L. Fraiberg (Ed.), *Selected writings of Selma Fraiberg* (pp. 100–136). Columbus: Ohio State University Press.

Fraiberg, L. (Ed.). (1987). *Selected writings of Selma Fraiberg.* Columbus: Ohio State University Press.

Freud, S. (1957). Five lectures on psychoanalysis. In J. Strachey (Ed. & Trans.), *The standard edition of the complete psychological works of Sigmund Freud* (Vol. 11, pp. 9–55). London: Hogarth Press. (Original work published 1910)

Gilliam, W. (2005). *Prekindergarteners left behind: Expulsion rates in state prekindergarten programs.* Foundation for Child Development Policy Brief Series no. 3. Retrieved from Foundation for Child Development website: *http://fcd-us.org/sites/default/files/ExpulsionPolicyBrief.pdf.*

Harmon, R. J., Wagonfeld, S., & Emde, R. N. (1982). Anaclitic depression: A follow-up from infancy to puberty. *Psychoanalytic Study of the Child, 37,* 67–94.

Johnson, B. (1998). *The feminist difference: Literature, psychoanalysis, race, and gender.* Cambridge, MA: Harvard University Press.

Johnston, K., & Brinamen, C. (2006). *Mental health consultation in child care: Transforming relationships among directors, staff, and families.* Washington, DC: Zero to Three Press.

Lane, C. (Ed.). (1998). *The psychoanalysis of race.* New York: Columbia University Press.

Lansford, J. E., Malone, P. S., Stevens, K. I., Dodge, K. A., Bates, J. E., & Pettit, G. S. (2006). Developmental trajectories of externalizing and internalizing behaviors: Factors underlying resilience in physically abused children. *Development and Psychopathology, 18,* 35–55.

Lieberman, A. F. (1983). Infant–parent psychotherapy during pregnancy. In S. Provence (Ed.), *Infants and parents: Clinical case reports* (pp. 84–141). New York: International Universities Press.

Lieberman, A. F. (1992). Infant–parent psychotherapy with toddlers. *Development and Psychopathology, 4,* 559–574.

Lieberman, A. F., & Blos, P. (1980). Make room for Paulie: Building attachment before birth. In S. Fraiberg (Ed.), *Studies in infant mental health: The first year of life* (pp. 242–259). New York: Basic Books.

Lieberman, A. F., Diaz, M., & Van Horn, P. (2010). Safer beginnings: Perinatal child–parent psychotherapy for newborns and mothers exposed to domestic violence. *Zero to Three Journal, 29*(5), 17–22.

Lieberman, A. F., Ghosh Ippen, C., & Marans, S. (2008). Psychodynamic treatment of child trauma. In E. B. Foa, T. M. Keane, M. J. Friedman, & J. A. Cohen (Eds.), *Effective treatments for PTSD: Practice guidelines from the International Society for Traumatic Stress Studies* (2nd ed., pp. 370–387). New York: Guilford Press.

Lieberman, A. F., Ghosh Ippen, C., & Van Horn, P. (2006). Child–parent psychotherapy: 6-month follow-up of a randomized controlled trial. *Journal of the American Academy of Child and Adolescent Psychiatry, 45*, 913–918.

Lieberman, A. F., & Harris, W. W. (2007). Still searching for the best interests of the child: Trauma treatment in infancy and early childhood. *Psychoanalytic Study of the Child, 62*, 211–238.

Lieberman, A. F., Silverman, R., & Pawl, J. H. (2000). Infant–parent psychotherapy: Core concepts and current approaches. In C. H. Zeanah (Ed.), *Handbook of infant mental health* (2nd ed., pp. 472–484). New York: Guilford Press.

Lieberman, A. F., & Van Horn, P. (2005). *Don't hit my mommy: A manual for child–parent psychotherapy with young witnesses of family violence.* Washington, DC: Zero to Three Press.

Lieberman, A. F., & Van Horn, P. (2008). *Psychotherapy with infants and young children: Repairing the effects of stress and trauma on early attachment.* New York: Guilford Press.

Lieberman, A. F., Van Horn, P. J., & Ghosh Ippen, C. (2005). Toward evidence-based treatment: Child–parent psychotherapy with preschoolers exposed to marital violence. *Journal of the American Academy of Child and Adolescent Psychiatry, 44*, 1241–1248.

Lieberman, A. F., Weston, D. R., & Pawl, J. H. (1991). Preventive intervention and outcome with anxiously attached dyads. *Child Development, 62*, 199–209.

MacDonald, H. Z., Geeghly, M., Grant-Knight, W., Augustyn, M., Woods, R. Y., Cabral, H., et al. (2008). Longitudinal association between infant disorganized attachment and childhood posttraumatic stress symptoms. *Development and Psychopathology, 20*, 493–508.

Maschinot, B. (2008). *The changing face of the United States: The influence of culture on child Development.* Washington, DC: Zero to Three Press.

Midgley, N. (2009). Research in child and adolescent psychotherapy: An overview. In M. Lanyado & A. Horne (Eds.), *Handbook of child and adolescent psychotherapy: Psychoanalytic approaches* (2nd ed., pp. 71–97). New York: Routledge.

National Research Council and Institute of Medicine. (2000). *From neurons to neighborhoods: The science of early childhood development* (J. P. Shonkoff & D. A. Phillips, Eds.). Washington, DC: National Academies Press.

Norman, J. (2001). The psychoanalyst and the baby: A new look at work with infants. *International Journal of Psychoanalysis, 82*, 83–100.

Norman, J. (2004). Transformations of early infantile experiences: A 6-month-old in psychoanalysis. *International Journal of Psychoanalysis, 85*, 1103–1122.

Pawl, J. H., & St. John, M. (1998). *How you are is as important as what you do in making a positive difference for infants, toddlers and their families.* Washington, DC: Zero to Three Press.

Pruett, K. (1997). How men and children affect each other's development. *Zero to Three Journal, 18*(1), 3–11.

Renschler, T. S. (2009). Sleeping on the couch: Interpretation-in-action in infant–parent psychotherapy. *Journal of Infant, Child, and Adolescent Psychotherapy, 8*, 145–155.

St. John, M. (2015). *Parent–child relationship competencies: A framework for tapping the power of parent–child relationships in guiding infant/family and early childhood mental health assessment, treatment planning and intervention.* Manuscript in preparation.

St. John, M., & Pawl, J. H. (2000). Inclusive interaction in infant–parent psychotherapy. In J. H. Pawl, C. A. Ahern, C. Grandison, K. Johnston, M. St. John, & A. Waldstein (Eds.), *Responding to infants and parents: Inclusive interaction in assessment, consultation, and treatment in infant/family practice.* Washington, DC: Zero to Three Press.

St. John, M., Thomas, K., & Noroña, C. (2012). Infant mental health professional development: Together in the struggle for social justice. In K. Thomas, J. D. Osofsky, & S. Powers (Eds.), Emerging issues in infant mental health from the Irving B. Harris Foundation Professional Development Network. *Zero to Three Journal, 33*(2), 13–22.

Salomonsson, B. (2010). *"Baby worries": A randomized controlled trial of mother–infant psychoanalytic treatment.* Stockholm, Sweden: Karolinska Institute.

Scaramella, L. V., Sohr-Preston, S. L., Callahan, K. L., & Mirabile, S. P. (2008). A test of the family stress model on toddler-aged children's adjustment among Hurricane Katrina impacted and nonimpacted low-income families. *Journal of Clinical Child and Adolescent Psychology, 37*, 530–541.

Seshadri-Crooks, K. (2000). *Desiring whiteness: A Lacanian analysis of race.* New York: Routledge.

Shedler, J. (2010). The efficacy of psychodynamic psychotherapy. *American Psychologist, 65*, 98–109.

Silverman, R., Lieberman, A. F., & Pekarsky, J. P. (1997). Anxiety disorder. In *DC:0–3 casebook: A guide to the use of Zero to Three's diagnostic classification of mental health and developmental disorders of infancy and early childhood in assessment and treatment planning* (pp. 47–59). Washington, DC: Zero to Three Press.

Spitz, R. A. (1946). Anaclitic depression: An inquiry into the genesis of psychiatric conditions in early childhood. *Psychoanalytic Study of the Child, 1*, 47–53.

Stern, D. (1995). *The motherhood constellation: A unified view of parent–infant psychotherapy.* New York: Basic Books.

Tandon, M., Cardeli, E., & Luby, J. (2009). Internalizing disorders in early childhood: A review of depressive and anxiety disorders. *Child and Adolescent Psychiatric Clinics of North America, 18*, 593–610.

Toth, S. L., Maughan, A., Manly, J. T., Spagnola, M., & Cicchetti, D. (2002). The relative efficacy of two interventions in altering maltreated preschool children's representational models: Implications for attachment theory. *Developmental Psychopathology, 14*, 877–908.

Toth, S. L., Rogosch, F. A., Manly, J. T., & Cicchetti, D. (2006). The efficacy of toddler–parent psychotherapy to reorganize attachment in the young offspring of mothers with major depressive disorder: A randomized preventive trial. *Journal of Consulting and Clinical Psychology 74*, 1006–1016.

Trentacosta, C. J., Hyde, L. W., Shaw, D. S., Dishion, T. J., Garden, F., & Wilson, M. (2008). The relations among cumulative risk, parenting, and behavior problems in early childhood. *Journal of Childhood Psychology and Psychiatry, 49*, 1211–1219.

U.S. Department of Health and Human Services, Administration of Child, Youth and Families. (2007). Child maltreatment. Retrieved from *www.acf.hhs.gov/programs/cb/pubs/cm07/cm07.pdf.*

Walton, J. (2001). *Fair sex, savage dreams: Race, psychoanalysis, sexual difference.* Durham, NC: Duke University Press.

Weatherston, D. (2002). *Case studies in infant mental health.* Washington, DC: Zero to Three Press.

Winnicott, D. W. (1971). The location of cultural experience. In *Playing and reality* (pp. 128–139). New York: Routledge.

Winnicott, D. W. (1975). *Through pediatrics to psychoanalysis.* London: Hogarth Press.

Zeanah, C. H., & Zeanah, P. D. (2009). The scope of infant mental health. In C. H. Zeanah (Ed.), *Handbook of infant mental health* (3rd ed., pp. 5–21). New York: Guilford Press.

Zero to Three. (2005). *Diagnostic classification of mental health and developmental disorders of infancy and early childhood: Revised edition (DC:0–3R).* Washington, DC: Zero to Three Press.

CHAPTER 19

Conduct Disorders

Jonathan Hill and Helen Sharp

Recurrent, serious problems of aggression and oppositionality are often referred to collectively as the conduct disorders (Hill, 2002). They are commonly first evident in early childhood, and carry a substantially increased risk of later criminality and psychiatric disorders, spanning depression, anxiety disorders, substance misuse, and personality disorders (Odgers et al., 2008). Our understanding of their nature and their origins has increased dramatically over the past 30 years as the result of high-quality research worldwide. However, it could be argued that psychodynamic perspectives have played very little part in the evolution of our empirical understanding of conduct disorders in children. Few researchers in the field would regard them as relevant, and explicit theorizing referring to psychoanalysis or psychodynamics is almost entirely absent from the research literature. In particular, even though many of the leading psychoanalytic theorists, such as Anna Freud and Melanie Klein, have provided detailed theories of normal and aberrant development, their views have rarely influenced empirical studies, despite continuing to underpin the therapeutic work of many dynamic therapists.

In this chapter we argue that the contemporary relevance of psychodynamic perspectives lies not so much in the developmental theory but in its modes of explanation and activity. Specifically, we present a theoretical approach that integrates psychodynamic perspectives with attachment theory and recent empirical findings, and discuss the potential relevance of reflective interpersonal therapy for children and parents (RICAP; Roff, 2008) in this regard.

A key element in psychodynamic approaches from Freud's early writings onwards has been the proposition that psychopathology may arise from attempts during childhood to deal with intolerable states of mind, such as intense fear, through mental processes. This is particularly likely to occur either in the presence of severe threat, such as that presented by maltreatment, or in the absence of sources of relief, or both. These attempts are described in psychoanalysis in terms of psychic defenses (see also Luyten, Mayes, Blatt, Target, & Fonagy, Chapter 1, and Waldinger & Schulz, Chapter 6, this volume). However, examples such as "over-general memories" can be found in contemporary cognitive science based on very similar principles. We have proposed that coping strategies in childhood that entail inhibition of the "intentional stance," whereby others' actions are interpreted in terms of their meaning, may also perform a similar function—"solving" a problem while at the same time creating the conditions for maladaptive behavior patterns (Hill, Fonagy, Lancaster, & Broyden, 2007; Hill, Murray, Leidecker, & Sharp, 2008). In the face of repeated threats, for example, of physical violence, dropping to the "physical stance," in which behaviors are interpreted merely as physical events, enables the child to avoid the emotional implications of others' behaviors, and hence in some respects brings relief. Penalties are, however, paid in adopting this strategy if it becomes generalized and limits the child's ability to interpret the meaning of others' actions, undermining effective social action, and increasing the likelihood of using coercive solutions to social challenges. Evidence for the contribution of these processes in the conduct disorders will be described later in the chapter. First, we review current empirically based hypotheses regarding the classification and origins of the conduct disorders and discuss psychodynamic explanations, contrasting them with other kinds.

CLASSIFICATION AND DIAGNOSIS

Problems of persistent disruptive and aggressive behaviors are the most common form of childhood psychiatric problems in the community and in referrals to child mental health services in the West (Hill, 2002). These behaviors lead to considerable distress in children and their families, and are associated with social and educational failure. Young children with these problems are at substantially increased risk for antisocial behaviors in adolescence and adult life, are likely to have impaired interpersonal and work functioning, often cross conventional thresholds for personality disorders, and have an increased rate of adult psychiatric disorders (Odgers et al., 2008). They are more likely to enter and contribute to violent marriages and cohabitations, hence putting the next generation at risk.

The conduct disorders are distinctive among mental disorders in that they are embedded in the patient's social context and have consequences for victims, apart from conferring harm on the individual patient. Many features of these disorders are seen in social interactions, notably, verbal and physical aggression, bullying, oppositional behavior, and lying. Thus, the symptoms of the disorders are also social behaviors that arise in the context of family, peer, educational, and wider social relationships, and in turn have a detrimental impact on these relationships. The origins, maintenance, and cessation of the symptoms cannot be understood independently of these contexts. Equally, the symptoms are not simply the product of social processes, in that individual vulnerabilities are known to play a prominent role. Biological, psychological, and social processes are all implicated in the etiology and treatment of the conduct disorders, through additive and interactive effects (Hill, 2002).

The two principal classification systems, DSM-5 (American Psychiatric Association [APA], 2013) and ICD-10 (World Health Organization [WHO], 1992), are quite similar in that both specify behaviors that must be present for diagnosis of a conduct disorder. Both emphasize the persistent duration of the symptom behaviors for some months. The principal difference is that, in DSM-5, oppositional defiant disorder (ODD) and conduct disorder (CD) are separated, whereas in ICD-10 the criterion set of items required for CD is very close to what would be obtained by combining the DSM-5 ODD and CD items (Costello, Mustillo, Erkanli, Keeler, & Angold, 2003). ODD is defined as a recurrent pattern of negativistic, defiant, angry, and hostile behaviors leading to impairment of day-to-day activities, and CD as the repetitive and persistent violation of the basic rights of others and societal norms.

Although the principal classification systems, DSM-5 and ICD-10, take a categorical approach, there is no natural category, and outcomes associated with ODD and CD are predicted best by scores. In a study that systematically examined the predictive validity of categorical diagnoses versus dimensional measures of ODD and CD (Fergusson & Horwood, 1995), the dimensional variables were better predictors of outcome than the categories. There appeared to be a dose–response relationship of increasing risk for juvenile offending and school dropout associated with increasing severity of disruptive behaviors. Furthermore, genetic influences appear to operate in a similar manner in relation to conduct problems, irrespective of whether they are assessed as dimensions or categories (Eaves et al., 1997). Although diagnoses are commonly used as categories in clinical settings, a major drawback of this categorical approach is that important differences in the severity or type of dysfunction below and above the cutoff are lost. In this chapter the term *conduct problems* is therefore used to refer to persistent problems of oppositional, destructive, or aggressive behaviors taken to be a broad phenotype that may be assessed categorically or dimensionally.

Estimates of the prevalence of conduct problems vary according to the criteria used. However, on the basis of the majority of epidemiological studies from the industrialized West, between 5 and 10% of children aged 8–16 years have significant persistent oppositional, disruptive, or aggressive behavior problems (Egger & Angold, 2006).

Disruptive and aggressive behavior problems with onset from around 2 years of age onward have been distinguished from those with adolescent onset on the basis both of risk factors and adult outcomes. Early-onset "life course persistent" (Moffitt, Caspi, Harrington, & Milne, 2002) problems are associated with multiple individual and family risks, including temperamental vulnerabilities, lower verbal IQ, impairments in executive function, history of parental criminality, family disruption, and child maltreatment. They strongly predict poor adult outcomes. By contrast, adolescent-onset, "adolescence-limited" problems are associated with fewer risk factors, and their adult outcomes are better than those of the life-course-persistent group.

Equally, though, their deviance is not limited to adolescence, and they do share some of the poor outcomes of the life-course-persistent group (Odgers et al., 2008).

While early-onset, life-course-persistent conduct problems share poor long-term outcomes, it is likely that there is heterogeneity in the vulnerability and risk factors and underlying processes. We do not yet know how much heterogeneity there is. However, at least three possible pathways can be envisaged. In the first, vulnerability arises from early temperamental emotional reactivity, sometimes referred to as *difficult temperament* (Lee & Bates, 1985). This refers to a temperamental profile characterized by a low threshold for becoming upset, with intense distress that is difficult to calm. Some longitudinal studies have found that emotional reactivity in infancy is predictive of later conduct problems, commonly when it occurs together with negative parenting or low parental guidance (Belsky, Hsieh, & Crnic, 1998; Smeekens, Riksen-Walraven, & van Bakel, 2007). These problems are thought to be mainly of proneness to aggression that is angry and reactive, although studies have yet to demonstrate this specific continuity. Physical abuse also contributes to the risk of childhood aggression (Jaffee, Caspi, Moffitt, & Taylor, 2004). The link between exposure to physical abuse and reactive aggression may be mediated, at least in part, via a proneness to interpret others' neutral or mildly angry behaviors as hostile or threatening, leading to easily triggered intensely angry responses (Dodge, Pettit, Bates, & Valente, 1995). Although the term *difficult temperament* is commonly used, with its implication that these infants are harder to parent, it is probably misleading in two important respects. First, it does not distinguish between anger proneness and fearfulness. These emotional states cannot be distinguished during the first weeks of life, but they certainly can by one year, and they perform quite different functions. Anger proneness is likely to contribute to the pathway to conduct problems, whereas fearfulness is more likely to lower the risk of such problems, for reasons including the inhibition of aggressive or disruptive behaviors and the promotion of fear conditioning (Hill, 2002). Second, infants with high levels of negative emotionality whose parents are able to respond calmly, without withdrawing or retaliating, may become the most skilled at emotion regulation, and hence well adapted (Belsky & Beaver, 2010).

A second potential pathway involved in conduct problems is related to the development of so-called callous–unemotional (CU) traits. There is much current interest in a possible subgroup of conduct-disordered children who show a lack of conscience or concern for others' feelings, particularly their distress, and whose aggression is predominantly instrumental and apparently not accompanied by anger. Compared to others with conduct problems, children with CU features have lower trait anxiety, are less likely to have experienced adverse parenting, and have higher verbal IQ (Frick & Viding, 2009). Genetic influences on CU traits may be different from those involved more generally in conduct disorders (Viding, Blair, Moffitt, & Plomin, 2005). It has been argued that CU traits arise from a deficit in fear recognition and processing, perhaps as the result of underactivity of the amygdala and without substantial contributions from environmental variations (Blair, 2008). Developmental studies have found that early fearfulness is associated with the development of conscience (Kochanska, 1997), and CU traits may therefore have their origins in fearlessness in early development. This possibility is supported by studies finding prospective associations between parent-reported fearlessness in infancy and later conduct problems, and predictions from observed fearlessness at age 2 to conduct problems at age 8 (Shaw, Gilliom, Ingoldsby, & Nagin, 2003). However, the prospective association between early fearlessness and CU traits has not been examined in published studies. This pathway may be explained by a neurobiological deficit acting independently of the environment rather than by reactivity to environmental stressors. On the other hand, some limited evidence would suggest that a warm, reciprocal, positive relationship may promote attachment security and conscience development in fearless children and hence reduce the risk for CU traits (Kochanska, 1997). Furthermore, harsh parenting may be to some degree associated with CU traits (Waller et al., 2012).

Thus far, we have considered two pathways in which the risk is thought to arise either from persistent adverse environments without a major contribution from adaptive mechanisms, or from a neurobiological deficit, neither of which is close to psychodynamic models. However, many developmental theories, not only those with strong psychodynamic influences, envisage forms of adaptation to adversity in which the child acquires strategies to downregulate negative emotions where the environment is either threatening or unsupportive. As the temperament researchers Derryberry and Rothbart (1997) noted, under these conditions the child "may come to rely upon primarily avoidant strategies, disengaging attention from the threatening situation without attending to sources of relief and available coping options" (p. 647). Derryberry and Rothbart are referring primarily to behavioral strategies, but the dilemma, and the form of the solution and its implications, are the same as those envisaged by Freud and Bowlby. Some states of fear or distress require a resolution, and if none is available, the child has to find a strategy to deal with them, and this strategy is likely to—or perhaps inevitably will—come at a cost. Within a psychodynamic framework, the cost is that an area of mental life becomes disconnected from the remainder, still emotionally charged and potentially threatening, but not available for review or understanding. Later in life, for example, as the individual meets the demands of adolescent sexual relationships, it is reactivated and again threatens the equilibrium of the person unless transformed into something else such as a symptom. From an information-processing perspective, the cost of an avoidant strategy may be that the child ceases to attend to the details of the threatening social encounter and other social experiences that to a greater or lesser extent resemble it. Thus, the child's attention to the details is diminished, and he or she is more likely to work from generalized inaccurate schemas, leading to a limited repertoire of social problem-solving options. Both psychodynamic and information-processing formulations envisage that the coping strategy is used to downregulate negative emotions. This is likely to have implications for functioning in relationships and for the regulation of aggression. Where the child uses an avoidant strategy, the negative emotions are not brought into the parent–child relationship, and hence the child is deprived of the experience, and does not practice the skills, of regulating emotions within close relationships. Downregulation of fear may inhibit anxious inhibition of antisocial or aggressive behaviors and reduce fear conditioning. In what follows, we expand on these formulations.

PSYCHODYNAMIC APPROACHES TO CDs

Attachment and CDs

Ever since Bowlby's (1944) original observations linking early separation experiences to juvenile delinquency, there has been an interest in the possible contribution of insecure attachment to the conduct disorders. In a meta-analysis from 69 samples ($N = 5,947$), moderate and significant associations were found between attachment status and externalizing problems (Fearon, Bakermans-Kranenburg, van IJzendoorn, Lapsley, & Roisman, 2010). However, as is evident from their review, studies have varied considerably in the methods used to ascertain attachment, and the findings have not been consistent. For example, some studies find main effects of attachment status (e.g., Moss et al., 2006), and others find effects only in interaction with other risk factors (e.g., Fearon & Belsky, 2011). It is also clear that many individual studies have examined the relationship between attachment status and conduct disorders without yielding strong evidence regarding either the extent or nature of the association. There have been three main reasons for this: small sample sizes, the modest stability of attachment status over time, and a lack of explicit theorizing regarding the link between attachment and aggression and oppositional behaviors. Attachment status in infancy is generally assessed using the Strange Situation, which yields a four-category classification: secure, insecure ambivalent, insecure avoidant, and disorganized (see Mikulincer & Shaver, Chapter 2, this volume). In general population samples, approximately 60% of infants are rated as secure, 15% disorganized, and the remainder ambivalent or avoidant (van IJzendoorn, Schuengel, & Bakermans-Kranenburg, 1999). Studies typically employ sample sizes in the range of 100–200, and thus the number of children in each insecure attachment subgroup ranges between 10 and 30, limiting statistical power. This commonly leads to insecure groups being collapsed, which has consequences for attempts to understand links to conduct disorders. In contrast to the theory, which predicts that early relationship experiences lay the foundations for later relationships, implying stability, children commonly move from one attachment category to another, even over quite short periods of time (Vondra, Shaw, Swearingen, Cohen, & Owens, 2001). Change of attachment status is commonly associated with environmental changes, raising the question of whether attachment status is primarily, or even solely, an index of recent psychosocial stressors (Thompson & Raikes, 2003).

Although few attempts have been made to integrate attachment processes into a broader model of conduct problems, three strands can be identified in the research literature. In the first, attachment processes are not thought to contribute to the psychopathology, but they do influence the child's ability to elicit or make use of support from caregivers in solving the problems posed by their behavior problems (Speltz, DeKlyen, & Greenberg, 1999). In the second, conduct problems are seen as a direct manifestation of insecure and, generally, either ambivalent or disorganized attachment (Moss et al., 2006). In the case of the ambivalent-dependent pattern, the child shows exaggerated dependency with parental figures, often accompanied by angry resistance and conflictual exchanges. This attention-seeking strategy may become increasingly maladaptive with age, as developmental expectations for autonomy increase. Disorganized attachment, characterized by a lack of a coherent emotion-regulation strategy with caregivers, may be "solved" in some children by the development of a "controlling-punitive" role-reversed attachment pattern with their parents. Communication between controlling-punitive children and their parents has been described as characterized by failed reciprocity and periods of very low engagement or hostile, conflictual interaction (NICHD Early Child Care Research Network, 2004). Conduct problems may arise where these interactions become generalized outside the family: "Disorganized and controlling children may not believe that they can master the challenges of engaging competently with others and see them as a potential threat, they may demonstrate fight or flight behaviors, that is aggression accompanied by fearful affect, in which children aggress to ward off perceived threats" (Moss et al., 2006, p. 439).

Finally, attachment processes may interact with other emotion-regulatory processes to create the risk for conduct problems. For example, avoidant attachment (in which emotionality is downregulated with attachment figures following separation) in combination with low temperamental fearfulness was found to predict conduct behaviors 2 years later (Burgess, Marshall, Rubin, & Fox, 2003). The difficulties in researching this area are illustrated by findings from the NICHD study, which has the largest sample size to date. In this study, over 1,000 infants were assessed using the Strange Situation, and nearly 800 were followed up at the age of 11 years. Disorganized attachment predicted increasing conduct problems, but only in boys who experienced high psychosocial risk. The total number of disorganized boys was 53, of whom only 13 were in the high-risk group (Fearon & Belsky, 2011).

Revival of Traditional Psychodynamic Approaches to Understanding CD

While the integration of traditional psychodynamic perspectives into a program of research into conduct disorders must be a long-term goal, these perspectives have never been envisaged as tied in any straightforward way to an empirical program. This is because traditional psychoanalysis has prioritized explanation over method. Psychoanalysis started with, and has preserved ambitions tightly linked to, physical medicine, where the characterization of the features or symptoms of the disorder is linked to the underlying processes and to concepts of function and dysfunction. This is in contrast to most empirical traditions in psychology and psychiatry, which have defined clinical problems in terms of behaviors and impairment, largely free of specification of underlying process, and lacking a clear method for demarcating function and dysfunction. To put it another way, phenotypes in the study of psychopathology are largely descriptive and probably map poorly on to mechanism. The problem is widely recognized, and there is general acceptance that a tighter link between disorder and mechanism will reveal that most so-called disorders, whether specified dimensionally or categorically, are heterogeneous (Arango, Kirkpatrick, & Buchanan, 2000; Hasler, Drevets, Manji, & Charney, 2004), and equally that there may be commonalities of mechanism across ostensibly different conditions (Conway, Hammen, & Brennan, 2012). Viewed in this context, psychoanalysis, paradoxically, while appearing to have become disconnected from the empirical agenda regarding psychopathology in general and conduct disorders in particular, adopts an approach that is more in tune with an empirical agenda to be set for the 21st century than the one that prevailed in the second half of the 20th century.

Psychodynamic perspectives are firmly committed to explaining symptoms in terms of meanings. Meanings are what we use in everyday life to explain our own and others' behaviors, for example, in terms of love, fear, rejection, or loss, and these have an important place in the currency of psychodynamic perspectives and treatments. This form of explanation stands in contrast to many of the prevailing perspectives in the empirical approaches to psychopathology of the late 20th century. These envisaged that explanations of psychopathology would resemble physical accounts of medical disorders, with causes such as pressure on the brain that would make no reference to meanings. Inasmuch as patients ascribed meaning to the origins of their problems, they would be simply displaying an "effort after meaning" in the way parents might blame themselves for their child's leukemia. This view envisaged a contrast, captured in Jaspers's (1923/1963) distinction between meaningful and causal connection. Late 20th-century empirical approaches to psychopathology commonly embraced Jaspers's distinction, and following him, envisaged that a troubling dualism would be resolved by redefining the meaningful in the currency of causal connections. Psychoanalysis asserts that meanings are causal! Furthermore, they cannot be redescribed in the terms of the "pressure on the brain" kind of causality. This approach paved the way for forms of treatment in which the meaning of an individual's thoughts, emotions, relationships, and life history were highly relevant.

This emphasis on meaning has probably contributed to the marginalization of psychodynamic perspectives within the scientific enterprise, because meanings seem to be so far from the "hard" causal mechanisms of biology. We have previously argued that meaning, as understood in everyday life, is a particularly elaborated form of intentionality, and intentional-causality is pervasive in biological processes irrespective of whether they are psychological (Bolton & Hill, 2004). The term *intentionality* is used here within a long philosophical tradition to refer to a quality of "aboutness" or directedness. Thus, states of mind such as elation or sadness have intentionality with respect to success or loss; the intentionality of the dance performed by bees on their return to the hive refers to the distance and direction of nectar; activations of the amygdala refer to threat; and impulse frequencies in nerves from baroreceptors to the brainstem have intentionality with respect to blood pressure. If we follow this line of argument, then meanings, as a subset of the wider arena of intentional causal processes, have a causal role within the biology of psychopathology without any implied loss of humanity. Meanings are embedded in narratives, and psychoanalytic treatments create the conditions for telling and reviewing personal stories. In psychoanalytic work with young children, for instance, play is a central medium of expression, and play-based research assessments have begun to contribute to our understanding of the conduct disorders.

The idea that meanings have a causal role in psychopathology leads to a major question: How can processes that explain adaptive or functional behaviors also explain symptomatic or dysfunctional behaviors? This issue concerns not only how such processes account for dysfunction, but also how they can give rise to symptoms experienced as coming "out of the blue" like a physical illness, and why they persist in the face of apparently favorable circumstances and when, generally, they are not in the best interests of the sufferer. Freud's answers are central to the contribution of psychodynamic perspectives and to their application to conduct disorders.

Before going on to discuss some psychodynamic perspectives in more detail, we feel it essential to emphasize that Freud himself revised many of his views, and that since his time there have been many debates and controversies resulting in multiple, and frequently contradictory, opinions. In many respects, Freud's earliest writings are some of the most illuminating in relation to psychopathology. In his essays with Breuer on the origins of hysteria and of obsessions, he wrestles with the questions of how a psychological disorder, arising from experiences with personal meaning, could in the same way as a physical condition have origins of which the sufferer is not aware, how early experiences could have effects that are evident only later in life, and how mental mechanisms could account for the specific symptoms of the disorder (Breuer & Freud, 1895). Crucially, in this early work, he concluded that hysteria has its origins in early sexual trauma—famously, he subsequently reversed this view because he did not believe that sexual abuse was sufficiently common to account for large numbers of cases. It is now clear that childhood traumas—not only sexual abuse, but also physical abuse and exposure to domestic violence—are common, and that they make a major contribution to many forms of psychopathology (Hill, 2002). Freud argued that sexual trauma in childhood was linked to hysteria via early coping strategies to deal with the distress or anxiety associated with the trauma.

The key elements of Freud's hypothesis were that even young children employ mental mechanisms to deal with trauma, and that these can alleviate distress and hence perform an adaptive function, but at a cost that is evident later in development. Symptoms of disorder therefore represent elements of both earlier and current attempts to find a solution to the problem of regulating emotions generated by severe threat. It is crucial to this hypothesis that the child does not have alternative solutions to the distress. In the case of sexual abuse, this is commonly because of the surrounding coercion and secrecy. Freud is uncompromising in his description of the horror of child maltreatment. In his lecture "The Aetiology of Hysteria" (Freud 1896/1962), he encapsulates the way the adult misuses his authority to gratify his needs, rendering the child helpless and confused.

Post-Freudian developments gave increasing emphasis to "object relations," the dynamics of early processes with caregivers and their role in shaping an individual's internal representations of relationships, which in turn are thought to influence later intimate relationships. The internalization of early caregiver–child relationships is also central to attachment theory. Attachment theory, like early Freudian theory, focuses on infant regulation of distress. However, in contrast to Freud, Bowlby's emphasis is on the implications for emotion regulation of a caregiver's availability to provide comfort and calm the infant (Bowlby, 1973). Both theories argue that when distress (fear, anxiety, or sadness) is intense, and hence likely to be intolerable, the infant has to find a way to reduce it. Under most circumstances, according to attachment theory, regulation is achieved through the parent's comfort. Regulation in the face of intense distress caused by maltreatment may not be achieved even with the comfort of a caregiver. Equally, more ordinary levels of distress may not be regulated where the caregiver is unpredictable or unavailable. In either case, according to psychoanalytic and attachment theories, the child will attempt to perform mental operations that lessen the mental pain, through defensive or avoidant maneuvers. Theories of disorganized attachment (see Steele & Steele, Chapter 20, this volume) bring together the Freudian emphasis on trauma with Bowlby's emphasis on parent–child interactions by hypothesizing that the infant's regulatory strategy is radically undermined where the caregiver is the source of the trauma; hence, there is no source of comfort.

Early Freudian theories of the child's efforts to manage intense distress, coupled with object relations and attachment theories, provide a fairly comprehensive model of distress regulation within close relationships. However, it is missing one key element, namely, individual differences in emotional reactivity. Children differ markedly from early infancy in temperament, how readily they become upset, the intensity and duration of their distressed states, and how easily they are soothed (Derryberry & Rothbart, 1997). Whether or not a traumatic experience gives rise to distress depends not only on the nature of the trauma but also on the child's emotional reactivity, and likewise the child's need for comfort in the face of everyday threats. Thus, a revised psychodynamic perspective on emotion regulation needs to take account of the child's emotionality, together with the extent of adversity or trauma to which the child is exposed, and the availability of comfort from caregivers. The likelihood that the infant will employ defensive strategies to deal with extreme distress will depend on all three factors.

Freud saw that a model of what maintains disorder is required, and he proposed a mechanism. The hypothesis is that psychopathology may arise from attempted solutions to problems that themselves involve sacrifices. It follows that the mechanism underlying the disorder is motivated, and not readily abandoned, unless alternative solutions are available. The mechanism entailed an adaptation early in life to deal with an intolerable state of mind, hypothezised to be associated with sexuality, which remained adaptive until adult life, when sexuality became a prominent issue. A similar mechanism has been hypothesized to account for adult-onset depression associated with childhood sexual abuse (Hill, Pickles, Rollinson, Davies, & Byatt, 2004).

Child sexual abuse is only one of a number of forms of maltreatment commonly faced by children that are associated with child and adult psychopathology and are very likely to have a causal role. To understand the developmental pathways, we focus on the dilemma of the threatened, frightened child lacking a source of relief. The psychodynamic perspective will tend to ask what it is like to be in that child's shoes and what psychological algorithms are available to the child. This will go something like this: he or she can either transform his or her perception of threat so that it becomes benign, and hence solve the problem of the emotional state, or change the emotional state so that it transforms the perception of the threat, or attempt to behave in a way that deals with the threat. We have explored one possible way in which reinterpreting threatening experiences may reduce fear or distress while at the same time creating the conditions for conduct disorders, using the concept of intentionality referred to earlier.

According to Dennett (1996), when interpreting others' behaviors we adopt the "intentional stance," meaning that we infer beliefs, wishes, plans, and emotions from their expressions, tones of voice, and actions. This permits rapid interpretation and underpins timely and effective social action. Where others' actions are threatening, at least three factors are likely to influence the child's emotional responses and regulation: the child's emotional reactivity, the severity of the threat, and the availability of comfort. The intentional stance is adaptive where the effects of these factors, singly or jointly, do not lead to overwhelming or intolerable distress. The alternative "physical stance," in which others' behaviors are interpreted in terms of their physical characteristics, without reference to interpersonal motives, is much less likely to provide an accurate sequence of information processing and emotional reaction leading to rapid, effective action. However, under conditions that lead to overwhelming or intolerable distress, use of the physical stance may have advantages. Although the intentionality of loud voices and raised arms, interpreted accurately as anger, and hence threatening, creates fear and anxiety, using the physical stance to interpret loud voices and raised arms as simply loud voices and raised arms enables the emotional accompaniments to be avoided. This kind of adaptation may, however, create problems in social understanding, and hence increase the likelihood that a child will attempt to resolve social challenges with coercive tactics.

Studies of abused children illustrate the penalties of not implementing coping strategies designed to reduce distress. Those exposed to high levels of parental anger expression and physical abuse become attuned to signals of threat in the social environment. They are faster to recognize anger as faces go from neutral to angry, and they attend to auditory anger cues more than nonmaltreated children do. The extent to which children attend to anger cues mediates the relationship between physical abuse and their reports of anxiety (Shackman, Shackman, & Pollak, 2007).

The idea that psychopathology may have its origins in early psychological adaptation now has its parallels in theories of the effects of early neurobiological adaptation. Fetal origins hypotheses argue that harmful long-term effects of fetal adversity arise from adaptations in utero that have advantageous consequences for physiological regulation later in life in some environments, but confer risk in others (Glover, 2011). This "developmental origins of health and disease" hypothesis was first developed to account for the relationship between low birth weight and cardiovascular disease in later life. The association between low birth weight and later disease is thought to arise from a predictive adaptive response of the fetus leading to the "thrifty" phenotype, which is suited to a poor nutritional environment later in life but not to high-carbohydrate Western diets. The long-term effects of low birth weight are not, however, confined to physical diseases. Recent studies have indicated that low birth weight predicts later psychiatric disorders, including depression and schizophrenia (Costello, Worthman, Erkanli, & Angold, 2007). The risk is amplified by major childhood adversities, implying that the vulnerability may arise where the child encounters more than the expectable level of threat, for example, in the form of child maltreatment.

Fetal-origins hypotheses have also been applied to the effects of prenatal stress. In animal models, prenatal stress is associated with a reduction in birth weight and subsequent increased likelihood of disorders of cardiovascular function and glucose homeostasis. The effects are mediated by excess exposure of the fetus to glucocorticoids, which result in low birth weight and hypothalamic–pituitary–adrenal axis dysregulation. Prenatal stress is also associated with behavioral and neuroendocrine indices of increased stress reactivity. Long-term effects of prenatal stress can also be seen as a predictive adaptive response in anticipation of a high-threat environment (Glover, 2011). In humans, indices of prenatal stress, such as maternal anxiety during pregnancy, are associated with later emotional and behavioral problems in children, and depression in adults, after accounting for postnatal exposures (O'Connor, Heron, Golding, & Glover, 2003). A challenge for the future is to explore how these contrasting forms of early adaptation may jointly contribute to later risks for psychopathology.

EMPIRICAL FINDINGS

A key feature of the psychoanalytic approach, as we saw at the beginning of the chapter, has been its close tie to therapy. In contrast to behavioral and cognitive-behavioral approaches, where therapy and research remained close, for many years psychoanalytic therapies and developmental research diverged. This gap has to some degree closed. Researchers who are also psychoanalysts have contributed to techniques that promise to bring the research closer to the clinical setting. This has, for example, been exemplified through the development of story stem techniques, in which children are invited to portray their inner world through play, within a setting that allows their responses to be quantified for research purposes (e.g., Emde, Oppenheim, & Wolf, 2003). Most of the pioneers of psychoanalytic work with children, including Anna Freud, Melanie Klein, and Donald Winnicott, viewed play as the vital medium of expression of children from around 2 to 10 years of age. They did not, however, agree on what play conveyed or on how to work with it in therapy. Story stem techniques allow the researcher to introduce some structure by standardizing the scenarios that the child is asked to address while leaving the child free to develop the story. Much of the pioneering work carried out by Bob Emde, Inge Bretherton, Denis Wolf, JoAnne Robinson, and David Oppenheim, and funded by the MacArthur Foundation, is described in the book *Revealing the Inner Worlds of Young Children: The Macarthur Story Stem Battery and Parent–Child Narratives* (Emde et al., 2003).

Many other variants of the technique have been developed, including those focusing on attachment (Green, Stanley, Smith, & Goldwyn, 2000) and on the child's portrayal of family life (Murray, 2007). The disagreements, especially those between Anna Freud and Melanie Klein, find echoes in dilemmas regarding how to use story stems for measurement. To what extent do children provide an account in play of their current life realities, and to what extent is play a visible manifestation of the way their minds work? The answer is impossible to quantify in the absence of external validation, but a range of coding systems reflect the fact that children probably engage in both Picking up from our initial consideration of the ways in which children may, in their minds, transform adverse experiences in order to make them tolerable, we focus on some ways in which this may be seen in their responses to story stems.

Intentionality can be rated from children's performance in story stem assessments. We illustrate this with the "Scary Dog" story from the MacArthur Story Stem Battery (MSSB). In MSSB story stems, there is a named child doll figure who is the same sex as the child being assessed, two parent figures, and sometimes other characters such as siblings or friends. In the Scary Dog story stem as told to a boy, Michael is in the park with his parents, and he is playing with his ball. The ball runs close to some bushes, and as Michael goes to fetch it a large dog emerges and barks loudly at him. The administrator makes the sound of a dog barking and then portrays Michael saying, "Oh, oh, I am so scared." The administrator then says, "Show me and tell me what happens next." A high intentionality score for portraying characters with feelings, wishes, plans, or beliefs would be given for a response along the lines of "Michael runs back to his mother and father, and his father picks him up and tells him not to worry, and Michael starts to feel better." Lower intentionality would be rated where the child replied using the physical stance, for example, "Now the dog is jumping on the ball, mom is talking to dad, and Michael is sitting on the ground," as behaviors are portrayed in which the explanatory states of mind are neither made clear nor implied.

Low intentionality, that is, adopting the physical stance in response to threat, has two-sided properties in the same way as denial. On the one hand, as outlined earlier, low intentionality can provide a way of responding to threat without generating the accompanying anxiety. On the other, it can contribute to conduct problems. First, by reducing anxious inhibition, it may remove the brake on antisocial behaviors and reduce fear conditioning and, hence, the effectiveness of punishment. Second, it will impair the child's ability to interpret others' behaviors in threatening social encounters, reducing the capacity to respond with appropriate assertiveness. The child then either runs the risk of repeated experiences of helplessness in social encounters or may attempt to deal with such encounters using coercive behaviors. Third, the child's awareness of the impact of his or her behaviors on others is likely to be reduced, also reducing social problem solving and creating a lack of responsiveness to others' suffering. Fourth, it may impair the child's ability to make use of previous experiences to modify future behaviors. This is because the intentional stance deals in broad cross-modal categories, so that previous experiences (e.g., of fear and comfort) can readily be generalized to other anticipated situations in which fear is caused for quite different reasons, or comfort provided in different ways. By contrast, physical stance memories of a dog jumping on a ball or of sitting on the ground are unlikely to inform events under different physical conditions. Finally, the child who employs the physical stance to interpret others' behaviors or others' experience of his or her behaviors may also apply it to his or her own mental life, thereby experiencing him- or herself as a physical object rather than a psychological being. The effect of adopting the physical stance to avoid fear may have particularly severe consequences where the child preserves the intentional stance in relation to situations associated with anger. This intentional stance is likely to be influenced by a sensitivity to anger cues and a low threshold for intense angry responses. Thus, the child will be prone to angry responses unmodified by the beneficial effects of fear or anxiety described earlier.

If low intentionality scores, representing the physical stance, are a means of dealing with fear or anxiety, and they contribute to conduct problems, then children with conduct problems should show reduced intentionality when responding specifically to story stem challenges that portray a distressed or frightened child. We compared a group of boys referred with conduct problems and a community control group, using four MSSB story stems (Hill et al., 2007). Two story stems portrayed fear/distress, "Scary Dog" and "Burnt Hand" (in which the child knocks a pan of soup over and burns his hand), and two portrayed conflicts (one in which the parents argue over lost keys, and the other in which friends have a dispute and get into a fight). The referred boys had lower mean intentionality scores for the fear/distress stories, consistent with their use of the physical stance to deal with distress. However, in response to the conflict stems, they did not show lower intentionality but did exhibit more aggression than control children. This suggested that the children did adopt the intentional stance in relation to conflict and aggression, leading, in their play, to heightened aggression. The effect of the combination of adopting the physical stance to avoid fear and preserving intentionality focused on anger-related hostile cues is illustrated in the case example provided later in this chapter.

We also examined the role of attachment security in the subsequent portrayal of intentionality in story stem assessments using data from Lynne Murray's study of children of women with postnatal depression. Attachment was assessed at 18 months in the Strange Situation, and story stems were administered at age 5 years (Hill, Murray, et al., 2008). Infants rated as insecure in the Strange Situation showed behavioral evidence of limitations in distress regulation with caregivers, in the form of either avoidance of emotional expression and regulation, or heightened emotionality. The avoidance may be the behavioral forerunner of a physical stance strategy, and the heightened emotionality a limitation in emotion regulation for which a physical stance strategy may be employed. We therefore predicted that insecure attachment in the Strange Situation would be associated with lower intentionality scores at age 5, indicating greater use of a physical stance strategy, specifically when tackling a story stem with a threatening theme. Unlike the MacArthur story stems, these stems included neutral (bedtime) and positive (happy and best time) contrasts to a high-threat story stem, "Show me what happens at a bad and nasty time." Compared with the secure group, the insecure children had significantly lower mean intentionality scores in their responses to the high-threat stem, but they did not differ in their responses to the neutral or positive story stems. The difference in the effects of security on high-threat versus low-threat story stems, tested as a statistical interaction, was significant ($p = .006$). Intentionality scores in response to the high-threat scenario mediated the link between insecure attachment and teacher-rated conduct problems, but only in the children of women with postnatal depression. It is not possible to tell from this study how the vulnerability in the children of the postnatally depressed mothers arose—whether it was genetic, or arose from the effects of prenatal depression or anxiety on the fetus or from postnatal experiences with their depressed mothers. Yet, there was evidence for a specific link between insecure attachment in infancy and the subsequent use of the physical stance in the face of threat, consistent with our proposal that the physical stance represents an attempt at adaptation where sources of comfort have not been successful in reducing distress. In turn, among children with a preexisting vulnerability, use of the physical stance, evidenced in lower intentionality scores, was associated with elevated conduct problems.

PSYCHODYNAMIC TREATMENT OF CDs: RICAP

The central premise of this chapter is that psychodynamic perspectives are concerned with the dynamics of adaptive mental processes and ways in which those dynamics may under some circumstances undermine psychological functioning. Therapeutically, the importance of this approach is that it points to the possibility that the child may not suffer from malfunction, or be repeatedly making mistakes, but in fact, through symptomatic behavior, is attempting to solve a problem. In that case, the task of the therapist is to see the problem, understand the child's attempts, and work with the child to find possible alternative adaptive behaviors that better meet the child's current psychological needs. Furthermore, intervention involving the current primary caregivers may bring further benefits. Changes in parental understanding of the child's communications may ensure that their own parenting behavior and conceptualization of the child's "problems" can promote healthy development and maintenance of adaptive alternative child understandings and behaviors over time.

Here we briefly describe a structured treatment for conduct disorders that integrates psychodynamic perspectives with attachment theory and recent empirical findings. RICAP (Roff, 2008) aims to help children with resistant conduct problems, particularly where there has been a complex interplay over time between child vulnerability, adult vulnerability, and adverse environment. These are the conditions under which parent training is less likely to be effective.

RICAP is a manualized therapy that involves two therapists working in parallel with the parent(s)/carer(s) and child separately. The focus is, first, on facilitating the child's capacity to think about his or her own emotions, thoughts, and behaviors, and those of others—in other words, to develop the capacity to reflect and self-reflect. The child is asked to draw pictures of topics such as "Draw you and your mom doing something together." The therapist sticks the drawings inside a book, together with a written summary of the conversations and reflections between the child and therapist about the drawings, between each session. The child and therapist review the book each week so that the drawings are available to form a narrative of the child's thoughts and feelings individually and in close relationships. The process of therapist completion between sessions provides the child with an experience of being held in mind. The experience of hearing another person's reflections about the drawings, and having a conversation about ideas, gives the child access to the mind of another. Understandings can be developed, reconsidered, and revised as the treatment progresses.

The parent(s) joins for 10 minutes at the start of the session to share one good time and one difficult time during the past week, and at the end they plan together for the next week. In parallel work, the second therapist and the parent(s) review recent events reflecting on the child's possible underlying feelings, intentions, and motives. This generates new understandings on which to base ideas for new parenting responses.

The drawings often reveal a much more coherent inner world than is apparent from the child's "mindless" behavior, and one in which the child is able to express a sense of self or explain what the portrayed figures are trying to do. For children prone to adopting the physical stance in the face of adversity, the conversations about the drawings enable the therapist and child to adopt the intentional stance, curious to explore what emotions and behaviors are about. Thus, the treatment, though influenced by attachment theory and research, also has strong links with psychoanalytic aims to replace symptoms with narrative—a narrative generated and owned by the child.

CLINICAL ILLUSTRATION

We briefly illustrate RICAP with an example,[1] described more fully by Roff (2008). Ollie, a 5-year-old boy, was referred because of his outbursts of angry destructive behavior, which had included pulling a door off its hinges and kicking a hole in a wall, and physical aggression including kicking, biting, and hitting. He had previously been abused and neglected by his natural parents, and now he lived with foster parents who were considering adopting him. He had been in nine care placements before the age of 3 years. His foster parents viewed his behaviors entirely in terms of opposition and anger when he could not get his own way. His first drawing in response to the therapist's request to "draw the problem" (in session 4) shows him smearing mud over the wall in response to his mother saying "No"' when he asked for a glass of lemonade. He entitles the drawing "Repmet" (Figure 19.1).

The therapist (Anne) wrote in the book:

> When Anne said it was strange how Ollie had no arms—how did the mud get on the wall—Ollie quickly drew them in.
> They are big arms.
> Anne wondered if Ollie felt important having a temper.
> Ollie said he felt powerful.

Anne wondered later if Ollie also felt upset, inside out and back to front like "repmet" ("temper" backwards).

Over time, and through the conversations between the therapist and Ollie written in the book, and the parallel work with both foster parents, two themes emerged: one

---

[1] From Roff (2008). Copyright 2008 by John Wiley & Sons, Ltd. Reprinted by permission.

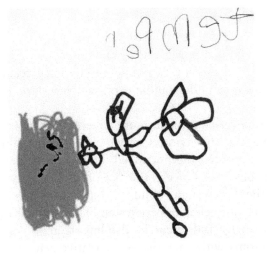

FIGURE 19.1. "Repmet." From Roff (2008). Copyright 2008 by John Wiley & Sons, Ltd. Reprinted by permission.

of anger in response to threat, and the other of fear, probably arising from his earlier experiences of powerlessness and loss. In this example, the foster parent's "No" sufficiently resembled his earlier experiences of threat to trigger an emotional response. While the anger was apparent to Ollie and his foster parents, the fear became apparent only through the conversations. In terms of the previous discussion of intentionality, the intentionality of Ollie's behaviors as "about" anger was evident to him and to his foster parents, while the role of fear and his attempts to avoid it became apparent only during the treatment. Once it was clarified, he became more able to show distress, to which his caregivers could respond by comforting him.

CONCLUSIONS AND FUTURE DIRECTIONS

Although psychodynamic perspectives have not so far contributed significantly to the rapidly expanding body of knowledge of the conduct disorders, they are highly relevant to the development of future work. This is likely to entail the demarcation of pathways based on an understanding of mechanisms, some of which will implicate threats to emotion regulation in infancy and during childhood.

The psychodynamic hypothesis that vulnerability to disorder arises from early adaptations to threat that have a later cost is highly relevant to the conduct disorders. Avoidant strategies such as repression or adopting the physical stance can be effective ways of dealing with intolerable distress, but also undermine adaptation later in life. Where threat continues in a child's life, avoidant strategies may continue to diminish fear, while heightened sensitivity to threat may lead to easily triggered aggression. Where threat does not continue, minor provocations that in some ways resemble previous, more serious adverse experiences may also trigger one or both of heightened anger or fear avoidance. Problems of destructiveness and aggression, no less than those of nonorganic physical symptoms or obsessions, may reflect, unobserved by the child or those who care for him, extreme distress coupled with his long-standing efforts to feel better. However, more research along these lines is needed, as well as studies investigating the efficacy and effectiveness of RICAP and other treatments in conduct disorders.

REFERENCES

American Psychiatric Association. (2013). *Diagnostic and statistical manual of mental disorders* (5th ed.). Arlington, VA: Author.

Arango, C., Kirkpatrick, B., & Buchanan, R. W. (2000). Neurological signs and the heterogeneity of schizophrenia. *American Journal of Psychiatry, 157,* 560–565.

Belsky, J., & Beaver, K. M. (2010). Cumulative-genetic plasticity, parenting and adolescent self-regulation. *Journal of Child Psychology and Psychiatry, 52,* 619–626.

Belsky, J., Hsieh, K. H., & Crnic, K. (1998). Mothering, fathering, and infant negativity as antecedents of boys' externalizing problems and inhibition at age 3 years: Differential susceptibility to rearing experience? *Development and Psychopathology, 10,* 301–319.

Blair, R. J. (2008). The amygdala and ventromedial prefrontal cortex: Functional contributions and dysfunction in psychopathy. *Philosophical Transactions of the Royal Society B: Biological Sciences, 363,* 2557–2565.

Bolton, D., & Hill, J. (2004). *Mind, meaning and mental disorder.* Oxford, UK: Oxford University Press.

Bowlby, J. (1944). Forty-four juvenile thieves: Their characters and home-life (II). *International Journal of Psycho-Analysis, 25,* 107–128.

Bowlby, J. (1973). *Attachment and loss: Vol. 2. Separation: Anxiety and anger.* London: Hogarth Press.

Breuer, J., & Freud, S. (1895). *Studies on hysteria.* Boston: Beacon Press.

Burgess, K. B., Marshall, P. J., Rubin, K. H., & Fox, N. A. (2003). Infant attachment and temperament as predictors of subsequent externalizing problems and cardiac physiology. *Journal of Child Psychology and Psychiatry, 44,* 819–831.

Conway, C. C., Hammen, C., & Brennan, P. A. (2012). Expanding stress generation theory: test of a transdiagnostic model. *Journal of Abnormal Psychology, 121,* 754–766.

Costello, E. J., Mustillo, S., Erkanli, A., Keeler, G., & Angold, A. (2003). Prevalence and development of psychiatric disorders in childhood and adolescence. *Archives of General Psychiatry, 60,* 837–844.

Costello, E. J., Worthman, C., Erkanli, A., & Angold, A. (2007). Prediction from low birth weight to female adolescent depression: A test of competing hypotheses. *Archives of General Psychiatry, 64,* 338–344.

Dennett, D. C. (1996). *The intentional stance.* Cambridge, MA: MIT Press.

Derryberry, D., & Rothbart, M. K. (1997). Reactive and effortful processes in the organization of temperament. *Development and Psychopathology, 9,* 633–652.

Dodge, K. A., Pettit, G. S., Bates, J. E., & Valente, E. (1995). Social information-processing patterns partially mediate the effect of early physical abuse on later conduct problems. *Journal of Abnormal Psychology, 104,* 632–643.

Eaves, L. J., Silberg, J. L., Meyer, J. M., Maes, H. H., Simonoff, E., Pickles, A., et al. (1997). Genetics and developmental psychopathology: 2. The main effects of genes and environment on behavioral problems in the Virginia Twin Study of Adolescent Behavioral Development. *Journal of Child Psychology and Psychiatry, 38,* 965–980.

Egger, H. L., & Angold, A. (2006). Common emotional and behavioral disorders in preschool children: Presentation, nosology, and epidemiology. *Journal of Child Psychology and Psychiatry, 47*, 313–337.

Emde, R. N., Oppenheim, D., & Wolf, D. P. (2003). *Revealing the inner worlds of young children: The Macarthur Story Stem Battery and Parent–Child Narratives.* New York: Oxford University Press.

Fearon, P. R. M., & Belsky, J. (2011). Infant–mother attachment and the growth of externalizing problems across the primary-school years. *Journal of Child Psychology and Psychiatry, 52*, 782–791.

Fearon, P. R. M., Bakermans-Kranenburg, M. J., van IJzendoorn, M. H., Lapsley, A.-M., & Roisman, G. I. (2010). The significance of insecure attachment and disorganization in the development of children's externalizing behavior: A meta-analytic study. *Child Development, 81*, 435–456.

Fergusson, D. M., & Horwood, L. J. (1995). Predictive validity of categorically and dimensionally scored measures of disruptive childhood behaviors. *Journal of the American Academy of Child and Adolescent Psychiatry, 34*, 477–485; discussion 485–477.

Freud, S. (1962). The aetiology of hysteria. In J. Strachey (Ed., & Trans.), *The standard edition of the complete psychological works of Sigmund Freud* (Vol. 3, pp. 187–221). London: Hogarth Press. (Original work published 1896)

Frick, P. J., & Viding, E. (2009). Antisocial behavior from a developmental psychopathology perspective. *Development and Psychopathology, 21*, 1111–1131.

Glover, V. (2011). Annual Research Review: Prenatal stress and the origins of psychopathology: an evolutionary perspective. *Journal of Child Psychology and Psychiatry, 52*, 356–367.

Green, J., Stanley, C., Smith, V., & Goldwyn, R. (2000). A new method of evaluating attachment representations in young school-age children: The Manchester Child Attachment Story Task. *Attachment and Human Development, 2*, 48–70.

Hasler, G., Drevets, W. C., Manji, H. K., & Charney, D. S. (2004). Discovering endophenotypes for major depression. *Neuropsychopharmacology, 29*, 1765–1781.

Hill, J. (2002). Biological, psychological and social processes in the conduct disorders. *Journal of Child Psychology and Psychiatry, 43*, 133–164.

Hill, J., Fonagy, P., Lancaster, G., & Broyden, N. (2007). Aggression and intentionality in narrative responses to conflict and distress story stems: An investigation of boys with disruptive behaviour problems. *Attachment and Human Development, 9*, 223–237.

Hill, J., Murray, L., Leidecker, V., & Sharp, H. (2008). The dynamics of threat, fear and intentionality in the conduct disorders: Longitudinal findings in the children of women with postnatal depression. *Philosophical Transactions of the Royal Society B: Biological Sciences, 363*, 2529–2541.

Hill, J., Pickles, A., Rollinson, L., Davies, R., & Byatt, M. (2004). Juvenile- versus adult-onset depression: Multiple differences imply different pathways. *Psychological Medicine, 34*, 1483–1493.

Jaffee, S. R., Caspi, A., Moffitt, T. E., & Taylor, A. (2004). Physical maltreatment victim to antisocial child: Evidence of an environmentally mediated process. *Journal of Abnormal Psychology, 113*, 44–55.

Jaspers, K. (1963). *General psychopathology* (J. Hoenig & M. W. Hamilton, Trans.). Manchester, UK: Manchester University. (Original work published 1923 as *Allgemeine Psychopathologie*. Berlin, Germany, Springer Verlag)

Kochanska, G. (1997). Multiple pathways to conscience for children with different temperaments: From toddlerhood to age 5. *Developmental Psychology, 33*, 228–240.

Lee, C. L., & Bates, J. E. (1985). Mother–child interaction at age two years and perceived difficult temperament. *Child Development, 56*, 1314–1325.

Moffitt, T. E., Caspi, A., Harrington, H., & Milne, B. J. (2002). Males on the life-course-persistent and adolescence-limited antisocial pathways: Follow-up at age 26 years. *Development and Psychopathology, 14*, 179–207.

Moss, E., Smolla, N., Cyr, C., Dubois-Comtois, K., Mazzarello, T., & Berthiaume, C. (2006). Attachment and behavior problems in middle childhood as reported by adult and child informants. *Development and Psychopathology, 18,* 425–444.

Murray, L. (2007). Future directions for doll play narrative research: A commentary. *Attachment and Human Development, 9,* 287–293.

NICHD Early Child Care Research Network. (2004). Affect dysregulation in the mother–child relationship in the toddler years: Antecedents and consequences. *Development and Psychopathology, 16,* 43–68.

O'Connor, T. G., Heron, J., Golding, J., & Glover, V. (2003). Maternal antenatal anxiety and behavioural/emotional problems in children: A test of a programming hypothesis. *Journal of Child Psychology and Psychiatry, 44,* 1025–1036.

Odgers, C. L., Moffitt, T. E., Broadbent, J. M., Dickson, N., Hancox, R. J., Harrington, H., et al. (2008). Female and male antisocial trajectories: From childhood origins to adult outcomes. *Development and Psychopathology, 20,* 673–716.

Roff, H. (2008). *Reflective interpersonal therapy for children and parents.* Chichester, UK: Wiley.

Shackman, J. E., Shackman, A. J., & Pollak, S. D. (2007). Physical abuse amplifies attention to threat and increases anxiety in children. *Emotion, 7,* 838–852.

Shaw, D. S., Gilliom, M., Ingoldsby, E. M., & Nagin, D. S. (2003). Trajectories leading to school-age conduct problems. *Developmental Psychology, 39,* 189–200.

Smeekens, S., Riksen-Walraven, J. M., & van Bakel, H. J. (2007). Multiple determinants of externalizing behavior in 5-year-olds: A longitudinal model. *Journal of Abnormal Child Psychology, 35,* 347–361.

Speltz, M. L., DeKlyen, M., & Greenberg, M. T. (1999). Attachment in boys with early onset conduct problems. *Development and Psychopathology, 11,* 269–285.

Thompson, R. A., & Raikes, H. A. (2003). Toward the next quarter-century: Conceptual and methodological challenges for attachment theory. *Development and Psychopathology, 15,* 691–718.

van IJzendoorn, M. H., Schuengel, C., & Bakermans-Kranenburg, M. J. (1999). Disorganized attachment in early childhood: Meta-analysis of precursors, concomitants, and sequelae. *Development and Psychopathology, 11,* 225–249.

Viding, E., Blair, R. J., Moffitt, T. E., & Plomin, R. (2005). Evidence for substantial genetic risk for psychopathy in 7-year-olds. *Journal of Child Psychology and Psychiatry, 46,* 592–597.

Vondra, J. I., Shaw, D. S., Swearingen, L., Cohen, M., & Owens, E. B. (2001). Attachment stability and emotional and behavioral regulation from infancy to preschool age. *Development and Psychopathology, 13,* 13–33.

Waller, R., Gardner, F., Hyde, L. W., Shaw, D. S., Dishion, T. J., & Wilson, M. N. (2012). Do harsh and positive parenting predict parent reports of deceitful-callous behavior in early childhood? *Journal of Child Psychology and Psychiatry, 53,* 946–953.

World Health Organization. (1992). *ICD-10 Classifications of Mental and Behavioural Disorder: Clinical descriptions and diagnostic guidelines.* Geneva, Switzerland: World Health Organization.

CHAPTER 20

Attachment Disorders

Miriam Steele and Howard Steele

Among the permanent damage done to the child we emphasized above all the impairment in the capacity for and quality of object relationships which can be observed in cases where repeated changes of mother figure have taken place. Under such circumstances the child either becomes withdrawn (disinclined to cathect objects) or shallow and superficial in his object relations (i.e., never reaches or recaptures object constancy). On this point agreement between Dr. Bowlby and us is complete.
—ANNA FREUD (1960, p. 60)

These words of Anna Freud from more than 50 years ago, reflecting her complete agreement with John Bowlby, speak to the heart of what is known in the clinical psychological and psychiatric literature as reactive attachment disorder (RAD). RAD formally entered the psychiatric literature with the third edition of the *Diagnostic and Statistical Manual* (DSM) of the American Psychiatric Association and became further reified over successive iterations of the DSM (American Psychiatric Association, 1980, 1994, 2000, 2013). RAD has been researched (and treated) in respect of waves of children who were adopted in large numbers to Western Europe and North America throughout the 1980s and 1990s out of childcare institutions or orphanages in the former Soviet Union, eastern Europe, China, and parts of Africa. Observations and clinical studies of these children confirmed Anna Freud's observation that two overarching types of troubled behavior deserve our attention: a withdrawn/inhibited type of RAD, where a selective attachment is expected but absent, and a more common disinhibited type, which may co-occur with selective attachments, yet is a marked social engagement disorder (Zeanah & Gleason, 2010). In DSM-5, these subtypes are defined as distinct disorders: reactive attachment disorder and disinhibited social engagement disorder. Both disorders are relatively rare in the population at large, but are very common among abandoned, previously institutionalized children (O'Connor & Zeanah, 2003).

This chapter approaches the topic of attachment disorders with the aim of integrating perspectives from attachment theory and other psychoanalytic theories, in an attempt to describe and *explain* the evolving literature on RAD. Although the overall prevalence of RAD is extremely low, with rates of less than 1% in the overall population (Richters & Volkmar, 1994), this number soars to 40% or more when ex-institutionalized children, who have been radically deprived of consistent and sensitive care, are studied (O'Connor & Zeanah, 2003). Also, some measures of attachment disturbances are noted in the wider literature on childhood psychopathology, where at any given time, approximately 20% of children experience the signs and symptoms that constitute a DSM disorder, with approximately 7% evidencing extreme functional impairment (Tolan & Dodge, 2005). For this latter reason, it is not surprising that the term *attachment disorders* is sometimes used as a general term for the whole range of emotional disturbances and psychopathology linked to attachment experiences, representations, and relationships (Brisch, 2012). While alluding to attachment phenomena in general, this chapter approaches the term *attachment disorder* in the narrow sense as it applies to children who have suffered extreme neglect and maltreatment, and manifest behaviors, as Anna Freud (1960) noted, indicating extreme withdrawal from the social world or a shallow and superficial investment in relations with multiple others.

This chapter, then, attempts to provide a comprehensive psychoanalytic perspective on attachment disorders by way of addressing three related questions: (1) In what sense did the early psychoanalytically inspired pioneers in observation of "attachment-disordered" children foreshadow the current interest in ex-institutionalized children and provide a level of understanding perhaps unrivalled in subsequent writings on the topic?; (2) correspondingly, are there specific psychodynamic concepts that may elucidate contemporary thinking about attachment disorders?; and (3) can contemporary research on RAD enhance a psychoanalytic understanding of children with RAD and their distraught parents struggling to cope? Furthermore, we address a fourth question: How can a psychoanalytic approach to RAD improve treatment options for children (and families) with these difficulties?

In the context of answering these questions, this chapter provides an overview and critique of both current psychiatric assumptions about RAD and psychoanalytic observations and thinking, with the aim of refining an effective research agenda and a competent range of treatment plans that can improve the lives of children with RAD and their families.

CLASSIFICATION AND DIAGNOSIS

RAD refers to a distinct class of adjustment problems, namely, challenging behavior underpinned by core deficits in self and social development, seemingly specific to children growing up in, or removed from, contexts of impersonal institutional rearing or chronically maltreating environments. Thus, the constellation of disturbed behavior known as RAD is assumed to be a response to an extreme variation from the average expectable environment.

DSM-IV-TR described RAD as having two subtypes: inhibited and disinhibited. The inhibited subtype is manifest as hypervigilant, excessively inhibited, highly ambivalent, and contradictory responses. The disinhibited type is characterized by diffuse attachments, marked by indiscriminate sociability, and inability to exhibit appropriate selective attachments. The classifications for both types stipulate that RAD should:

- Be differentiated from pervasive developmental disorders.
- Be likely to occur in relation to abusive or radically impoverished child care.
- Have age of onset before 5 years.
- Manifest markedly disturbed and developmentally inappropriate social relatedness fitting the inhibited or disinhibited behavior pattern (and assuming this follows the experience of impoverished or abusive care).

The term *RAD*, as mentioned earlier, is firmly established in the psychiatric classification schemes (DSM and ICD), where the term has existed since 1980. The phenomenon is also reified in the Diagnostic Classification of Mental Health and Developmental Disorders in Infancy and Early Childhood (Zero to Three, 2005). In DSM-5 (American Psychiatric Association [APA], 2013), as noted, both subtypes of RAD are now defined as distinct disorders (reactive attachment disorder and disinhibited social engagement disorder) because of purported differences in correlates, course, and response to intervention. Yet, despite their distinctness, DSM-5 stresses their common background in terms of serious social neglect and deprivation. In the most recent infant/child psychiatry publication, the terms *deprivation/maltreatment disorder* and *reactive attachment disorder* are linked as twin diagnostic concepts, underlining the close connection between gross deviations from the average expectable environment and consequent disturbances in the domain of social relations with accompanying disturbances in emotion regulation and attention (Zeanah & Gleason, 2010). This calls to mind the argument advanced by Anna Freud (1965) in her account of developmental lines when she posited that the object relationship line is the central unifying thread in development. Yet, the psychiatric literature on RAD is relatively devoid of attention to the meaning of the behaviors displayed by the child so diagnosed, or, indeed, the meaning of any behaviors identified in DSM as qualifying one for belonging to a diagnostic category. As Balbernie (2010, p. 266) recently put it, "The DSM classification is a description of visible behaviors clustered together, a Flora of symptoms, and has little to say about the meaning of the mental disorders." For an appreciation of the meaning of behavior, one turns naturally to the psychoanalytic literature. And, in respect of the behaviors taken to indicate RAD, one finds attention to their presence *and meaning for the individual child* in detailed notes and writings from over 70 years ago.

PSYCHODYNAMIC APPROACHES TO ATTACHMENT DISORDERS

The Original Psychoanalytic "Baby Observers"

Psychoanalysts and pediatricians noted the *behaviors* that would later come to comprise the diagnosis of RAD in various writings dating from the mid-20th century (e.g., Freud & Burlingham, 1944; Goldfarb, 1947; Spitz, 1945). It is indeed a distinguished list of contributors who were first intrigued and motivated to write about their compelling observations of children whose early experiences deviated markedly from an "average expectable environment" (Hartmann, 1939/1958). It could be that the practice of careful observations of children, and specifically of the early parent–child relationship, began with the practice of watching these children develop in such unusual conditions. One might imagine that observing children in these extreme contexts or "natural experiments" (Cicchetti, 2003) would have provoked the "baby watchers" to hone their observational skills in a way that would not have been possible in more typical parent–child relationship contexts. It cannot have been coincidental that in 1944/1945, Rene Spitz, Anna Freud, and John Bowlby published works outlining their astute observations of distressed children who were at the mercy of an environment devoid of typical parental care (Bowlby, 1944; Freud & Burlingham, 1944; Spitz, 1945). What motivated them? World War II, with the trauma, separation, and disruption it wrought? The psychoanalytic interest, set in motion by Freud, regarding the powerful influence of earliest experiences? Factors in their own early relational experience? Whatever the reasons for their inspired observations, the psychoanalytic literature and domain of clinical practice, the mental health field broadly, and the wider world are richer for the efforts of these foundational figures in psychoanalysis. Their work continues to resonate, especially in respect of the topic of attachment disorders.

Spitz (1945), struck by the terrible statistics on infant mortality rates among institutionalized infants, sometimes as high as 70%, undertook a long-term study of 164 infants residing in low-socioeconomic-status homes with their mothers, a "Penal Nursery" where infants resided with their mothers, and a "Foundling Home," most reminiscent of orphanage/institutional care. Aside from the large sample he recruited, and the structured assessments of development he administered, Spitz was ahead of his time by including a total of 31,500 feet of film of abandoned children living in institutional settings or foundling homes. Spitz concluded:

> It is true that the children in the Foundling Home are condemned to solitary confinement in their cots. But we do not think that it is the lack of perceptual stimulation in general that counts in their deprivation. We believe that they suffer because their perceptual world is emptied of human partners, that their isolation cuts them off from any stimulation by any persons who could signify mother-representatives. (p. 68)

The agreement then is clear: There is something uniquely damaging to the human character (what Bowlby might later refer to as "the attachment system") in spending the first years of life in an environment devoid of typical parental care.

During and immediately after World War II, Anna Freud and colleagues provided long-lasting insights into how very young children cope when their caregiving environment is radically changed from a birth family to a larger institutional group without parents. This "natural experiment" arose in London during World War II in the Hampstead War Nurseries, which provided care to children who were temporarily and/or permanently orphaned. As Midgley (2007) comments, although Anna Freud herself saw her efforts mainly as her contribution to the war effort, she did much more than that. In particular, her efforts brought the advent of formulating the crucial role of observing children in situ, and this had a profound impact on developmental psychology and on the development of technique in psychoanalytic treatment. Our understanding of children living in institutional care, albeit a high-quality setting such as that provided by Anna Freud and her colleagues, was enhanced by the pages upon pages of carefully construed observations of children assembled by Anna Freud and Dorothy Burlingham (1944). The technique of writing up these observations could be seen to lay some of the groundwork for later psychoanalytic training and technique, in that they require an education in the theory that guides the observer's attention to notable behaviors, acts showing empathy, frustration, aggression, caring, responsiveness or lack thereof—carefully noting what is seen and heard, who initiates an action, who responds, and how, with what follow-on consequences. Anna Freud championed the view that very young children's behaviors, nonverbal and verbal, convey essential meaning about the nature of human motivation, social interactions, and self or ego development.

Bowlby's seminal study *44 Juvenile Thieves* (1944) reports on an early clinical research study carried out at the London Child Guidance Clinic during the years 1936–1939. The report included not only 44 youths who had been caught stealing and were seen for psychotherapy, but also an additional 44 youths who were part of a nonthieving comparison group. Bowlby highlights a personality pattern he labeled the "affectionless character." With astute clinical observation, Bowlby describes how

> fourteen of the 44 thieves were distinguished from the remainder by their remarkable lack of affection or warmth of feeling for anyone. . . . In this they differed from the children who had apparently never since infancy shown normal affection to anyone and were, consequently, conspicuously solitary, undemonstrative and unresponsive. Many of their parents and foster-parents remarked how nothing you said or did to them made any difference. They responded neither to kindness nor to punishment. (p. 38)

This paper and the work it describes are often highlighted as the tipping point in the development of attachment theory, with Bowlby paying special attention to the role of the caregiving environment in the development of psychopathology. Later, in the 1960s, Bowlby advanced the idea of childhood grief and mourning concerning actual or feared loss of the loved-for mother figure, embracing Freud's (1926/1959) listing of the sources of signal anxiety. Bowlby's (1969/1982) focus would become that of describing the normal ontogeny of attachment behavior in the human (and other) animals, in the context of a radical psychoanalytic object relations framework, where the motivation for attachment behaviors and feelings was seen to come from an evolutionarily determined attachment system housed in the central nervous system.

Normative Attachment Relationships from a Developmental Research Perspective

Attachment is a term with multiple meanings, including biological, social, and psychological processes present in the human and other animals from birth, if not before (Bowlby, 1969/1982; see also Mikulincer & Shaver, Chapter 2, this volume). The term *attachment* is applied both to observable behavior and to unseen internal mental and affective processes (the "internal working model" of self and attachment figures assumed to become consolidated, organized, and stable in the final quarter of the first year). In the 1-year-old child there is robust evidence that individual differences in attachment patterns are observable in the context of the Strange Situation—a filmed 20-minute sequence involving the child and parent in a playroom-like setting, including a stranger, with two separations from, followed by two reunions with, the parent (Ainsworth, Blehar, Waters, & Wall, 1978).

The normal developmental trajectory from birth onward includes an initial period (up to about 6 months) when an infant's bids for contact/comfort are nonselective (he or she will accept sensitive ministrations from an unfamiliar person), followed by the establishment of selective attachments (from 8–9 months the healthy infant shows stranger anxiety, as noted by Spitz [1950] and crystallized in Bowlby's [1969/1982] attachment theory). By the age of 1 year, signs of typical selective secure or insecure (avoidant/resistant) attachments are apparent in the Strange Situation, as well as the extent of disorganized/disoriented behavioral responses and attachment-disordered behavior.

The four main patterns of response to separation and reunion are shown in Figure 20.1, where security is shown to result from sensitive and responsive care, and insecurity (either avoidance or resistance) is linked to insensitive or unresponsive care. Figure 20.1 depicts a continuum showing the range of attachment patterns from secure, through avoidant and resistant, to their momentary collapse in disorganized/disoriented attachments and, at the most extreme clinical end, attachment disorders linked to gross deviations from normative care.

As Figure 20.1 shows, secure attachments (depicted to the far left) are a response to optimally sensitive and responsive care, consistently seen in 55% of community samples (van IJzendoorn & Kroonenberg, 1988). Notably, a central feature of this optimal care is the caretaker's prompt responsiveness to infant distress, where the infant has had the common experience of repair following rupture, recovery following distress. To the right of the secure pattern in Figure 20.1 are the insecure patterns

Attachment Pattern	Secure	Avoidant	Resistant	Disorganized	Disordered
Quality of caregiving	Sensitive and responsive	Insensitive (overly neglectful)	Insensitive (overly intrusive)	Fearful or frightening; abusive	Absent; profoundly neglectful

FIGURE 20.1. The continuum of attachment: From security to disorder.

(avoidance and resistance) consistently found in approximately 30% of community samples, where familiarity with disappointment (in response to unduly neglectful or intrusive care) seems to be the normative childhood experience (van IJzendoorn & Kroonenberg, 1988). In the avoidant case, the child opts for *flight* in the face of distress; in analytic terms, the strategy adopted is denial and isolation of affect. In the resistant case, the child opts for *fight* in the face of distress, protesting loudly either with anger or passivity—a choice to fight or protest. While the proportion of security (55–65%) is stable across cultures, insecurity (avoidance vs. resistance) tends to vary somewhat across cultures, with avoidance being more prevalent in northern Europe and America but resistance being more prevalent in Japan and Israel (van IJzendoorn & Sagi-Schwartz, 2008).

As to which insecure strategy the child chooses in response to suboptimal care, there is some suggestion that, as well as culture, endogenous temperamental factors play a role. Resistance—literally, resistance to being settled—seems more compatible with a child who is highly inhibited and easily given to crying. In contrast, avoidance is more compatible with a child who lacks inhibition and bravely explores outward. And, although children with avoidant attachments tend not to cry at all during separation, salivary cortisol assays (obtained prior to and 15 and 30 minutes after the Strange Situation observation) have long confirmed that they are nonetheless distressed inside (Spangler & Grossmann, 1993).

To the center right of Figure 20.1 we see disorganized/disoriented attachments, which are linked to frightened or frightening caregiving (and/or abusive) behavior. This anomalous response is seen in 15% of community samples but in 40–80% of clinical samples (e.g., depressed mothers, or infants where maltreatment is suspected; Lyons-Ruth & Jacobvitz, 2008). Interestingly, it is usually possible to readily assign a best-fitting alternative attachment strategy (avoidant, resistant, or secure) for toddlers who show disorganized/disoriented behavior in the Strange Situation, pointing again to the robustness of the attachment system and the inherent wish to form organized attachments.

For all these patterns of response to the Strange Situation observed in both community and clinical samples—secure, avoidant, resistant, and disorganized—a selective attachment to the observed caregiver can normally be assumed. This is often not the case for infants living in institutional settings where serious questions have been raised about the extent of attachment formation. These children show a curious absence of attachment behaviors that would otherwise be expected, initially identified by Elizabeth Carlson in her work scoring Strange Situation responses among infants living in Romanian orphanages (Zeanah, Smyke, Koga, Carlson, & Bucharest Group, 2005). In other words, early maltreatment and neglect appear to be capable of disrupting the normal biological, social, and psychological process from nonselective to selective attachments, keeping a child "stuck," as it were, in the nonselective phase. Balbernie (2010, pp. 274–275), in his evolutionary account of RAD, refers to this as "diffusing the attachment system," enabling "an abandoned child to move among a pool of caregivers on a brief encounter basis," and concludes that "even if this desperate tactic worked for only a minority of children, the genes enabling the activation of that behavior would be retained and thus remain as a potential within the population." Among abandoned, institutionalized, and then adopted children with an activated pattern of uninhibited nonselective or multiple-choice attachment, "a new parent who is trying to create a healthy relationship is likely to be the person most rebuffed as they menace the status quo" (Balbernie, 2010, p. 275).

A nuanced understanding of the evolutionary and psychoanalytic meaning of RAD was not available to the authors of DSM-III in the late 1970s, as this was a time when they were deliberately moving away from the perceived conflation of explanation and description that typified DSM-I and -II, pursuing instead with zeal the task of reliable description as an end in itself. Thus, when RAD was introduced into DSM-III in 1980, it was irrevocably limited to descriptions of behavior, yet it also included a firm reference to causation. To this day, it is only the stress disorders, RAD, and DSED (see below) for which the diagnostic criteria include the requirement that a significant trauma rests in the individual's past. The DSM (prior to DSM-5) specified that the child's pattern of social behavior will take the form of either extremely withdrawn or indiscriminately friendly behavior *in the context of a history of highly pathogenic care*. DSM-5 (APA, 2013) separates out indiscriminately friendly behavior and calls it disinhibited social engagement disorder (DSED). Yet both the inhibited RAD and disinhibited forms are seen as reactions to pathogenic care, and should be seen from a psychoanalytic perspective, as two sides of the same coin.

RAD and the Surge in International Adoptions from Institutional Settings

Institutional rearing, due to its regimented nature, high child-to-caregiver ratios, multiple shifts, and frequent changes of caregivers, almost inevitably deprives children of reciprocal interactions with stable caregivers. In this respect, institutional care implies structural neglect. A considerable number of studies have shown that children growing up in orphanages are at risk in various domains of functioning, including their physical, socioemotional, and cognitive development—findings that have recently been summarized and evaluated (Bakermans-Kranenburg et al., 2011; McCall, van IJzendoorn, Juffer, Groark, & Groza, 2011).

"Catch-up" rates following adoption into a typical family arrangement after early institutional rearing have been studied extensively in recent years, and meta-analytic reviews have been published (Juffer & van IJzendoorn, 2009; van IJzendoorn & Juffer, 2006). At the risk of simplification, the following summary of catch-up rates can be made. Catch-up is observed first in the domain of physical development, with children assuming a place on normal growth curves within 6 months of receiving appropriate nutrition and stimulation. Developmental catch-up typically takes longer in the domain of cognition, with some persisting language and cognitive delays being evident for years in a substantial group of children adopted out of institutions. Finally, the slowest catch-up occurs in the social domain, which may be seen as testament to the relevance of the diagnostic term *RAD*. As many as 10 years postadoption, fully one-third of adoptees show signs of RAD. This means, of course, that the majority of adoptees do *not* present with RAD. These consequences of early institutional rearing are most marked in children who remained for longer during infancy (and beyond in some cases) in the institution from which they were adopted.

In other words, there is a dose–response relationship between length of time in early institutional living and later postadoption developmental delays. Rutter and Sonuga-Barke (2010) summarized results from their 15-year follow-up of children adopted in the United Kingdom out of Romanian orphanages at the end of the communist regime, compared with English adoptees. This well-controlled study found a range of specific long-term developmental deficits persisting for the adoptees from Romania who spent more than their first six months in the institution.

This literature on catch-up rates has arisen comparatively recently, from the late 1980s, when profoundly neglected orphans from Romania were adopted to homes in the United Kingdom, the United States, and Canada, where some participated in systematic longitudinal studies. These and other studies of internationally adopted children from countries in the former communist sphere (e.g., Russia and China) or the developing world (e.g., Ethiopia) have helped to illuminate the nature of RAD, while also demonstrating the immense resilience of the attachment process. Attachment difficulties were readily seen in many of the tens of thousands of children adopted out of orphanages in China, Russia, Romania, Ethiopia, and other countries with large numbers of abandoned children (Bakermans-Kranenburg et al., 2011).

Notably, most adoptees do not meet the diagnostic criteria for RAD, yet a sizable minority of adoptive parents have been strident in seeking therapeutic help for the "affectless psychopathy" (as Bowlby would have predicted) shown by their adopted children. The mental health industry has responded with a range of treatments, most infamously "holding therapy," all largely untested in terms of their efficacy (Steele, 2003). Since holding therapy led to the tragic deaths by suffocation of a number of children in the late 1990s and the early part of the 21st century, somewhat more (but still insufficient) support has been made available to adoptive parents, and caution has been sounded by responsible mental health providers (Chaffin et al., 2006).

The American child psychiatrist who has published most extensively on attachment disorders, Charles Zeanah, and his colleagues have been strident in cautioning against overuse of the term *RAD*. They recommend a distinction between children in whom the primary and exclusive difficulty is one of attachment disorder and other children with primary difficulties of attention-deficit/hyperactivity disorder (ADHD) or conduct disorder, with a secondary difficulty concerning pathogenic care and attachment difficulties (Gleason et al., 2011). This approach holds much promise in terms of delineating the specificity and sensitivity of the RAD diagnosis. A recent report contributing to this effort, based on longitudinal study of the Bucharest Early Intervention Project, concluded that evidence-derived criteria for indiscriminately social/disinhibited and emotionally withdrawn/inhibited RAD define two statistically and clinically cohesive syndromes (Gleason et al., 2011). Gleason and colleagues report on over 120 children observed at four time periods through the intervention, beginning in the second year of life and studied systematically at 30, 42 and 54 months. Interestingly, 40 (32%) of the children initially met criteria for indiscriminately social/disinhibited RAD, but this number diminished by half by 30 months and remained stable to 54 months. These children with the disinhibited form of RAD had some ADHD symptoms but were *not*, on the whole, a group with diagnostic criteria for ADHD. Interestingly, over half of the children with disinhibited RAD had organized secure or insecure (avoidant/resistant) attachments. By contrast, the emotionally withdrawn/inhibited form of RAD was observed in only six (4%) of the children and remained stable for five children throughout the study period. Most of these children were securely attached and, while a few met the criteria for childhood depression at 54 months, two children did not. Both types of RAD in the study of Gleason and colleagues (2011) contributed independently to functional impairment and were stable over time. This is the most detailed study offering discriminant and predictive validity of the two types of RAD.

At the same time, this work highlights a conceptual challenge: How do we understand the phenomenon whereby a child can both exhibit behaviors consistent with RAD and be securely attached to the caregiver? This question speaks to a long-standing psychoanalytic interest: That is, what in the patient's current functioning reflects earliest experiences? And what in the patient's functioning reflects current experiences? RAD may reflect what is earliest and persisting in a child's inner world, while that inner world may also hold (in a segregated or fragile fashion) representations of current, more secure interactions with the adoptive (or foster) parent. Put differently, but consistent with this picture, RAD is thought to reside within the child whose early experiences of neglect and maltreatment constitute profound deprivation, and the consequences of this adversity are fairly pervasive. Yet the very same child may still be open to responding to positive secure qualities of the present (adoptive) parent–child relationship and, when distressed, will be able to turn to the (new) caregiver for protection, inhibiting or setting aside the concerns that lead him or her to show RAD-like symptoms at other times.

Psychodynamic Concepts Relevant to Understanding Attachment Disorders

While a plethora of psychodynamic theoretical and therapeutic constructs are relevant to the understanding of children with attachment disorders, this chapter comments on two that seem vital: (1) mental representations and the representational world and (2) defense mechanisms, specifically turning passive into active. In the next section, we discuss the importance of therapeutic work aimed at helping the child metabolize intensely negative affect.

Mental Representations

Many fields within psychology and cognitive science are concerned with the development of mental representations, but their study has been a constant in psychoanalytic theory and research from Freud's day forward. This is perhaps because, from a psychoanalytic perspective, we are always living in two worlds: (1) the shared interpersonal world, and (2) the inner personal world where fantasy and reality meet and coalesce into sometimes fleeting, often enduring mental representations of self and others that serve as a guide for regulating arousal, interpreting others' behavior, and determining one's own behavior (Fonagy, Gergley, Jurist, & Target, 2002; Sandler & Rosenblatt, 1962). Bowlby's (1969/1982) focus on *actual* interactions between parent and infant differentiated him from many in the psychoanalytic community who focused more on the role of fantasy in the development of mental representations and, ultimately, personality. Bowlby's internal working model, by contrast, refers to the process by which children arrive at internal representations of their emotional experiences and significant relationships. Within the context of attachment disorders, internal working models play a crucial role, as they can help us understand what might be at play as we observe the behavior of the child as he or she moves from the context of institution or maltreating environment to the hopefully positive, or at least benign, context provided by the adoptive or foster parent.

Mental representations of attachment are the appropriate focus of inquiry when working, either clinically or in research, with preschool-age or older children and their caregivers (foster/adoptive parents) where language is intact and more or less functional. The classic tool of child psychoanalysis, doll play, has been extensively applied in this work in relation to the children (e.g. Steele et al., 2009). In respect of the adoptive or foster parents and the contribution they are, or can be, making to the children placed with them, there is no better set of tools than the Adult Attachment Interview (AAI; George, Kaplan, & Main, 1996) and its associated method of analysis (Main, Hesse, & Goldwyn, 2008). Work comparing adoptive parents' AAIs with their adopted children's doll play and story-completion responses has robustly revealed the positive organizing influence that a secure and resolved (with regard to past trauma or loss) adoptive parent can have on a child with a history of maltreatment and multiple foster placements (Steele et al., 2003, 2008). The AAI coding system is a veritable list of how the ego's defense mechanisms manifest in language used to describe and evaluate one's childhood attachment experiences. Is the speaker prone to isolation of affect and grandiosity? Or is he or she inclined toward rationalization, humor, and other "mature" defenses? Alternatively, might the speaker be overly reliant on intellectualization and displacement? One or more of these patterns are readily identified in responses to the AAI and will be predictive of specific types of difficulties in the parenting role. Administering the AAI at the beginning of treatment is likely to help a parent perceive how his or her thoughts and feelings regarding the past may be powerfully influencing their thoughts, feelings, and behavior in the present.

Defense Mechanisms: Turning Passive Into Active and Identification with the Aggressor

One of the often-observed behaviors that adoptive parents cite, especially for children removed from maltreating contexts, is that the child behaves toward the new attachment figures as if they were the *old* figures. The aggressive, provocative treatment of the new caregivers is often hard for the adoptive or foster parent to manage, even if they have some understanding of where the provocation originally came from. The behavior is akin to the classical analytic construct of "turning active into passive" or, in other words, the child communicating by their behavior the message, "I will turn on you before you have a chance to turn on me." Juliet Hopkins (2006) comments that this is a potentially dangerous defensive strategy, as one of the risks of adopting children in care is that they may perpetuate their deprivation by rejecting the loving care offered them; the literature on adoption breakdown, perhaps unsurprisingly, is significant. Bowlby (1979) offers a conceptual understanding of why a child might adopt such a strategy, drawing on his notion of internal working models:

> It seems necessary to postulate that whatever representational models of attachment figures and of self an individual builds during his childhood and adolescence, tend to persist relatively unchanged into and throughout adult life. As a result he tends to assimilate any new person with whom he may form a bond, to an existing model and often continue to do so despite repeat evidence that the model is inappropriate. Similarly he expects to be perceived and treated by them in ways that would be appropriate to his self models and to continue with such expectations despite contrary evidence. (p. 141)

Clinicians and social workers can readily verify that many maltreated children show a strong tendency to provoke new caregivers (either foster or adoptive) to behave negatively and often punitively toward them. While often perplexing to the parent, this makes sense if one puts into context the child's troubled representations of previous attachment figures that guide the child's expectations of future attachment interactions. John Bowlby (1979, p. 6) comments similarly when he says that "the aggressive child acts on the basis that attack is the best means of defense." This construct does not fit neatly into the nosology of RAD, as it is neither an inhibited nor a disinhibited type of behavior. In fact, such aggression may rule out a pure diagnosis of RAD, as a primary diagnosis of childhood conduct disorder may be called for. This comorbid pattern does, however, describe a good many children who have suffered from deprived and/or maltreating environments. Drawing on psychoanalytic renderings of the meaning of the child's behavior, adoptive parents may be brought some relief and encouraged toward tolerance of their challenging children. Much patience and vigilance with respect to their own reactions to repeated rejections from the child will be required. "Time-out," for example, a standard behavioral approach to discipline that has been argued as appropriate for the treatment of RAD (e.g., Buckner, Lopez, Dunkel, & Joiner, 2008), is likely to trigger powerful fears of abandonment, rooted in real experiences. Other discipline strategies are called for in respect of children with a history of deprivation or maltreatment—for example, "time-in," where a parent calmly and deliberately focuses on the child's mental states, modeling empathy and understanding.

A further psychoanalytic construct that elucidates our understanding of what might be underlying some of the specific issues at work with children with attachment disorders is Bowlby's notion of multiple models, and specifically the defensive processes that lead to segregation of models in children (and adults) with loss and trauma histories where the posttrauma experience has been unsupportive and misleading. Bowlby (1988) describes environments that breed in the child mental representations that are confused and confusing to the child. The caregiver induces these multiple models via a range of pathogenic caregiving strategies—for example, frightening the child and then offering nurturance, and thus confusing the child by rewriting the meaning of the fearful experiences—encouraging a narrative of experience that is a sanitized, alternate, and fictional version. For instance, Bowlby cites clinical research involving children of parents who committed suicide. In one case, a child was told that the parent had gone on a trip, and in another case that the parent had died in a car accident despite the child having witnessed the actual suicide. In such cases, maintaining competing actual and fictional representations leads to multiple models in the child's mind that require more psychic energy than would be the case if a singular, well-functioning internal world made up of coherent, tolerably accurate representations had formed.

Alternatively, multiple models may be seen to arise within the internal world of a child who had many different caregivers, most of whom did not make their mark as being especially connected to the child—as would be the case in institutional care—or, for cases that arise among children in foster care, the children may have had the experience of being perpetually in transition. Jenny Kenrick (2006, p. 70), a psychodynamic clinician with special expertise in therapeutic work with children in transition, commented: "The repeated and often very abrupt moves that children seem to have to make while in transitional placements become cumulatively so damaging. They are effectively traumatic and extremely prejudicial to the development of the child." Their representational worlds may contain elements including a range of diverse and possibly conflicting representations from many and often abrupt changes of caregivers, often occurring in a context of confusion and fear. It could well be that in such cases we are witnessing the child who demonstrates elements of both RAD and secure attachment.

Turning passive into active, identifying with the aggressor, and segregating mental models as described by Bowlby all serve the purpose of minimizing psychic pain, at the expense of a coherent, integrated inner world capable of processing pain through interactions with supportive others who provide clarification, communication, and reparation. Achieving the transmutation of defenses and fragmented inner worlds, from (in Freud's words) neurotic suffering to ordinary human misery or, more hopefully, into other more socially valued, and ultimately more joyful, adaptations, is the business of psychoanalytic treatment.

PSYCHODYNAMIC TREATMENT APPROACHES: HELPING THE INDIVIDUAL WITH ATTACHMENT DISORDER METABOLIZE EXTREMELY NEGATIVE AFFECT

Much has been said in relation to the issue of how *not to treat* children who are diagnosed with RAD (Chaffin et al., 2006; O'Connor & Zeanah, 2003; Steele, 2003). We wholeheartedly agree that "attachment therapy" of the kind that involves forceful holding, humiliation, or other coercive methods has no place in the psychological treatment of any child. Instead, we are proponents of a range of treatments (individual psychodynamic treatment, family therapy, video interaction psychotherapy). All of these treatments have a place in the efforts of experienced and well-trained clinicians to assist these families, many of whom are at the point of desperation and are contemplating relinquishing the care of their children.

Psychodynamic clinicians have amassed a huge wealth of clinical experience in treating children, especially if we look to the Fostering and Adoption team at the Tavistock Clinic and the Adoption Research Group at the Anna Freud Centre that thrived some 30 years ago. As an avid member of the Tavistock's Adoption and Fostering workshop, one of us (MS) had the pleasure of learning from the inspiring clinical work of Jenny Kenrick, Lorraine Tollemache, Caroline Lindsay, and others. Many of the clinicians who participated in the specialist work were convinced of the utility of engaging a child "in transition" in therapeutic work as a way of bolstering the child, so that a subsequent placement might become permanent. Rather than seeing the children as unable to make use of individual treatment, these clinicians would often comment on and bring examples of how hard these children seemed to work at making meaning out of their disjointed and confusing life trajectories, and so made good use of their access to the therapeutic context. Fundamental to any psychodynamic treatment is the need to pay attention to both the internal world and external forces, as these are the essence of mental health and so too in cases of children in transition. A challenge for the psychoanalyst skilled in delivering treatment to children with RAD and related profound difficulties is the vital task of documenting and manualizing the treatment work so that others can learn the art of the trade.

Kenrick (2006, p. 80) comments that much progress can be made if the child experiences the therapist as "someone able to understand the impact of their rage and despair," as someone who "could bring a thoughtful mind to the child's emotional predicaments and dilemmas." To do this is no easy feat, however, as clinicians working with this population all agree that the challenges are great, as is the skill required in conducting the therapeutic work. There is no underestimating the therapist's need to closely observe the child's behavior—*and the therapist's actions*—in the "here-and-now" context, as this permits a mapping of the child's internal and external worlds. Kenrick (2006) eloquently comments on the task at hand:

> A concomitant of the need to monitor closely what one's patient is able to explore emotionally in today's session or in a specific part of the session is the need to think carefully about both timing and wording of what the therapist says in the sessions. A particular way of wording a thought or interpretation could be taken as criticism by the child and would instantly increase levels of persecutory anxiety. . . . It may be preferable initially to describe what is happening in the child's play—in the transitional area of play. That is to say, there may be a description or observation of how the baby pigs are being attacked by the lions. Then it may be possible to comment on the fierce and terrifying feelings while this is happening. That may be as much as a particular child can manage. But a language of emotions is being developed. (p. 81)

But how does a psychodynamic approach to treating children with traumatized histories, and often in foster care, proceed, with the goal of enhancing future attachment relationships? Of central help to the child in forging ahead with a new attachment relationship is the therapist's availability to contain the negative affect and help the child recognize and label it, so that it can be tolerated in more adaptive ways. Juliet Hopkins sums up what is needed for these children to succeed in making use of therapeutic input:

Although new attachments can develop without the need to talk about the past, much effort in therapy is directed towards talking about the "here and now." Current feelings and intentions are put gradually into words. Clinical tact is needed to find acceptable ways to verbalize what needs to be understood. . . . Therapy provides a trial ground where children can integrate painful emotions in small doses. New developments can be explored before they are taken safely home. (2006, p. 106)

Psychoanalytically oriented clinical research encouraging foster parents to take on this stabilizing and caring task for the previously maltreated child suggests that slow and clearly paced communications that underscore the new relationship, via calm use of the child's name and references to recent shared (positive) past experiences, have an attachment-facilitating effect (Steele et al., 2007). Attachment-facilitating interventions can and have been planned, and successfully implemented, in analytically informed work with birth parents at risk of losing their babies or toddlers to care (Steele, Murphy, & Steele, 2010). Privileging the parent–child relationship and focusing on consolidating relationship strengths in the "here and now" may be the best buttress against the intrusive effects of past trauma or the pressing worries about what the future may bring.

CONCLUSIONS AND FUTURE DIRECTIONS

In many ways, we have come a long way to understanding the pernicious impact on children's development that comes about as a result of the "experiments in nature" that comprise the experience of institutionalized and maltreated children. The move from deprived environments to more benign or positive caregiving contexts is mostly, it should be said, achieved. Research studies of both foster parents (Dozier, 2003) and adoptive parents (Steele et al., 2008) point to characteristics of parents that facilitate radical changes toward organization and security for children. These are an autonomous secure state of mind as indexed by the AAI (designed to "surprise the unconscious"), not disabled by unresolved loss regarding past loss or trauma experienced by the parent (Main et al., 2008; Steele & Steele, 2008). Yet research also points to characteristics of individual children that make some of them more, and others less, susceptible to the environmental context (e.g., Belsky & Pleuss, 2009). The argument is that from an evolutionary perspective, it makes survival sense to equip some children with extreme sensitivity to the environment (as it may change) and others with much less sensitivity to small variations in the environment (as these may be misleading given the overall stability of the environment). With respect to differential susceptibility, which may affect parents as much as children, we are only at the early stages of knowing how to identify those most and least at risk. And what if we could reliably distinguish between them? Would we leave in the orphanage the child who is *less* impacted by the environment and favor for "early release" the child who is *more* impacted? Clearly, efforts must be invested in improving the lot of all children and in helping as best we can every parent and every child in emotional turmoil or despair.

The careful work of clinicians aiming to shift the fractured internal worlds of individuals with attachment disorders should continue to be informed by state-of-the-art research that combines many facets of development, including physical, social, emotional, and psychophysiological. Some exemplar efforts, considering the phenomenon of differential susceptibility to the caregiving environment and significantly moving the field forward, have been published recently (e.g., De Schipper, Oosterman, & Scheungel, 2012). Specifically, these authors found that shy children who had more sensitive foster parents were more likely to be securely attached, while, for non-shy children, differing levels of parental sensitivity had no noticeable effects on attachment security. This speaks to the long-puzzling matter of why some children react to adverse caregiving with marked insecurity, perhaps even RAD, while other children exposed to the same adversity are not so deleteriously affected.

Ultimately, the value of a psychoanalytic perspective on attachment disorders is to be realized, revisited, and learned anew in the detailed, careful attention analytic thinkers and clinicians give to the range of possible internal meanings resting at the foundation and underpinning character development and functioning. For the psychoanalytic perspective to achieve the influence it deserves on both research and treatment of clinical problems linked to RAD, existing bridges between psychoanalysts and psychiatrists/psychologists need to be strengthened and new bridges need to be established so that children (and families) with RAD may be better understood and more effectively treated. There may be no better set of building materials and tools to advance this task than can be found in attachment theory and research (Steele, 2006). Single case studies (e.g., Baradon & Steele, 2008) and narrative reviews (e.g., Steele & Steele, 2008) contribute much, but policy changes are driven by empirical findings arising from pragmatic clinical trials, including random assignment to treatment group(s) or comparison group(s). Only then can a requisite level of confidence in the results be assured. Both psychoanalysis and psychiatry/psychology have been remiss in writing about the constellation of problems known as RAD without sufficient investment in such pragmatic clinical trials. We do not expect any "quick fix" for children with RAD, but at the same time it is not acceptable to say that deep disturbances arising from chronic trauma require unlimited ongoing psychoanalytic treatment. It must be possible to identify the minimum clinical investment required to launch a maltreated child with RAD toward normative attachments and a socially secure future.

Given what we are coming to know about differential susceptibility, how can we best target types and amounts of treatment? Now is the time to vigorously research these questions, from an empirical, psychoanalytically informed position, so that children in need and their families may receive effective support and treatments. The psychological, social, and economic costs of delay or inaction are substantial.

REFERENCES

Ainsworth, M. D., Blehar, M. C., Waters, E., & Wall, S. (1978). *Patterns of attachment: Assessed in the strange situation and at home.* Hillsdale, NJ: Erlbaum.
American Psychiatric Association. (1980). *Diagnostic and statistical manual of mental disorders* (3rd ed.). Washington, DC: Author.

American Psychiatric Association. (1994). *Diagnostic and statistical manual of mental disorders* (4th ed.). Washington, DC: Author.

American Psychiatric Association. (2000). *Diagnostic and statistical manual of mental disorders* (4th ed., text rev.). Washington, DC: Author.

American Psychiatric Association. (2013). *Diagnostic and statistical manual of mental disorders* (5th ed.). Arlington, VA: Author.

Bakermans-Kranenburg, M. J., Steele, H., Zeanah, C. H. Muhamedrahimov, R. J., Vorria, P., Dobrova-Krol, N. A., et al. (2011). Attachment and emotional development in institutional care: Characteristics and catch-up. In R. McCall, M. H. van IJzendoorn, F. Juffer, C. J. Groark, & V. K. Groza (Eds.), Children without permanent parents: Research, practice and policy. *Monographs of the Society for Research of Child Development, 76,* 62–91.

Balbernie, R. (2010). Reactive attachment disorder as an evolutionary adaptation. *Attachment and Human Development, 12,* 265–282.

Baradon, T., & Steele, M. (2008). Integrating the AAI in the clinical process of psychoanalytic parent–infant psychotherapy in a case of relational trauma. In H. Steele & M. Steele (Eds.), *Clinical applications of the Adult Attachment Interview* (pp. 195–212). New York: Guilford Press.

Belsky, J., & Pluess, M. (2009). Beyond diathesis stress: Differential susceptibility to environmental influences. *Psychological Bulletin, 135,* 885–908.

Bowlby, J. (1944). Forty-four juvenile thieves: Their characters and home-life. *International Journal of Psycho-Analysis, 25,* 19–53.

Bowlby, J. (1979). *The making and breaking of affectional bonds.* London: Tavistock.

Bowlby, J. (1982). *Attachment and loss: Vol. 1. Attachment.* London: Hogarth Press and the Institute of Psychoanalysis. (Original work published 1969)

Bowlby, J. (1988). *A secure base: Clinical applications of attachment theory.* London: Routledge.

Brisch, K. H. (2012). *Treating attachment disorders: From theory to therapy* (2nd ed.). New York: Guilford Press.

Buckner, J. D., Lopez, C., Dunkel, S., & Joiner, T. E., Jr. (2008). Behavior management training for the treatment of Reactive Attachment Disorder. *Child Maltreatment, 13,* 289–296.

Chaffin, M., Hanson, R., Saunders, B. E., Nichols, T., Barnett, D., Zeanah, C. H., et al. (2006). Report of the APSAC Task Force on attachment therapy, reactive attachment disorder, and attachment problems. *Child Maltreatment, 11,* 76–89.

Cicchetti, D. (2003). Experiments of nature: Contributions to developmental theory [Editorial]. *Development and Psychopathology, 15,* 833–835.

De Schipper, J. C., Oosterman, M., & Scheungel, C. (2012). Temperament, disordered attachment and parental sensitivity in foster care: Differential findings on attachment security for shy children. *Attachment and Human Development, 14,* 349–365.

Dozier, M. (2003). Attachment-based treatment for vulnerable children. *Attachment and Human Development, 5,* 253–257.

Fonagy, P., Gergely, G., Jurist, E., & Target, M. (2002). *Affect regulation, mentalization, and the development of the self.* New York: Other Press.

Freud, A. (1960). Discussion of Dr. John Bowlby's paper. *Psychoanalytic Study of the Child, 15,* 53–62.

Freud, A. (1965). *Normality and pathology in childhood.* New York: International Universities Press.

Freud, A., & Burlingham, D. (1944). *Infants without families.* New York: International Universities Press.

Freud, S. (1959). Inhibitions, symptoms and anxiety. In J. Strachey (Ed. & Trans.), *The standard edition of the complete psychological works of Sigmund Freud* (Vol. 14, pp. 146–158). London: Hogarth Press. (Original work published 1926)

George, C., Kaplan, N., & Main, M. (1996). *Adult Attachment Interview* (3rd ed.). Unpublished manuscript, University of California, Berkeley.

Gleason, M. M., Fox, N. A., Dury, S., Smyke, A., Egger, H. L., Nelson, C. A., 3rd, et al. (2011). Validity of evidence-derived criteria for reactive attachment disorder: Indiscriminately social/ disinhibited and emotionally withdrawn/inhibited subtypes. *Journal of the American Academy of Child and Adolescent Psychiatry, 50,* 216–231.

Goldfarb, W. (1947). Variations in adolescent adjustment in institutionally reared children. *American Journal of Orthopsychiatry, 17,* 449–457.

Hartmann, H. (1958). *Ego psychology and the problem of adaptation.* New York: International Universities Press, as English translation of Ich-Psychologie und Anpaussungs-problem. (Original work published 1939)

Hopkins, J. (2006). Individual psychotherapy for late-adopted children: How one new attachment can facilitate another. In J. Kenrick, C. Lindsey, & L. Tollemache (Eds.), *Creating new families: Therapeutic approaches to fostering, adoption, and kinship care* (pp. 95–106). London: Karnac Books.

Juffer, F., & van IJzendoorn, M. H. (2009). International adoption comes of age: Development of international adoptees from a longitudinal and meta-analytic perspective. In G. M. Wrobel & E. Neil (Eds.), *International advances in adoption research for practice* (pp. 169–192). Chichester, UK: Wiley-Blackwell.

Kenrick, J. (2006). Work with children in transition. In J. Kenrick, C. Lindsey, & L. Tollemache (Eds.), *Creating new families: Therapeutic approaches to fostering, adoption, and kinship care* (pp. 67–83). London: Karnac Books.

Lyons-Ruth, K., & Jacobvitz, D. (2008). Attachment disorganization: Genetic factors, parenting contexts, and developmental transformation from infancy to adulthood. In J. Cassidy & P. R. Shaver (Eds.), *Handbook of attachment: Theory, research, and clinical applications* (2nd ed., pp. 666–697). New York: Guilford Press.

Main, M., Hesse, E., & Goldwyn, R. (2008). Studying differences in language use in recounting attachment history: An introduction to the Adult Attachment Interview. In H. Steele & M. Steele (Eds.), *Clinical applications of the Adult Attachment Interview* (pp. 31–68). New York: Guilford Press.

McCall, R. B., van IJzendoorn, M. H., Juffer, F., Groark, C. J., & Groza, V. K. (2011). Children without permanent parents: Research, practice, and policy. *Monographs of the Society for Research in Child Development, 76,* 1–7.

Midgley, N. (2007). Anna Freud: The Hampstead War Nurseries and the role of the direct observation of children for psychoanalysis. *International Journal of Psychoanalysis, 88,* 939–959.

O'Connor, T., & Zeanah, C. H. (2003). Attachment disorders: Assessment strategies and treatment approaches. *Attachment and Human Development, 5,* 223–244.

Richters, M., & Volkmar, F. (1994). Reactive attachment disorder of infancy or early childhood. *Journal of the American Academy of Child and Adolescent Psychiatry, 33,* 328–332.

Rutter, M., & Sonuga-Barke, E. J. (2010). Conclusions: Overview of findings from the ERA study, inferences, and research implications. In M. Rutter, E. J. Sonuga-Barke, C. Beckett, J. Kreppner, R. Kumsta, W. Schlotz, et al. (Eds.), Deprivation-specific psychological patterns: Effects of institutional deprivation. *Monographs of the Society for Research in Child Development, 75,* 232–247.

Sandler, J., & Rosenblatt, B. (1962). The concept of the representational world. *Psychoanalytic study of the Child, 17,* 128–188.

Spangler, G., & Grossmann, K. E. (1993). Biobehavioral organization in securely and insecurely attached infants. *Child Development, 64,* 1439–1450.

Spitz, R. (1945). Hospitalism: An inquiry into the genesis of psychiatric conditions in early childhood. *Psychoanalytic Study of the Child, 1,* 53–73.

Spitz, R. (1950). Anxiety in infancy: A study of its manifestations in the first year of life. *International Journal of Psychoanalysis, 31,* 138–143.

Steele, H. (2003). Holding therapy is not attachment therapy. *Attachment and Human Development, 5,* 219.

Steele, H., & Steele, M. (2008). Ten clinical uses of the Adult Attachment Interview. In H. Steele & M. Steele (Eds.), *Clinical applications of the Adult Attachment Interview* (pp. 3–30). New York: Guilford Press.

Steele, M. (2006). The added value of attachment theory and research for clinical work in adoption and foster care. In J. Kenrick, C. Lindsey, & L. Tollemache (Eds.), *Creating new families: Therapeutic approaches to fostering, adoption, and kinship care* (pp. 33–42). London: Karnac Books.

Steele, M., Hodges, J., Kaniuk, J., Hillman, S., & Henderson, K. (2003). Attachment representations in newly adopted maltreated children and their adoptive parents: Implications for placement and support. *Journal of Child Psychotherapy. 29*, 187–205.

Steele, M., Hodges, J., Kaniuk, J., Steele, H., Asquith, K., & Hillman, S. (2009). Attachment representations and adoption outcome: On the use of narrative assessments to track the adaptation of previously maltreated children in their new families. In B. Neil & G. Wrobel (Eds.), *International advances in adoption research for practice* (pp. 193–216). New York: Wiley.

Steele, M., Hodges, J., Kaniuk, J., Steele, H., D'Agostino, D., Blom, I., et al. (2007). Intervening with maltreated children and their adoptive families: Identifying attachment-facilitative behavior. In D. Oppenheim & D. F. Goldsmith (Eds.), *Attachment theory in clinical work with children: Bridging the gap between research and practice* (pp. 58–89). New York: Guilford Press.

Steele, M., Hodges, J., Kaniuk, J., Steele, H., Hillman, S., & Asquith, K. (2008). Forecasting outcomes in previously maltreated children: The use of the AAI in a longitudinal attachment study. In H. Steele & M. Steele (Eds.). *Clinical applications of the Adult Attachment Interview* (pp. 427–451). New York: Guilford Press.

Steele, M., Murphy, A., & Steele, H. (2010). Identifying therapeutic action in an attachment-based intervention with high-risk families. *Clinical Social Work Journal, 38*, 61–72.

Tolan, P., & Dodge, K. (2005). Children's mental health as a primary care concern: A system for comprehensive support and service. *American Psychologist, 60*, 601–614.

van IJzendoorn, M. H., & Juffer, F. (2006). The Emanuel Miller Memorial Lecture 2006: Adoption as intervention. Meta-analytic evidence of massive catch-up and plasticity in physical, socio-emotional, and cognitive development. *Journal of Child Psychology and Psychiatry, 47*, 1228–1245.

van IJzendoorn, M. H., & Kroonenberg, P. M. (1988). Cross-cultural patterns of attachment: A meta-analysis of the strange situation. *Child Development, 59*, 147–156.

van IJzendoorn, M. H., & Sagi-Schwartz, A. (2008). Cross-cultural patterns of attachment: Universal and contextual dimensions. In J. Cassidy & P. R. Shaver (Eds.), *Handbook of attachment theory, research and clinical applications* (2nd ed., pp. 713–734). New York: Guilford Press.

Zeanah, C. H., & Gleason, M. M. (2010). *Reactive attachment disorder: A review for DSM-V.* Washington, DC: American Psychiatric Association.

Zeanah, C. H., Smyke, A. T., Koga, S., Carlson, E., & Bucharest Early Intervention Project Core Group. (2005). Attachment in institutionalized and community children in Romania. *Child Development, 76*, 1015–1028.

Zero to Three. (2005). *Diagnostic classification of mental health and developmental disorders of infancy and early childhood: Revised edition (DC:0–3R).* Washington, DC: Zero to Three Press.

CHAPTER 21

Reflective and Mindful Parenting
A NEW RELATIONAL MODEL OF ASSESSMENT, PREVENTION, AND EARLY INTERVENTION

John Grienenberger, Wendy Denham, and Diane Reynolds

> Collaborative and flexible parent–infant dialogues have been termed *open communication* in the developmental attachment literature but this term is subject to misinterpretation. Coherent, or "open" dialogue is characterized not by parental "openness" in the sense of unmonitored parental self-disclosure, but by parental "openness" to the state of mind of the child, including an entire array of the child's communications, so that particular affective or motive states of the child (anger, passion, distress) are not foreclosed from intersubjective sharing and regulation. . . . Collaborative dialogue, then, is about getting to know another's mind and taking it into account in constructing and regulating interactions. . . . Another's mind is a terrain that can never be fully known. . . . Thus, empathy should not be viewed as a simple apprehension of one person's state by another but as a complex outcome of a number of skilled communicative procedures for querying and decoding another's subjective reality.
> —LYONS-RUTH (1999, pp. 583–584)

These statements highlight some of the most significant implications that have emerged from developmental theory and research aimed at uncovering the intersubjective foundations of early cognitive and emotional development. Recent theories emphasize the importance of the parental capacity to comprehend the developing mind of the child and to respond in a manner that gives the child a sense of his own mind.[1] Lyons-Ruth has tied parental "openness" to the child's state of mind to the quality of the regulatory functions provided by the parent. Thus, the parent must rely on an emerging understanding of the child's mind in order to engage effectively with the child at the level of behavior.

This involves great challenges to the parent, including both the attempt to understand the child and in terms of self-reflection or mindful awareness. For many parents,

---

[1] In the pages that follow, for the purposes of clarity, we have chosen to refer to the child as "he" and to the parent/caregiver or group leader as "she."

the birth of a child can lead to the healthy reorganization of previously established beliefs, defenses, and definitions of self. However, parents are not equally prepared to meet the psychological burdens of parenthood. Thus, there is a great range in the degree to which the parent–child relationship is dominated by the emotions or defenses of the parent versus the developmental needs of the child.

The majority of parenting and early intervention programs have sought to help caregivers by providing both specific behavioral techniques and general information about child development. These models often fail to influence the deeper dynamics and intergenerational patterns of relatedness that powerfully impact the overall quality of parent–child interactions. Therefore, it is important to address each parent–child dyad as a unique entity, characterized by particular strengths and vulnerabilities at the level of intersubjective relatedness. The provision of proscriptive behavioral techniques often fails to take such factors into consideration. It may also serve to undermine a parent's development of an emergent capacity to reflect on her child's developing mind, as she attempts to fit a given child or child-rearing situation into a general behavioral approach. By telling parents what to do, rather than helping them tolerate the experience of "not knowing," we may be undermining the reflective and regulatory processes that can emerge as caregivers attempt to make sense of the confusing, chaotic, and distressing interactions that are an inevitable part of parenthood.

In this chapter, we describe a model of early intervention and prevention that seeks to minimize such pitfalls. This model emphasizes the cultivation of the emotional and cognitive processing mechanisms that underlie affect regulation and form the basis for attachment security in children. It utilizes interventions derived from the assessment of the reflective capacities and attachment dynamics of each caregiver on a case-by-case basis. It is a strength-building approach that allows space for differences in cultural and familial values while enhancing the reflective processes that can be extended into a wide range of parenting issues or relational dynamics.

This approach is explicitly nondidactic. Instead, it engages parents in a process of exploration, curiosity, imagination, and mindfulness. Parents attempt to sort through and become more sensitive to the internal states within their children and themselves, then begin to make links between these "inside stories" and the behaviors being expressed externally. We call this approach "reflective and mindful parenting." It is rooted in contemporary psychodynamic theory, attachment research, and mindfulness practice, with a particular emphasis on the role of parental mentalization as it contributes to the emotional development of young children.

PSYCHODYNAMIC APPROACHES TO EARLY PREVENTION AND INTERVENTION

One goal of this volume is to examine the disease mechanisms that underlie a range of psychological disorders across the developmental spectrum, with the hope of contributing to the emergence of treatment models that can address the underlying causes of psychological suffering. It is a timely volume, as evaluation researchers (e.g., Kazdin & Nock, 2003) have increasingly demanded that treatment approaches be based on clearly defined models of psychopathology that include consideration for underlying change mechanisms (Fonagy & Target, 2005). The two early intervention models described next meet these criteria, as they utilize case-specific assessment of the strengths and limitations of a given caregiver's capacity for mentalization as it relates to her ability to respond in developmentally appropriate ways to her child's attachment cues. In utilizing a nuanced assessment of parental mentalization, clinicians are afforded the opportunity to develop interventions that specifically target the blind spots or areas of vulnerability that the parent is experiencing in relation to her child, while also highlighting and consolidating any inherent parenting strength that may exist.

Mentalization

Mentalization is a construct with roots in multiple disciplines, including cognitive psychology (Baron-Cohen, 1995; Dennett, 1987), attachment theory (Main, 1991), and psychoanalytic theory (Bion, 1962; Winnicott, 1960). In the present context, we are most concerned with the seminal ideas introduced by Peter Fonagy and his colleagues (Fonagy, Steele, Steele, Moran, & Higgitt, 1991) that have been expanded in recent years and extended to a wide range of clinical applications (e.g., Allen & Fonagy, 2006). Fonagy and Target (2008, p. 17) define mentalization as "a form of mostly preconscious *imaginative* mental activity, namely, interpreting people's actions in terms of 'intentional' mental states." Fonagy and his colleagues have elaborated on Main's concept of metacognitive monitoring to include not only the capacity to observe one's own representational processes, but also the ability to reflect on the mental states of one's attachment objects. Their research considers the developmental achievement of the capacity for mentalization as involving an awareness of the nature of complex mental states, including attitudes, feelings, beliefs, intentions, desires, and plans (Fonagy & Target, 1998). Mentalization is first developed within the context of early attachment relationships, as the parent relates to the child as an intentional being. As children internalize this process, they begin to see other people's behavior as predictable. Mentalization underlies affect regulation, impulse control, and self-agency. Individuals lacking in this capacity struggle to step back from their experience to consider the symbolic aspects of other people's thoughts and feelings.

Mentalization theory also considers the concept of containment (Bion, 1962)—the idea that the parent not only reflects the infant's internal state but also represents it as a manageable experience. In doing so, the parent demonstrates that she understands the child's feelings and communicates this in a way that indicates that the child can have a similar experience of mastery (Fonagy & Target, 1998). Fonagy, Gergely, Jurist, and Target (2002) have described this process as "marked mirroring," whereby the caregiver is able to contingently respond to the child's internal state while adding something that makes it clear to the child that her internal state is not a direct equivalent of his own. This "re-presentation" of the child's state of mind may involve a softening or heightening of affect, or a cross-modal response in which the caregiver uses tone of voice to mirror the infant's gestures, or a facial expression to mirror a child's words. This complex multimodal dialogue operates largely outside the conscious awareness of the caregiver. However, it is crucial to the child's emerging capacity for symbolic representation and his developing sense of self. It also forms the basis of the child's representations of attachment.

In fact, Fonagy has suggested that secure attachment is the direct outcome of successful containment, while insecure attachment evidences failures of containment that differ in terms of the defensive compromises adopted by the caregiver (Fonagy, 1996). In the case of dismissing attachment, there is a failure of affect mirroring but some evidence of stability and mastery. In the case of preoccupied attachment, there is an abundance of affect mirroring but a dearth of calmness and confidence on the part of the caregiver.

The caregiver's capacity for mentalization is particularly critical in cases of deprivation, loss, or abuse, as it provides a protective measure against the intergenerational transmission of trauma (Fonagy, 1996). However, if the parent is lacking in mentalization, she will not be able to accurately attend to the child's painful reactions to stressful situations and will thereby misrepresent the child's affect and intentions. For these children, it is too painful to consider the apparently malevolent intentions of one's caregivers. As a result, the developmental acquisition of mentalization within the child may become severely impaired.

Parental Mentalization

The original reflective functioning measure (Fonagy, Target, Steele, & Steele, 1998) was designed for application to the Adult Attachment Interview (AAI; George, Kaplan, & Main, 1985). Thus, it referred to the parent's capacity to reflect on her childhood experiences with her own parents. More recently, Slade and her colleagues have extended mentalization research into the context of parents' current relationships with their children (Grienenberger, Kelly, & Slade, 2005; Slade, Grienenberger, Bernbach, Levy, & Locker, 2005). These studies have utilized the Parent Development Interview (PDI; Aber, Slade, Berger, Bresgi, & Kaplan, 1985) to focus on the capacity of parents to reflect upon their children's internal experiences and upon their own experiences as parents. Unlike the AAI, which assesses representations of past experiences, the PDI elicits representations derived from a current, ongoing relationship with one's child. Thus, child development, and the caregiver's capacity to reflect upon the child's ever-changing abilities and upon the constantly evolving parent–child relationship, all provide the backdrop to the assessment of parental mentalization.

The PDI studies, as well as others using related measures (e.g., Meins, Fernyhough, Fradley, & Tuckey, 2001; Oppenheim & Koren-Karie, 2002) have shown that parental mentalization is strongly predictive of child attachment (Sharp & Fonagy, 2008). Parental mentalization has also been demonstrated to be inversely related to disruptions in mother–infant affective communication in response to infant distress (Grienenberger et al., 2005). More specifically, reflective mothers were found to have fewer and less severe behaviors that evidenced affective communication errors, role or boundary confusion, fearful, disoriented, or dissociated behavior, withdrawal, or intrusiveness and negativity.

The Transmission Gap and Implications for Early Intervention

Attachment theorists have long emphasized the role of "maternal sensitivity" in the intergenerational transmission of attachment from caregivers to their children. They have hypothesized that caregivers who are themselves secure in their attachment will be more able to respond to their children in ways that are warm, sensitive, and responsive. However, a meta-analytic review of the attachment literature (van IJzendoorn, 1995) has identified a "transmission gap," as behavioral measures of maternal sensitivity failed to account adequately for the strong link between adult attachment and infant attachment.

The studies by Slade and colleagues (Grienenberger et al., 2005; Slade et al., 2005) have helped to close this gap and suggest that maternal mentalization, rather than maternal sensitivity per se, may be the critical mediator between the parent's attachment style, parental behavior in response to infant distress, and child attachment. These findings provide further support for the need to target parental mentalization directly in order to have a significant impact on child attachment security. They also suggest that more sensitive, positive, or warm parental behavior in general, in the absence of a reflective stance in relation to the child, is likely to have a limited impact on child outcomes.

In fact, the maternal behaviors likely to be the most salient in terms of child attachment security are those occurring during times of distress within the child, the parent, or both. It is also during such moments of heightened affective and physiological arousal that mentalizing efforts are the most difficult to sustain. Fonagy (2008) has reviewed a growing body of research on the neurobiology of attachment and mentalization that "suggests that being in an emotionally attached state inhibits or suppresses aspects of social cognition, including mentalizing and the capacity to accurately see the attachment figure as a person" (p. 12). One of the most useful aspects of the PDI as an assessment measure is that it requires parents to reflect on some of the painful, distressing, and uncomfortable mental states occurring within themselves and within their children, and to make links between these states and what is being expressed behaviorally. It is this point of interface between the mentalizing efforts of the caregiver and the heightened affective arousal that characterizes the activation of the attachment system with which we are most concerned. Following from the PDI, our early intervention model is focused on helping parents identify and navigate elements of the parent–child relationship that involve conflict, distress, anger, and other uncomfortable feelings. As parents begin to see such experiences as inevitable, ordinary aspects of parenting, they often shift toward a more reflective stance and are better able to regulate emotions within themselves and within their children.

Current Models of Early Intervention

Current models of early intervention primarily target the parent–child relationship utilizing parental representations, or parental behavior, as ports of entry, due in large part to the theoretical or contextual environments from which they have emerged

(Stern, 1995). A number of approaches have evolved from the educational and behavioral world (e.g., Field, 1982; McDonough, 2004) that target parent–child interactive behavior using mothers' behavior as the overt port of entry. In contrast, a core concept guiding psychodynamic models of early intervention is that change in the child depends on change in caregiver representations of the child and of the caregiver–child relationship (Lieberman, Silverman, & Pawl, 2000).

Models such as McDonough's "Interaction Guidance" (2004), which begin with the observable parent–infant behaviors as the therapeutic focus, also understand caregiver interactions as a reflection of the caregiver's and infant's representational world, although this is not the therapeutic port of entry. Other popular group approaches such as "The Incredible Years" (Webster-Stratton, 2005) utilize stricter behavioral models that provide parents with behavioral tools as well as child development information, but do not consider parental representations.

Literally hundreds of studies have shown attachment to be a critical variable that has been linked to multiple measures of social and emotional functioning, psychopathology, and resiliency across the lifespan (Cassidy & Shaver, 1999; Sroufe, 2005). Thus, it could be argued that attachment security should be the primary early intervention target. Berlin, Zeanah, and Lieberman (2008) propose that the main focus of attachment-based early intervention should include both parents' internal working models and parenting behaviors, specifically in relation to how they respond to their children's desire for contact, along with their desire for autonomy. It is clear that models of early intervention need to account for the reciprocal and bidirectional influence that occurs between representation and behavior (Griencnberger & Slade, 2002).

Since 2005, several attachment-based programs have demonstrated success in supporting children's early attachment security (for a review, see Berlin et al., 2008). These programs start from the premise that while behavioral tools may be helpful in managing interactive behaviors, the underlying intentions that drive and motivate behavior need to be addressed in order to most effectively target the quality of parent–child attachment and child developmental outcomes. Furthermore, several authors have argued that shifting internal working models of attachment depends on parental reflective capacity. Thus, parental mentalization is perhaps the critical intervention target in and of itself (Grienenberger, 2007; Sadler, Slade, & Mayes, 2006; Suchman, McMahon, Slade, & Luthar, 2005). When therapists give voice to the intentions behind children's behavior, it can allow for shifts within parents' internal working models (Berlin et al., 2008). As parents acknowledge their children's intentions, it also has the effect of reducing the frequency and duration of children's dysregulated or disruptive behavior.

Other early intervention programs that specifically target parental mentalization include the Mothers and Toddlers Program (Suchman, DeCoste, Castiglioni, Legow, & Mayes, 2008), a 20-week individual therapy intervention for substance-abusing mothers; the Minding the Baby project (Sadler et al., 2006), an interdisciplinary home visiting program for high-risk mothers that combines nursing intervention with mental health support; and the Circle of Security Project (Hoffman, Marvin, Cooper, & Powell, 2006), a group treatment model that utilizes video feedback, parent education, and psychotherapy to target insecure and disorganized attachment patterns. All three of these psychodynamic/attachment-based intervention programs have reported pilot data that include favorable outcomes. For example, the Mothers and Toddlers Program found that mothers who completed the program showed moderate improvement in maternal behavior and improved capacity to foster their children's socioemotional development. The Circle of Security project found significant within-subject shifts whereby the majority of children moved from disorganized to organized attachment classifications following the intervention. However, while these studies are promising, randomized control trials are an important next step in establishing the validity of mentalization-based models of early intervention. In addition, further replications at additional sites are needed to ensure that these models are transferable beyond work implemented under the direct involvement of the program developers.

The PDI as Assessment Tool and Outcome Measure

During the past two decades, there has been a significant growth in clinical applications of attachment theory to a variety of treatment contexts, including adult psychotherapy (Wallin, 2007), child therapy (Slade, 2004), and family therapy (Fearon et al., 2006). Even more recently, research tools such as the Strange Situation and the AAI are being directly integrated into clinical interventions across a range of treatment modalities (e.g., Powell, Cooper, Hoffman, & Marvin, 2009; Steele & Steele, 2008). The programs at the Center for Reflective Communities are part of this next wave in the clinical application of attachment research. Both programs use the Reflective Functioning coding system (Slade et al., 2002) for use with the PDI (Aber et al., 1985) as both an outcome measure and a tool for case formulation. A key element of the intake process is that the PDI is administered by one of the clinicians facilitating the group. This allows for a one-on-one meeting that engages the parent in the therapeutic process and facilitates the development of a therapeutic relationship with the clinician. It also affords the group leader an opportunity to begin to develop a working formulation of the parent's attachment dynamics in terms of her capacity to mentalize around various issues.

More specifically, the PDI asks questions about a range of mental states and behaviors, with an emphasis on the challenging emotions and interactions that are central to issues of affect regulation within parent–child attachment. For example, there are questions that ask the caregiver to speak about her own pain, anger, guilt, or neediness in her parenting role and the impact of these feelings on her child. Other questions focus on the child's negative affects, such as times when he may feel upset, rejected, or distressed about separation, as well as the impact that the child's affective experience may have on the parent. There are also questions that ask about the role of the parent–child relationship in the child's emerging personality or development, and the impact of the parent's own early history on her current experience as a parent.

Parental reflective functioning is scored for several passages on the PDI on a scale ranging from –1 to 9 (Slade et al., 2002). An aggregate score is also provided for the interview as a whole. A score of –1 is indicative of antireflective, unintegrated, bizarre, distorted, or self-serving responses. A rating of 5 indicates ordinary reflective functioning, such as a response that links affect to behavior or to another mental state. A score of 9 indicates exceptional mentalizing capacity.

The majority of clinicians undergoing training at the Center for Reflective Communities do not receive formal training in the reflective functioning coding system for the PDI; however, they are all trained to administer the interview. They also learn to recognize the range of mentalization within parents' speech as it exists along a continuum from low to high. This allows group leaders to utilize the PDI as an assessment tool even if they will not be scoring it as an outcome measure. Trainees learn to listen for mental state language within parents' communications and to notice when parents are able to link mental states to behaviors and to other mental states in themselves and their children. They are trained to listen for the following "building blocks of reflective functioning," which can be understood as indicating increasingly complex or sophisticated indications of parental mentalization: (1) recognizing and labeling basic mental states (e.g., sad, angry, worried, afraid, etc.) in self, child, or other family members; (2) enhancing the understanding that one's overt behavior, or that of others, is motivated by underlying mental states (e.g., "I feel guilty because I have to work so much, so sometimes I think I have trouble saying no to my daughter"); (3) fostering links between mental states (e.g., "I feel guilty because I have to work so much, and sometimes I think she picks up on that and is confused"); and (4) an awareness of the interconnectedness of minds—the notion that one's own mental states and behaviors impact and are impacted by the mental states and behaviors of one's child (e.g., "I feel guilty because I have to work so much, and sometimes I think she picks up on that and is confused. She may even play off of my guilt a bit and try and push limits with me, knowing that I may have a hard time saying no after I have been traveling for work"). We have found that clinicians can be trained, in a relatively short amount of time, to identify these building blocks, to evaluate the range of parental mentalization, and to listen for those areas where a parent may be more or less able to reflect on their children's attachment needs.

States of Mind with Respect to Attachment

The intervention models we have developed integrate traditional attachment theory, with its focus on internal working models of attachment or attachment categories, and mentalization theory. Mentalization theory has tended to emphasize the range of mentalizing capacities, from low to high, rather than focusing on particular patterns of representation, as was the focus of Main's original coding system for the AAI (Main & Goldwyn, 1998). We view attachment organization as representative of various positions existing upon a continuum (Slade, 2004). These positions are seen as indications of the dominant mode of affect regulation and defense for a parent at a particular time and in relation to a specific child. In other words, we focus on "states of mind" with respect to attachment, and we see these states as somewhat fluid as they develop in relationship to a range of parenting issues and parent–child interactions. In translating the findings of attachment research to clinical intervention, we concur with Slade (2004), who argues that it is more important to sensitize clinicians to identify attachment phenomena within their patients' behavior and narratives than to try to assign them to attachment categories. By focusing on states of mind within a specific parent–child context, rather than seeing each parent or child in a categorical way, clinicians are freed from the limitations that have sometimes been associated with the application of attachment theory to clinical work.

We have found that it is useful to think of dismissing states of mind and preoccupied states of mind as simply opposite ways of defending against the same experience: the challenge of managing strong affect within the context of intimate relationships. On the preoccupied side of the continuum are states of mind characterized by feelings of enmeshment, dependency, and uncontained affect. Moving further in this direction are states of mind influenced by unresolved loss or trauma, leading to the development of a "helpless/fearful" parenting style, as child distress re-stimulates dissociated memories or affect (Lyons-Ruth, Bronfman, & Atwood, 1999). On the dismissing side of the continuum are states of mind that may be intellectualized or concrete, minimizing of emotions, and characterized by detachment from others. At the extreme of this end of the continuum are states of mind that are unresolved with respect to loss or trauma in which the caregiver may have developed a "hostile/intrusive" parenting style, as her child's vulnerability stimulates an identification with past aggressors as a means of warding off dissociated feelings of vulnerability (Lyons-Ruth et al., 1999). In contrast to the two ends of the continuum, free or secure states of mind can be understood as existing in the middle of the attachment continuum. These states involve a balance between thinking and feeling, autonomy and intimacy, separateness and connection with others (see also Mikulincer & Shaver, Chapter 2, and Luyten & Blatt, Chapter 5, this volume).

As we consider this continuum, it is helpful to examine the implications that are posed regarding the impact of states of mind on a given caregiver's ability to mentalize. For example, mentalization is often more limited within dismissing states of mind around issues of dependency, intimacy, and the experience of distress, shame, or uncertainty. The caregiver may be able to think of her child as having a separate mind; however, she may fail to see the impact of her thoughts, feelings, and behaviors on her child's emotions. By contrast, preoccupied states of mind are often characterized by breakdowns in mentalization fueled by feelings of anxiety, insecurity, or fear of loss. The primary challenge to the caregiver involves seeing her child as having a separate mind that is not the equivalent of her own.

Figure 21.1 illustrates an integration of the continuum of attachment states of mind with the role of parental mentalization within parent–child relationships.

In this model, secure states of mind are thought of as evidencing the highest levels of mentalization; both hostile/intrusive and helpless/fearful states are seen as being the least reflective; and preoccupied and dismissive states fall somewhere in the middle to low range. This model has preliminary empirical support from a study that found the highest level of reflective functioning in mothers of securely attached children, the lowest in mothers of children with disorganized attachment, and moderately low reflective functioning in mothers of children with insecure/organized attachment (i.e., the anxious-resistant and avoidant groups) (Grienenberger et al., 2005). It is often helpful for clinicians to consider this continuum as they attempt to formulate interventions that target the specific areas of strength and vulnerability of the parents within their groups. This approach to assessing states of mind with respect to attachment and the impact such states have on mentalization fits well

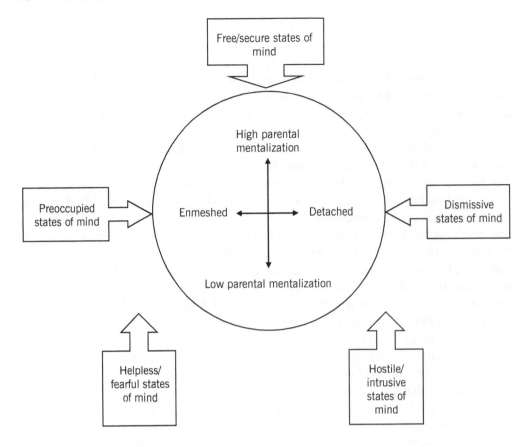

FIGURE 21.1. Parental mentalization and states of mind with respect to attachment.

within recent work that has increasingly seen mentalization as a multidimensional construct that requires the evaluation of a "mentalizing profile" in order to most effectively target areas of weakness and to formulate appropriate interventions (Luyten, Fonagy, Lowyck, & Vermote, 2012).

PSYCHODYNAMIC APPROACHES TO EARLY INTERVENTION: MENTALIZATION-BASED EARLY INTERVENTION PROGRAMS AT THE CENTER FOR REFLECTIVE COMMUNITIES

The Center for Reflective Communities is a nonprofit organization established in Los Angeles in 2009, whose mission is to (1) promote the development of secure parent–child attachment through increasing parental mentalization and (2) provide training to clinicians in the facilitation and development of parental mentalization through the use of the Reflective Parenting Program Parent Workshops and Mindful Parenting Group models. The Center is actively engaged in the empirical evaluation of these programs.

The Reflective Parenting Program is a manualized intervention. Preliminary outcome data indicate that after completing the program, parents reported significantly less stress, fewer depressive symptoms, and fewer behavior problems in their children (all ps <.001). More specifically, there was a 28% decrease in depressive symptoms on the Beck Depression Inventory with a medium effect size (.39) ($n = 89$), a 7% decrease in the Parenting Stress Index with a small effect size (.29), and a 12% decrease in Total Problems on the Achenbach Child Behavior Checklist, which represents a medium effect size (.45) ($n = 71$). Such findings suggest that interventions aimed at improving parental mentalization may be effective in improving both parental and child functioning, and thereby reduce some of the risks conferred upon children of parents who are compromised in some way, including those with mental health problems. A manual for Mindful Parenting Groups is currently under development. Both programs have been qualified as "Community Defined Evidence Based Treatments" by the California Institute of Mental Health. A large-scale randomized control trial study has recently been submitted for a federal grant that would include evaluation of the Reflective Parenting Program model with both Spanish- and English-speaking parents among families participating in community-based Head Start preschool.

Certification training is available for both programs that includes the following: (1) training in the building blocks of parental mentalization; (2) training in group dynamics and ways of interacting with parents and infants that attend to both verbal and also the more subtle, nonverbal, procedural level of communications; (3) engaging facilitators-in-training through an experiential learning process that involves holding and containing complex, difficult, emotionally charged case examples; and (4) group supervision experiences through which trainees learn to develop dynamic case formulations of the parents they are working with. These formulations include an integration of attachment dynamics with an understanding of parental mentalization.

The training is heavily experiential, actively facilitating the development of the reflective capacities of facilitators in training. The Mindful Parenting Group facilitator training includes a demonstration group led by a senior trainer in which trainees are supervised as they sit in a "participant-observer" role; the Reflective Parenting Program utilizes role-playing and review of videotaped groups to facilitate the trainee's development of a reflective stance in relation to parents with a wide range of mentalizing strengths and limitations. Watching experienced senior trainers make interventions from a mentalizing perspective, and then having the opportunity to practice through role-playing, or through the experience of being supervised while leading groups, maximizes procedural learning. Our training model is consistent with other mentalization-based programs that have noted the importance of using exercises that immerse trainees in the challenges of mentalizing in the face of intensely emotional dynamics (Williams et al., 2006).

Recent research into attachment-based programs supports the idea that the parent's relationship with the therapist or intervener is a major facilitator of change (Berlin et al., 2008). We believe that it is the observational and reflective stance of *both* the therapist *and* the other group members that is the agent of change. Thomson-Salo and Paul (2001) suggest that the benefits of a group experience may include a lessening of mothers' feelings of blame and persecution as they listen to each other weather the struggles with their children. Furthermore, other group members provide rich sources of material for therapeutic identification. Reynolds (2003) refers to the meaningful and regulating social contact that groups can provide for parents and infants. Grienenberger (2007) describes how the group process creates a secure base and a holding environment that is containing and facilitative of mentalization, as well as accelerating the therapeutic process by providing parents with a chance to observe the strengths and limitations of a range of parenting styles seen among various group members.

Both the Reflective Parenting Workshops and Mindful Parenting Groups foster the development of careful, detailed observation as the foundation for building reflective capacity. Infant observation was pioneered by Esther Bick (1964) at the Tavistock Clinic as a training tool for child psychotherapists to develop their ability to nonjudgmentally attend to the minute details of infant experience and bear witness, rather than react to, intense affects. Formal infant observation traditionally consists of weekly visits to a family during the first year of the baby's life. During these visits, the therapist maintains an observational stance, tracking the moment-to-moment experience of the infant's and mother's states and behaviors, alongside the therapist's own emotional experience.

The training builds on Bion's (1962) notion of "reverie," emphasizing the willingness of the therapist to be permeated by the infant's state as much as possible, allowing the infant to "find a place inside us" (Sternberg, 2005, p. 49). The ability to experience and observe simultaneously develops the internal flexibility of the observer, along with the ability to think and feel at the same time (Sternberg, 2005). While intervention is not the focus of this method, the observer's mind may provide the family an unseen digestive function—what Bion described as "alpha function." Reynolds (2003) built on the idea of formal infant observation in introducing child-centered observation in Mindful Parenting Groups. She describes a "profound bidirectional, relational, and regulatory utility in strengthening a parent's capacity to come as close as possible to a child's subjective, affective experiences" (p. 362). Both Reflective Parenting Program parent workshops and Mindful Parenting Groups include structured observational components as a way of developing parental mentalization. Reynolds describes this process as "the accumulated practice of directing quieted, patient, curious, alive attention to both child and self, through learning to respect and follow the child's lead in contact-seeking and exploratory behaviors" (p. 362). This slowed-down focus on moment-to-moment experience helps to develop parents' curiosity and wonder, their ability to think and feel at the same time, and their ability to sit with the uncertainty that is a fundamental part of building reflective capacity and mindfulness.

The Reflective Parenting Program Workshop Structure

The Reflective Parenting Program parent workshops provide a developmentally scaled, 12-week workshop series for parents. These workshops are curriculum-based but process-focused. Multiple curricula are available, including workshop series for expectant mothers and for parents of 0- to 2-year-olds, 3- to 6-year-olds, and elementary-school-aged children. A curriculum for parents of adolescents is currently under development. The workshops have also been applied to specific, diverse populations, including Spanish-speaking parents, teenage mothers, and parents adopting children from the foster care system.

Each curriculum focuses on specific topics that are used as the context within which to explore parents' capacity to reflect on their children and their experiences as parents. Topics include areas such as temperament, responding to children's emotions, rupture and repair, and limit-setting. Each workshop begins with a structured mindfulness exercise that engages parents in an experience of observation and provides a transition into the reflective space of the group experience. Exercises such as role-playing are utilized in order to stimulate parents' engagement in making sense of children's feelings and behavior and to help parents examine their characteristic, often automatic, ways of responding. "Take-home reflections" are employed as a way for parents to practice observational, mindful ways of relating to their children. The workshops are led by co-facilitators who model a collaborative, reflective approach for parents, offering containment and support, as well as boundaries and limit-setting. Facilitators help group members expand and explore by asking questions that elicit reflection, and they reinforce reflective comments by explicitly noting when links are made. Interventions are tailored to each parent's mentalizing capacity and parenting style.

Mindful Parenting Group Structure

Mindful Parenting Groups are experiential, observation-based, development-driven groups for infants or toddlers and their parents. Each group consists of three primary components: child-centered observation of the children at play, modeling of respectful parenting practices through facilitation of social interactions, and parent-centered reflection on what is observed, as well as time for questions and discussion (Reynolds, 2003). During child-centered observation, parents are asked to sit back quietly while they follow their children's lead and pay attention to both their children's feelings and behaviors and what arises inside themselves. The facilitator then poses an open question to the group about their observations to facilitate a process of inquiry and wonder (Reynolds, 2003). At times, facilitators actively draw the attention of the group back to an affect-laden moment, such as one between two toddlers, to explore both the parents' experiences and what they imagined about the nature of the toddlers' mental states and behaviors. The inquiries are bidirectional, looking always at the flow of mental states and behaviors between the parents and children. Facilitators work to enhance mentalization about affect-laden moments in the here-and-now between parents and their children, as well as making links between the present and past family histories.

Parents commonly inquire about practical concerns around behavioral and emotional issues, such as sleeping, eating, fears, tantrums, and other challenges typical of infants and toddlers. Facilitators hold these questions in a lively way, and the group is challenged to wrestle with uncertainty and complexity, as all group members are invited to share their unique perspectives. For older toddlers, a group snack and a circle time with songs and games are added. This provides opportunities for the children to participate in a school-readiness activity at their own pace, experiencing the joys and challenges of navigating structure and turn-taking (Reynolds, 2003). The groups have been facilitated with a number of diverse populations, including teenage mothers, Spanish-speaking parents, and parents adopting from foster care.

The next section provides two case examples, the first from a Mindful Parenting Group and the second from a Reflective Parenting Program workshop. The examples illustrate a theoretical model that is based in an understanding of states of mind with respect to attachment as contributing to the creation of case-specific profiles of mentalization. These profiles, in turn, allow for the highly individualized treatment planning that forms the foundation of these unique approaches to early intervention and prevention.

CLINICAL ILLUSTRATIONS

The following examples represent two parents who were struggling with states of mind at opposite ends of the attachment continuum. In both cases we describe some of the personal histories gathered at intake, and we use excerpts from the PDI, administered pre- and postintervention, to illustrate changes in each parent's mentalizing capacity and states of mind in relation to specific attachment-related contexts. Interventions based on our case formulations are also presented. These examples can be understood as cases in which there were breakdowns in parental mentalization triggered by histories of unresolved loss or trauma. Both parents, however, exhibited average reflective capacity in the context of nontriggering attachment-related affects. The mentalizing deficits that were observed related to out-of-control feelings involving fear, anger, intense need, loss, or vulnerability in relation to their children, but these manifested themselves in two very different parenting styles: a dismissive/hostile/intrusive parenting style in the first example and an enmeshed/helpless/fearful style in the second.

Samantha and Billy: A Parent–Toddler Case
Illustrating Dismissive/Hostile/Intrusive States of Mind

Billy, a 26-month-old toddler who had been prenatally substance exposed, was in the process of being adopted from the foster care system by Samantha, a single woman in her mid-40s, when they were referred to a Mindful Parenting Group. He had been placed with her 3 months before the start of the group after experiencing a disrupted and chaotic foster care environment from which he had been precipitously removed. During the PDI at intake, Samantha demonstrated an intermittent capacity for reflection; however, questions inquiring about more challenging affect states and difficult interactions revealed moments of uncontained hostility, distortion of its impact on Billy, and lapses of narrative coherence. An example is her response to the question "Can you tell me about a time in the last week when you felt really angry as a parent?"

"He began yelling when I was going to change the diaper and, and . . . I, um [long pause] grabbed him sort of, you know [pause] on the arm [laughs] [*uncontained hostility?*] and then I was like, OK, let's get this over with. But I was over it. I am a completely, a pretty calm sort of mom [*incoherent*]. Sometimes I grab him, but I decided not to yell at him, so I grab him by the arm instead. You know I wasn't pissed off, I was frustrated [*incoherent*]. Sometimes I have to be forceful, although usually he's already sobbing so I don't think it really matters what I do, as he is just going to cry it out on his own [*minimizing*].

The interviewer then asked Samantha a follow-up question about the impact of her anger on Billy, and she responded:

"He is who he is, and I could do it four different ways and it isn't going to matter that much. I was expressing my annoyance nicely [*incongruent*] and he was fine with it [*self-serving, minimizing impact on child*]."

This example illustrates the role of uncontained, unmentalized hostility within Samantha's narrative that is likely related to unresolved trauma from her own early history. Parents with unresolved/intrusive attachment strategies often pose some of the greatest challenges to group leaders because of their inherent difficulties with self-regulation. There is often a tendency to externalize affect, and parental behavior may be characterized by criticism, detachment, and rejection of the child. It is clear that Samantha is finding the experience of parenting to be highly provocative, and she is having great difficulty seeing the ways in which her own mental states (in particular anger) are impacting her behavior and subsequently Billy's internal experience. Samantha's narrative in the PDI foreshadows some of the disrupted behavioral interactions that would later be observed during the Mindful Parenting Groups.

Armed with this kind of information, group leaders are able to develop interventions for working with parents who struggle with dismissive or hostile/intrusive states of mind by helping them to slow down and begin to make links between their mental states and their behavior in relation to their children. Parents may benefit from interventions that help to clarify misperceptions of their children and the impact of their responses to their children's behavior. It is also important to track countertransference closely, as feelings of annoyance, rejection, rage, helplessness, and even dissociation may be felt by the therapist. Group leaders should seek to avoid overreaction to such feelings, which can manifest as intrusiveness, boundary violations, or power struggles. Interventions should seek to stop the action and allow for the gradual integration of difficult material. It is also important to help parents struggling with dismissive or hostile states of mind to become more aware of and sensitive to their children's needs for comfort and contact. These parents often fail to see that their child's apparently provocative or disruptive behavior may in fact be his way of seeking proximity and connection (Slade, 2004).

Samantha and Billy joined a Mindful Parenting Group for families with toddlers being adopted from foster care. Billy typically entered the group independently of Samantha, and initially he rarely made eye contact or returned to her during the

90-minute group experience. If something happened that upset him, he would stand or sit alone in the room and cry. At these times, Samantha would not respond, commenting frequently to the facilitator that he "isn't usually so emotional." She frequently described Billy as "a bruiser" and "rough."

During the fifth group, Samantha disclosed that Billy had frequently hit her during the previous week. When asked for her thoughts about this, she said she believed it was "good for him to be able to be tough." The facilitator gently inquired as to whether she knew anything about that from her own history. Samantha then shared that she was the youngest of four, that her eldest sister had been physically abusive, and that her parents had done nothing to protect her. While she was speaking, Billy initiated several conflicts with other toddlers. Suddenly, Samantha stood up and lurched across the room saying, "That's it! I can't handle this! I will not let him hurt other kids!" She grabbed Billy roughly by the arms and pushed him hard toward the facilitator, saying angrily, "I want you to pay attention." The facilitator, a trainee, later reported in supervision that she had felt frightened by Samantha's behavior, as well as significant dread as to how Samantha might respond to any intervention. She noted that during the group, she was unclear whether Samantha was speaking to her or to Billy when she said, "I want you to pay attention," and she reported a countertransference reaction in which she had felt criticized for having "allowed" Billy's aggression. This led to a deeper understanding of the confusion that existed between Samantha and Billy in terms of the ownership and source of anger and aggressive impulses.

During the group, the facilitator had recognized the need to slow things down. She told Samantha that she could see that she was very upset by Billy's behavior, and that she would be available during group to help her manage things. Samantha continued to struggle with the urge to punish Billy for his behavior, but she was able to take direction. During parent-centered reflection, the facilitator commented that Samantha had been talking about something important and relevant from her personal history when she had responded to Billy's behavior. Samantha, who had become very quiet, said that she realized she had been aggressive with Billy. She had worried that if she was too focused on trying to understand the meaning behind Billy's behavior, she would not be able to set limits on his aggressiveness. This led to a discussion of how difficult it is to "hold the feeling" while also "holding the line" in relation to children's aggression.

Over the course of the next several weeks, Billy began to occasionally check in with his mother during group sessions, facing her as he sat in her lap, looking into her eyes with a smile. He began to express more warmth, which Samantha was very responsive to. At times, Billy would cry, and Samantha would express concern and console him. During the observation period of the 15th group, Billy was struggling with another child over a toy when he hit the child. It was unclear whether this had been intentional. The facilitator moved in close and narrated for both the children. Billy was obviously curious about what was going on with the other little boy, who was crying, and he continued to look at the child with curiosity. When the incident had been resolved, the facilitators asked the group for their thoughts and feelings about what had happened. Samantha, who had been observing relatively calmly during the entire incident, stated that she didn't believe that Billy had intended to seriously hurt the child, and she wondered whether a child his age had the ability to anticipate the outcome of his actions. A turning point seemed to have been Samantha's experience of reflecting on her unresolved traumatic history with her sister, which had been projected on to her relationship with Billy.

Samantha's ability to mentalize had grown through the course of the group, with her overall reflective functioning score improving from 2 at the time of intake to 5 during the posttest, a significant increase. This enhanced reflective capacity was also evident in her improved ability to regulate her anger and feelings of helplessness, to accurately identify Billy's intentions, and to recognize both her own aggressive impulses and feelings and their impact on Billy. As an example, in answer to the question "Can you tell me about a time in the last week that you felt really guilty as a parent?" Samantha responded:

> "Yes, it was related to toilet training of course. He wet his pants again, and I was starting to get annoyed. So I made him sit on the toilet and I said very sternly, 'Billy, I want you to go potty on the toilet right now.' I think I was being harsh, and I knew it wasn't helpful to him. I started to feel guilty, and that I was being the critical mom again. He is not going to figure out toilet training if he is feeling pressured by me. [*Interviewer*: '*What kind of effect did these feelings have on Billy?*'] Well, I don't know if he was aware of my guilty feelings, but he definitely is aware of my anger. When he was first placed with me, I know I was not managing my anger well. I think I was too rough with him, you know, when I would grab him by the arm and walk him to where I wanted him to be. He is sensitive, and I remember the one time that it all began to change. It was when I could see by his expression that he was scared. It really changed my whole tone, I remember thinking, 'I don't want my kid to fear me.' I am working on all of that now, but it is hard. With the toilet training incident that I mentioned, I did feel pretty guilty, and I also realized I was making things worse, by causing him to feel pressure from me. The guilty feelings have actually been good to notice, and this has made me more sensitive to how my feelings, especially my anger, are impacting Billy."

This example highlights the way in which targeted assessment tools such as the PDI can aid clinicians in their attempts to facilitate parental mentalization precisely in those areas where the parent is most challenged. Samantha entered the adoption process with Billy with a history of relational trauma that was manifesting in her current experience around issues of aggression and uncontained anger. She was not conflicted about setting limits, but, rather, she had a tendency to do so in ways that were aggressive, controlling, and punitive. The group facilitators were able to intervene in this dynamic through a careful process of slowing down and attending to Samantha's mental states, and to Billy's, in a manner that helped her to begin to form a more contained and containing way of responding to Billy's behavior that was grounded in an increased awareness of his underlying intentions and motivations.

Joanne: A Case Study Illustrating Preoccupied/Helpless/Fearful/Enmeshed States of Mind

Joanne, the mother of a 4-year-old girl, joined a Reflective Parenting Program workshop offered at her daughter's Head Start preschool. During the intake, Joanne disclosed that her daughter had become gravely ill due to complications surrounding her birth. Joanne described the first year as very difficult but said that as a result of these experiences, she and her daughter "had become insanely close." The fear related to the possible loss of her daughter to illness seemed to have exacerbated already existing difficulties that Joanne had tolerating separation. The following excerpt is taken from the PDI administered at intake.

> "We don't have to talk for her to know what I am feeling. All I have to do is put it out there and she gets it. The same for her, I can always read her mind. And I am exactly like that with my mom. If I am having a bad day, she will turn up at my doorstep. It is a sixth sense. It is like we are always connected, me with my mom, and my daughter with me."

The PDI revealed that Joanne seemed to be struggling with, and fearful of, the growing evidence of her daughter's separate mind. She said she was motivated to join the Reflective Parenting Program group because in the past 18 months she had started to feel more helpless as her daughter began to test the limits and assert her independence. While this behavior may have been developmentally appropriate, Joanne described her daughter's desire to try to do things her own way as disturbing. Joanne's PDI responses further suggested that she often felt flooded with affect and that her daughter was playing an important regulatory function for these feelings. The following example illustrates the role reversal that was occurring in this parent–child dyad.

> "We are super tight. She has my back and I have hers. She also knows that I, I need [long pause] Papa. I don't want to feel scared or um, worried, and I don't think she feels like she's not safe, she helps me feel safe. Sometimes I fear things I don't want to have to hear, I mean fear. We can face my fears together, hers, you know, with Papa. You know honestly I've made it, we're a very tight family, nothing can hurt us."

This example illustrates the fear that Joanne was living with, and the confusion she sometimes has between her own experience and her daughter's. The incoherence in her response makes it difficult to know whose fear she is speaking about. This kind of response alerts the interviewer to the possibility of unresolved loss or trauma, as her narrative reads as if she were a young girl needing containment and regulation, rather than a mother responsible for providing these functions for her child. Parents presenting with unresolved trauma sometimes exhibit more helpless or fearful ways of interacting within groups. They may pose a challenge to group leaders as they become flooded with uncontained affect or dissociated memories, and may often demand much of the time and resources from the group by their overt needs and their intense search for solutions. Paradoxically, solution-focused interventions are often not particularly helpful, due to the "leaky bucket" nature of their internal psychic structure. Instead, interventions that promote slowing down, containment, and integration of affect in order to facilitate thinking, particularly in regard to the separateness of others' mental states, often serve to assist the development of self-regulation and mentalization.

During the Reflective Parenting Program workshops, Joanne repeatedly demonstrated her difficulty tolerating and being sensitive to separate states of mind in others. For example, during the first group, she made several intrusive comments about some of the other parents, with whom she was acquainted from school. This included the assertion that she was intuitive and therefore knew the reasons they had joined the group. She proceeded to provide these specific reasons; however, her explanations were unrelated to anything the other parents had said. The group facilitators felt ambushed and described in supervision experiencing feelings of helplessness related to containing Joanne's hijacking of the group process. Joanne did not respond well to the group leaders' attempts to redirect her during the initial sessions and often interrupted the group process with emotional pleas for help, along with contradictory statements saying that there was nothing that could help her, as she already understood her daughter so well.

During supervision, the facilitators worked with the trainers to devise several intervention strategies. First, they would seek to model their own separate states of mind and their ability to provide boundaries by letting Joanne know, if she interrupted, that she would need to wait until later in the group when there would be time for her to share. They also sought to address her feelings of helplessness by facilitating the development of more structured narratives as they slowed her down and provided containment of the feelings that seemed to interfere with her ability to think. The facilitators spoke directly to her ambivalence about taking a strong authoritative role in relation to her daughter. They were able to link this ambivalence to the fear of loss that she had associated with her daughter's increasing autonomy.

In the workshop focused on "Responding to Children's Distress," the facilitators asked the group what they knew about this topic from their own experiences of being parented. Joanne disclosed that her mother, whom she'd been very close to as a child, had a mental breakdown when Joanne was 11. The group leaders gently facilitated a reflective process about how this had impacted her, and she was able to state that without her mother's presence, she had felt completely adrift, with no emotional anchor. The facilitators helped Joanne to differentiate this experience from what was happening currently with her daughter. They helped her to see that her daughter was developing not just a mind that was connected to her mother's, but one that was most definitely her own, as evidenced by the behaviors that were leaving Joanne feeling worried and unsettled. This reframed the benefits of having a separate mind and opened the door for Joanne to be less threatened by her daughter's autonomy. In her post-group PDI, Joanne stated:

"I think I have learned to see her more clearly through this group. [*Interviewer: 'How do you see that?'*] Well, just learning that it's important to slow it down and check out what she is feeling. Before, I believed that I always knew what she needed or felt, but I don't think I always did. I have slowed down and started to really pay attention to what she is saying to me, like when she wants to do something her way. I am realizing that she is trying to be her own person, and I don't feel so worried about that any more. Sometimes we can do things her way, and sometimes I have to say no, and she doesn't like that. But I am feeling calmer when I need to say no to her, and she is handling it better when I do."

This example illustrates the decrease in anxiety that Joanne began to feel in relation to her daughter's autonomy. Rather than experiencing these behaviors as merely confrontational, she began to internalize a model that more accurately linked her daughter's behavior to the normal developmental strivings of a 4-year-old child. This reflective stance had helped her to become less influenced by her own early trauma and more grounded in her current relationship with her daughter. Also evidenced was a growing capacity to set limits, as she viewed her daughter's upset feelings as not necessarily destructive to their connection, but as the normal conflict experienced between two people whose minds are interconnected yet separate.

CONCLUSIONS AND FUTURE DIRECTIONS

The PDI was originally designed to help researchers better understand the processes involved in the intergenerational transmission of attachment. The programs at the Center for Reflective Communities have extended the use of this measure and are part of a new wave of treatment approaches that utilize attachment measures for the purposes of assessment and intervention. We have found that clinicians can be effectively trained to use the PDI during the intake process to informally assess a given parent's capacity for reflective functioning by evaluating "the building blocks of mentalization."

The PDI is also an ideal tool for understanding attachment dynamics because it has many questions that require parents to reflect on negative affect or times of relational strain, which we know to be central to the issues of affect regulation that are involved when the attachment system is activated. By focusing on "states of mind with respect to attachment," clinicians are able to evaluate areas of strength and vulnerability within the parent's narrative that may be linked to key parenting issues. This integration of mentalization with attachment patterns provides a rich source of information that can be used for case formulation and intervention planning. It also helps group facilitators to use attachment concepts in a manner that is flexible and nimble.

This fluid way of conceptualizing parenting allows clinicians to track moments of reflection and moments where parents become reactive and concrete. By focusing on the waxing and waning of mentalization within a given parent or within the group, facilitators are able to engage parents in a manner that can be understood as a parallel process to the dynamics that occur in the parent–child relationship. By creating a safe holding experience, parents are more likely to be reflective during the day-to-day interactions that occur with their children.

All caregivers, regardless of what attachment category might be assigned to them in a formal research study, are nonetheless capable of moments that might be characterized as exhibiting dismissing, hostile, preoccupied, helpless, or secure states of mind. By moving away from attachment categories and toward attachment processes, group leaders are able to engage with parents in a manner that is empathic, flexible, and hopeful. In this model, attachment patterns and mentalization are viewed not only as representing stable patterns of relatedness, but also as capable of adaptation and change.

Mentalization-based programs such as the Reflective Parenting Program and Mindful Parenting Groups represent a depth approach to early intervention. Preliminary findings suggest that these models are effective in changing both parent and child outcomes. However, future research should include randomized control trials as well as additional replications to make sure that these models are transferable and therefore capable of wider dissemination for children and families facing the intergenerational and current risk factors that increase the likelihood of insecure and disorganized attachment styles in children. The Reflective Parenting Program is currently being evaluated in a federally funded randomized control trial promoting school readiness skills through parent workshops within Head Start preschools.

REFERENCES

Aber, J., Slade, A., Berger, B., Bresgi, I., & Kaplan, M. (1985). *The Parent Development Interview.* Unpublished protocol, City University of New York.

Allen, J. G., & Fonagy, P. (2006). *Handbook of mentalization-based treatment.* New York: Wiley.

Baron-Cohen, S. (1995). *Mindblindness: An essay on autism and theory of mind.* Cambridge, MA: MIT Press.

Berlin, L. J., Zeanah, C. H., & Lieberman, A. F. (2008). Prevention and intervention programs for supporting early attachment security. In J. Cassidy & P. R. Shaver (Eds.), *Handbook of attachment: Theory, research and clinical applications* (2nd ed., pp. 745–761). New York: Guilford Press.

Bick, E. (1964). Notes on infant observation in psychoanalytic training. In M. H. Williams (Ed.), *Collected papers of Martha Harris and Esther Bick.* Strath Tay, UK: Clunie Press.

Bion, W. R. (1962). *Learning from experience.* London: Heinemann.

Cassidy, J., & Shaver, P. R. (Eds.). (1999). *Handbook of attachment: Theory, research, and clinical applications.* New York: Guilford Press.

Dennett, D. (1987). *The intentional stance.* Cambridge, MA: MIT Press.

Fearon, P., Target, M., Sargent, J., Williams, L., McGregor, J., Bleiberg, E., et al. (2006). Short-term mentalization and relational therapy (SMART): An integrative family therapy for children and adolescents. In P. Fonagy (Ed), *Handbook of mentalization-based treatment* (pp. 201–222). Hoboken, NJ: Wiley.

Field, T. (1982). Interaction coaching for high-risk infants and their parents. In H. Moss, R. Hess, & C. Swift (Eds.), *Prevention in human services* (Vol. 1, pp. 5–24). New York: Hayworth Press.

Fonagy, P. (1996). The significance of the development of metacognitive control over mental representations in parenting and infant development. *Journal of Clinical Psychoanalysis, 5,* 67–86.

Fonagy, P. (2008). Mentalization-focused approach to social development. In F. N. Busch (Ed.), *Mentalization: Theoretical considerations, research findings, and clinical implications* (pp. 15–49). New York: Analytic Press.

Fonagy, P., Gergely, G., Jurist, E., & Target, M., (2002). *Affect regulation, mentalization, and the development of the self.* New York: Other Press.

Fonagy, P., Steele, M., Steele, H., Moran, G., & Higgitt, A. (1991). The capacity for understanding mental states: The reflective self in parent and child and its significance for security of attachment. *Infant Mental Health Journal, 12,* 201–218.

Fonagy, P., & Target, M. (1998). Mentalization and the changing aims of child psychoanalysis. *Psychoanalytic Dialogues, 8,* 87–114.

Fonagy, P., & Target, M. (2005). Bridging the transmission gap: An end to an important mystery of attachment research? *Attachment and Human Development, 7,* 333–343.

Fonagy, P., & Target, M. (2008). Attachment, trauma, and psychoanalysis: Where psychoanalysis meets neuroscience. In E. L. Jurist, A. Slade, & S. Bergner (Eds.), *Mind to mind: Infant research, neuroscience, and psychoanalysis* (pp. 15–49). New York: Other Press.

Fonagy, P., Target, M., Steele, H., & Steele, M. (1998). *Reflective-functioning manual, Version 5.* Unpublished manuscript.

George, C., Kaplan, N., & Main, M. (1985). *The Adult Attachment Interview.* Unpublished manuscript, Department of Psychology University of California, Berkeley.

Grienenberger, J. (2007). Group process as a holding environment facilitating the development of parental reflective functioning: Commentary on paper by Arietta Slade. *Psychoanalytic Inquiry, 26,* 668–675.

Grienenberger, J., Kelly, K., & Slade, A. (2005). Maternal reflective functioning, mother–infant affective communication, and infant attachment: Exploring the link between mental states and observed caregiving behavior in the intergenerational transmission of attachment. *Attachment and Human Development, 7,* 299–311.

Grienenberger, J., & Slade, A. (2002). Maternal reflective functioning, mother–infant affective communication, and infant attachment: Implications for psychodynamic treatment with children and families. *Psychologist-Psychoanalyst, 12*(3), 20–24.

Hoffman, K., Marvin, R. S., Cooper, G., & Powell, B. (2006). Changing toddlers' and preschoolers' attachment classifications: The circle of security intervention. *Journal of Consulting and Clinical Psychology, 74,* 1017–1026.

Kazdin, A. E., & Nock, M. K. (2003). Delineating mechanisms of change in child and adolescent therapy: Methodological issues and research recommendations. *Journal of Child Psychology and Psychiatry, 44,* 1116–1129.

Lieberman, A. F, Silverman, R., & Pawl, J. H. (2000). Infant–parent psychotherapy: Core concepts and current approaches. In C. H. Zeanah, Jr. (Ed.), *Handbook of infant mental health* (2nd ed., pp. 472–484). New York: Guilford Press.

Luyten, P., Fonagy, P., Lowyck, B., & Vermote, R. (2012). Assessment of mentalization. In A. W. Bateman & P. Fonagy (Eds.), *Handbook of mentalizing in mental health practice* (pp. 43–65). Washington, DC: American Psychiatric Publishing.

Lyons-Ruth, K. (1999). The two-person unconscious: Intersubjective dialogue, enactive representation, and the emergence of new forms of relational organization. *Psychoanalytic Inquiry, 19,* 576–617.

Lyons-Ruth, K., Bronfman, E., & Atwood, G. (1999). A relational diathesis model of hostile-helpless states of mind: Expressions in mother–infant interaction. In J. Solomon & C. George (Eds.), *Attachment disorganization* (pp. 33–70). New York: Guilford Press.

Main, M. (1991). Metacognitive knowledge, metacognitive monitoring, and singular (coherent) versus multiple (incoherent) models of attachment: Findings and directions for future research. In C. M. Parkes, J. Stevenson-Hinde, & P. Marris (Eds.), *Attachment across the life cycle* (pp. 127–159). London: Routledge.

Main, M., & Goldwyn, R. (1998). *Adult attachment scoring and classification systems* (2nd ed.). Unpublished manuscript, University of California at Berkeley.

McDonough, S. C. (2004). Interaction guidance: Promoting and nurturing the caregiving relationship. In A. J. Sameroff, S. C. McDonough, & K. L. Rosenblum (Eds.), *Treating parent–infant relationship problems: Strategies for intervention* (pp. 79–96). New York: Guilford Press.

Meins, E., Fernyhough, C., Fradley, E., & Tuckey, M. (2001). Rethinking maternal sensitivity: Mothers' comments on infants' mental processes predict security of attachment at 12 months. *Journal of Child Psychology and Psychiatry, 42*, 637–648.

Oppenheim, D., & Koren-Karie, N. (2002). Mothers' insightfulness regarding their children's internal worlds: The capacity underlying secure child–mother relationships. *Infant Mental Health Journal, 23*, 593–605.

Powell, B., Cooper, G., Hoffman, K., & Marvin, R. S. (2009). The circle of security. In C. H. Zeanah (Ed.), *Handbook of infant mental health* (3rd ed., pp. 450–467). New York: Guilford Press.

Reynolds, D. (2003). Mindful parenting: A group approach to enhancing reflective capacity in parents and infants. *Journal of Child Psychotherapy, 29*, 357–374.

Sadler, L. S., Slade, A., & Mayes, L. C. (2006). Minding the baby: A mentalization-based parenting program. In J. G. Allen & P. Fonagy (Eds.), *The handbook of mentalization-based treatment* (pp. 271–288). Hoboken, NJ: Wiley.

Sharp, C., & Fonagy, P. (2008). The parent's capacity to treat the child as a psychological agent: Constructs, measures and implications for developmental psychopathology. *Social Development, 17(3)*, 737–754.

Slade, A. (2004). The movement from categories to process: Attachment phenomena and clinical evaluation. *Infant Mental Health Journal, 25*, 269–283.

Slade, A., Bernbach, E., Grienenberger, J., Wohlgemuth Levy, D., & Locker, A. (2002). *Addendum to Reflective Functioning Scoring Manual: For use with the Parent Development Interview.* Unpublished manuscript, City College and Graduate Center of the City University of New York.

Slade, A., Grienenberger, J., Bernbach, E., Levy, D., & Locker, A. (2005). Maternal reflective functioning, attachment, and the transmission gap: A preliminary study. *Attachment and Human Development, 7*, 283–298.

Sroufe, A. (2005). Attachment and development: A prospective, longitudinal study from birth to adulthood. *Attachment and Human Development, 7*, 349–367.

Steele, H., & Steele, M. (2008). *Clinical applications of the Adult Attachment Interview.* New York: Guilford Press.

Stern, D. N. (1995). *The motherhood constellation.* New York: Basic Books.

Sternberg, J. (2005). *Infant observation at the heart of training.* London: Karnac Books.

Suchman, N., DeCoste, C., Castiglioni, N., Legow, N., & Mayes, L. (2008). The mothers and toddlers program: Preliminary findings from an attachment-based parenting intervention for substance-abusing mothers. *Psychoanalytic Psychology, 25*, 499–517.

Suchman, N., McMahon, T., Slade, A., & Luthar, S. (2005). How early bonding, depression, illicit drug use, and perceived support work together to influence drug-dependent mothers' caregiving. *American Journal of Orthopsychiatry, 75*, 431–445.

Thomson-Salo, F., & Paul, C. (2001, January–June). Some principles of infant–parent psychotherapy: Ann Morgan's contribution. *The Signal, World Association for Infant Mental Health*, pp. 14–19.

van IJzendoorn, M. (1995). Adult attachment representations, parental responsiveness, and infant attachment: A meta-analysis on the predictive validity of the Adult Attachment Interview. *Psychological Bulletin, 117*, 387–403.

Wallin, D. (2007). *Attachment in Psychotherapy.* New York: Guilford Press.

Webster-Stratton, C. (2005). The incredible years: A training series for the prevention and treatment of conduct problems in young children. In E. D. Hibbs & P. S. Jensen (Eds.), *Psychosocial treatments for child and adolescent disorders: Empirically based strategies for clinical practice* (2nd ed., pp. 507–555). Washington, DC: American Psychological Association.

Williams, L. L., Fonagy, P., Target, M., Fearon, P., Sargent, J., Bleiberg, E., et al. (2006). Training psychiatry residents in mentalization-based therapy. In J. G. Allen & P. Fonagy (Eds.), *Handbook of mentalization-based treatment* (pp. 223–232), Chichester, UK: Wiley.

Winnicott, D. W. (1960). The theory of the parent infant relationship. *International Journal of Psychoanalysis, 41,* 585–595.

CHAPTER 22

Working with Families

Trudie Rossouw

I am Sisyphus, and today I stopped on my journey and rested in the shade of a tree, and then, as I reflected upon my life, it occurred to me that I was busy doing something quite peculiar: I was repeating the same task again and again. How strange. Why do I do that?

How strange to us that he did not stop and reflect, but instead carried on repeating himself, seemingly oblivious to the predictable outcome each time. Yet, most intimate relationships seem to repeat elements of the same dance in which familiar patterns are retraced. These patterns are intricately layered interactional loops that we inhabit, just as we inhabit "home" without "seeing" it. Like Sisyphus's journey, we have little awareness of these patterns, their scope, architecture, and intricacy, or how they shape us as we co-create and co-perpetuate them. This mutual shaping is the "familiarness" of intimacy. Even when the familiar is filled with pain, we cannot get outside the familiar and change the repetition of the dance. Hence, we end up in multiple binds outside our awareness, perpetuating similar scripts in our loving relationships with parents, children, and siblings.

This chapter first reviews psychodynamic approaches to working with families with focus on mentalization-based approaches (see also Clarkin, Fonagy, Levy, & Bateman, Chapter 17, this volume). Mentalization-based treatment for families (MBT-F) is discussed as an example of this approach.

PSYCHODYNAMIC APPROACHES TO WORKING WITH FAMILIES

A Brief Historical Review

The dance of intimacy just described is never clearer than in psychodynamic work with children and families. All psychodynamic theories are underpinned by a developmental framework in which the development of the psyche is, at least in part, dependent on the early attachment relationships the infant experiences with his or her caregivers. Melanie Klein explored the interpersonal aspect of the structural model introduced by Freud. Unlike Freud, she believed that the infant could relate to the mother from birth and that the baby internalized aspects of his or her experience of the relationship. Klein (1932) described these aspects as internalized part-objects, distinguished as "good" and "bad." In contrast, Anna Freud felt that the infant did not arrive in the world with such ego capabilities; instead, she believed that the infant emerges gradually from a state of primary narcissism through its responses to environmental impingements. Anna Freud also conceived of the early defense mechanisms as possessing a wider relational repertoire than Klein's concept of the limited archaic defenses (Freud, 1936). Winnicott's contributions to theory emphasize the helplessness of the infant's ego, which, he suggested, can be brought in to being only in the context of the mother–child relationship (Winnicott, 1965). Bion expanded these ideas further with his theory on thinking and the containing role of the mother in the development of the baby's mind (Bion, 1962).

Pioneering work in the 1950s by John Bowlby (1969) in the United Kingdom and John Bell (1961) in the United States demonstrated that working with the dynamic relationships within a family brought about change in the index child. They focused not on the referred child's unconscious fantasies, but instead on the relationships in the family and the effect of these relationships on the child.

In describing family therapy with a psychodynamic focus, a multisystems model may offer the best depiction. Each member of the family has an "internal family" based on internal object relationships while simultaneously being influenced by the "external/real family"; the two systems, internal and external, continuously influence one another. Fraiberg, Adelson, and Shapiro (1975) described, very powerfully, the influence of "ghosts in the nursery" by which they refer to the unconscious influences of the mother's past that suddenly appear to haunt her and interfere with her relationship with her baby. These "ghosts," which belong to the "internal family," do not arrive only in the nursery; we see their appearance in many situations of difficulty in family lives. As strong as the influence of the ghosts from the unconscious can be on family relations, so too can the direct, real-life interactions be, as illustrated by the careful observations of Beatrice Beebe (2003), who describes the moment-by-moment adjustment that each partner in a mother–baby dyad makes to the behaviors of the other. Her micro-moment observation of the intimacy between mother and baby highlighted the exquisite sensitivity of each to the other and illustrated how their behaviors are shaped by one another within the partnership. This interplay was similarly described by Stern (1977). Winnicott's (1965) description of the in-tune, "good enough" mother provides a similar depiction of this dyad. Winnicott also drew attention to the early importance of the father–infant/child dyad as an alternative to the intensity of the mother–infant dyad with its potential fears of merger.

Psychodynamic family work perhaps began in a rudimentary form in the 1940s, when Anna Freud started the Hampstead War Nurseries (now known as the Anna Freud Centre) in London with the aim of providing treatment to traumatized young children. This work often involved the treatment of the relationship between the child and his or her mother. Similarly, the Hanna Perkins Center in Cleveland, Ohio, which originated in 1880 as a nursery and later developed into a teaching and child development center, was staffed by child analysts who were keenly influenced by Anna Freud's work and who published extensively, describing their work with the relationship between young children and their parents.

During the 1950s, what is now conceived of as the school of systemic family therapy began to develop; simultaneously, a variety of different movements that contributed to its conception emerged in a number of different countries (Balint, 1957; Bateson, 1958; Jackson, 1957). The uniting feature of these movements was the view that emotional problems were essentially interpersonal/relational in nature, as opposed to predominantly intrapsychic. Thus, the primary method in resolving psychological problems was to focus on the relationships within families as well as with their social network. In the 1970s, Bateson (1972) offered an overarching theoretical framework for family therapy based on communications theory, systems theory, and cybernetics, which changed family therapy thereafter. In this framework, the cause of problems within family systems was viewed as circular and involving patterns of mutual influence. Family therapy has since developed as a broad psychotherapeutic modality that contains within it many different schools of thought regarding the origin of psychological distress, including problem-maintaining behavior patterns, problematic belief systems, and historical predisposing factors (Carr, 2000). Heavily influenced by concurrent social and political climates, developments in systemic therapy accommodated social constructionist and constructivist ideologies.

Under the umbrella term of *systemic family therapy* there exists a number of distinct approaches, such as structural family therapy (Minuchin, 1974), strategic therapy (Haley, 1963), the Milan approach (Palazzoli, Boscolo, Cecchin, & Prata, 1980), functional family therapy (Alexander & Parsons, 1982), narrative approaches (White & Epston, 1990), and brief solution-focused therapy (de Shazer, 1982). More recent developments have emphasized the importance of attachment theory in systemic work (Akister & Reibstein, 2004; Byng-Hall, 1991; Dallos, 2006; Diamond, Diamond, & Levy, 2013; Diamond, Reis, Diamond, Siqueland, & Isaacs, 2002; Diamond & Siqueland, 1998; Hughes, 2007; Powell, Cooper, Hoffman, & Marvin, 2014; Siegel, 1999) as well as some direct attempts to bridge the systemic and psychodynamic worlds to form hybrid ways of working (Flaskas & Pocock, 2009). Those working from a systemic perspective will see many techniques familiar to them, from "joining" (Minuchin, 1974) to focusing on exceptions to symptomatic behaviors (de Shazer, 1982) and including the importance of "curiosity" (Cecchin, 1987) and "circular questioning" (Palazzoli et al., 1980).

Recent additions to the practice of psychodynamic family work have been the development of attachment-based family therapy (ABFT) and mentalization-based treatment for families (MBT-F). Great similarities exist between ABFT and MBT-F. In ABFT, the therapist works with the parents to improve emotional attunement and responsiveness toward their adolescent. In both ABFT and MBT-F, the focus of the work is aimed at the relationship between the parents and the adolescent, and both modalities emphasize the fostering of an alliance with all members of the family. MBT-F is not a novel treatment per se. It has many origins in systemic practice; however, its conceptualization of distress, and how to intervene, incorporates both the internal psychodynamic and the external systemic worlds of family members. It specifically integrates attachment theory with systemic practice, making links between external relationships and inner worlds and connecting behavior and interaction patterns with meaning-making (Asen & Fonagy, 2012).

Mentalization-Based Model for Understanding Family Pathology

Mentalization, the capacity for self-awareness and sensitivity to others, is a skill that develops in the context of an attachment relationship (Fonagy, 2000) (see also Clarkin et al., Chapter 17, this volume). It is therefore directly influenced by and dependent on family relations and highly influenced by family pathology.

The Development of Mentalization and Nonmentalization

Our ability to make sense of ourselves and those around us depends on our original caregiver's ability to make sense of our internal states. When a mother (or any primary caregiver) makes sense of what her baby is experiencing, she forms an internal representation in her mind of what the baby is going through; this representation is communicated back to the baby with her entire demeanor, her voice, her tone, her body, and the expression on her face. The baby finds its own state reflected in the mother's response, but in a modified and contained form, which gives it meaning. This experience is internalized by the baby and forms a secondary representation of the baby's original affect. This contributes to the baby's development of a core sense of self, and it is this ability that helps the baby make future sense of him- or herself as well as those around him or her (Fonagy, Gergely, Jurist, & Target, 2002; Fonagy, Target, & Gergely, 2000).

The mother's ability to form a representation in her mind that is congruent with the baby's affect is highly dependent on how she feels about herself as a woman/mother, how supported she is by her partner, and what "ghosts" she has in the "nursery" of her own childhood that may come out and haunt her with persecution and terror. If her mind is filled with persecutions, she could very easily hear the baby's cry as an accusation and attack. Hence, her response may be one of hostility or fear, which in turn will be internalized by the baby. This state or object relation that the baby is internalizing is alien to the authentic state of the baby; Fonagy and colleagues (2000, 2002) termed it the "alien self." The inner experience of the alien self is akin to the experience of an inner tormentor—it is the constant experience of inner criticism, self-hatred, lack of internal validation, and expectation of failure. The self is hated, and, through the projected lens of the alien self, the external world can be perceived as potentially hostile, humiliating, and attacking.

In an internal state dominated by the alien self, where the inner representations are alien to the self, representations of others that are generated will, similarly, be inaccurate, leading to the experience that the relational world does not make sense and is unpredictable. In this way, the alien self will interfere in the development of mentalization of both self and other. Mentalization failures can also arise from other causes, such as constitutional factors, factors that interfere in brain development, or any other organic factors.

Figure 22.1 illustrates how the alien self expresses itself in the clinical context in the presence of nonmentalizing cycles.

The following example illustrates this cycle.

• *Feeling*: Sally starts to feel anxious because she had a bad day at school and felt bullied by the other children. When she feels anxious, she starts to believe there is something wrong with her body, such as that she might be having a heart attack, and she then feels terrified that she may die.

• *Action*: She rushes to her mother and insists on being taken to hospital.

• *Impact*: Her mother feels irritated by this demand as she has learned over time that there is nothing physically wrong with Sally, and no matter how many times she and the doctor have told Sally this, she does not listen. Her mother thinks Sally is just attention-seeking.

• *Action*: Sally's mother tells her to go away and that she is imagining it.

• *Feeling*: Sally feels that her mother was not listening to her, which makes her furious.

• *Action*: Sally goes to her room and starts throwing things out of the window.

• *Impact*: Sally's mother becomes angry and frightened that the situation is going to get out of hand.

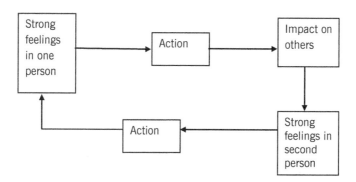

FIGURE 22.1. Expression of the alien self in the presence of nonmentalizing cycles of interpersonal interaction.

- *Action*: She tells Sally to go into the garden and locks her out of the house.

- *Feeling*: Sally feels that her mother does not love her, and she feels desperate. She feels horrible, bad, and unlovable, and she starts to panic.

- *Action*: Sally starts throwing bricks at the window to be let in.

- *Impact*: Now Sally's mother starts to feel frightened of her daughter. She is afraid Sally will break a window and hurt her two younger children; she feels helpless and does not know what to do. She starts to panic and finally calls the police. At this stage she feels incompetent as a parent, helpless, and frightened.

At the climactic moment of such an escalating cycle, both parties feel like victims. Not only do both parties feel attacked by the other, but both have terribly bad feelings about themselves. They feel bad, incompetent, and unlovable. Nonmentalization in one individual rarely exists in isolation; it very soon migrates into the interpersonal world of family relations and can cause a "domino effect" of nonmentalizing in the family.

Specific Examples of Nonmentalizing in Families

Maladaptive behavior patterns and/or escalating family conflicts regularly result from a failure in mentalization. Failures in mentalization can instigate affect dysregulation within an individual, which in turn produces further mentalization failure as affect storms derail thinking capacity further. This can lead to an inability to make sense of the behavior of others and a desire to control others in order to have some control over a world that feels incomprehensible. Such emotional dysregulation in one individual rarely exists in a bubble of isolation in which all others are spared; instead, the mounting dysregulation and mentalization failure spread into the individual's interpersonal world, where many relationships fall prey to mentalization failure characterized by escalating interpersonal misunderstanding and conflict. Furthermore, the spread of mentalization failure often culminates in some form of concrete act, or "acting out" behavior, exhibited by one or more of the individuals involved—be it through self-harm, physical violence, slamming doors, breaking things, taking drugs, or running away. It is because of this process that the emphasis of MBT-F is not on managing the symptomatic, overt behaviors, but rather on understanding the multitude of ways in which mentalization has broken down and the ways in which this affects the people within an individual's social system. To this end, an important endeavor of MBT-F is to track back to the moment before the breakdown in mentalization in order to explore and understand the emotional and interpersonal context in which the failure originated.

Mentalization failure in a family is usually not a constant state of affairs. Failure to mentalize frequently occurs in the context of increased emotional arousal; for example, a mother may be capable of mentalizing her child, but after an argument with her husband, when she may be overwhelmed by her own emotional state, she may be less able to mentalize the child's mental state during the argument.

The most common form of mentalization failure is what has been described as *concrete mentalization* (Bateman & Fonagy, 2004). Concrete explanations are found to explain behavior or experiences, as exemplified in the statements: "You are such a typical . . ." or "When you came into the room, you made the atmosphere toxic." Constant blame or self-blame in families are other examples of mentalization failures; "Of course it is your fault, it's always your fault"; "He did not do the work because he is lazy"; or "It's my fault, it is all my fault; if I die, you will all feel better." Seeking concrete solutions for mental anguish also finds clear expression in eating disorders and somatization disorders. Impulsive actions and behaviors can also be seen as concretizations of internal states, as are requests by families for clinicians to come up with concrete solutions to problems, such as medication.

Trauma needs specific reference in this context, as the reexperience of trauma in the form of flashbacks, and the consequential confusion between what is present and what is past, is an example of *psychic equivalence* (equating what is in the mind with external reality), which is part of concrete mentalizing. The impact of this phenomenon on family relations is familiar to clinicians. One example is the mother who was abused in her past, who now flinches each time her child reaches out to her as she experiences his ordinary need for affection as a dangerous demand. This in turn leads to an experience in the child of himself as "bad" and may later lead to an escalation of hostile behavior from him. In a similar vein, the mental state of a parent with a mental illness can impact upon mentalizing failure in a family—for example, the persecutory world of a paranoid parent or the despairing, hostile world of a parent with depression.

Another form of nonmentalizing is *pseudomentalization* (Bateman & Fonagy, 2004). This form of nonmentalizing is often dominated by a sense of certainty about the mental states of others—for instance, the parent who told his or her child what the child felt or what his or her motives were without trying to understand what the child was actually feeling or thinking. Another example is a mother who complained that her child was deliberately behaving in an angry way because the child's father was aggressive and, hence, the child was "like his father." In this case, only very careful work revealed that the child's anger was related to his feeling that his mother blamed and misunderstood him, and that whatever he did seemed to make her angry. A few sessions alone with the mother revealed her unresolved anger toward her ex-husband for leaving her for someone else, and her deeper feelings of humiliation and rejection. Once her feelings were understood, she was more able to see how she had confused her son in her mind with her ex-husband. In enmeshed families with poor boundaries between the generations, forms of intrusive mentalizing are commonplace—one member of the family readily believes that he or she knows what someone else is feeling or thinking.

Lastly, the most extreme and malignant form of mentalizing failure is *misuse of mentalization* (Bateman & Fonagy, 2004). In this form of nonmentalization, the "perpetrator" is capable of mentalization of the child, but instead of using this skill to help, it is used to exploit or humiliate the child. Extreme examples of this are the pedophile who correctly perceives a child's vulnerabilities and exploits them to his own gain, or the parent who claims in front of the child that the child fell down the stairs when in fact he or she had abused the child. Another example is coercion against the child's thoughts, such as humiliating the child for his or her feelings. Misuse of mentalization can also be seen in the context of acrimonious divorce situations, such as the mother who says to the father: "Johnny was so upset when you were late to pick him up; I think it will be best if you don't come again."

MBT-F: PSYCHODYNAMIC TREATMENT FOR FAMILIES DOMINATED BY NONMENTALIZATION

Although MBT-F is discussed here as an example of an innovative form of psychodynamic family work, it must be highlighted and acknowledged that this intervention is but one form of psychodynamic family work.[1] Many of those working in child and family mental health services work with families in psychodynamic ways (see also St. John & Lieberman, Chapter 18; Hill & Sharp, Chapter 19; and Grienenberger, Denham, & Reynolds, Chapter 21, this volume).

The specific aim of MBT-F is to enhance mentalization in family relations and to reduce impulsive enactments, coercion, nonmentalizing interactions, and escalating affective storms. MBT-F focuses on emotions as cues to what goes on within individual family members and pays specific attention to emotional regulation. A key goal of the approach is to increase the empathic understanding that parents and caregivers have for their children and, depending on the developmental stages of the children, vice versa (Asen & Fonagy, 2012).

As the focus of the work is on emotional cues, the therapist continually thinks about and comments on the thoughts and feelings of the members of the family and the relationships between them. The therapist positively notes the different perspectives in the family and praises their spontaneous attempts to understand what someone is feeling or thinking. The therapist repeatedly checks whether they have understood what someone means, modeling the importance of curiosity and an awareness of the opaque nature of mental states. At times the therapist helps the family members to express what they feel by pausing the conversation with a "naive" question about what someone may be feeling (Asen & Fonagy, 2012). The therapist aims to strike a balance between allowing the family to interact naturally and intervening actively when there are critical or nonmentalizing moments. He or she may actively encourage family members to name their own feelings and to reflect openly on how they may be affected by these feelings and how they might affect others.

When explaining this model, Asen and Fonagy (2012) describe the treatment intervention as an MBT-F "loop," which involves working with the family as collaborators to identify a moment of nonmentalization. The moment is then highlighted and given a name (which externalizes it). Then, great care is taken to mentalize the moment and to see what everyone experienced in the moment. This may highlight aspects of the interplay between the inner and external representations of the family in each member of the family. This moment can often be generalized to other moments. In this work, the emphasis is on thinking about feelings before planning actions or thinking about how to do things differently next time.

Use of the MBT-F loop is demonstrated in the following example.

---

[1]MBT-F is manualized, and the manual is available at *http://mbtf.tiddlyspace.com*.

CLINICAL ILLUSTRATION

Sarah, who is 16, came to the clinic with her parents because they "could no longer cope" with her defiant and acting-out behavior. She would stay out all night, she started taking drugs and drinking, and, when confronted, she would storm out of the house and might not return for a day. Her parents became particularly concerned about her when they noticed that she had started to harm herself. Her father was suffering from cancer, for which he was receiving treatment, and her mother, the breadwinner of the family, was burdened by helplessness and anxiety. In the first session, it became clear that Sarah's mother swung from blaming herself to blaming Sarah's father for Sarah's behavior, while Sarah's father was angry and wanted the therapist to force Sarah to "admit" what her problem was. Sarah was uncommunicative; she refused to answer questions with more than a dismissive shrug of her shoulders. What seemed like an approaching dead end and possibly even a young person storming out of the room was turned around when the therapist used a "mentalizing game" to help with opening up the MBT-F loop.

The therapist asked Sarah whether she thought her parents knew what she was feeling. Sarah indicated that they did not. The therapist then gave Sarah a microphone as a prop and asked her to interview her parents and ask them to describe what she looks like when she is in different states—happy, sad, angry, depressed. They described their perceptions. Sarah then had the opportunity to comment on their accuracy; she told them that they were wrong and that when she feels depressed and sad, she appears happy. The therapist wondered with the parents why Sarah needed to hide her depressed feelings. Sarah then mentioned that if her pain was hidden then it would not burden someone else.

This opened up a possibility to use the MBT-F loop. "So, are you speaking about feeling a deep worry that you may cause pain or suffering?" the therapist asked.

"Yes, I always do, that is why I don't want to be here, then I won't disappoint or hurt people," Sarah said.

"Gosh, that sounds really painful; Mom and Dad, did you know that Sarah felt like that?"

The parents mentioned that Sarah often feels that things are her fault. The father then mentioned that he at times made it worse by blaming her too, and the mother admitted that she often blamed the father for the situation. The therapist then said that this appeared to be a painful occurrence that seemed to happen to them as a family: "This occurrence in which there seems to be a lot of blame, would you agree that this sort of situation happens a lot?" When the family affirmed that it did happen a lot, the therapist suggested that they give the situation a name, and eventually they named it the "blame-thing."

Then, the therapist paid great attention to mentalizing the "blame-thing" by trying to understand what happened for each member of the family in the situation. With regard to Sarah she felt overwhelmed and burdened by her father's complaints about his illness as well as her concern that he might die. His illness made him depressed and short-tempered, which meant that he became quite quick to experience her as out of control, and hence quick to blame and accuse her. This made her feel guilty and hopeless, and hence she coped by running away and getting drunk, which further increased her sense of guilt and finally led to her harming herself as a form of punishment. Her mother, on the other hand, had recently lost her own father and found that any experience of Sarah being out of the house or harming herself induced in her a state of fear that she would lose her daughter too. In her attempt to manage her anxiety, she argued with Sarah's father, and in her attempt to keep Sarah at home, she tried to control her through guilt-inducing statements.

By exploring the MBT-F loop, the family was able to adopt a more reflective stance, which helped them to understand one another's behavior as well as their own responses. This humanization of the self and the other led to less coercive behavior, greater mastery, and more reciprocity over time.

EMPIRICAL FINDINGS

Although the practice of working with families is commonplace in all child and adolescent mental health services, research into the effectiveness of such interventions is limited. Several meta-analytic studies have concluded that family therapies were significantly more effective than no treatment and at least as effective as other forms of psychotherapy, with an overall effect size of $d = 0.53$ (Shadish & Baldwin, 2002; Stanton & Shadish, 1997).

As noted earlier, Diamond and colleagues (2002) developed and tested ABFT for depressed adolescents. In their study, a 12-week treatment was compared with a 6-week waitlist. Remission occurred in 84% of the adolescents treated with ABFT and in 36% of the patients in the control group. ABFT also produced more significant reductions in anxiety, hopelessness, and family conflict, and improved adolescent attachment to parents.

Mentalization-based treatment for adolescents (MBT-A) presenting with self-harm is a combination of MBT-F plus individual MBT sessions for the adolescent. Rossouw and Fonagy (2012) compared MBT-A against treatment as usual for adolescents who harmed themselves. The sample size was 80 youths between ages 12 and 18, and the treatment duration was one year. Rossouw and Fonagy found that the MBT/MBT-F combination group showed a significant effect size in terms of depression, reduction in self-harm, and borderline features. Attachment avoidance ratings decreased pre- to posttest in the MBT/MBTF group only. In addition, mentalization scores improved in the MBT/MBT-F group only.

An initial outcome evaluation of the MBT-F study at the Anna Freud Centre indicated that young people receiving the intervention showed an improved sense of well-being and found that they displayed fewer symptoms at the end of treatment and had improved global functioning (Keaveny et al., 2012). Much more research, however, is needed, particularly to determine whether or not the family component is essential.

Trowell and colleagues (2007) compared individual psychodynamic psychotherapy against systemic family therapy in depressed adolescents, and both interventions demonstrated significant reductions in symptoms. Clearly, although these studies suggest that psychodynamic work with families may be effective, more research is needed to substantiate this claim.

CONCLUSIONS AND FUTURE DIRECTIONS

Historically, psychoanalytic practitioners have been working with families since the 1940s; early examples include the work of John Bowlby and Anna Freud and the psychotherapists and analysts of the Hanna Perkins Center. These early pioneers began to focus on the interrelational impact of family members on one another. Psychoanalytic theory, too, started to incorporate more explicitly a focus on the relational, in particular the dyadic relationship between a mother and her baby.

The 1950s saw the development of family therapy as an approach and discipline in its own right. Although originally instigated by psychoanalytically informed practitioners, its theoretical foundations were predominantly based on systems theory, and as such this modality is referred to as systemic family therapy. In recent years, an attempt has been made to integrate the two worlds of systemic and psychoanalytic thinking with an interest in both the internal and the external family. One catalyst to this integration has been the body of empirical research into attachment theory that has so influenced our clinical understanding of mental health. Common examples of psychodynamic family work within health services include family sessions convened alongside individual work to support a child's experience of child psychotherapy, work with children in the presence of their adoptive or foster parents to facilitate making sense of a child's disrupted relational experiences, and parent–infant work in cases with very early relational difficulties. More recently, the development of MBT-F represents the first psychodynamic family therapy model to be made explicit and to be subject to research for the treatment of vulnerable adolescents, with promising results.

Unfortunately, the research evidence for family work is surprisingly limited. In the systemic field some evidence is emerging, most notably that reported by Judith Trowell and colleagues (2007), who demonstrate that systemic family therapy can be an effective treatment for children diagnosed with depression. Further evidence of the effectiveness of systemic work has been illustrated in studies in which systemic work was combined with other forms of intervention (Brent et al., 1997; Godart et al., 2012; Liddle, Rowe, Dakof, Henderson, & Greenbaum, 2009). Recently, MBT has been shown to be effective in the treatment of violent youths as well as victims of sexual abuse and neglect. However, the family work in this model was only one of several components of the intervention, and the emphasis of this intervention was solution-focused, with strong leanings toward behavior therapy concepts (Sawyer & Borduin, 2011; Swenson et al., 2010).

Although psychodynamic family work may be practiced widely, at the time of writing the only research evidence of its effectiveness is the study by Rossouw and Fonagy (2012) with young people who self-harm. This study reported that the intervention was associated with reductions in self-harm, depression, and borderline traits as well as an improvement in attachment security and mentalization. Clearly, more research is needed in the field of psychodynamic work with families.

REFERENCES

Akister, J., & Reibstein, J. (2004). Links between attachment theory and systemic practice: Some proposals. *Journal of Family Therapy, 26*, 2–16.

Alexander, J., & Parsons, B. V. (1982). Special family phases, structures, and themes. In *Functional family therapy* (pp. 123–145). Monterey, CA: Brooks/Cole.

Asen, E., & Fonagy, P. (2012). Mentalization-based family therapy. In A. Bateman & P. Fonagy (Eds.), *Handbook of mentalizing in mental health practice* (pp. 107–128). Arlington, VA: American Psychiatric Publishing.

Balint, M. (1957). *The doctor, his patient and the illness.* London: Pitman Medical.

Bateman, A. W., & Fonagy, P. (2004). *Psychotherapy for borderline personality disorder: Mentalization-based treatment.* Oxford, UK: Oxford University Press.

Bateson, G. (1958). *Naven.* Stanford, CA: Stanford University Press.

Bateson, G. (1972). *Steps to an ecology of mind.* New York: Ballantine Books.

Beebe, B. (2003). Brief mother–infant treatment: Psychoanalytically informed video feedback. *Infant Mental Health Journal, 24*, 24–52.

Bell, J. (1961). *Family group therapy* [Public Health Monograph No. 64]. Washington, DC: U.S. Government Printing Office.

Bion, W. R. (1962). The psycho-analytic study of thinking. *International Journal of Psycho-Analysis, 43*, 306–310.

Bowlby, J. (1969). *Attachment and loss, Vol. 1: Attachment.* New York: Basic Books.

Brent, D., Holder, D., Kolko, D., Birmaher, B., Baugher, M., Roth, C., et al. (1997). A clinical psychotherapy trial for adolescent depression comparing cognitive, family, and supportive therapy. *Archives of General Psychiatry, 54*, 877–885.

Byng-Hall, J. (1991). The application of attachment theory to understanding and treatment in family therapy. In C. M. Parkes, J. Stevenson-Hinde, & P. Marris (Eds.), *Attachment across the life cycle* (pp. 199–215). New York: Routledge.

Carr, A. (2000). *Family therapy: Concepts, process and practice.* New York: Wiley.

Cecchin, G. (1987). Hypothesizing, circularity, and neutrality revisited: An invitation to curiosity. *Family Process, 26*, 405–413.

Dallos, R. (2006). *Attachment narrative therapy: Integrating systemic, narrative and attachment approaches.* Maidenhead, UK: Open University Press.

de Shazer, S. (1982). *Patterns of brief family therapy: An ecosystemic approach.* New York: Guilford Press.

Diamond, G. S., Diamond, G. M., & Levy, S. A. (2013). *Attachment-based family therapy for depressed adolescents.* Washington, DC: Magination Press/American Psychological Association.

Diamond, G. S., Reis, B. F., Diamond, G. M., Siqueland, L., & Isaacs, L. (2002). Attachment-based family therapy for depressed adolescents: A treatment development study. *Journal of the American Academy of Child and Adolescent Psychiatry, 41*, 1190–1196.

Diamond, G. S., & Siqueland, L. (1998). Emotions, attachment and the relational reframe: The first session. *Journal of Systemic Therapies, 17*, 36–50.

Flaskas, C., & Pocock, D. (2009). *Systems and psycho-analysis: Contemporary integration in family therapy.* London: Karnac Books.

Fonagy, P. (2000). Attachment and borderline personality disorder. *Journal of the American Psychoanalytic Association, 48*, 1129–1146.

Fonagy, P., Gergely, G., Jurist, E., & Target, M. (2002). *Affect regulation, mentalization, and the development of the self.* New York: Other Press.

Fonagy, P., Target, M., & Gergely, G. (2000). Attachment and borderline personality disorder: A theory and some evidence. *Psychiatric Clinics of North America. 23*, 103–122.

Fraiberg, S., Adelson, E., & Shapiro, V. (1975). Ghosts in the nursery: A psychoanalytic approach to problems of impaired infant–mother relationships. *Journal of the American Academy of Child Psychiatry, 14*, 387–422.

Freud, A. (1936). *Ego and the mechanisms of defense*. London: Hogarth Press.

Godart, N., Berthoz, S., Curt, F., Perdereau, F., Rein, Z., Wallier, J., et al. (2012). A randomized controlled trial of adjunctive family therapy and treatment as usual following inpatient treatment for anorexia nervosa adolescents. *PLoS ONE, 7*, e28249.

Haley, J. (1963). *Strategies of psychotherapy*. New York: Grune & Stratton.

Hughes, D. A. (2007). *Attachment-focused family therapy*. New York: Norton.

Jackson, D. (1957). The question of family homeostasis. *Psychiatric Quarterly, 31*(Suppl. 1), 79–90.

Keaveny, E., Midgley, N., Asen, E., Bevington, D., Fearon P, Fonagy, P., et al. (2012). Minding the family mind: The development and initial evaluation of mentalization-based treatment for families. In N. Midgely & I. Vrouva (Eds.), *Minding the child: Mentalization-based interventions with children, young people and their families* (pp. 98–112). Hove, UK: Routledge.

Klein, M. (1932). *The psycho-analysis of children*. London: Hogarth Press.

Liddle, H. A., Rowe, C. L., Dakof, G., Henderson, C. E., & Greenbaum, P. E. (2009). Multidimensional family therapy for young adolescent substance abuse: Twelve-month outcomes of a randomized controlled trial. *Journal of Consulting and Clinical Psychology, 77*, 12–25.

Minuchin, S. (1974). *Families and family therapy*. Cambridge, MA: Harvard University Press.

Palazzoli, S., Boscolo, M., Cecchin, M., & Prata, G. (1980). Hypothesising—circularity—neutrality: Three guidelines for the conductor of the session. *Family Process, 19*, 3–12.

Powell, B., Cooper, G., Hoffman, K., & Marvin, B. (2014). *The circle of security intervention: Enhancing attachment in early parent–child relationships*. New York: Guilford Press.

Rossouw, T. I., & Fonagy, P. (2012). Mentalization-based treatment for self-harm in adolescents: A randomized controlled trial. *Journal of the American Academy of Child and Adolescent Psychiatry, 51*, 1304–1313.

Sawyer, A. M., & Borduin, C. M. (2011). Effects of multisystemic therapy through midlife: A 21.9-year follow-up to a randomized clinical trial with serious and violent juvenile offenders. *Journal of Consulting and Clinical Psychology, 79*, 643–652.

Shadish, W. R., & Baldwin, S. A. (2002). Meta-analysis of MFT interventions. In D. H. Sprenkle (Ed.), *Effectiveness research in marriage and family therapy* (pp. 339–370). Alexandria, VA: American Association for Marital and Family Therapy.

Siegel, D. J. (1999). *The developing mind: How relationships and the brain interact to shape who we are* (2nd ed.). New York: Guilford Press.

Stanton, M. D., & Shadish, W. R. (1997). Outcome, attrition, and family-couples treatment for drug abuse: A meta-analysis and review of controlled, comparative studies. *Psychological Bulletin, 122*, 170–191.

Stern, D. (1977). *The first relationship: Infant and mother*. Cambridge, MA: Harvard University Press.

Swenson, C. C., Schaeffer, C. M., Henggeler, S. W., Faldowski, R., & Mayhew, A. M. (2010). Multisystemic therapy for child abuse and neglect: A randomized effectiveness trial. *Journal of Family Psychology, 24*, 497–507.

Trowell, J., Joffe, I., Campbell, J., Clemente, C., Almqvist, F., Soininen, M., et al. (2007). Childhood depression: A place for psychotherapy. An outcome study comparing individual psychodynamic psychotherapy and family therapy. *European Child and Adolescent Psychiatry, 16*, 157–167.

White, M., & Epston, D. (1990). *Narrative means to therapeutic ends*. New York: Norton.

Winnicott, D. W. (1965). *The maturational process and the early facilitating environment*. London: Karnac Books.

PART IV

PROCESS AND OUTCOME IN PSYCHODYNAMIC PSYCHOTHERAPIES

CHAPTER 23

Efficacy of Psychodynamic Psychotherapy in Specific Mental Disorders
AN UPDATE

Falk Leichsenring, Johannes Kruse, and Sven Rabung

There is a need for empirical outcome research in psychodynamic and psycho-analytic therapy (Gunderson & Gabbard, 1999). This chapter reviews the available evidence for psychodynamic psychotherapy (PDT) in adults. The first section discusses the procedures of evidence-based medicine and empirically supported treatments with regard to their applicability to psychotherapy. The second section presents a review of the available evidence for PDT in specific mental disorders in adults. The focus is on randomized controlled trials (RCTs).

EVIDENCE-BASED MEDICINE AND EMPIRICALLY SUPPORTED TREATMENTS

Several proposals have been made to grade the available evidence for both medical and psychotherapeutic treatments (Chambless & Hollon, 1998; Guyatt et al., 1995). Apart from other differences, all available proposals regard RCTs (efficacy studies) as the "gold standard" for demonstrating that a treatment is effective. According to this view, only RCTs can provide level I evidence, that is, the highest level of evidence. RCTs are conducted under controlled experimental conditions; thus, they allow control for variables systematically influencing the outcome apart from the treatment. The defining feature of an RCT is the random assignment of subjects to the different conditions of treatment (Shadish, Cook, & Campbell, 2002). Randomization is regarded as indispensable in order to ensure that a priori existing differences between subjects are equally distributed. The goal of randomization is to attribute the observed effects exclusively to the applied therapy. Thus, randomization is used to ensure the internal validity of a study (Shadish et al., 2002). Gabbard, Gunderson, and Fonagy (2002) discuss different types of RCTs that provide different levels of evidence. The most stringent test of efficacy is achieved by comparison with rival treatments, thus controlling for specific and nonspecific therapeutic factors (Chambless & Hollon, 1998, p. 8). Furthermore, such comparisons provide explicit information regarding the relative benefits of competing treatments. Treatments that are found to be superior to rival treatments are more highly valued. Gabbard and colleagues regard RCTs in which a treatment is compared with a psychological placebo as the second most rigorous variant within RCTs. In our view, however, comparisons with treatment as usual (TAU) can provide more stringent tests than placebo-controlled studies because they control for both common factors (e.g., attention) and treatment effects of TAU. However, a frequent problem in TAU-controlled studies is that TAU is poorly defined and differs from one study to another. In one study, for example, TAU may be routine outpatient psychotherapy in clinical practice; in another study, it may be a pure psychopharmacological treatment; and in a third study, it may include counseling or other forms of health care. The fourth most rigorous forms of RCTs use wait-list controls. However, in this type of study, it is not clear whether the observed effect in the treatment group is to be attributed to specific or nonspecific therapeutic factors (Gabbard et al., 2002). The next level of evidence is provided by prospective pre–post studies, followed by case series, and finally by case reports.

The exclusive position of RCTs in psychotherapy research, however, has recently been questioned (Leichsenring, 2004; Rothwell, 2005; Westen, Novotny, & Thompson-Brenner, 2004). In psychotherapy research, the defining features of RCTs, such as randomization, the use of treatment manuals, focus on specific mental disorder, and, frequently, excluding patients with a poor prognosis, raise the question as to whether RCTs are sufficiently representative of clinical practice (Leichsenring, 2004; Rothwell, 2005; Westen et al., 2004). Furthermore, the methodology of an RCT, with its use of treatment manuals and randomized control conditions, is hardly applicable to long-term psychotherapy lasting several years (Seligman, 1995; Wallerstein, 1999). Another debatable aspect of the empirically supported treatments approach is the emphasis on disorders and on symptoms (Blatt, 1995). As Henry (1998, p. 129) put it: "EVTs [Empirically Validated Treatments] place the emphasis on the disorder . . . and not on the individual . . . who seeks our services." Furthermore, a method of psychotherapy that has been shown to work under controlled conditions will not necessarily work equally well under the conditions of clinical practice (Leichsenring, 2004). The main reason for this gap is that psychotherapy is not a drug that works the same way under different conditions. Difficult-to-quantify factors in the therapist–patient match may influence the outcome. Thus, it is questionable whether the methodology of pharmacological research is adequate for psychotherapy research of mental disorders, at least if the effectiveness of a treatment in clinical practice is to be studied. After all, RCTs serve only a limited function (Roth & Parry, 1997, p. 370): "RCTs are . . . an imperfect tool; almost certainly their results are best seen as one part of a research cycle."

In contrast to RCTs, naturalistic studies (effectiveness studies) are conducted under the conditions of clinical practice. Thus, their results are more representative of clinical practice with regard to patients, therapists, and treatments (external validity; Shadish, Matt, Navarro, & Phillips, 2000). Effectiveness studies cannot control for factors affecting the outcome to the same extent as RCTs (internal validity). However, the internal validity of effectiveness studies can be improved by quasi-experimental designs using methods other than randomization to rule out alternative explanations of the results (Leichsenring, 2004; Shadish et al., 2002).

Paradoxically, naturalistic studies are not accepted by, for example, the American Psychological Association as methods for demonstrating that a therapy is effective (Chambless & Hollon, 1998). The main argument against naturalistic studies refers to threats to the internal validity, that is, to the reduced possibility of controlling factors influencing outcome apart from therapy. However, according to several studies, effectiveness studies do not seem to overestimate effect sizes compared with RCTs (Benson & Hartz, 2000; Concato, Shah, & Horwitz, 2000; Shadish et al., 2000).

Following these considerations, efficacy studies and effectiveness studies address different research questions: RCTs examine the efficacy of a treatment under controlled experimental conditions, whereas effectiveness studies address the effectiveness under clinical practice conditions (Leichsenring, 2004). As a consequence, the results of an efficacy study cannot be directly transferred to clinical practice and vice versa. From this perspective, a distinction is required between empirically supported therapies and RCT methodology (Leichsenring, 2004; Westen et al., 2004). RCTs and effectiveness studies are not rivals; rather, they are complementary approaches to testing the value of clinical interventions.

EVIDENCE FOR PDT IN SPECIFIC MENTAL DISORDERS

The aim of this review is to identify for which mental disorders RCTs are available that provide evidence for the efficacy of PDT. Here, the criteria proposed by the Task Force on Promotion and Dissemination of Psychological Procedures of the American Psychological Association, modified by Chambless and Hollon (1998) to define efficacious treatments, have been applied. Only RCTs were included in which PDT was compared with either (1) no treatment (waiting list, minimal contact), placebo, or TAU, or (2) pharmacotherapy or other (nonpsychodynamic) forms of psychotherapy. Studies examining the combination of PDT and medication were not included; concomitant medication in both treatment arms, however, was allowed (for previous reviews, see Fonagy, Roth, & Higgitt, 2005; Leichsenring, 2005).

Definition of Psychodynamic Psychotherapy

PDT operates on an interpretive-supportive continuum (Gunderson & Gabbard, 1999; Wallerstein, 1989). Interpretive interventions enhance the patient's insight about repetitive conflicts sustaining his or her problems (Gabbard, 2004; Luborsky, 1984). Supportive interventions aim to strengthen abilities ("ego functions") that are either temporarily not accessible to a patient due to acute stress (e.g., traumatic events) or have not been sufficiently developed (e.g., impulse control in borderline personality disorder). Thus, supportive interventions maintain or build ego functions (Wallerstein, 1989). Supportive interventions include fostering a therapeutic alliance, setting goals, or strengthening ego functions such as reality testing or impulse control (Luborsky, 1984).

The use of more supportive or more interpretive (insight-enhancing) interventions depends on the patient's needs. The more severely disturbed a patient is or the more acute his or her problem is, the more supportive and the less interpretive interventions are required, and vice versa (Luborsky, 1984; Wallerstein, 1989). Borderline patients, as well as healthy subjects in an acute crisis or after a traumatic event, may need more supportive interventions (e.g., stabilization, providing a safe and supportive environment). Thus, a broad spectrum of psychiatric problems and disorders can be treated with PDT, ranging from milder adjustment disorders or stress reactions to severe personality disorders such as borderline personality disorder or psychotic conditions.

Efficacy Studies of PDT in Specific Mental Disorders

Forty-six RCTs providing evidence for the efficacy of PDT in specific mental disorders were identified and included in this review. These studies are presented in Table 23.1. In the studies identified, different forms of PDT were applied. The models developed by Luborsky (1984), Shapiro and Firth (1985), or Malan (1976) were used most frequently.

From a psychodynamic perspective, the results of a therapy for a specific psychiatric disorder (e.g., depression, agoraphobia) are influenced by the underlying psychodynamic features (e.g., conflicts, defenses, personality organization), which may vary considerably within one category of psychiatric disorder (Kernberg, 1996). These psychodynamic factors may affect treatment outcome and may have a greater impact on outcome than descriptive DSM diagnoses (Piper, McCallum, Joyce, & Ogrodniczuk, 2001).

Depressive Disorders

Cognitive-behavioral therapists activate patients and focus on depressive cognitions. Psychodynamic therapists focus on the conflicts or ego functions associated with depressive symptoms and often address the interpersonal origin of these conflicts. At present, four RCTs are available that provide evidence for the efficacy of PDT compared with cognitive-behavioral therapy (CBT) in major depressive disorder (Barkham et al., 1996; Gallagher-Thompson & Steffen, 1994; Shapiro et al., 1994; Thompson, Gallagher, & Breckenridge, 1987). Different models of PDT were applied (Table 23.1). For these studies, a meta-analysis found PDT and CBT to be equally effective with regard to depressive symptoms, general psychiatric symptoms, and social functioning (Leichsenring, 2001). In this meta-analysis, PDT achieved large pre–post effect sizes in depressive symptoms, general psychiatric symptoms, and social functioning (Leichsenring, 2001). The results proved to be stable in follow-up studies (Gallagher-Thompson, Hanley-Peterson, & Thompson, 1990; Shapiro et al., 1995). These results are consistent with the findings of the meta-analysis by Wampold, Minami, Baskin, and Tierney (2002), who did not find significant differences between CBT and "other therapies" in the treatment of depression.

TABLE 23.1. Randomized Controlled Trials of Psychodynamic Psychotherapy in Specific Psychiatric Disorders

Study	Disorder	n (PDT)	Comparison group	Concept of PDT	Treatment duration
Depressive disorders					
Barber et al. (2012)	Major depression	51	Pharmacotherapy: n = 55 Placebo: n = 50	Luborsky (1984)	20 sessions; 16 weeks
Barkham et al. (1996)	Major depression	18	CBT: n = 18	Shapiro & Firth (1985)	8 vs. 16 sessions
Gallagher-Thompson & Steffen (1994)	Major, minor, or intermittent depression	30	CBT: n = 36	Mann (1973); Rose & DelMaestro (1990)	16–20 sessions
Johansson et al. (2012)	Major depression	46	Structured support treatment: n = 46	Internet-guided PDT; Silverberg (2005)	10 weeks
Maina et al. (2005)	Dysthymic disorder	10	Brief supportive therapy: n = 10 Waiting list: n = 10	Malan (1976)	15–30 sessions; M = 19.6
Salminen et al. (2008)	Major depression	26	Fluoxetine: n = 25	Malan (1976a); Mann (1973)	16 sessions
Shapiro et al. (1994)	Major depression	58	CBT: n = 59	Shapiro & Firth (1985)	8 vs. 16 sessions
Thompson et al. (1987)	Major depression	24	Behavioral therapy: n = 25 CBT: n = 27 Waiting list: n = 19	Horowitz & Kaltreider (1979)	16–20 sessions
Anxiety disorders					
Andersson et al. (2012)	Generalized anxiety disorder	27	Internet-guided CBT: n = 27 Waiting list: n = 27	Internet-guided PDT; Silverberg (2005)	8 weeks
Bögels et al. (2003)	Social phobia	22	CBT: n = 27	Malan (1976a)	36 sessions

(continued)

TABLE 23.1. *(continued)*

Study	Disorder	*n* (PDT)	Comparison group	Concept of PDT	Treatment duration
Anxiety disorders (continued)					
Crits-Christoph et al. (2005)	Generalized anxiety disorder	15	Supportive therapy: *n* = 16	Crits-Christoph et al. (1995); Luborsky (1984)	16 sessions
Knijnik et al. (2004)	Social phobia	15	Credible placebo control group: *n* = 15	Knijnik et al. (2004)	12 sessions
Leichsenring et al. (2009)	Generalized anxiety disorder	28	CBT: *n* = 29	Crits-Christoph et al. (1995); Luborsky (1984)	30 sessions
Leichsenring et al. (2012)	Social phobia	207	Cognitive therapy: *n* = 209 Waiting list: *n* = 79	Leichsenring, Beutel, & Leibing (2007); Luborsky (1984)	Up to 30 sessions
Milrod et al. (2007)	Panic disorder	26	CBT (applied relaxation): *n* = 23	Milrod et al. (1997)	24 sessions
Mixed samples of depressive and anxiety disorders					
Bressi et al. (2010)	Depression and anxiety disorders	30	TAU: *n* = 30	Malan (1976)	40 sessions; 1 year
Knekt et al. (2008)	Depressive and anxiety disorders	128; 101	Solution-focused therapy: *n* = 97	Gabbard (2004); Malan (1976a); Sifneos (1978)	232 sessions; 18.5 sessions
Posttraumatic stress disorder					
Brom et al. (1989)	Posttraumatic stress disorder	29	Desensitization: *n* = 31 Hypnotherapy: *n* = 29	Horowitz (1976)	18.8 session

Somatoform disorders

Study	Disorder	n	Conditions	Manual	Dose
Creed et al. (2003)	Irritable bowel syndrome	59	Paroxetine: n = 43; TAU: n = 86	Hobson (1985); Shapiro & Firth (1985)	8 sessions
Guthrie et al. (1991)	Irritable bowel syndrome	50	Supportive listening: n = 46	Hobson (1985); Shapiro & Firth (1985)	8 sessions
Hamilton et al. (2000)	Functional dyspepsia	37	Supportive therapy: n = 36	Shapiro & Firth (1985)	7 sessions
Monsen & Monsen (2000)	Somatoform pain disorder	20	TAU/no therapy: n = 20	Monsen & Monsen (1999)	33 sessions
Sattel et al. (2012)	Multisomatoform disorder	107	Enhanced medical care: n = 107	Hardy et al. (2014)	12 sessions

Eating disorders

Study	Disorder	n	Conditions	Manual	Dose
Bachar et al. (1999)	Anorexia nervosa, Bulimia nervosa	17	Cognitive therapy: n = 17; Nutritional counseling: n = 10	Barth (1991); Geist (1989); Goodsitt (1985)	46 sessions
Dare et al. (2001)	Anorexia nervosa	21	Cognitive analytic therapy (Ryle): n = 22; Family therapy: n = 22; Routine treatment: n = 19	Dare (1995); Malan (1976)	M = 24.9 sessions
Fairburn et al. (1986)	Bulimia nervosa	11	CBT: n = 11	Bruch (1973); Rosen (1979); Stunkard (1976)	19 sessions
Garner et al. (1993)	Bulimia nervosa	25	CBT: n = 25	Luborsky (1984)	19 sessions
Gowers et al. (1993)	Anorexia nervosa	20	TAU: n = 20	Crisp (1980)	12 sessions
Tasca et al. (2006)	Binge-eating disorder	48	Group CBT: n = 47; Waiting list: n = 40	Tasca et al. (2002)	16 sessions

(continued)

TABLE 23.1. *[continued]*

Study	Disorder	n (PDT)	Comparison group	Concept of PDT	Treatment duration
Substance-related disorders					
Crits-Christoph et al. (1999, 2001)	Cocaine dependence	124	CBT + group DC: $n = 97$ Individual DC: $n = 92$ Individual DC + group DC: $n = 96$	Mark & Luborsky (1992) + group DC	Up to 36 individual and 24 group sessions; 4 months
Sandahl et al. (1998)	Alcohol dependence	25	CBT: $n = 24$	Foulkes (1964)	15 sessions ($M = 8.9$)
Woody et al. (1983, 1990)	Opiate dependence	31	DC: $n = 35$ CBT + DC: $n = 34$	Luborsky (1984) + DC	12 sessions
Woody et al. (1995)	Opiate dependence	57	DC: $n = 27$	Luborsky (1984) + DC	26 sessions
Borderline personality disorder					
Bateman & Fonagy (1999, 2001)	Borderline personality disorder	19	TAU: $n = 19$	Bateman (1995)	18 months
Bateman & Fonagy (2009)	Borderline personality disorder	71	Structured clinical management: $n = 63$	Bateman & Fonagy (2004)	18 months
Clarkin et al. (2007)	Borderline personality disorder	30	Dialectical behavioral therapy: $n = 30$ Supportive therapy: $n = 30$	Clarkin et al. (1999); Kernberg (1984)	12 months
Doering et al. (2010)	Borderline personality disorder	43	Treatment by experienced community therapists: $n = 29$	Clarkin et al. (1999)	Assessment after 1 year
Giesen-Bloo et al. (2006)	Borderline personality disorder	42	CBT: $n = 44$	Clarkin et al. (1999); Kernberg (1984)	3 years with sessions twice a week

Study	Personality disorder	n	Treatment conditions	Manual	Dose
Gregory et al. (2008)	Borderline personality disorder	15	TAU: n = 15	Gregory & Remen (2008)	24.9 sessions
Munroe-Blum & Marziali (1995)	Borderline personality disorder	31	Interpersonal group therapy: n = 25	Kernberg (1984)	17 sessions
Cluster C personality disorders					
Muran et al. (2005)	Cluster C personality disorders	22	Brief relational therapy: n = 33; CBT: n = 29	Pollack et al. (1992)	30 sessions
Svartberg et al. (2004)	Cluster C personality disorders	25	CBT: n = 25	Malan (1976); McCullough Vaillant (1997)	40 sessions
Avoidant personality disorder					
Emmelkamp et al. (2006)	Avoidant personality disorder	23	CBT: n = 21; Waiting list: n = 18	Luborsky (1984); Luborsky & Mark (1991); Malan (1976a); Pinsker et al. (1991)	20 sessions
Samples of mixed personality disorders					
Abbass et al. (2008)	Heterogeneous personality disorders	14	Minimal contact: n = 14	Davanloo (1980)	M = 27.7 sessions
Hellerstein et al. (1998)	Primarily Cluster C personality disorders	25	Brief supportive psychotherapy: n = 24	Davanloo (1980)	40 sessions
Winston et al. (1994)	Heterogeneous personality disorders	25	Brief adaptive psychotherapy: n = 30; Waiting list: n = 26	Davanloo (1980)	40 weeks; M = 40.3 sessions

CBT, cognitive-behavioral therapy; DC, drug counseling; PDT, psychodynamic psychotherapy; TAU, treatment as usual.

In an RCT by Salminen and colleagues (2008), PDT was found to be of equal efficacy to fluoxetine in reducing symptoms of depression and improving functional ability. However, with sample sizes of $n_1 = 26$ and $n_2 = 25$, statistical power may have not been sufficient to detect possible differences between treatments. Testing for noninferiority, $n_1 = n_2 = 86$ patients are required to detect an at least medium difference (effect size $d = 0.5$) between two treatments with a sufficient power (alpha = 0.05, two-tailed test, $1 - $ beta $= 0.90$; Cohen, 1988). In a small RCT, Maina, Forner, and Bogetto (2005) examined the efficacy of PDT and brief supportive therapy in the treatment of minor depressive disorders (dysthymic disorder, depressive disorder not otherwise specified, or adjustment disorder with depressed mood). Both treatments were superior to a wait-list condition at the end of treatment. At 6-month follow-up, PDT was superior to brief supportive therapy. In a recent study by Barber, Barrett, Gallop, Rynn, and Rickels (2012), PDT and pharmacotherapy were equally effective in the treatment of depression. However, in this trial, neither PDT nor pharmacotherapy was superior to placebo.

Internet-guided self-help based on PDT is also available. In a recent RCT, Johansson and colleagues (2012) found this type of Internet-guided self-help to be significantly more efficacious than a structured support intervention (psychoeducation and scheduled weekly contact online) in patients with major depressive disorder. Treatment effects were maintained at 10-month follow-up. Psychodynamically oriented self-help was based on formulations by Silverberg (2005). Internet-guided self-help based on PDT is a promising approach, especially for patients who do not receive psychotherapy. Future studies should further investigate its efficacy.

A recent meta-analysis, which examined the effects of CBT, PDT, interpersonal therapy, and other forms of psychotherapy in adult depression, did not find one treatment significantly superior to others, with the exception of interpersonal therapy (Cuijpers, van Straten, Andersson, & van Oppen, 2008). Another recent meta-analysis examined the effects of PDT in depression (Driessen et al., 2010). The authors found PDT to be significantly superior to control conditions. If group therapy was included, PDT was less efficacious compared to other treatments at the end of therapy. If only individual therapy was included, there were no significant differences between PDT and other treatments (Abbass & Driessen, 2010). At 3-month and 9-month follow-ups, no significant differences between treatments were found. In another meta-analysis, PDT was found to be as effective as other psychotherapies in patients with depression and comorbid personality disorders (Abbass, Town, & Driessen, 2001).

Pathological Grief

The treatment of prolonged or complicated grief by short-term psychodynamic group therapy was studied in two RCTs by McCallum and Piper (1990) and Piper and colleagues (2001). In the first study, short-term psychodynamic group therapy was significantly superior to a wait-list condition (McCallum & Piper, 1990). In the second study, a significant interaction was found. With regard to grief symptoms, patients with high-quality object relations improved more in interpretive therapy, and patients with low-quality object relations improved more in supportive therapy. For general symptoms, clinical significance favored interpretive therapy over supportive therapy (Piper et al., 2001).

Anxiety Disorders

For anxiety disorders, a small number of RCTs are presently available (Table 23.1). With regard to *panic disorder* (with or without agoraphobia), Milrod and colleagues (2007) showed that PDT was superior to applied relaxation.

For *social phobia*, three RCTs of PDT exist. In the first study, a short-term psychodynamic group treatment for generalized social phobia was superior to a credible placebo control (Knijnik, Kapczinski, Chachamovich, Margis, & Eizirik, 2004). In the second RCT, PDT proved to be as effective as CBT in the treatment of generalized social phobia (Bögels, Wijts, & Sallaerts, 2003). However, with sample sizes of $n = 22$ and $n = 27$, statistical power may have not been sufficient to detect possible differences between treatments.

In a large-scale multicenter RCT, the efficacy of PDT and cognitive therapy in the treatment of social phobia was studied (Leichsenring et al., 2012). In an outpatient setting, 495 patients with a primary diagnosis of social phobia were randomly assigned to CBT, PDT, or a waiting-list condition. This study is one of the few trials that are sufficiently powered for a noninferiority (equivalence) trial. Treatments were carried out according to manuals, and treatment fidelity was carefully controlled for. Both treatments were significantly superior to the waiting list. Thus, this trial provides evidence that PDT is effective in the treatment of social phobia according to the criteria proposed by Chambless and Hollon (1998). There were no differences between PDT and CBT with regard to response rates (52% vs. 60%) and reduction of depression. There were significant differences between CBT and PDT in favor of CBT, however, with regard to remission rates (36% vs. 26%), self-reported symptoms of social phobia, and reduction of interpersonal problems. Differences in terms of between-group effect sizes, however, were small (Leichsenring et al., 2013).

In a randomized controlled feasibility study of *generalized anxiety disorder*, PDT was equally as effective as a supportive therapy with regard to continuous measures of anxiety, but significantly superior on symptomatic remission rates (Crits-Christoph, Connolly Gibbons, Narducci, Schamberger, & Gallop, 2005). However, sample sizes in this study were relatively small ($n = 15$ vs. $n = 16$), and the study was not sufficiently powered to detect possible differences between treatments. In another RCT of generalized anxiety disorder, PDT was compared with CBT (Leichsenring et al., 2009). PDT and CBT were equally effective with regard to the primary outcome measure. However, in some secondary outcome measures, CBT was found to be superior both at the end of therapy and at the 6-month follow-up. Other differences may exist that were not detected due to the limited sample size and power (CBT: $n = 29$; PDT: $n = 28$). The results of the one-year follow-up will soon be available. A core element in the applied method of CBT, in contrast to short-term PDT, was a modification of worrying. This specific difference between the treatments may explain the superiority of CBT in the Penn State Worry Questionnaire and in part also in the

State-Trait Anxiety Inventory (trait measure). The latter also contains several items related to worrying. The results of this study may suggest that the outcome of short-term PDT in generalized anxiety disorder may be further optimized by employing a stronger focus on the process of worrying. In PDT, worrying can be conceptualized as a defense mechanism that protects the subject from fantasies or feelings that are even more threatening than the contents of his or her worries (Crits-Christoph, Crits-Christoph, Wolf-Palacio, Fichter, & Rudick, 1995).

A study of Internet-based therapy showed no differences in outcome between PDT, CBT, and a waiting-list condition at the end of treatment. At 3-month follow-up, however, both PDT and CBT were superior to a waiting list (Andersson et al., 2012). No significant differences were found between PDT and CBT. For PDT, CBT, and a waiting list, remission rates were, respectively, 54.5%, 35%, and 16% at the end of treatment, and 72.7, 66.7%, and 61.9% at 18-month follow-up. According to these results, PDT delivered over the Internet appears to be as efficacious as CBT in generalized anxiety disorder.

Mixed Samples of Depressive and Anxiety Disorders

Knekt and colleagues compared short-term PDT (STPP), long-term PDT (LTPP), and solution-focused therapy (SFT) in patients with depressive or anxiety disorders (Knekt, Lindfors, Harkanen, et al., 2008; Knekt, Lindfors, Laaksonen, et al., 2008). STPP was more effective than LTPP during the first year. During the second year of follow-up, no significant differences were found between long-term and short-term treatments. At 3-year follow-up, LTPP was more effective; no significant differences were found between the short-term treatments. With regard to specific mental disorders, it is of note that after 3 years significantly more patients recovered from anxiety disorders in the LTPP group (90%) compared with the STPP (67%) and SFT (65%) groups. For depressive disorders, no such differences occurred. In an RCT by Bressi, Porcellana, Marinaccio, Nocito, and Magri (2010), PDT was superior to TAU in a sample of patients with depressive or anxiety disorders.

Posttraumatic Stress Disorder

In an RCT by Brom, Kleber, and Defares (1989), the effects of PDT, behavioral therapy, and hypnotherapy in patients with posttraumatic stress disorder (PTSD) were studied. All of the treatments proved to be equally effective. The results reported by Brom and colleagues are consistent with those of a more recent meta-analysis by Benish, Imel, and Wampold (2008), which found no significant differences between bona fide therapies for the treatment of PTSD. In a response to the meta-analysis by Benish and colleagues, Ehlers and colleagues (2010) critically reviewed the study by Brom and colleagues, arguing that "in this study, neither hypnotherapy nor PDT was consistently more effective than the waiting list control condition across the analyses used. . . . In addition, Brom and colleagues pointed out that patients in PDT showed slower overall change than those in the other two treatment conditions, and did *not* improve in intrusive symptoms significantly" (for a rebuttal, see Wampold et al., 2012). Results were different for different outcome measures. For the avoidance scale and the total score of the Impact of Event Scale, PDT was significantly superior to the waiting-list condition, both after therapy and at follow-up (Brom et al., 1989, p. 610; Table 23.1). While effect sizes for PDT were somewhat smaller at posttreatment (avoidance: 0.66, total: 1.10), PDT achieved the largest effect sizes at follow-up (avoidance: 0.92, total: 1.56) compared with CBT (0.73, 1.30) and hypnotherapy (0.88, 1.54).[1] For the Intrusion Scale of the Impact of Event Scale, the primary outcome measure, PDT was not superior to waiting list at posttest and at 3-month follow-up. Pre–post differences of PDT, however, were significant, and the pre–post and pre–follow-up effect sizes were large (0.95 and 1.55, respectively). In contrast, the pre–post effect size for the waiting list was small (0.34). For the CBT condition (trauma desensitization), the pre–post and pre–follow-up effect sizes were 1.66 and 1.43, respectively. Thus, at follow-up, PDT achieved larger effect sizes than CBT. While the effect size of CBT tended to decrease at follow-up, it tended to increase for PDT. As is shown below, this is true for the avoidance scale and the total score of the Impact of Event Scale.[2] For this reason, it is strange that Brom and colleagues reported the difference between PDT and the control condition to be not significant at follow-up. For intrusion, PDT achieved the lowest score of all conditions at follow-up. These results, however, were not reported by Ehlers and colleagues. The data presented by Ehlers and colleagues (p. 273, Figure 2) included only the pre–post effect sizes and not the pre–follow-up effect sizes, for which PDT achieved larger effect sizes as shown above. In a critical review, the results of all analyses should be presented, not only the results that support the authors' own perspective. Furthermore, for general symptoms, Brom and colleagues noted that PDT "seems to withstand the comparison [with waiting list] best" (p. 610). Thus, after all, it seems to take a longer period of time (3 months) for PDT to achieve its effects, but these effects are at least as large as those of CBT.

It is clear that further studies of PDT in PTSD are required. To date, only one RCT of PDT in PTSD is available.

Somatoform Disorders

At present, five RCTs of PDT in somatoform disorders that fulfill the inclusion criteria are available (Table 23.1). In the RCT by Guthrie, Creed, Dawson, and Tomenson (1991), patients with irritable bowel syndrome, who had not responded to standard medical treatment over the previous 6 months, were treated with PDT in addition to standard medical treatment. This treatment was compared to standard medical treatment alone. PDT was effective in two-thirds of the patients. In another RCT, PDT was significantly more effective than routine care and as effective as medication (paroxetine) in the treatment of severe irritable bowel syndrome (Creed et al., 2003). During the follow-up period, PDT, but not paroxetine, was associated with a significant

---

[1] Effect sizes assessed by FL.

[2] Brom and colleagues (1989) did not report means and standard deviations for the waiting-list condition at follow-up, only for posttreatment. For this reason, no effect sizes for follow-up can be calculated.

reduction in health care costs compared with TAU. In an RCT by Hamilton and colleagues (2000), PDT was compared with supportive therapy in the treatment of patients with chronic intractable functional dyspepsia who had failed to respond to conventional pharmacological treatments. At the end of treatment, PDT was significantly superior to the control condition. The effects were stable at the 12-month follow-up. Monsen and Monsen (2000) compared 33 sessions of PDT with a control condition (no treatment or TAU) in the treatment of patients with chronic pain. PDT was significantly superior to the control condition on measures of pain, psychiatric symptoms, interpersonal problems, and affect consciousness. These results remained stable or even improved at the 12-month follow-up. In a recent RCT, Sattel and colleagues (2012) compared PDT with enhanced medical care in patients with multisomatoform disorders. At follow-up, PDT was superior to enhanced medical care with regard to improvements in patients' physical quality of life.

Thus, specific variants of PDT appear to be effective in the treatment of somatoform disorders. Abbass, Kisely, and Kroenke (2009) carried out a review and meta-analysis on the effects of PDT in somatic disorders. They included both RCTs and controlled before-and-after studies. Meta-analysis was possible for 14 studies, revealing significant effects on physical symptoms, psychiatric symptoms, and social adjustment, which were maintained at long-term follow-up.

Bulimia Nervosa

Three RCTs of PDT for the treatment of bulimia nervosa are available (Table 23.1). Significant and stable improvements in bulimia nervosa after PDT were demonstrated in RCTs by Fairburn, Kirk, O'Connor, and Cooper (1986), Fairburn and colleagues (1995), and Garner and colleagues (1993). In the primary disorder-specific measures (bulimic episodes, self-induced vomiting), PDT was as effective as CBT (Fairburn et al., 1986, 1995; Garner et al., 1993). However, the studies were not sufficiently powered to detect possible differences (see Table 23.1 for sample sizes). Apart from this, CBT was superior to PDT in some specific measures of psychopathology (Fairburn et al., 1986). However, in a long-term follow-up of the Fairburn and colleagues study, both forms of therapy proved to be equally effective and were partly superior to a behavioral form of therapy (Fairburn et al., 1995). Accordingly, for a valid evaluation of the efficacy of PDT in bulimia nervosa, longer-term follow-up studies are necessary. In another RCT, PDT was significantly superior to both a nutritional counseling group and cognitive therapy (Bachar, Latzer, Kreitler, & Berry, 1999). This was true of patients with bulimia nervosa and a mixed sample of patients with bulimia nervosa or anorexia nervosa.

Anorexia Nervosa

In contrast to bulimia nervosa, evidence-based treatments for anorexia nervosa are scarce (Fairburn, 2005). This applies to both PDT and CBT. In an RCT by Gowers, Norton, Halek, and Vrisp (1994), PDT combined with four sessions of nutritional advice yielded significant improvements in patients with anorexia nervosa (Table 23.1). Weight and BMI changes were significantly more improved than in a control condition (TAU). Dare, Eisler, Russel, Treasure, and Dodge (2001) compared PDT (with a mean duration of 24.9 sessions) with cognitive analytic therapy, family therapy, and routine treatment in the treatment of anorexia nervosa (Table 23.1). PDT yielded significant symptomatic improvements, and PDT and family therapy were significantly superior to the routine treatment with regard to weight gain. However, the improvements were modest; several patients remained undernourished at the follow-up. Thus, the treatment of anorexia nervosa remains a challenge, and more effective treatment models are required.

Binge-Eating Disorder

In an RCT by Tasca and colleagues (2006), a psychodynamic group treatment was as efficacious as CBT and superior to a waiting-list condition in binge-eating disorder (e.g., in terms of days binged, interpersonal problems). For the comparison of PDT with CBT, again the question of statistical power arises ($n_1 = 48$, $n_2 = 47$, $n_3 = 40$).

Substance-Related Disorders

Woody and colleagues (Woody, Luborsky, McLellan, & O'Brien, 1990; Woody et al., 1983) studied the effects of PDT and CBT in addition to drug counseling in the treatment of opiate dependence (Table 23.1). PDT plus drug counseling yielded significant improvements on measures of drug-related symptoms and general psychiatric symptoms. At 7-month follow-up, PDT and CBT plus drug counseling were equally effective, and both conditions were superior to drug counseling alone. In another RCT, 26 sessions of PDT in addition to drug counseling was also superior to drug counseling alone in the treatment of opiate dependence (Woody, Luborsky, McLellan, & O'Brien, 1995). At 6-month follow-up, most of the gains made by the patients who had received PDT remained. In an RCT conducted by Crits-Christoph and colleagues (1999, 2001), up to 36 individual sessions of PDT were combined with 24 sessions of group drug counseling in the treatment of cocaine dependence. The combined treatment yielded significant improvements and was as effective as CBT combined with group drug counseling. However, neither CBT plus group drug counseling nor PDT plus group drug counseling was more effective than group drug counseling alone. Furthermore, individual drug counseling was significantly superior to both forms of therapy in terms of measures of drug abuse. With regard to psychological and social outcome variables, all treatments were equally effective (Crits-Christoph et al., 1999, 2001). In an RCT by Sandahl, Herlitz, Ahlin, and Rönnberg (1998), the efficacy of PDT and CBT in the treatment of alcohol abuse was compared. PDT yielded significant improvements on measures of alcohol abuse, which were stable at 15-month follow-up. PDT was significantly superior to CBT in the number of abstinent days and in the improvement of general psychiatric symptoms.

Borderline Personality Disorder

At the time of writing, seven RCTs are available of PDT in borderline personality disorder (Bateman & Fonagy, 1999, 2009; Clarkin, Levy, Lenzenweger, & Kernberg,

2007; Doering et al., 2010; Giesen-Bloo et al., 2006; Gregory et al., 2008; Munroe-Blum & Marziali, 1995). Of these, several showed that PDT was superior to TAU (Bateman & Fonagy, 1999; Doering et al., 2010; Gregory et al., 2008). Bateman and Fonagy (1999, 2001) studied mentalization-based treatment (MBT) in a psychoanalytically oriented partial hospitalization treatment program for patients with borderline personality disorder. The major difference between the treatment group and the control group was the provision of individual and group psychotherapy in the treatment group. The treatment lasted a maximum of 18 months. MBT was significantly superior to standard psychiatric care both at the end of therapy and at the 18-month and 8-year follow-up (Bateman & Fonagy, 2001, 2008). In a recent RCT, transference-focused psychotherapy (TFP) was compared with a treatment carried out by experienced community psychotherapists in borderline outpatients (Doering et al., 2010). TFP was superior with regard to borderline psychopathology, psychosocial functioning, personality organization, inpatient admission, and dropouts. Another RCT compared PDT ("dynamic deconstructive psychotherapy") with TAU in the treatment of patients with BPD and co-occurring alcohol use disorder (Gregory & Remen, 2008). In this study, PDT but not TAU achieved significant improvements in outcome measures of parasuicide, alcohol misuse, and institutional care. Furthermore, PDT was superior with regard to improvements in borderline psychopathology, depression, and social support. No difference was found in dissociation. This was true, although TAU participants received a higher average treatment intensity. Another recent RCT found outpatient MBT to be superior to manual-driven structured clinical management with regard to the primary (suicidal and self-injurious behaviors, hospitalization) and secondary (e.g., depression, general symptom distress, interpersonal functioning) outcome measures (Bateman & Fonagy, 2009).

With regard to the comparison of PDT with specific forms of psychotherapy, one RCT reported PDT to be equally as effective as interpersonal group therapy (Munroe-Blum & Marziali, 1995). PDT yielded significant improvements on measures of borderline-related symptoms, general psychiatric symptoms, and depression, and was as effective as the interpersonal group therapy. However, the power of the study may not have been sufficient to detect differences between treatments ($n_1 = 22$, $n_2 = 26$). Giesen-Bloo and colleagues (2006) compared PDT (TFP) based on Kernberg's model (Clarkin, Yeomans, & Kernberg, 1999) with schema-focused therapy (SFT), a form of CBT. Treatment duration was 3 years, with two sessions a week. The authors reported statistically and clinically significant improvements for both treatments. However, SFT was found to be superior to TFP in several outcome measures. Furthermore, a significantly higher dropout rate for TFP was reported. This study, however, has serious methodological flaws. The authors used scales for adherence and competence for both treatments, for which they adopted an identical cutoff score of 60, indicating competent application. According to the data published by the authors (Giesen-Bloo et al., 2006; p. 651), the median competence level was 85.67 for SFT but only 65.6 for TFP. While the competence level for SFT clearly exceeded the cutoff, the competence level for TFP only just surpassed it. This indicates that there were major differences between the two treatments in terms of therapist competence. Thus, the results of the study are questionable. The difference in competence was not taken into account by the authors either in the analyses of the data or in the discussion of the results. This study therefore raises serious concerns about an investigator allegiance effect (Luborsky et al., 1999).

Another RCT compared PDT (TFP), dialectical behavior therapy (DBT), and psychodynamic supportive psychotherapy (SPT; Clarkin et al., 2007). Patients treated with all three modalities showed general improvement in the study. However, TFP was shown to produce improvements not demonstrated by either DBT or SBT. Those participants who received TFP were more likely to move from an insecure attachment classification to a secure one. They also showed significantly greater changes in mentalizing capacity and narrative coherence compared with the other two groups. TFP was associated with significant improvement in 10 of the 12 variables across the six symptomatic domains, compared with six for SBT and five for DBT. Only TFP was associated with significant changes in impulsivity, irritability, verbal assault, and direct assault. TFP and DBT reduced suicidality to the same extent. Here, too, power may have been not sufficient to detect further possible differences ($n_1 = 23$, $n_2 = 17$, $n_3 = 22$). Thus, for TFP, two RCTs carried out in independent research settings are available providing evidence that TFP is an efficacious and specific treatment for BPD, according to the criteria of empirically supported treatments proposed by Chambless and Hollon (1998; see also Leichsenring, Leibing, Kruse, New, & Leweke, 2011).

Cluster C Personality Disorders

There is also evidence for the efficacy of PDT in the treatment of Cluster C personality disorders. In an RCT conducted by Svartberg, Stiles, and Seltzer (2004), PDT of 40 sessions in length was compared with CBT (Table 23.1). Both PDT and CBT yielded significant improvements in patients with DSM-IV Cluster C personality disorders (i.e., avoidant, compulsive, or dependent personality disorder). The improvements refer to symptoms, interpersonal problems, and core personality pathology. The results were stable at 24-month follow-up. No significant differences were found between PDT and CBT with regard to efficacy. However, once again, this study was not sufficiently powered to detect possible differences ($n_1 = 25$, $n_2 = 25$). Muran, Safran, Samstag, and Winston (2005) compared the efficacy of PDT ($n = 22$), brief relational therapy ($n = 33$), and CBT ($n = 29$) in the treatment of Cluster C personality disorders and personality disorders not otherwise specified. Treatments lasted for 30 sessions. No significant differences were found between the treatment conditions either at termination or at follow-up on all outcome measures. Furthermore, there were no significant differences between the treatments with regard to the percentage of patients achieving clinically significant change in symptoms, interpersonal problems, features of personality disorders, or therapist ratings of target complaints. At termination, CBT and brief relational therapy were superior to PDT in one outcome measure (patient ratings of target complaints). However, this difference did not persist at follow-up. With regard to the percentage of patients showing change, no significant differences were found either at termination or at follow-up, except in one comparison: At termination, CBT was superior to PDT on the Inventory of Interpersonal Problems (Horowitz, Alden, Wiggins, & Pincus, 2000). Again, this difference did not persist at follow-up. The conclusion is that only a few significant differences were found between the treatments, which did not persist at follow-up.

Avoidant Personality Disorder

Avoidant personality disorder is among the above-mentioned Cluster C personality disorders. In an RCT, Emmelkamp and colleagues (2006) compared CBT to PDT and a wait-list condition in the treatment of avoidant personality disorder. The authors reported CBT as being more effective than the wait-list control and PDT. However, the study suffers from several methodological shortcomings (Leichsenring & Leibing, 2007). Design, statistical analyses, and the reporting of the results raise serious concerns about an investigator allegiance effect (Luborsky et al., 1999).

Heterogeneous Samples of Patients with Personality Disorders

Winston and colleagues (1994) compared PDT with brief adaptive psychotherapy or waiting list in a heterogeneous group of patients with personality disorders. Most of the patients showed a Cluster C personality disorder. Patients with paranoid, schizoid, schizotypal, borderline, or narcissistic personality disorders were excluded. Mean treatment duration was 40 weeks. Patients in both treatment groups showed significantly more improvements than the patients on the waiting list. No differences in outcome were found between the two forms of psychotherapy. Hellerstein and colleagues (1998) compared PDT with brief supportive therapy in a heterogeneous sample of patients with personality disorders. Again, most of the patients showed a Cluster C personality disorder. The authors reported similar degrees of improvement both at termination and at 6-month follow-up. However, the studies by Winston and colleagues and Hellerstein and colleagues were not sufficiently powered to detect possible differences (see Table 23.1 for sample sizes). Abbass, Sheldon, Gyra, and Kalpin (2008) compared PDT (intensive short-term dynamic psychotherapy; ISTDP) with a minimal-contact group in a heterogeneous group of patients with personality disorders. The most common Axis II diagnoses were borderline personality disorder (44%), obsessive–compulsive disorder (37%), and avoidant personality disorder (33%). Average treatment duration was 27.7 sessions. PDT was significantly superior to the control condition in all primary outcome measures. When control patients were treated, they experienced benefits similar to those seen in the initial treatment group. At long-term follow-up 2 years after the end of treatment, the whole group maintained their gains and had an 83% reduction of personality disorder diagnoses. In addition, treatment costs were offset threefold by reductions in medication and disability payments. This preliminary study of ISTDP suggests it is efficacious and cost-effective in the treatment of personality disorders.

At present, two meta-analyses on the effects of PDT in personality disorders are available (Leichsenring & Leibing, 2003, Town, Abbass, & Hardy, 2011). A meta-analysis addressing the effects of PDT and CBT in personality disorders reported that PDT yielded large effect sizes not only for comorbid symptoms, but also for core personality pathology (Leichsenring & Leibing, 2003). This was true especially for BPD.

A more recent meta-analysis by Town and colleagues (2011) included seven RCTs on short-term PDT in personality disorders. Although it is difficult to draw strong conclusions given the relatively small number of studies, this meta-analysis suggests that PDT is efficacious for a wide range of personality disorders, producing significant and medium- to long-term improvements for a large percentage of patients.

Complex Mental Disorders

The majority of available RCTs addressing the efficacy of PDT have focused on short-term treatments. Evidence, however, demonstrates that short-term treatments are not sufficiently helpful for a considerable proportion of patients with more complex mental disorders, such as personality disorders or other chronic mental disorders (Kopta, Howard, Lowry, & Beutler, 1994; Perry, Banon, & Floriana, 1999). Some studies suggest that longer-term psychotherapy may be helpful for these patients (Bateman & Fonagy, 1999; Clarkin et al., 2007; Linehan et al., 2006; Linehan, Tutek, Heard, & Armstrong, 1994). As stated earlier, the RCT methodology may be of limited utility for the study of longer-term psychotherapies lasting 1 year or longer (Seligman, 1995; Wallerstein, 1999). In such cases, observational studies using quasi-experimental designs may be more appropriate (Shadish et al., 2002). Consequently, a meta-analysis of LTPP included 11 RCTs and 12 observational studies (Leichsenring & Rabung, 2008). According to the results, LTPP (defined as lasting at least one year or 50 sessions) yielded large and stable effects in patients with complex mental disorders (defined as personality disorders, multiple mental disorders, and chronic mental disorders). For overall outcome, the effect sizes even increased significantly between treatment termination and follow-up. The comparison of RCTs versus observational studies revealed no significant differences in outcome, suggesting that the outcome data of the RCTs included in this meta-analysis were representative for clinical practice. The results also showed that the data of the observational studies did not systematically over- or underestimate the effects of LTPP. When compared with other methods of psychotherapy which were predominantly less intensive or briefer, LTPP proved to be significantly superior with regard to overall outcome, target problems, and personality functioning. This meta-analysis was met by considerable criticism (Bhar et al., 2010). A rebuttal has addressed these concerns (Leichsenring & Rabung, 2011a), and a recent update of the meta-analysis, taking into account earlier criticism, essentially corroborated findings from the original 2008 meta-analysis (Leichsenring & Rabung, 2011b). Nevertheless, further studies are required to allow for more refined analyses that will address the effects of LTPP in specific complex disorders, including comparison to other specific forms of therapies.

CONCLUSIONS AND FUTURE DIRECTIONS

Under the requirements of the criteria proposed by the Task Force on Promotion and Dissemination of Psychological Procedures modified by Chambless and Hollon (1998), 46 RCTs are presently available that provide evidence for the efficacy of PDT in specific mental disorders. In these studies, either PDT was more effective than placebo therapy, supportive therapy, or TAU, or there were generally no differences between PDT and CBT or between PDT and pharmacotherapy. These results are consistent with those of an earlier meta-analysis of PDT reporting that PDT was superior to wait-list conditions or TAU and equally as effective as other psychotherapies (Leichsenring, Rabung, & Leibing, 2004). This meta-analysis reported large effect sizes for PDT in target problems, general psychiatric problems, and social functioning, which were stable at follow-up and tended to increase (Leichsenring et al., 2004). In a few studies, PDT was superior to a method of CBT (Milrod et al., 2007), and in another study it was superior at least in some outcome measures (Clarkin et al., 2007). Most of the studies that found no differences in efficacy between PDT and another bona fide treatment were not sufficiently powered. As reported above, testing for noninferiority (i.e., equivalence) requires $n_1 = n_2 = 86$ patients to detect an at least medium difference (effect size $d = 0.5$) between two treatments with a sufficient power (alpha = 0.05, two-tailed test, $1 -$ beta = 0.90; Cohen, 1988). At present, only three RCTs comparing PDT with a bona fide treatment fulfill this criterion (Crits-Christoph et al., 1999; Knekt, Lindfors, Harkanen et al., 2008; Leichsenring et al., 2012). However, for comparisons of PDT with bona fide therapies, the between-group effect sizes were found to be small (Leichsenring et al., 2004). Thus, it is an open question whether studies with more statistical power will find significant differences and whether these (possibly small) differences are clinically relevant or significant (Jacobson & Truax, 1991).

The issue of small sample size studies, however, is not specific to studies of PDT, since many studies of CBT are not sufficiently powered as well (Leichsenring & Rabung, 2011a). It is important, furthermore, to realize that there are several mental disorders for which no RCTs of PDT are available. This is true, for example, for dissociative disorders or for some specific forms of personality disorders (e.g., narcissistic personality disorder). For PTSD, only one RCT is presently available (Brom et al., 1989).

Some studies reported differences, at least in some measures, in favor of CBT. This is true, for example, for the studies by Fairburn and colleagues (1986) and Garner and colleagues (1993) on bulimia nervosa, and for the study of Leichsenring and colleagues (2009) on generalized anxiety disorder. For the study on generalized anxiety disorder, we have already noted that a stronger focus on the process of worrying could perhaps improve the effects of PDT. More generally, researchers should address the question of whether the efficacy of PDT can be improved by focusing in more detail on the specific mechanisms involved in the course of different disorders. MBT or TFP may serve as good examples for psychodynamic treatments that focus on purported underlying mechanisms in a specific disorder.

Further research concerning the efficacy and effectiveness of PDT in specific mental disorders is necessary, and there is also a strong need for studies addressing the mechanisms of change in these treatments. This will necessarily entail the inclusion not only of symptomatic measures and DSM criteria, but also measures more specific to PDT. Future studies should also examine whether there are gains achieved only by PDT, that is, the question of "added value." Furthermore, studies should address the translation of psychotherapies that have been tested under experimental conditions ("efficacy") to routine clinical practice ("effectiveness").

REFERENCES

Abbass, A., & Driessen, E. (2010). The efficacy of short-term psychodynamic psychotherapy for depression: A summary of recent findings. *Acta Psychiatrica Scandinavica, 121*, 398–399.

Abbass, A. A., Kisely, S., & Kroenke, K. (2009). Short-term psychodynamic psychotherapy for somatic disorders. Systematic review and meta-analysis of clinical trials. *Psychotherapy and Psychosomatics, 78*, 265–274.

Abbass, A. A., Sheldon, A., Gyra, J., & Kalpin, A. (2008). Intensive short-term dynamic psychotherapy for DSM-IV personality disorders: A randomized controlled trial. *Journal of Nervous and Mental Disease, 196*, 211–216.

Abbass, A., Town, J., & Driessen, E. (2011). The efficacy of short-term psychodynamic psychotherapy for depressive disorders with comorbid personality disorder. *Psychiatry, 74*, 58–71.

Andersson, G., Paxling, B., Roch-Norlund, P., Ostman, G., Norgren, A., Almlöv, J., et al. (2012). Internet-based psychodynamic versus cognitive behavioral guided self-help for generalized anxiety disorder: A randomized controlled trial. *Psychotherapy and Psychosomatics, 81*, 344–355.

Bachar, E., Latzer, Y., Kreitler, S., & Berry, E. M. (1999). Empirical comparison of two psychological therapies. Self psychology and cognitive orientation in the treatment of anorexia and bulimia. *Journal of Psychotherapy Practice and Research, 8*, 115–128.

Barber, J. P., Barrett, M. S., Gallop, R., Rynn, M. A., & Rickels, K. (2012). Short-term dynamic psychotherapy versus pharmacotherapy for major depressive disorder: A randomized, placebo-controlled trial. *Journal of Clinical Psychiatry, 73*, 66–73.

Barkham, M., Rees, A., Shapiro, D. A., Stiles, W. B., Agnew, R. M., Halstead, J., et al. (1996). Outcomes of time-limited psychotherapy in applied settings: Replicating the Second Sheffield Psychotherapy Project. *Journal of Consulting and Clinical Psychology, 64*, 1079–1085.

Barth, D. (1991). When the patient abuses food. In H. Jackson (Ed.), *Using self-psychology in psychotherapy* (pp. 223–242). Northvale, NJ: Jason Aronson.

Bateman, A. (1995). The treatment of borderline patients in a day hospital setting. *Psychoanalytic Psychotherapy, 91*, 3–16.

Bateman, A., & Fonagy, P. (1999). Effectiveness of partial hospitalization in the treatment of borderline personality disorder: A randomized controlled trial. *American Journal of Psychiatry, 156*, 1563–1569.

Bateman, A., & Fonagy, P. (2001). Treatment of borderline personality disorder with psychoanalytically oriented partial hospitalization: An 18-month follow-up. *American Journal of Psychiatry, 158*, 36–42.

Bateman, A., & Fonagy, P. (2004). *Psychotherapy for borderline personality disorder: Mentalization-based treatment.* Oxford, UK: Oxford University Press.

Bateman, A., & Fonagy, P. (2008). 8-year follow-up of patients treated for borderline personality disorder: Mentalization-based treatment versus treatment as usual *American Journal of Psychiatry, 165*, 631–638.

Bateman, A., & Fonagy, P. (2009). Randomized controlled trial of outpatient mentalization-based treatment versus structured clinical management for borderline personality disorder *American Journal of Psychiatry, 166*, 1355–1364.

Benish, S. G., Imel, Z. E., & Wampold, B. E. (2008). The relative efficacy of bona fide psychotherapies for treating post-traumatic stress disorder: A meta-analysis of direct comparisons. *Clinical Psychology Review, 28*, 746–758.

Benson, K., & Hartz, A. J. (2000). A comparison of observational studies and randomized, controlled trials. *New England Journal of Medicine, 342*, 1878–1886.

Bhar, S. S., Thombs, B. D., Pignotti, M., Bassel, M., Jewett, L., Coyne, J. C., et al. (2010). Is longer-term psychodynamic psychotherapy more effective than shorter-term therapies? Review and critique of the evidence. *Psychotherapy and Psychosomatics, 79*, 208–216.

Blatt, S. (1995). Why the gap between psychotherapy research and clinical practice: A response to Barry Wolfe. *Journal of Psychotherapy Integration, 5*, 73–76.

Bögels, S. M., Wijts, P., & Sallaerts, S. (2003, September). *Analytic psychotherapy versus cognitive-behavioral therapy for social phobia.* Paper presented at the European Association for Behavioural and Cognitive Therapies Congress, Prague, Czech Republic.

Bressi, C., Porcellana, M., Marinaccio, P. M., Nocito, E. P., & Magri, L. (2010). Short-term psychodynamic psychotherapy versus treatment as usual for depressive and anxiety disorders: A randomized clinical trial of efficacy. *Journal of Nervous and Mental Disease, 198*, 647–652.

Brom, D., Kleber, R. J., & Defares, P. B. (1989). Brief psychotherapy for posttraumatic stress disorders. *Journal of Consulting and Clinical Psychology, 57*, 607–612.

Bruch, H. (1973). *Eating disorders: Obesity, anorexia nervosa, and the person within.* New York: Basic Books.

Chambless, D. L., & Hollon, S. D. (1998). Defining empirically supported therapies. *Journal of Consulting and Clinical Psychology, 66*, 7–18.

Clarkin, J. F., Levy, K. N., Lenzenweger, M. F., & Kernberg, O. F. (2007). Evaluating three treatments for borderline personality disorder: A multiwave study. *American Journal of Psychiatry, 164*, 922–928.

Clarkin, J. F., Yeomans, F. E., & Kernberg, O. F. (1999). *Psychotherapy for borderline personality.* New York: Wiley.

Cohen, J. (1988). *Statistical power analysis for the behavioral sciences.* Hillsdale, NJ: Erlbaum.

Concato, J., Shah, N., & Horwitz, R. I. (2000). Randomized, controlled trials, observational studies, and the hierarchy of research designs. *New England Journal of Medicine, 342*, 1887–1892.

Creed, F., Fernandes, L., Guthrie, E., Palmer, S., Ratcliffe, J., Read, N., et al. (2003). The cost-effectiveness of psychotherapy and paroxetine for severe irritable bowel syndrome. *Gastroenterology, 124*, 303–317.

Crisp, A. H. (1980). *Anorexia nervosa: Let me be.* London: Academic Press.

Crits-Christoph, P., Connolly Gibbons, M. B., Narducci, J., Schamberger, M., & Gallop, R. (2005). Interpersonal problems and the outcome of interpersonally oriented psychodynamic treatment of GAD. *Psychotherapy: Theory, Research, Practice, Training, 42*, 211–224.

Crits-Christoph, P., Crits-Christoph, K., Wolf-Palacio, D., Fichter, M., & Rudick, D. (1995). Brief supportive-expressive dynamic psychotherapy for generalized anxiety disorder. In J. P. Barber & P. Crits-Christoph (Eds.), *Dynamic therapies for psychiatric disorders (Axis I)* (pp. 43–83). New York: Basic Books.

Crits-Christoph, P., Siqueland, L., Blaine, J., Frank, A., Luborsky, L., Onken, L. S., et al. (1999). Psychosocial treatments for cocaine dependence: National Institute on Drug Abuse Collaborative Cocaine Treatment Study. *Archives of General Psychiatry, 56*, 493–502.

Crits-Christoph, P., Siqueland, L., McCalmont, E., Weiss, R. D., Gastfriend, D. R., Frank, A., et al. (2001). Impact of psychosocial treatments on associated problems of cocaine-dependent patients. *Journal of Consulting and Clinical Psychology, 69*, 825–830.

Cuijpers, P., van Straten, A., Andersson, G., & van Oppen, P. (2008). Psychotherapy for depression in adults: A meta-analysis of comparative outcome studies. *Journal of Consulting and Clinical Psychology, 76*, 909–922.

Dare, C. (1995). Psychoanalytic psychotherapy (of eating disorders). In G. O. Gabbard (Ed.), *Treatment of psychiatric disorders* (pp. 2129–2151). Washington, DC: American Psychiatric Press.

Dare, C., Eisler, I., Russel, G., Treasure, J., & Dodge, L. (2001). Psychological therapies for adults with anorexia nervosa. Randomised controlled trial of out-patient treatments. *British Journal of Psychiatry, 178*, 216–221.

Davanloo, H. (1980). *Short-term dynamic psychotherapy.* New York: Jason Aronson.

Doering, S., Horz, S., Rentrop, M., Fischer-Kern, M., Schuster, P., Benecke, C., et al. (2010).

Transference-focused psychotherapy v. treatment by community psychotherapists for border-line personality disorder: Randomised controlled trial. *British Journal of Psychiatry, 196,* 389–395.

Driessen, E., Cuipers, P., deMaat, S. C. M., Abbass, A., deJonghe, F., & Dekker, J. J. M. (2010). The efficacy of short-term psychodynamic psychotherapy for depression. A meta-analysis. *Clinical Psychology Review, 30,* 25–36.

Ehlers, A., Bisson, J., Clark, D. M., Creamer, M., Pilling, S., Richards, D., et al. (2010). Do all psychological treatments really work the same in posttraumatic stress disorder? *Clinical Psychology Review, 30,* 269–276.

Emmelkamp, P. M. G., Benner, A., Kuipers, A., Feiertag, G. A., Koster, H. C., & van Apeldoorn, F. J. (2006). Comparison of brief dynamic and cognitive-behavioral therapies in avoidant personality disorder. *British Journal of Psychiatry, 189,* 60–64.

Fairburn, C. G. (2005). Evidence-based treatment of anorexia nervosa. *International Journal of Eating Disorders, 37*(Suppl.), 26–30.

Fairburn, C. G., Kirk, J., O'Connor, M., & Cooper, P. J. (1986). A comparison of two psychological treatments for bulimia nervosa. *Behaviour Research and Therapy, 24,* 629–643.

Fairburn, C. G., Norman, P. A., Welch, S. L., O'Connor, M. E., Doll, H. A., & Peveler, R. C. (1995). A prospective study of outcome in bulimia nervosa and the long-term effects of three psychological treatments. *Archives of General Psychiatry, 52,* 304–312.

Fonagy, P., Roth, A., & Higgitt, A. (2005). Psychodynamic therapies, evidence-based practice and clinical wisdom. *Bulletin of the Menninger Clinic, 69,* 1–58.

Foulkes, S. H. (1964). *Therapeutic group analysis.* London: Allen & Urwin.

Gabbard, G. O. (2004). *Long-term psychodynamic psychotherapy.* Washington, DC: American Psychiatric Publishing.

Gabbard, G. O., Gunderson, J. G., & Fonagy, P. (2002). The place of psychoanalytic treatments within psychiatry. *Archives of General Psychiatry, 59,* 505–510.

Gallagher-Thompson, D. E., Hanley-Peterson, P., & Thompson, L. W. (1990). Maintenance of gains versus relapse following brief psychotherapy for depression. *Journal of Consulting and Clinical Psychology, 58,* 371–374.

Gallagher-Thompson, D. E., & Steffen, A. M. (1994). Comparative effects of cognitive-behavioral and brief psychodynamic psychotherapies for depressed family caregivers. *Journal of Consulting and Clinical Psychology, 62,* 543–549.

Garner, D. M., Rockert, W., Davis, R., Garner, M. V., Olmsted, M. P., & Eagle, M. (1993). Comparison of cognitive-behavioral and supportive-expressive therapy for bulimia nervosa. *American Journal of Psychiatry, 150,* 37–46.

Geist, R. A. (1989). Self psychological reflections on the origins of eating disorders. *Journal of the American Academy of Psychoanalysis, 17,* 5–28.

Giesen-Bloo, J., van Dyck, R., Spinhoven, P., van Tilburg, W., Dirksen, C., van Asselt, T., et al. (2006). Outpatient psychotherapy for borderline personality disorder: Randomized trial of schema-focused therapy vs transference-focused psychotherapy. *Archives of General Psychiatry, 63,* 649–658.

Goodsitt, A. (1985). Self psychology and the treatment of anorexia nervosa. In D. M. Garner & P. E. Garfinkel (Eds.), *Handbook of psychotherapy for anorexia nervosa and bulimia* (pp. 55–82). New York: Guilford Press.

Gowers, D., Norton, K., Halek, C., & Vrisp, A. H. (1994). Outcome of outpatient psychotherapy in a random allocation treatment study of anorexia nervosa. *International Journal of Eating Disorders, 15,* 165–177.

Gregory, R. J., Chlebowski, S., Kang, D., Remen, A. L., Soderberg, M. G., Stepkovitch, J., et al. (2008). A controlled trial of psychodynamic psychotherapy for co-occurring borderline personality disorder and alcohol use disorder. *Psychotherapy: Theory, Research, Practice, Training, 45,* 28–41.

Gregory, R. J., & Remen, A. L. (2008). A manual-based psychodynamic therapy for treatment-resistant borderline personality disorder. *Psychotherapy: Theory, Research, Practice, Training, 45,* 14–26.

Gunderson, J. G., & Gabbard, G. O. (1999). Making the case for psychoanalytic therapies in the current psychiatric environment. *Journal of the American Psychoanalytic Association, 47*, 679–704.

Guthrie, E., Creed, F., Dawson, D., & Tomenson, B. (1991). A controlled trial of psychological treatment for the irritable bowel syndrome. *Gastroenetrology, 100*, 450–457.

Guyatt, G. H., Sacket, D. L., Sinclair, J. C., Hayward, R., Cook, D. J., & Cook, R. (1995). User's guides to the medical literature. IX. A method for grading health care recommendations. *Journal of the American Medical Association, 274*, 1800–1804.

Hamilton, J., Guthrie, E., Creed, F., Thompson, D., Tomenson, B., Bennett, R., et al. (2000). A randomized controlled trial of psychotherapy in patients with chronic functional dyspepsia. *Gastroenterology, 119*, 661–669.

Hardy, G., Barkham, M., Shapiro, D., Guthrie, E., & Margison, F. (Eds.). (2014). *Psychodynamic-interpersonal psychotherapy*. Thousand Oaks, CA: Sage.

Hellerstein, D. J., Rosenthal, R. N., Pinsker, H., Wallner Samstag, L., Muran, J. C., & Winston, A. (1998). A randomized prospective study comparing supportive and dynamic therapies. Outcome and alliance. *Journal of Psychotherapy Research and Practice, 7*, 261–271.

Henry, W. (1998). Science, politics, and the politics of science: The use and misuse of empirically validated treatment research. *Psychotherapy Research, 8*, 126–140.

Hobson, R. F. (1985). *Forms of feeling: The heart of psychotherapy*. London: Tavistock.

Horowitz, L. M., Alden, L. E., Wiggins, J. S., & Pincus, A. L. (2000). *Inventory of Interpersonal Problems: Manual*. Odessa, FL: Psychological Corporation.

Horowitz, M. (1976). *Stress response syndromes*. New York: Jason Aronson.

Horowitz, M., & Kaltreider, N. (1979). Brief therapy of the stress response syndrome. *Psychiatric Clinics of North America, 2*, 365–377.

Jacobson, N. S., & Truax, P. (1991). Clinical significance: A statistical approach to defining meaningful change in psychotherapy research. *Journal of Consulting and Clinical Psychology, 59*, 12–19.

Johansson, R., Ekbladh, S., Hebert, A., Lindstrom, M., Moller, S., Petitt, E., et al. (2012). Psychodynamic guided self-help for adult depression through the internet: A randomised controlled trial. *PLoS ONE, 7*, e38021.

Kernberg, O. F. (1984). *Severe personality disorders: Psychotherapeutic strategies*. New Haven, CT: Yale University Press.

Kernberg, O. F. (1996). A psychoanalytic model for the classification of personality disorders. In M. Achenheil, B. Bondy, R. Engel, M. Ermann, & N. Nedopil (Eds.), *Implications of psychopharmacology to psychiatry*. New York: Springer.

Knekt, P., Lindfors, O., Harkanen, T., Valikoski, M., Virtala, E., Laaksonen, M. A., et al. (2008). Randomized trial on the effectiveness of long-and short-term psychodynamic psychotherapy and solution-focused therapy on psychiatric symptoms during a 3-year follow-up. *Psychological Medicine, 38*, 689–703.

Knekt, P., Lindfors, O., Laaksonen, M. A., Raitasalo, R., Haaramo, P., Järvikoski, A., et al. (2008). Effectiveness of short-term and long-term psychotherapy on work ability and functional capacity: A randomized clinical trial on depressive and anxiety disorders. *Journal of Affective Disorders, 107*, 95–106.

Knijnik, D. Z., Kapczinski, F., Chachamovich, E., Margis, R., & Eizirik, C. L. (2004). Psychodynamic group treatment for generalized social phobia. *Revista Brasileira de Psiquiatria, 26*, 77–781.

Kopta, S. M., Howard, K. I., Lowry, J. L., & Beutler, L. E. (1994). Patterns of symptomatic recovery in psychotherapy. *Journal of Consulting and Clinical Psychology, 62*, 1009–1016.

Leichsenring, F. (2001). Comparative effects of short-term psychodynamic psychotherapy and cognitive-behavioral therapy in depression. A meta-analytic approach. *Clinical Psychology Review, 21*, 401–419.

Leichsenring, F. (2004). Randomized controlled vs. naturalistic studies. A new research agenda. *Bulletin of the Menninger Clinic, 68*, 115–129.

Leichsenring, F. (2005). Are psychoanalytic and psychodynamic psychotherapies effective? A review of empirical data. *International Journal of Psychoanalysis, 86*, 1–26.

Leichsenring, F., Beutel, M., & Leibing, E. (2007). Psychodynamic psychotherapy for social phobia: A treatment manual based on supportive-expressive therapy. *Bulletin of the Menninger Clinic, 71*, 56–83.

Leichsenring, F., & Leibing, E. (2003). The effectiveness of psychodynamic therapy and cognitive behavior therapy in the treatment of personality disorders: A meta-analysis. *American Journal of Psychiatry, 160*, 1223–1232.

Leichsenring, F., & Leibing, E. (2007). Cognitive–behavioural therapy for avoidant personality disorder. *British Journal of Psychiatry, 190*, 80.

Leichsenring, F., Leibing, E., Kruse, J., New, A. S., & Leweke, F. (2011). Borderline personality disorder. *Lancet, 377*, 74–84.

Leichsenring, F., & Rabung, S. (2008). The effectiveness of long-term psychodynamic psychotherapy: A meta-analysis. *Journal of the American Medical Association, 300*, 1551–1564.

Leichsenring, F., & Rabung, S. (2011a). Double standards in psychotherapy research. *Psychotherapy and Psychosomatics, 80*, 48–51.

Leichsenring, F., & Rabung, S. (2011b). Long-term psychodynamic psychotherapy in complex mental disorders: Update of a meta-analysis. *British Journal of Psychiatry, 199*, 15–22.

Leichsenring, F., Rabung, S., & Leibing, E. (2004). The efficacy of short-term psychodynamic therapy in specific psychiatric disorders: A meta-analysis. *Archives of General Psychiatry, 61*, 1208–1216.

Leichsenring, F., Salzer, S., Jager, U., Kächele, U., Kreische, R., Leweke, F., et al. (2009). Short-term psychodynamic psychotherapy and cognitive-behavioral therapy in generalized anxiety disorder: A randomized controlled trial. *American Journal of Psychiatry, 166*, 875–881.

Leichsenring, F., Salzer, S., Beutel, M. E., Herpertz, S., Hiller, W., Hoyer, J., et al. (2013). Psychodynamic therapy and cognitive-behavioral therapy in social anxiety disorder: A multicenter randomized controlled trial. *American Journal of Psychiatry, 170*, 759–767.

Linehan, M. M., Comtois, K. A., Murray, A. M., Brown, M. Z., Gallop, R. J., Heard, H. L., et al. (2006). Two-year randomized trial and follow-up of dialectical behavior therapy vs therapy by experts for suicidal behaviors and borderline personality disorder. *Archives of General Psychiatry, 63*, 757–766.

Linehan, M. M., Tutek, D. A., Heard, H. L., & Armstrong, H. E. (1994). Interpersonal outcome of cognitive behavioral treatment for chronically suicidal borderline patients. *American Journal of Psychiatry, 151*, 1771–1776.

Luborsky, L. (1984). *Principles of psychoanalytic psychotherapy. Manual for supportive-expressive treatment.* New York: Basic Books.

Luborsky, L., Diguer, L., Seligman, D. A., Rosenthal, R., Krause, E. D., Johnson, S., et al. (1999). The researcher's own allegiances: A "wild" card in comparison of treatment efficacy. *Clinical Psychology: Science and Practice, 6*, 95–106.

Luborsky, L., & Mark, D. (1991) Short term supportive-expressive psychoanalytic psychotherapy. In P. Crits-Christoph & J. P. Barber (Eds.), *Handbook of short-term dynamic psychotherapy* (pp. 110–136). New York: Basic Books.

Maina, G., Forner, F., & Bogetto, F. (2005). Randomized controlled trial comparing brief dynamic and supportive therapy with waiting list condition in minor depressive disorders. *Psychotherapy and Psychosomatics, 74*, 3–50.

Malan, D. H. (1976a). *The frontier of brief psychotherapy: An example of the convergence of research and clinical practice.* New York: Plenum Medical Book Company.

Malan, D. H. (1976b). *Toward the validation of dynamic psychotherapy: A replication.* New York: Plenum Medical Book Company.

Mann, J. (1973). *Time-limited psychotherapy.* Cambridge, MA: Harvard University Press.

Mark, D., & Luborsky, L. (1992). *A manual for the use of supportive-expressive psychotherapy in the treatment of cocaine abuse.* Philadelphia: Department of Psychiatry, University of Pennsylvania.

McCallum, M., & Piper, W. E. (1990). A controlled study of effectiveness and patient suitability for short-term group psychotherapy. *International Journal of Group Psychotherapy, 40,* 431–452.

McCullough Vaillant, L. (1997). *Changing character.* New York: Basic Books.

Milrod, B., Busch, F., Cooper, A., & Shapiro, T. (1997). *Manual of panic-focused psychodynamic psychotherapy.* Arlington, VA: American Psychiatric Publishing.

Milrod, B., Leon, A. C., Busch, F., Rudden, M., Schwalberg, M., Clarkin, J., et al. (2007). A randomized controlled clinical trial of psychoanalytic psychotherapy for panic disorder. *American Journal of Psychiatry, 164,* 265–272.

Monsen, J. T., & Monsen, K. (1999). Affects and affect consciousness: A psychotherapy model integrating Silvan Tomkins' affect and script theory within the framework of self-psychology. *Progress in Self-Psychology, 15,* 287–306.

Monsen, K., & Monsen, J. T. (2000). Chronic pain and psychodynamic body therapy. *Psychotherapy, 37,* 257–269.

Munroe-Blum, H., & Marziali, E. (1995). A controlled trial of short-term group treatment for borderline personality disorder. *Journal of Personality Disorders, 9,* 190–198.

Muran, J. C., Safran, J. D., Samstag, L. W., & Winston, A. (2005). Evaluating an alliance-focused treatment for personality disorders. *Psychotherapy: Theory, Research, Practice, Training, 42,* 532–545.

Perry, J. C., Banon, E., & Floriana, I. (1999). Effectiveness of psychotherapy for personality disorders. *American Journal of Psychiatry, 156,* 1312–1321.

Pinsker, H., Rosenthal, R., & McCullough, L. (1991). Dynamic supportive psychotherapy. In P. Crits-Christoph & J. P. Barber (Eds.), *Handbook of short-term dynamic psychotherapy* (pp. 220–247). New York: Basic Books.

Piper, W. E., McCallum, M., Joyce, A. S., & Ogrodniczuk, J. S. (2001). Patient personality and time-limited group psychotherapy for complicated grief. *International Journal of Group Psychotherapy, 51,* 525–552.

Pollack, J., Flegenheimer, W., Kaufman, J., & Sadow, J. (1992). *Brief adaptive psychotherapy for personality disorders: A treatment manual.* San Diego, CA: Social and Behavioral Documents.

Rose, J., & DelMaestro, S. (1990). Separation–individuation conflict as a model for understanding distressed caregivers: Psychodynamic and cognitive case studies. *The Gerontologist, 30,* 693–697.

Rosen, B. (1979). A method of structured brief psychotherapy. *British Journal of Medical Psychology, 52,* 157–162.

Roth, A. D., & Parry, G. (1997). The implications of psychotherapy research for clinical practice and service development: Lessons and limitations. *Journal of Mental Health, 6,* 367–380.

Rothwell, P. M. (2005). External validity of randomized controlled trials. To whom do the results of this trial apply? *Lancet, 365,* 82–92.

Salminen, J. K., Karlsson, H., Hietala, J., Kajander, J., Aalto, S., Markkula, J., et al. (2008). Short-term psychodynamic psychotherapy and fluoxetine in major depressive disorder: A randomized comparative study. *Psychotherapy and Psychosomatics, 77,* 351–357.

Sandahl, C., Herlitz, K., Ahlin, G., & Rönnberg, S. (1998). Time-limited group psychotherapy for moderately alcohol dependent patients: A randomized controlled clinical trial. *Psychotherapy Research, 8,* 361–378.

Sattel, H., Lahmann, C., Gundel, H., Guthrie, E., Kruse, J., Noll-Hussong, M., et al. (2012). Brief psychodynamic interpersonal psychotherapy for patients with multisomatoform disorder: Randomised controlled trial. *British Journal of Psychiatry, 200,* 60–67.

Seligman, M. E. P. (1995). The effectiveness of psychotherapy. The Consumer Reports study. *American Psychologist, 50,* 965–974.

Shadish, W. R., Cook, T. D., & Campbell, D. T. (2002). *Experimental and quasi-experimental designs for generalized causal inference.* Boston: Houghton Mifflin.

Shadish, W. R., Matt, G., Navarro, A., & Phillips, G. (2000). The effects of psychological therapies under clinically representative conditions: A meta-analysis. *Journal of Consulting and Clinical Psychology, 126*, 512–529.

Shapiro, D. A., Barkham, M., Rees, A., Hardy, G. E., Reynolds, S., & Startup, M. (1994). Effects of treatment duration and severity of depression on the effectiveness of cognitive-behavioral and psychodynamic-interpersonal psychotherapy. *Journal of Consulting and Clinical Psychology, 62*, 522–534.

Shapiro, D. A., & Firth, J. A. (1985). *Exploratory therapy manual for the Sheffield Psychotherapy Project (SAPU Memo 733)*. Sheffield, UK: University of Sheffield.

Shapiro, D. A., Rees, A., Barkham, M., & Hardy, G. E. (1995). Effects of treatment duration and severity of depression on the maintenance of gains after cognitive-behavioral and psychodynamic-interpersonal psychotherapy. *Journal of Consulting and Clinical Psychology, 63*, 378–387.

Sifneos, P. E. (1978). Short-term anxiety provoking psychotherapy. In H. Davanloo (Ed.), *Short-term dynamic psychotherapy* (pp. 35–42). New York: Spectrum.

Silverberg, F. (2005). *Make the leap: A practical guide to breaking the patterns that hold you back*. New York: Marlowe.

Stunkard, A. J. (1976). *The pain of obesity*. PaloAlto, CA: Bull Publishing.

Svartberg, M., Stiles, T., & Seltzer, M. (2004). Randomized, controlled trial of the effectiveness of short-term dynamic psychotherapy and cognitive therapy for Cluster C personality disorders. *American Journal of Psychiatry, 161*, 810–817.

Tasca, G. A., Mikail, S., & Hewitt, P. (2002). *Group psychodynamic interpersonal psychotherapy: A manual for time limited treatment of binge eating disorder*. Unpublished manuscript.

Tasca, G. A., Ritchie, K., Conrad, G., Balfour, L., Gayrton, J., Lybanon, V., et al. (2006). Attachment scales predict outcome in a randomized clinical trial of group psychotherapy for binge eating disorder: An aptitude by treatment interaction. *Psychotherapy Research, 16*, 106–121.

Thompson, L. W., Gallagher, D., & Breckenridge, J. S. (1987). Comparative effectiveness of psychotherapies for depressed elders. *Journal of Consulting and Clinical Psychology, 55*, 385–390.

Town, J. M., Abbass, A., & Hardy, G. (2011). Short-term psychodynamic psychotherapy for personality disorders: A critical review of randomized controlled trials. *Journal of Personality Disorders, 25*, 723–740.

Wallerstein, R. (1989). The psychotherapy research project of the Menninger Foundation: An overview. *Journal of Consulting and Clinical Psychology, 57*, 195–205.

Wallerstein, R. (1999). Comment on Gunderson and Gabbard. *Journal of the American Psychoanalytic Association, 47*, 728–734.

Wampold, B. E., Minami, T., Baskin, T. W., & Tierney, S. C. (2002). A meta-(re)analysis of the effects of cognitive therapy versus "other therapies" for depression. *Journal of Affective Disorders, 68*, 159–165.

Westen, D., Novotny, C. M., & Thompson-Brenner, H. (2004). The empirical status of empirically supported psychotherapies: Assumptions, findings, and reporting in controlled clinical trials. *Psychological Bulletin, 130*, 631–663.

Winston, A., Laikin, M., Pollack, J., Samstag, L. W., McCullough, L., & Muran, J. C. (1994). Short-term psychotherapy of personality disorders. *American Journal of Psychiatry, 151*, 190–194.

Woody, G. E., Luborsky, L., McLellan, A. T., & O'Brien, C. P. (1990). Corrections and revised analyses for psychotherapy in methadone maintenance patients. *Archives of General Psychiatry, 47*, 788–789.

Woody, G. E., Luborsky, L., McLellan, A. T., & O'Brien, C. P. (1995). Psychotherapy in community methadone programs: A validation study. *American Journal of Psychiatry, 152*, 1302–1308.

Woody, G. E., Luborsky, L., McLellan, A. T., O'Brien, C. P., Beck, A. T., Blaine, J., et al. (1983). Psychotherapy for opiate addicts: Does it help? *Archives of General Psychiatry, 40*, 639–645.

CHAPTER 24

Beyond Transference
FOSTERING GROWTH THROUGH THERAPEUTIC IMMEDIACY

Jared A. DeFife, Mark J. Hilsenroth, and Klara Kuutmann

The nature of transference in psychodynamic thinking and practice is somewhat unclear. On the one hand, transference manifestations and interpretations are seen by many to be central elements of the dynamic treatment process (e.g., Clarkin, Yeomans, & Kernberg, 2006; Davanloo, 1978; Malan, 1976; Sifneos, 1971; Yeomans, Clarkin, & Kernberg, 2002). On the other hand, it is hard to find consensus on exactly what transference is (Ehrenreich, 1989), what a transference interpretation actually sounds like, and when such interpretations are appropriate to foster adaptive change (Høglend & Gabbard, 2012). This is a sticky problem for the field, creating problems for implementing effective therapeutic technique, disseminating psychodynamic ideas, and passing on clinical and empirical wisdom to the next generation.

The traditional psychoanalytic attitude toward the empirical investigation of transference is reflected in the following statement by David Rapaport: "There is a temptation to mix up terms denoting empirical observations with those denoting theoretical constructs . . . transference and resistance are not empirical observations . . . they are concepts, which condense a set of dynamic variations of phenomena into a theoretical construction" (1967, p. 202). Unfortunately, some in the field still cling to this viewpoint. Hoffman (2009) recently wrote that "the carrying out and empowering of systematic quantitative research . . . is flawed epistemologically and . . . threatens to embody yet a new form of prescriptive, authoritarian objectivism" (p. 1045).

However, there is an inherent contradiction (perhaps even hypocrisy) in the belief that clinical phenomena such as transference can be observed, formulated, and responded to during a session, yet are somehow not amenable to quantitative observation and evaluation. If we are to follow such logic, being ultimately unable to observe, quantify, and label manifest cognitive, affective, behavioral, and relational processes in therapy, then it seems that the field of psychoanalysis is fated to be a Dark Ages zeitgeist passed over by an Enlightenment era of nondynamically informed empirical wisdom and evidence-based practice. Fortunately, the true outlook is not so bleak. Whether approaching the problem phenomenologically or quantitatively, the clinician and the researcher have similar roles to play in respect of transference: to observe it, classify it, and identify the most effective manner of working with it.

The aim of this chapter is threefold: to examine a clinical and research-informed conceptualization of the transference construct; to evaluate the extant research on the efficacy of transference interpretation use in psychodynamic therapy; and to review what psychotherapy research offers to inform the process component of in-session focus on the patient–therapist relationship. We hope to demonstrate that our contemporary conceptualization of the transference construct (highlighting relational/interactional elements of the ongoing therapeutic relationship) is widely divergent from how it was originally operationalized (where transference represents the patient's contemporary distortion of old neurotic conflicts, which must be identified and divorced from the person of the clinician), and to offer a revised, experience-near definition and terminology (exploration of in-session affective/relational processes). Furthermore, we seek to advance the view that research on the practice of highly interpretive techniques in dynamic therapy is not as promising as commonly believed, whereas process research on supportive attention to in-session relational interactions suggests an additionally effective road to therapeutic success.

TRANSFERENCE MISINTERPRETATION

One of the enduring dilemmas in talking about transference is whether to conceptualize transference phenomena as fantasized distortions of the therapeutic process or legitimately responsive evaluations of the interactive "here-and-now" relationship.

In their initial formulation of the transference phenomenon, Breuer and Freud (1895/1957) described transference as a "false connection" (p. 302) between patient and clinician. Freud's (1917/1963) continued position on the issue was quite clear: "We overcome the transference by pointing out to the patient that *his feelings do not arise from the present situation and do not apply to the person of the doctor*" (pp. 443–444; emphasis added). Freud observed transferences as haunting specters of the past that were "something analogous [to], but immeasurably more important" than the circumstances of the present (1905/1953, p. 109). This view held across decades. Greenson, for example, wrote that "transference reactions are always inappropriate" (1967, p. 52). Gelso, Hill, and Kivlighan (1991) concluded that a typical definition of transference "involves unconscious processes, implicates a number of internal states, requires the deployment of defense mechanisms, and is basically an error in perception" (p. 428). More recently, however, psychoanalytic authors have suggested that the transference concept should include more relational (and more conscious) aspects of the interaction between the therapist and client, which also take into account the contribution of the therapist (Cooper, 1987; Gabbard, 2005; Gill, 1984; Gill & Hoffman, 1982a, 1982b; Høglend & Gabbard, 2012).

Despite its complexity, researchers have attempted to operationalize the construct of transference from a variety of perspectives. Gelso, Hill, Mohr, Rochlen, and Zack (1999) distinguished two models of transference measurement: direct measurement (in which patient in-session reactions and emotions are assessed as explicitly *unrealistic* to the treatment situation) or indirect measurement (assessing patients' common relational patterns and affects as they arise in treatment, but without inferring the justification of such reactions).

The Missouri Identifying Transference Scale (MITS; Multon, Patton, & Kivlighan, 1996) is one such "direct" measure of transference. It asks therapists to rate adjectives describing their patients' *extreme and unrealistic* emotional or behavioral reactions. Initial validation of the MITS yielded factors of negative transference (e.g., annoyance, distrust, argumentativeness, withdrawal) and positive transference (e.g., dependence, clinging, infatuation, flirtatiousness). The authors found partial supporting evidence that the client's self-reported view of his or her mother (but not father) was significantly related to counselor-identified transference reactions. Specifically, a client viewing his or her mother as controlling, untrustworthy, cold, and distant was more likely to exhibit therapist-identified negative transference reactions. Conversely, but to a lesser degree, the more positively the mother was viewed, the more positive in-session transference reactions were noted. This finding was later replicated by Woodhouse, Schlosser, Crook, Ligiéro, and Gelso (2003), as therapists observed more negative transference reactions in clients who had perceived their maternal care as cold and rejecting.

Multon and colleagues' (1996) results also suggested some direct linkage between a client's in-session reactions and his or her negative perceptions of the counselor. When the client perceived his or her therapist to be more controlling and less sociable, the counselor observed more negative transference reactions in the client. Without the addition of independent observer ratings of the therapeutic process, it is difficult to formulate whether these negative transference reactions were based on the clients' *unrealistic misinterpretations* of the counselor or their *realistic* assessment of a counselor's interactional stance.

Overall ratings of negative transference were low, and only counselors' ratings of positive transference were significantly related to their perceptions of the overall "amount" of transference occurring in a session. If internal distortions of relational interactions (epitomized by the distortion of the patient–therapist relationship) are theorized to be at the core of problems bringing patients to treatment, one would reasonably expect that the bulk of transference reactions would be negative, particularly early in the therapeutic encounter. At the same time, this finding might possibly reflect a tendency of some therapists (particularly those in training) to attribute their patients' negative therapeutic reactions as justifiably warranted to the situation, whereas positive emotional reactions to the therapist are attributed to distorted transference manifestations (e.g., McWilliams, 1994).

Similarly, a number of authors have used Graff and Luborsky's (1977) single-item measurements of positive, negative, and amount of transference as observed by therapist raters. These ratings exhibit modest psychometric qualities, converging with Multon and colleagues' positive and negative transference scales, correlating significantly between raters ($r = .67$, Kivlighan, 1995) and showing temporal stability across early psychotherapy sessions (alpha = .66–.86; Gelso, Kivlighan, Wine, Jones, & Friedman, 1997). However, one study failed to find evidence supporting the hypothesis that single-item transference ratings would be associated with patients' perceptions of their parents' empathy, regard, and unconditionality (Arachtingi & Lichtenberg, 1998). Furthermore, findings related to the course of transference scores across treatment are inconsistent, with studies suggesting that transference increases throughout successful psychoanalytic work (Graff & Luborsky, 1977; Patton & Kivlighan, 1997) but diminishes in the latter part of successful nonanalytic or theoretically heterogeneous treatment (Gelso et al., 1997). Finally, despite the fact that these transference measurement instruments are explicitly designed to assess *unrealistic* and *extreme* relational reactions, they do not evidence consistently significant inverse relationships with client and therapist ratings of genuineness and realism in the therapeutic relationship (Gelso, 2002; Marmarosh et al., 2009).

To date, there is little empirical evidence to support the assertion that transference manifestations reflect a highly unrealistic perspective of the therapeutic relationship seen through a glass, darkly. This is not to say, however, that patients enter psychotherapy as a relational tabula rasa. Individuals do exhibit characteristic patterns of thinking and relating with others, which are observable and stable across relational contexts, including psychotherapy. Luborsky (1977; Luborsky & Crits-Christoph, 1998) classified these relational templates as Core Conflictual Relationship Themes (CCRTs), composed of three elements: interpersonal wishes, real or fantasized responses of others, and responses of self. The CCRT scales show internal consistency and can be reliably scored (Barber, Foltz, & Weinryb, 1998; Crits-Christoph, Cooper, & Luborsky, 1988) by independent raters. Patients' common CCRT patterns with significant others in their lives are to some degree related to similar interaction components that emerge with the therapist across psychotherapy interactions (Barber, Foltz, DeRubeis, & Landis, 2002; Connolly et al., 1996). On the other hand, some evidence suggests that patients have more satisfying interactions with their therapists than in their other relationships. In a small sample of pedophile sexual abusers, Drapeau (2006) reported clear differences in relational responses between the abusers and their parents compared with relational interactions with their therapists. Whereas parents reacted to the patient's desire for closeness with rejection, distance, or domination, therapists responded to this same wish by being helpful. These "corrective emotional experiences" with the therapist resulted in these patients feeling greater degrees of self-control and self-confidence.

Bradley, Heim, and Westen (2005) set out to quantify and categorize the structure of patients' interactions specifically rooted in the patient–therapist relationship. Therapist ratings of their Psychotherapy Relationship Questionnaire (Bradley et al., 2005) yielded a five-factor structure encompassing cognitive, affective, and behavioral patterns and dynamics occurring across a range of therapeutic orientations and technical intervention strategies. The first factor, labeled *angry/entitled*, captured interactions characterized by a patient making excessive demands of the therapist while simultaneously being angry and dismissive. Angry/entitled patterns were characteristic of the psychotherapy hours spent treating patients with cluster

B personality disorders, particularly narcissistic and borderline personality disorders. A second factor, *anxious/preoccupied*, was marked by the patient's fears of the therapist's disapproval and rejection, and consequent dependent behaviors such as overcompliance or excessive reassurance-seeking. A *secure/engaged* factor reflected positive working alliance experiences in which patients talked openly and reflectively about the therapeutic relationship and about difficult material, and felt fond of, helped by, and nurtured by the therapist. Other transference pattern factors were marked by *avoidance/counterdependence* behaviors or *sexualization* of the therapeutic relationship.

One might say that our thinking about transference has undergone a radical change since (or perhaps distortion of) its early historical manifestations. A contemporary, empirically informed conceptualization of transference phenomena supports the view of the therapeutic relationship as a unique and novel relational experience, influenced by personality styles rooted in developmental history but not fermented in the distorted bonds of past reminiscences. While the relational patterns enacted during psychotherapy may not always be consciously articulated or attended to, the studies we have discussed illustrate that such interactions can be reliably operationalized and assessed through careful observation.

"IS THAT A TRANSFERENCE REACTION, OR ARE YOU JUST HAPPY TO SEE ME?"

Reconceptualizing transference as a patterned response to the experience of the present versus a misperceived manifestation of the past involves a fundamental reexamination of the role and effectiveness of "transference-based" technique. Some suggest that insight gained through the therapist's interpretation of transference may be particularly valuable in that it facilitates integration of cognition and affect more effectively, while a focus exclusively on relationships outside of therapy may invite more intellectual speculation (Kernberg et al., 2008; Messer & McWilliams, 2007; Strachey, 1934/1999). In recent years, psychotherapy researchers have attempted to isolate and examine the impact of transference interpretation as a therapeutic technique.

To do this, researchers must agree first on what types of therapist statements constitute a transference interpretation and then on how to reliably quantify them. Because a therapeutic interpretation can be conceptualized as the explicit linking of implicit patterns and because transference manifests itself through the intersection of internal states and external experiences, three main transference interpretation "routes" are possible. Interpretations can be made establishing links to past figures (genetic interpretations), current relationships outside of psychotherapy (extratransference interpretations), and/or the patient–therapist interaction (transference interpretation) (Høglend & Gabbard, 2012; Malan, 1979; McCullough et al., 2003). In 1999, Bøgwald, Høglend, and Sørbye (1999) first reported on the Specific Therapeutic Technique scale (STT; Høglend, 1994), a brief and efficient psychotherapy process scale for measuring the frequency of therapist interventions that address the patient–therapist interaction and transference phenomena. Only one aspect of the STT scale relates to genetic transference interpretations as traditionally understood (i.e., "therapist attempts to explore interpersonal repetitive patterns with important others and/or parents and link these patterns to transactions between the patient and therapist"). The remaining elements focus more exclusively on the patient–therapist relationship (e.g., "therapist addresses transactions in the patient therapist relationship," "therapist actively encourages the patient to explore thoughts and feelings about the therapist, therapy, and/or the patient therapist relationship," and "therapist encourages the patient to discuss how the therapist might feel or think about the patient").

The conventional clinical wisdom has been that patients with greater psychological resources and more mature relationships will benefit from the depth and complexity of transference interpretation (Gabbard, 2006; Sifneos, 1992). Several studies, however, have demonstrated that the interactions among patient quality of object relations (QOR), exploration of the treatment relationship (under the purview of transference interpretations as measured by the STT), and outcome are mixed and difficult to interpret.

For instance, some studies have demonstrated that a greater number of transference interpretations have led to negative outcome effects for high-QOR patients (Høglend, 1993, 2004; Piper et al., 1991), whereas some studies have found positive effects for high-QOR patients (Connolly et al., 1999; Ogrodniczuk, Piper, Joyce, & McCallum, 1999). In an experimental study, high-QOR patients benefited equally from treatments with and without transference interpretations, whereas patients with low QOR were found to benefit more from treatment including transference interpretations, an effect that was sustained during long-term follow-up (Høglend et al., 2006, 2008; Høglend, Johansson, Marble, Bøgwald, & Amlo, 2007). These authors have suggested that this discrepancy results from differences in the frequency of transference interpretations utilized, with the former studies having high levels per session (i.e., five to six) whereas later studies utilized low to moderate levels per session (i.e., one to four; Høglend, 2004; Piper, Ogrodniczuk, & Joyce, 2004).

A recent large-scale dismantling clinical trial examined links between transference interpretations, insight, and outcome in psychodynamic therapy (Johansson et al., 2010), with transference interpretation defined as "an interpretation with explicit linking to the patient–therapist interaction" (p. 439). The effect of transference interpretation on insight during treatment for the average (typical) high QOR patient was almost zero and nonsignificant. Yet, the authors found between-group differences, leading to a conclusion that "patients with a life-long pattern of low quality of object relations and personality disorder pathology profited more from therapy with transference interpretation than from therapy with no transference interpretation" (p. 438). Within the low QOR transference group, however, there was a large negative correlation between the level of transference interpretations used in-session and subsequent outcome ($r = -0.56$, $p = .003$). These findings further reinforce the position that while transference interpretations may be useful in a subset of patients, they should be selectively utilized and limited in frequency.

As prior empirical studies have traditionally examined the frequency and not necessarily the competence in delivery of transference interpretations, the mixed results described above may suggest that treatments containing higher degrees of transference interpretation could reflect therapists' attempts to force interpretive elements or inaccurate conceptualizations that simply do not fit the situation. Therapeutic wrong turns, miscues, and case corrections are an inevitable part of treatment, but interpretive work raises a unique hazard: patients who rightfully reject or dismiss inaccurate interpretations may be viewed as "resistant" or "defensive," leading some therapists to amplify their interpretive stance. According to Høglend and Gabbard (2012), "it seems fair to conclude that clinicians should be aware that a high dosage level of transference interpretations (on average four–six or more per session) does not seem to overcome patient resistance and defensiveness and may in fact contribute to a negative therapeutic process" (p. 454). These results are also consistent with emerging data that suggest that an in-session focus on the therapeutic relationship is most effective when the alliance has been found to be high (Ryum, Stiles, Svartberg, & McCullough, 2010; Schut et al., 2005).

Transference-focused psychotherapy (TFP) is a treatment modality centrally focused on the use of transference attendance and interpretation as the lever of therapeutic change. Designed for patients with significant personality pathology, TFP focuses on the reduction of symptomatology and self-destructive behavior through modifying representations of self and others as they are enacted in the treatment (Clarkin, Yeomans, & Kernberg, 1999; Clarkin et al., 2006). This highly interpretive form of psychodynamic therapy is hypothesized to be more efficacious in patients with low QOR than other, more supportive approaches. However, in a randomized controlled trial, supportive dynamic psychotherapy was equally as efficacious as TFP and dialectical behavioral therapy on the study's primary (i.e., global psychopathology, depression, anxiety, social adjustment) and secondary (impulsivity and anger) outcome variables (Clarkin, Levy, Lenzenweger, & Kernberg, 2007). The lack of significant differences in outcome with TFP and DBT was observed despite the fact that supportive psychodynamic therapy occurred only once a week, whereas TFP and DBT sessions occurred twice weekly (TFP had two individual sessions, and DBT had one individual and one group session). These are far from inconsequential procedural differences, as prior research has demonstrated that twice-weekly sessions produce significant effects over single sessions, both in general treatment and within psychodynamic approaches (Freedman, Hoffenberg, Vorus, & Frosch, 1999; Leichsenring & Rabung, 2008).

As reviewed above, evidence supporting the effectiveness of transference interpretations is variable dependent on patient characteristics. On the other hand, supportive forms of dynamic therapy or dynamic therapies that integrate both supportive and interpretive (i.e., expressive) components have been found to be as highly effective and efficacious in comparison with more interpretive forms of dynamic treatment (e.g., de Maat, de Jonghe, Schoevers, & Dekker, 2009; Piper, Joyce, McCallum, & Azim, 1998; Stevenson, Meares, & D'Angelo, 2005) (even for patients with borderline personality disorder; Bateman & Fonagy, 2004; Hilsenroth & Slavin, 2008; McMain et al., 2009). Like Gabbard and Horowitz (2009), we believe that a singular interpretive treatment focus and prohibition of supportive techniques represents a false dichotomy of practice that appears inconsistent with the available data on the optimal use of techniques exploring the patient–therapist relationship. Consistent with the findings reviewed here, an optimal approach to interpretive work seems to exist at a low to moderate number (one to four) of interventions per session examining the patient–therapist relationship, and in the context of a strong therapeutic alliance (see Kuutmann & Hilsenroth, 2012; Ryum et al., 2010; Schut et al., 2005).

As the therapeutic relationship is often experienced as an intimate, emotionally charged, asymmetrical, and typically nurturant relationship, psychotherapy is likely to activate many attachment-related patterns of thought, feeling, and conflict (Fonagy et al., 1996; Seligman & Csikszentmihalyi, 2000). As opposed to viewing the treatment situation as an interpretive stimulus field to be deconstructed, the therapeutic relationship instead offers an active experimental arena in which in vivo examination of patient–therapist relational experiences provides insight into some of the patient's familiar patterns in close interpersonal relationships. By extension, it presents a unique relational training ground to brainstorm and attempt new models of thinking and relating, which may generalize to lasting personal changes (e.g., Blatt, 1990; Safran & Muran, 2000b).

EMBRACING THE ELEPHANT IN THE ROOM: THERAPEUTIC IMMEDIACY AND IN-SESSION RELATIONAL PROCESSING

A focus on in-session patient–therapist interaction is a central component of psychodynamic therapy (Blagys & Hilsenroth, 2000; Hilsenroth, Blagys, Ackerman, Bonge, & Blais, 2006). The focus on the therapeutic relationship becomes increasingly important during times of conflict in the relationship, known as treatment ruptures, and identifying and disseminating strategies for solving treatment ruptures is important for improving effectiveness in psychotherapy (Hill et al., 2008; Muran et al., 2009). For instance, Rhodes, Hill, Thompson, and Elliott (1994) found that focus on the therapeutic relationship, attentiveness to patients' negative experiences, and willingness to discuss clients' feelings of being misunderstood were important factors in the resolution of patient–therapist ruptures and continuation of therapy. Safran, Muran, and colleagues have also presented group research that provides some support for advocating a focus on the therapeutic relationship as being effective in rupture resolution (Muran et al., 2009; Safran, Muran, Samstag, & Winston, 2005). Another recent study found that a greater focus on the therapeutic relationship was significantly related to patients' indirect rupture markers and to patient collaborative processes (Colli & Lingiardi, 2009). Other treatment research examining an explicit focus on the therapeutic relationship has also shown positive outcomes (Bennett, Parry, & Ryle, 2006; Constantino et al., 2008).

To overcome the definitional ambiguity of these perspectives, Hill (2004) makes a distinction between transference interpretations and what she refers to as *therapist immediacy* ("disclosure within the therapy session of how the therapist is feeling about the client, him- or herself in relation to the client, or about the therapeutic relationship"). Recently, in order to capture the more interactive and dyadic nature of the therapeutic relationship this definition has been broadened to also reflect any client-initiated disclosures of feelings about the therapist or the client–therapist relationship, and the revised term of *therapeutic immediacy* has been suggested (Kuutmann & Hilsenroth, 2012). Thus, therapeutic immediacy involves any discussion within the therapy session about the relationship between therapist and patient that occurs in the here-and-now, as well as processing what occurs in the here-and-now client–therapist relationship. Typical examples of therapeutic immediacy include: exploring parallels between external relationships and the therapeutic relationship; client or therapist expressing in-session emotional reactions; inquiring about the client's reactions to therapy; the therapist commenting on his or her experience of the patient; supporting, affirming, and validating the client's feelings in the therapeutic relationship; and expressing gratitude. The use of therapeutic immediacy to resolve conflicts in the therapeutic relationship can then act as a template for interpersonal functioning in the client's outside relationships. Thus, therapeutic immediacy seeks to create a corrective emotional experience for the patient by a focus on here-and-now awareness, whereas transference interpretations are used to help the patient discover and understand the origin of the displaced interactional patterns enacted during the session. Therefore, the ultimate endpoint of transference–interpretation interventions is focused on previous relationships.

In a recent study exploring therapeutic immediacy across the treatment process, Kuutmann and Hilsenroth (2012) found that higher levels of pretreatment personality pathology and interpersonal problems were positively correlated to a greater focus on the patient–therapist relationship early in treatment. This was especially true for patients with a cold/distant interpersonal style and low self-esteem. Moreover, these two patient pretreatment characteristics demonstrated a significant change over the course of therapy. These posttreatment changes also demonstrated a significant relationship with greater early treatment focus on the patient–therapist relationship. In addition, the results from this study found an interaction effect between QOR (i.e., higher levels of object relations) and greater early treatment focus on the patient–therapist relationship with subsequent changes in patients' cold/distant interpersonal problems. In contrast to these significant effects, surprisingly, a greater in-session focus on the therapeutic relationship was not significantly related to patient ratings of session process (i.e., alliance and session experience).

The focus on the therapeutic relationship variable used in the study was much broader than the specific focus on transference interpretations and encompassed any in-session discussion of the patient–therapist interaction, any observations, clarifications, explorations, or questions about the therapeutic relationship, regardless of whether these were interpretive. Genetic transference interpretations as classically understood (i.e., an explicit link between a historic caretaker and the therapist) occurred very rarely in the study. Given the paucity of explicit, clinically verbatim examples in the area of transference interpretation, we wanted to provide relevant applied examples of specific interventions that therapists might make that are examples of therapeutic immediacy. For instance, while therapists would often interpret or explore how interpersonal and affective themes covered during a session might play out in the therapeutic relationship (e.g., "You know we've talked a lot about the issue of _____ today, and I wonder how that might play out in here between the two of us?"; "How do you understand that issue in regard to our relationship?"), they would also frequently encourage perspective-taking in this relationship and about the therapy, as observed in a mentalizing therapeutic stance (Allen, Fonagy, & Bateman, 2008), (e.g., "How do you imagine I feel after hearing your story?"; "What do you imagine I might be thinking about you?"; "That certainly makes sense, but I wonder if there could be any other reason why I might do that other than just being upset with you?"; "I wonder if you can imagine any other way I might feel?"). Also importantly, clinicians in the study viewed the therapeutic relationship as an arena where more adaptive relating was first practiced and explored, rather than just a place to repeat prior behavior. Therefore, adaptive relational changes, no matter how small, were underlined and supported (e.g., "I think it's important to point out that you were just able to express this issue in here with me; what do you think helps to do that in here as opposed to your other relationships?"; "What do you think has changed the most in our relationship that allows you to say that to me now as opposed to in the past?"). Likewise, clinicians affirmed, validated, and supported patients' involvement or experience in the therapeutic relationship (e.g., "Given your history it only seems reasonable that you'd be cautious in allowing yourself to become emotionally open with me, a man"; "Recognizing the reasons for that caution, I feel privileged you're sharing those feelings with me now").

Furthermore, clinicians in the study, who were working from a short-term dynamic therapy framework, would often sustain focus on the therapeutic relationship with follow-up inquiry of patients' experience of the in-session process (e.g., "What's it like to share that out loud, in here with me?"; "What's it like to hear me say that?"; "How does it feel to tell me about having accomplished this?"). This exploration of in-session affective experience about the therapeutic relationship also extended to the clinicians (e.g., "As I listen to the story you just told me I also feel a deep sense of hopelessness and despair."), as well as observing the "emotional temperature" in the therapeutic space (e.g., "It seems like something has changed in the room the last minutes between us. Things have become more quiet and it feels like we are more distant from each other than we were earlier."; "As you were speaking about that, it seems like the room has filled with joy and excitement."). Such interventions sharing the in-session affective experience of clinicians have been described as "self-involving" statements and very often lead to further exploration of the therapeutic relationship (McCarthy, 1982; Reynolds & Fischer, 1983; Teyber & McClure, 2000). Similarly, therapists helped patients to recognize and explore emotional experiences in the relationship that might have been avoided or gone unrecognized (e.g., "You seemed to become tearful just now when I noticed the positive things you've accomplished, can we try to understand that more together?"; "It seems right now that it's easier to describe others' feelings for you than the way I might feel for you?"). In sum, the whole range of interventions under the purview of in-session therapeutic interactions is used to help create an adaptive, observing, affectively engaged relational interaction that might provide a template for patients to apply to other relationships in their lives.

We would also note the consistency between several of the interventions described above and the provision of an actively supportive milieu, as well as the rupture-and-repair model of Safran and Muran (2000a), with attachment-theory-based strategies for decreasing psychological/emotional distance from others. These distance-decreasing attachment strategies include (1) acknowledging or considering the other's message, (2) showing an intention or willingness to share information with the other, (3) perceiving similarity or shared experience with the other, and (4) expressing positive feeling and support for the other (Hess, 2002).

Therefore, the need for more adaptive (i.e., corrective) relational experiences with the therapist may be particularly true for patients with a cold/distant relational style. In sum, consistent with the work of Hess (2002), Hill (2004), Wachtel (1993, 2008), McCullough and colleagues (2003), as well as Safran and Muran (2000a), we would suggest that perhaps the most curative aspect of "here-and-now" in-session processing of the therapeutic relationship, rather than links to archaic or genetic associations, is the opportunity for an examined "in vivo" emotional-relational interaction that can provide a much-needed template for more adaptive attachment strategies and interpersonal functioning.

CONCLUSIONS AND FUTURE DIRECTIONS

Our contemporary understanding of and approach to working with the transference construct has significantly evolved from its roots in psychoanalytic theory. An empirically informed approach has moved away from the conceptualization of "transference reactions" as distortions of old neurotic conflicts that must be identified, divorced from the person of the clinician, and exorcised from the therapeutic encounter. Instead, the patient–therapist interactions that occur during the course of treatment are seen to be rooted in the experiential present and accessible to (even if not always attended by) conscious experience. We would suggest that the time has come to jettison the outdated and variably defined meta-psychological term *transference* in favor of more contemporary articulations of relational schemas and internal working models. As such, we would offer the term *therapeutic immediacy* as a more experience-near alternative to many current clinical uses of the construct "transference" in the psychodynamic lexicon. In effect, this may allow psychodynamic researchers and clinicians to communicate more accurately and effectively across disciplines.

Based on the evidence reviewed above, transference interpretations are most likely not the only or even the primary mechanism of change in psychodynamic psychotherapy. The effectiveness of transference interpretation as a therapeutic technique is not yet well established and appears to be variable based on various patient characteristics such as QOR or insight and the context of the therapeutic relationship (i.e., therapeutic alliance). However, the integration of supportive-expressive interventions used within dynamic treatments appears to be helpful in a variety of therapeutic situations.

In contrast to traditional transference interpretations, therapists might seek to make *therapeutically immediate interventions* one to four times during a session when relevant and within an optimally responsive context (Stiles, Agnew-Davies, Hardy, Barkham, & Shapiro, 1998). These therapeutic immediacy interventions can be reliably classified into the following categories: (1) exploring how interpersonal and affective themes covered during a session might be expressed or occur in the therapeutic relationship, (2) addressing a rupture event, (3) asking the patient to take the perspective of the therapist (thoughts or feelings), (4) expressing an immediate affect or association to the relationship with the patient in a self-involving manner, (5) asking the patient to reflect on/process what is happening in the immediate therapeutic interaction or feeling in the room, (6) exploring emotional experiences in the relationship that might have been avoided or gone unrecognized, (7) recognizing adaptive changes in functioning that occur in relation to the therapist or therapeutic relationship, (8) validating and supporting the patient's involvement or experience in the therapeutic relationship, and (9) processing the termination of the therapeutic relationship.

Combined with a supportive and attentive approach, the collaborative exploration of patient–therapist relational experiences tills fertile ground for therapeutic insight and relational growth. Such relational investigations (occurring within the context of a supportive relational milieu) may shed light on a patient's characteristic attachment patterns and methods of interpersonal relatedness. Furthermore, the therapeutic encounter provides a protected testing ground for experimenting with new ways of thinking, feeling, and relating. Focusing on the in-session affective and relational experiences that emerge in the patient–therapist interaction is an attempt to foster therapeutic depth, working toward the development and maintenance of a collaborative, observing, affectively engaged relationship that might serve as a template for new adaptive relational experiences in a patient's life.

REFERENCES

Allen, J. G., Fonagy, P., & Bateman, A. W. (2008). *Mentalizing in clinical practice.* Washington, DC: American Psychiatric Publishing.

Arachtingi, B. M., & Lichtenberg, J. W. (1998). The relationship between clients' perceptions of therapist–parent similarity with respect to empathy, regard, and unconditionality and therapists' rating of client transference. *Journal of Counseling Psychology, 45,* 143–149.

Barber, J. P., Foltz, C., DeRubeis, R. J., & Landis, J. R. (2002). Consistency in interpersonal themes in narratives about relationships. *Psychotherapy Research, 12,* 139–159.

Barber, J. P., Foltz, C., & Weinryb, R. M. (1998). The central relationship questionnaire: Initial report. *Journal of Counseling Psychology, 45,* 131–142.

Bateman, A., & Fonagy, P. (2004). *Psychotherapy for borderline personality disorder: Mentalization-based treatment.* Oxford, UK: Oxford University Press.

Bennett, D., Parry, G., & Ryle, A. (2006). Resolving threats to the therapeutic alliance in cognitive analytic therapy of borderline personality disorder: A task analysis. *Psychology and Psychotherapy: Theory, Research and Practice, 79,* 395–418.

Beretta, V., Despland, J. N., Drapeau, M., Michel, L., Kramer, U., Stigler, M., et al. (2007). Are relationship patterns with significant others reenacted with the therapist?: A study of early transference reactions. *Journal of Nervous and Mental Disease, 195,* 443.

Blagys, M. D., & Hilsenroth, M. J. (2000). Distinctive features of short term psychodynamic interpersonal psychotherapy: A review of the comparative psychotherapy process literature. *Clinical Psychology: Science and Practice, 7,* 167–188.

Blatt, S. J. (1990). Interpersonal relatedness and self-definition: Two personality configurations and their implications for psychopathology and psychotherapy. In J. L. Singer (Ed.), *Repression and dissociation: Implications for personality theory, psychopathology and health* (pp. 299–335). Chicago: University of Chicago Press.

Bøgwald, K. P., Høglend, P., & Sorbye, O. (1999). Measurement of transference interpretations. *Journal of Psychotherapy Practice and Research, 8,* 264–273.

Bradley, R., Heim, A., & Westen, D. (2005). Transference patterns in the psychotherapy of personality disorders: An empirical investigation. *British Journal of Psychiatry, 186,* 342–349.

Breuer, J., & Freud, S. (1957). *Studies on hysteria.* New York: Basic Books. (Original work published 1895)

Clarkin, J. F., Levy, K. N., Lenzenweger, M. F., & Kernberg, O. F. (2007). Evaluating three treatments for borderline personality disorder: A multiwave study. *American Journal of Psychiatry, 164,* 922–928.

Clarkin, J. F., Yeomans, F. E., & Kernberg, O. F. (1999). *Psychotherapy for borderline personality.* New York: Wiley.

Clarkin, J. F., Yeomans, F. E., & Kernberg, O. F. (2006). *Psychotherapy for borderline personality: Focusing on object relations.* Washington, DC: American Psychiatric Publishing.

Colli, A., & Lingiardi, V. (2009). The Collaborative Interactions Scale: A new transcript-based method for the assessment of therapeutic alliance ruptures and resolutions in psychotherapy. *Psychotherapy Research, 19,* 718–734.

Connolly, M., Crits-Christoph, P., Shappell, S., Barber, J., Luborsky, L., & Shaffer, C. (1999). Relation of transference interpretations to outcome in the early sessions of brief supportive-expressive psychotherapy. *Psychotherapy Research, 9,* 485–495.

Connolly, M. B., Crits-Christoph, P., Demorest, A., Azarian, K., Muenz, L., & Chittams, J. (1996). Varieties of transference patterns in psychotherapy. *Journal of Consulting and Clinical Psychology, 64,* 1213–1221.

Constantino, M. J., Marnell, M., Haile, A. J., Kanther-Sista, S. N., Wolman, K., Zappert, L., et al. (2008). Integrative cognitive therapy for depression: A randomized pilot comparison. *Psychotherapy, 45,* 122–134.

Cooper, A. M. (1987). Changes in psychoanalytic ideas: Transference interpretation. *Journal of the American Psychoanalytic Association, 35,* 77–98.

Crits-Christoph, P., Cooper, A., & Luborsky, L. (1988). The accuracy of therapists' interpretations and the outcome of dynamic psychotherapy. *Journal of Consulting and Clinical Psychology, 56,* 490–495.

Davanloo, H. (1978). *Basic principles and techniques in short-term dynamic psychotherapy.* New York: Jason Aronson.

de Maat, S., de Jonghe, F., Schoevers, R., & Dekker, J. (2009). The effectiveness of long-term psychoanalytic therapy: A systematic review of empirical studies. *Harvard Review of Psychiatry, 17,* 1–23.

Drapeau, M. (2006). Repetition or reparation?: An exploratory study of the relationship schemas of child molesters in treatment. *Journal of Interpersonal Violence, 21,* 1224–1233.

Ehrenreich, J. H. (1989). Transference: One concept or many? *Psychoanalytic Review, 76,* 37–65.

Fonagy, P., Leigh, T., Steele, M., Steele, H., Kennedy, R., Mattoon, G., et al. (1996). The relation of attachment status, psychiatric classification, and response to psychotherapy. *Journal of Consulting and Clinical Psychology, 64,* 22–31.

Freedman, N., Hoffenberg, J. D., Vorus, N., & Frosch, A. (1999). The effectiveness of psychoanalytic psychotherapy: The role of treatment duration, frequency of sessions, and the therapeutic relationship. *Journal of the American Psychoanalytic Association, 47,* 741.

Freud, S. (1953). Dora: Fragments of an analysis of a case of hysteria. In J. Strachey (Ed. &

Trans.), *The standard edition of the complete psychological works of Sigmund Freud* (Vol. 7, pp. 1–122). London: Hogarth Press. (Original work published 1905)

Freud, S. (1963). Introductory lectures on psycho-analysis: Part III. General theory of the neuroses. In J. Strachey (Ed. & Trans.), *The standard edition of the complete psychological works of Sigmund Freud* (Vol. 16, pp. 241–463). London: Hogarth Press/Institute of Psycho-Analysis. (Original work published 1917)

Gabbard, G. O. (2005). *Psychodynamic psychiatry in clinical practice.* Washington, DC: American Psychiatric Publishing.

Gabbard, G. O. (2006). When is transference work useful in dynamic psychotherapy? *American Journal of Psychiatry, 163,* 1667–1669.

Gabbard, G. O., & Horowitz, M. J. (2009). Insight, transference interpretation, and therapeutic change in the dynamic psychotherapy of borderline personality disorder. *American Journal of Psychiatry, 166,* 517–521.

Gelso, C. J. (2002). Real relationship: The "something more" of psychotherapy. *Journal of Contemporary Psychotherapy, 32,* 35–40.

Gelso, C. J., Hill, C. E., & Kivlighan, D. M., Jr. (1991). Transference, insight, and the counselor's intentions during a counseling hour. *Journal of Counseling and Development, 69,* 428.

Gelso, C. J., Hill, C. E., Mohr, J. J., Rochlen, A. B., & Zack, J. (1999). Describing the face of transference: Psychodynamic therapists' recollections about transference in cases of successful long-term therapy. *Journal of Counseling Psychology, 46,* 257–267.

Gelso, C. J., Kivlighan, D. M., Wine, B., Jones, A., & Friedman, S. C. (1997). Transference, insight, and the course of time-limited therapy. *Journal of Counseling Psychology, 44,* 209–217.

Gill, M. M. (1984). Psychoanalysis and psychotherapy: A revision. *International Review of Psychoanalysis, 11,* 161–179.

Gill, M. M., & Hoffman, I. Z. (1982a). *Analysis of transference: Theory and technique.* New York: International Universities Press.

Gill, M. M., & Hoffman, I. Z. (1982b). A method for studying the analysis of aspects of the patient's experience of the relationship in psychoanalysis and psychotherapy. *Journal of the American Psychoanalytic Association, 30,* 137–167.

Graff, H., & Luborsky, L. (1977). Long-term trends in transference and resistance: A report on a quantitative-analytic method applied to four psychoanalyses. *Journal of the American Psychoanalytic Association, 25,* 471–490.

Greenson, R. R. (1967). *The technique and practice of psychoanalysis.* New York: International Universities Press.

Hess, J. A. (2002). Distance regulation in personal relationships: The development of a conceptual model and a test of representational validity. *Journal of Social and Personal Relationships, 19,* 663–683.

Hill, C. E. (2004). *Helping skills: Facilitating exploration, insight, and action.* Washington, DC: American Psychological Association.

Hill, C. E., Sim, W., Spangler, P., Stahl, J., Sullivan, C., & Teyber, E. (2008). Therapist immediacy in brief psychotherapy: Case study II. *Psychotherapy: Theory, Research, Practice, Training, 45,* 298–315.

Hilsenroth, M. J., Blagys, M. D., Ackerman, S. J., Bonge, D. R., & Blais, M. A. (2006). Measuring psychodynamic-interpersonal and cognitive-behavioral techniques: Development of the Comparative Psychotherapy Process Scale. *Psychotherapy: Theory, Research, Practice, Training, 42,* 340–356.

Hilsenroth, M. J., & Slavin, J. M. (2008). Integrative dynamic treatment for comorbid depression and borderline conditions. *Journal of Psychotherapy Integration, 18,* 377–409.

Hoffman, I. Z. (2009). Doublethinking our way to "scientific" legitimacy: The desiccation of human experience. *Journal of the American Psychoanalytic Association, 57,* 1043–1069.

Høglend, P. (1993). Transference interpretations and long-term change after dynamic psychotherapy of brief to moderate length. *American Journal of Psychotherapy, 47,* 494–507.

Høglend, P. (1994). *Manual for process ratings of general skill, supportive interventions and specific techniques. Unpublished manual.* Oslo, Norway: Department of Psychiatry, University of Oslo.

Høglend, P. (2004). Analysis of transference in psychodynamic psychotherapy: A review of empirical research. *Canadian Journal of Psychoanalysis, 12,* 279–300.

Høglend, P., Amlo, S., Marble, A., Bogwald, K. P., Sorbye, O., Sjaastad, M. C., et al. (2006). Analysis of the patient–therapist relationship in dynamic psychotherapy: An experimental study of transference interpretations. *American Journal of Psychiatry, 163,* 1739–1746.

Høglend, P., Bøgwald, K. P., Amlo, S., Marble, A., Ulberg, R., Sjaastad, M. C., et al. (2008). Transference interpretations in dynamic psychotherapy: Do they really yield sustained effects? *American Journal of Psychiatry, 165,* 763–771.

Høglend, P., & Gabbard, G. O. (2012). When is transference work useful in psychodynamic psychotherapy?: A review of empirical research. In R. A. Levy, J. S. Ablon, & H. Kächele (Eds.), *Psychodynamic psychotherapy research: Evidence-based practice and practice-based evidence* (pp. 449–470). Totowa, NJ: Springer.

Høglend, P., Johansson, P., Marble, A., Bøgwald, J., & Amlo, S. (2007). Moderators of the effects of transference interpretations in brief dynamic psychotherapy. *Psychotherapy Research, 17,* 162–174.

Johansson, P., Høglend, P., Ulberg, R., Amlo, S., Marble, A., Bøgwald, K. P., et al. (2010). The mediating role of insight for long-term improvements in psychodynamic therapy. *Journal of Consulting and Clinical Psychology, 78,* 438–448.

Kernberg, O. F., Yeomans, F. E., Clarkin, J. F., & Levy, K. N. (2008). Transference focused psychotherapy: Overview and update. *International Journal of Psychoanalysis, 89,* 601–620.

Kivlighan, D. M. (1995). *Similarities and differences among counselor, supervisor and observer ratings of individual counseling process.* Unpublished manuscript, University of Missouri—Columbia.

Kuutmann, K., & Hilsenroth, M. J. (2012). Exploring in-session focus on the patient–therapist relationship: Patient characteristics, process, and outcome. *Clinical Psychology and Psychotherapy, 19,* 187–202.

Leichsenring, F., & Rabung, S. (2008). Effectiveness of long-term psychodynamic psychotherapy: A meta-analysis. *Journal of the American Medical Association, 300,* 1551.

Luborsky, L. (1977). Measuring a pervasive psychic structure in psychotherapy: The core conflictual relationship theme. In N. Freedman & S. Grand (Eds.), *Communicative structures and psychic structures* (pp. 367–395). New York: Plenum Press.

Luborsky, L., & Crits-Christoph, P. (1998). *Understanding transference: The core conflictual relationship theme method.* Washington, DC: American Psychological Association.

Malan, D. (1976). *The frontier of brief psychotherapy: An example of the convergence of research and clinical practice.* New York: Plenum Press.

Malan, D. H. (1979). *Individual psychotherapy and the science of psychodynamics.* London: Butterworths.

Marmarosh, C. L., Gelso, C. J., Markin, R. D., Majors, R., Mallery, C., & Choi, J. (2009). The real relationship in psychotherapy: Relationships to adult attachments, working alliance, transference, and therapy outcome. *Journal of Counseling Psychology, 56,* 337–350.

McCarthy, P. (1982). Differential effects of self-disclosing versus self-involving counselor statements across counselor–client gender pairings. *Journal of Counseling Psychology, 26,* 538–541.

McCullough, L., Kuhn, N., Andrews, S., Kaplan, A., Wolf, J., & Hurley, C. L. (2003). *Treating affect phobia : A manual for short-term dynamic psychotherapy.* New York: Guilford Press.

McMain, S. F., Links, P. S., Gnam, W. H., Guimond, T., Cardish, R. J., Korman, L., et al. (2009). A randomized trial of dialectical behavior therapy versus general psychiatric management for borderline personality disorder. *American Journal of Psychiatry, 166,* 1365–1374.

McWilliams, N. (1994). *Psychoanalytic diagnosis.* New York: Guilford Press.

Messer, S. B., & McWilliams, N. (2007). Insight in psychodynamic therapy: Theory and assessment. In L. G. Castonguay & C. E. Hill (Eds.), *Insight in psychotherapy*. Washington, DC: American Psychological Association.

Multon, K. D., Patton, M. J., & Kivlighan, D. M., Jr. (1996). Development of the Missouri Identifying Transference Scale. *Journal of Counseling Psychology, 43*, 243–252.

Muran, J. C., Safran, J. D., Gorman, B. S., Samstag, L. W., Eubanks-Carter, C., & Winston, A. (2009). The relationship of early alliance ruptures and their resolution to process and outcome in three time-limited psychotherapies for personality disorders. *Psychotherapy: Theory, Research, Practice, Training, 46*, 233–248.

Ogrodniczuk, J. S., Piper, W. E., Joyce, A. S., & McCallum, M. (1999). Transference interpretations in short-term dynamic psychotherapy. *Journal of Nervous and Mental Disease, 187,* 571–578.

Patton, M. J., & Kivlighan, D. M. (1997). The Missouri Psychoanalytic Counseling Research Project: Relation of changes in counseling process to client outcomes. *Journal of Counseling Psychology, 44*, 189–208.

Piper, W. E., Azim, H. F., Joyce, A. S., McCallum, M., Nixon, G. W., & Segal, P. S. (1991). Quality of object relations versus interpersonal functioning as predictors of therapeutic alliance and psychotherapy outcome. *Journal of Nervous and Mental Disease, 179*, 432–438.

Piper, W. E., Joyce, A. S., McCallum, M., & Azim, H. F. (1998). Interpretive and supportive forms of psychotherapy and patient personality variables. *Journal of Consulting and Clinical Psychology, 66*, 558–567.

Piper, W. E., Ogrodniczuk, J. S., & Joyce, A. (2004). Quality of object relations as a moderator of the relationship between pattern of alliance and outcome in short-term individual psychotherapy. *Journal of Personality Assessment, 83*, 345–356.

Rapaport, D. (1967). The scientific methodology of psychoanalysis. In M. Gill (Ed.), *The collected papers of David Rapaport* (pp. 165–221). New York: Jason Aronson.

Reynolds, C. L., & Fischer, C. H. (1983). Personal versus professional evaluations of self-disclosing and self-involving counselors. *Journal of Counseling Psychology, 41*, 473–483.

Rhodes, R. H., Hill, C. E., Thompson, B. J., & Elliott, R. (1994). Client retrospective recall of resolved and unresolved misunderstanding events. *Journal of Counseling Psychology, 41*, 473–483.

Ryum, T., Stiles, T. C., Svartberg, M., & McCullough, L. (2010). The role of transference work, the therapeutic alliance, and their interaction in reducing interpersonal problems among psychotherapy patients with Cluster C personality disorders. *Psychotherapy: Theory, Research, Practice, Training, 47*, 442–453.

Safran, J. D., & Muran, J. C. (2000a). *Negotiating the therapeutic alliance: A relational treatment guide*. New York: Guilford Press.

Safran, J. D., & Muran, J. C. (2000b). Resolving therapeutic alliance ruptures: Diversity and integration. *Journal of Clinical Psychology, 56*, 233–243.

Safran, J. D., Muran, J. C., Samstag, L. W., & Winston, A. (2005). Evaluating alliance-focused intervention for potential treatment failures: A feasibility study and descriptive analysis. *Psychotherapy: Theory, Research, Practice, Training, 42*, 512–531.

Schut, A. J., Castonguay, L. G., Flanagan, K. M., Yamasaki, A. S., Barber, J. P., Bedics, J. D., et al. (2005). Therapist interpretation, patient–therapist interpersonal process, and outcome in psychodynamic psychotherapy for avoidant personality disorder. *Psychotherapy: Theory, Research, Practice, Training, 42*, 494–511.

Seligman, M. E., & Csikszentmihalyi, M. (2000). Positive psychology. An introduction. *American Psychologist, 55*, 5–14.

Sifneos, P. (1971). *Short-term dynamic psychotherapy: Evaluation and technique*. New York: Plenum Press.

Sifneos, P. (1992). *Short-term anxiety-provoking psychotherapy: A treatment manual*. New York: Basic Books.

Stevenson, J., Meares, R., & D'Angelo, R. (2005). Five-year outcome of outpatient psychotherapy with borderline patients. *Psychological Medicine, 35,* 79–87.

Stiles, W. B., Agnew-Davies, R., Hardy, G. E., Barkham, M., & Shapiro, D. A. (1998). Relations of the alliance with psychotherapy outcome: Findings in the second Sheffield Psychotherapy Project. *Journal of Consulting and Clinical Psychology, 66,* 791–802.

Strachey, J. (1999). The nature of the therapeutic action of psycho-analysis. *Journal of Psychotherapy Practice and Research, 8*(1), 66–82 (Original work published 1934; reprinted from *International Journal of Psycho-Analysis,* 15, 1934, 1127–1159)

Teyber, E., & McClure, F. (2000). Therapist variables. In C. R. Snyder & I. E. Ingram (Eds.), *Handbook of psychological change* (pp. 62–86). New York: Wiley.

Wachtel, P. L. (1993). *Therapeutic communication.* New York: Guilford Press.

Wachtel, P. L. (2008). *Relational theory and the practice of psychotherapy.* New York: Guilford Press.

Woodhouse, S. S., Schlosser, L. Z., Crook, R. E., Ligiéro, D. P., & Gelso, C. J. (2003). Client attachment to therapist: Relations to transference and client recollections of parental caregiving. *Journal of Counseling Psychology, 50,* 395–408.

Yeomans, F. E., Clarkin, J. F., & Kernberg, O. F. (2002). *A primer of transference-focused psychotherapy for the borderline patient.* Northvale, NJ: Jason Aronson.

CHAPTER 25

Future Perspectives

Linda C. Mayes, Patrick Luyten, Sidney J. Blatt,
Peter Fonagy, and Mary Target

The pessimist complains about the wind;
The optimist expects it to change;
The realist adjusts the sails
                    —WILLIAM ARTHUR WARD

The body of research summarized in this volume suggests that we may be witnessing the birth of a new brand of psychodynamic psychology and psychiatry:

- The language of psychodynamic thought has become more relational and experience-near.
- Diagnostic concepts are increasingly more integrative, transdiagnostic, and developmental.
- There has been a greater openness to an empirical approach in dialogue with other fields of scientific research.
- There is an increasing evidence base supporting the efficacy and effectiveness of psychodynamic treatments.

Without exception, the chapters in this volume exemplify these trends, integrating theoretical views and empirical findings from fields as diverse as personality and social psychology, attachment theory, cognitive-behavioral approaches, and the neurosciences, without losing touch with the broader orientation of the psychoanalytic approach, which is informed by cultural considerations, intensive clinical practice, and research in the humanities. The future is likely to see more efforts to balance knowledge from these diverse fields in the pursuit of ever-broader and more comprehensive theories of human functioning. Indeed, the future is likely to see a redefining of the boundaries of some of these fields and the emergence of new, transdisciplinary fields focusing on how treatments change functioning from the level of the genome to interpersonal relations and self-definition. At the same time, it is clear that contemporary psychodynamic approaches are shedding their sometimes overly cautious, sometimes near-phobic attitude toward systematic empirical research and the dogmatism and orthodoxy that often accompanied this attitude.

This shift in attitude and action also has important implications for the future of psychodynamic therapy and psychotherapy more generally, as the chapters in this volume demonstrate. Psychodynamic therapy has become more integrative as well. For instance, in Chapter 10, Doron, Mikulincer, Kyrios, and Sar-El discuss "attachment-based cognitive-behavioral therapy" (Doron & Moulding, 2009), which explores attachment-related internal models within the therapeutic context based on an integration of psychodynamic and cognitive-behavioral views. Clarkin, Fonagy, Levy, and Bateman (Chapter 17) describe the influence of neuroscientific findings and cognitive-behavioral formulations on the development of transference-focused psychotherapy and mentalization-based treatment for patients with personality disorders, and Harder and Rosenbaum (Chapter 13) describe similar influences on current psychodynamic treatments for patients with psychotic features.

Here we discuss what we believe to be six major common themes that emerge from the chapters in this volume. The primary goals of our discussion of these themes are to set an agenda for future research and to foster a dialogue that attempts to stimulate integration with other theoretical approaches.

THE THEORETICAL LANGUAGE OF PSYCHOANALYSIS AND THE NEED FOR INTEGRATIVE THEORIES

The chapters in this volume illustrate the richness and productivity of the psychodynamic approach, with its emphasis on the role of unconscious factors, conflict/defense, and its person-centered, developmental understanding of the nature and course of psychopathology across the lifespan (see Luyten, Mayes, Blatt, Target, & Fonagy, Chapter 1). At the same time, it is clear that contemporary psychodynamic approaches are freeing themselves from what has historically been less helpful: the often highly metaphorical language characteristic of psychodynamic theory, which provided sophisticated descriptions rather than explanations, often leading to the illusion of shared meaning. These descriptions were also difficult for scientists and clinicians from other fields to access and similarly difficult to operationalize into testable hypotheses and study designs. Much has already been written on the problems related to the theoretical language of psychoanalysis, such as it being too far removed from clinical and experiential reality (Gill, 1976; Rapaport & Gill, 1959). Furthermore, there has been a strong reluctance within psychoanalysis to develop a more experience-driven language, despite Freud's (1925, pp. 32–33) own famous admonition that theoretical concepts were merely a "speculative superstructure" ("spekulativer Überbau") that could be abandoned in the light of new knowledge. In our opinion, however, with the growing realization that many of these concepts are actually descriptions disguised as explanations (Fonagy, Target, & Gergely, 2006) that hamper integration and dialogue with other sciences, a marked shift is happening within the psychodynamic literature.

Shahar (2010) has in this context introduced a helpful distinction between the clinical language of *poetics* and the scientific language of *schematics*. Much of the theoretical language of psychoanalysis does indeed belong to the realm of poetics: It uses metaphors (such as ego, id, superego, self, self objects, transitional space, the Symbolic) in an attempt to capture and understand psychological processes. These concepts have almost invariably emerged in the context of the clinical encounter, and they are, in this context, tremendously helpful: The language of poetics provides us with an often deeply felt, embodied understanding of the clinical encounter. In this respect, it is clearly superior to the language of empirical science—the language of schematics that aims to explain phenomena as parsimoniously and clearly as possible.

Both languages are needed if we really want to understand psychological phenomena, but we need to redress the balance within psychoanalysis, as in the past we tended almost exclusively to speak the language of poetics. This had two undesired effects (Luyten, 2015). First, as mentioned above, it resulted in descriptions that were sophisticated but lacking in explanatory power. Second, it hampered integration with other strands of research. Metaphorical concepts such as ego and superego are largely meaningless for neuroscientists, as they do not map neatly on to what we know about brain functioning. Likewise, developmental psychopathology has rendered many psychoanalytic speculations about early developmental stages improbable, as children lack the cognitive capacities attributed to them by many of these theories (Fonagy et al., 2006; Luyten, Mayes, Target, & Fonagy, 2012). This is true even for more post-Freudian theoretical approaches such as object relations theory. For instance, do we really believe that a representation is split in two or more parts in splitting? Or that one part of a mental representation is kept unconscious (i.e., is defended against)?

A more parsimonious explanation of splitting is that the individual lacks the capacity to generate a more differentiated representation or that this capacity is defensively inhibited (e.g., to prevent feelings of anxiety) such that in different contexts, the individual behaves differently toward another person with different desired goals for the interaction. If the complexity of contemporary psychoanalytic concepts and metaphors is to be seen as useful outside clinical psychoanalysis (where it remains of clear value), ways need to be found to link central embodied concepts such as splitting with what is becoming known of the actual body—and especially the brain—and with other sciences of mental functioning. If clinicians feel that meaning has been lost through such a "translation," say, between "splitting" and the "failure of generating an integrated multifaceted representation," this should be an occasion for celebration rather than remorse. We should join with renewed vigor to scrutinize the gap between preconscious metaphoric intuition of a mental process and the empirically approachable description as a potential further key area for empirical inquiry (Fonagy & Target, 2007).

Psychodynamic theorists and researchers thus have the task of developing a more appropriate theoretical language that combines the language of poetics to capture the lived experience of the clinical encounter, with the language of schematics that seeks to explain phenomena as parsimoniously as possible in a way that can be empirically operationalized. As many of the chapters in this volume attest, once stripped of their metaphorical overtones, many psychoanalytic assumptions in fact show much overlap with concepts and assumptions in other theoretical approaches. This is perhaps one of the key reasons why, despite much criticism, a number of psychoanalytic concepts have endured and are embedded in culture as a whole, and also why recent decades have seen such an increase in dialogue between psychodynamic and other approaches. Changes in our theoretical language thus promise to lead to more dialogue and perhaps also to more willingness by scientists from other orientations to acknowledge psychoanalytic influences. Indeed, one reason why some of our colleagues may have been so reluctant to acknowledge the obvious influences of psychoanalytic theory on their views may have been psychoanalysis's highly metaphoric and sometimes even mythical-sounding theoretical language, which is met with strong skepticism in many scientific circles.

THE NEED FOR A TRANSDIAGNOSTIC APPROACH

A second theme that emerges from the chapters in this volume concerns the move away from a focus on discrete disorders to a broader dimensional and transdiagnostic approach to psychopathology, in both its conceptualization and treatment.

Psychiatry and clinical psychology have for decades been dominated by a largely descriptive, atheoretical and disorder-centered approach that conceptualizes psychiatric disorders in terms of discrete entities that are categorically distinct from normality. As a consequence, specific treatments for these purportedly discrete disorders were developed, empirically evaluated, and their dissemination promoted by treatment guidelines and health care and governmental agencies. This static, categorical and nondevelopmental approach markedly contrasts with the psychoanalytic emphasis on the dynamic, dimensional, and developmental nature of psychopathology (Blatt & Luyten, 2010; Kernberg & Caligor, 2005; McWilliams, 2011; PDM Task Force, 2006; Westen, Shedler, & Bradley, 2006) (see also Luyten et al., Chapter 1; Luyten & Blatt, Chapter 5; Meehan & Levy, Chapter 15). It also markedly contrasts with the spectrum approach that is typical of psychoanalytic treatments of psychopathology. Rather than developing specific treatments for specific disorders, psychoanalysis, guided by the view that different clusters of psychopathology are intrinsically related, traditionally developed treatments for broad groups of patients, such as people with neurotic problems, or children with emotional or externalizing problems (Target & Fonagy, 1994). As a result of this very different approach, psychoanalysis was relegated to a secondary role in research on the causes of specific psychological/psychiatric disorders and their classification and treatment. However, there is a growing consensus that some of the fundamental assumptions of psychoanalytic approaches toward the nature, classification, and treatment of psychopathology contain a strong kernel of truth (see Luyten et al., Chapter 1, for a more detailed discussion of this issue). First, the dynamic or functional nature of psychopathology—that is, that many disorders involve attempts, however maladaptive, to establish an equilibrium—is increasingly recognized, particularly in cognitive-behavioral and personality-based approaches (Luyten & Blatt, 2011).

Second, a dimensional view of psychopathology is now recognized to be superior in many ways to categorical approaches to psychopathology. This is most clearly recognized in extant personality-based models of the nature and classification of psychological disorders, such as the Five-Factor Model (Costa & McCrae, 2010) and the tripartite model (Watson, Clark, & Chmielewski, 2008), which assume the existence of a fundamental continuity between normal and disrupted personality development. This has led to renewed attention to psychodynamic approaches to personality or character difficulties. Psychodynamic views and research concerning the dimensionality of personality pathology, for instance, now play a major role in proposed reformulations of the classification of personality disorders (Luyten & Blatt, 2013; Skodol et al., 2011). Psychoanalysis is in good company in this context. The recently launched Research Domain Criteria (RDoC) initiative of the National Institute of Mental Health, though more biological in orientation, similarly proposed that future research should focus on systems that underlie basic psychological capacities (such as reward neurocircuitry and the neural systems implicated in self-representation, theory of mind, attachment/separation fear, and positive and negative valence systems), rather than on discrete disorders (Casey et al., 2013; Cuthbert & Insel, 2013; Cuthbert & Kozak, 2013). It is very unlikely, as Eapen (2012, p. 1) recently noted, that "neurodevelopmental genes have . . . read the DSM." As in other dimensional approaches, including the psychoanalytic approach, the RDoC project starts from the assumption that current descriptive diagnoses are extremely unlikely to lead to insights into the neurobiological and psychosocial underpinnings of these disorders, and thus that our understandings of behavior–brain relationships should begin with the study of basic behavioral systems *across* disorders.

Third, there is increasing recognition that disorders share many etiological features and can be (hierarchically) organized in clusters or spectra of related disorders that share important etiological features (Caspi et al., 2013; Krueger, Skodol, Livesley, Shrout, & Huang, 2007; Lahey et al., 2008)—an assumption that is at the heart of psychoanalytic approaches to psychopathology (Blatt, 2008; Kernberg & Caligor, 2005; McWilliams, 2011; PDM Task Force, 2006; Shedler & Westen, 2010). The suggestion that future episodes of mental disorder are best predicted by a single overarching "p" (*psychopathology*) score (Caspi et al., 2013), rather than by the severity of an individual diagnostic condition, is aligned well with notions of ego weakness and its converse, resilience.

Finally, as a result of these major shifts, there is a clear move away from a focus on the development of treatments for specific disorders to the idea that treatments should target broad categories of patients. Barlow and colleagues, for instance, developed a Unified Protocol for Transdiagnostic Treatment of Emotional Disorders (UP) from a cognitive-behavioral perspective (Wilamowska et al., 2010), which contrasts markedly with the more traditional emphasis in cognitive-behavioral therapy on manualized protocols for specific disorders. Similarly, mindfulness-based therapy and dialectical behavior therapy are now used in a broad array of conditions characterized, respectively, by stress/emotional problems and by affective dysregulation (Kahl, Winter, & Schweiger, 2012).

The same trend is observable within the psychodynamic approach. Busch and Milrod, for instance, in Chapter 8, describe a transdiagnostic treatment, Panic-Focused Psychodynamic Psychotherapy, eXtended Range (PFPP-XR), for a *spectrum* of patients presenting with anxiety problems. In Chapter 18, St. John and Lieberman present a flexible, broad psychodynamic treatment approach for infants, toddlers, and preschoolers who enter treatment with a wide range of presenting problems that include internalizing and externalizing disorders, and show symptom presentations that defy neat categorization. Clarkin and colleagues, in Chapter 17, discuss how transference-focused psychotherapy and mentalization-based treatment, originally developed for the treatment of patients with marked borderline personality disorder features, have been adapted for patients with less severe personality problems. Grienenberger and colleagues, in Chapter 21, and Rossouw, in Chapter 22, describe a spectrum of mentalization-based interventions for at-risk children and their parents and families. Similarly, Hill and Sharp (Chapter 19) and the Steeles (Chapter 20) present broad psychodynamic interventions for the spectra of children and adolescents with externalizing and attachment disorders, respectively.

This does not mean, paradoxically, that we should give up on the development and evaluation of treatment protocols for specific disorders or psychological problems. Careful manualization and evaluation of specific treatments remains an important target for future research, as we do not want to return to a "one-size-fits-all" approach, nor do we want to leave decisions concerning the choice of treatment completely in the hands of clinicians who are commonly trained in a single approach. However, we do need to rethink the development, dissemination, training, and assessment of adherence to treatment protocols. Weisz and colleagues (2012), for instance, found that a modular approach, with clinicians being trained in different treatment modules that they could flexibly use in their treatments, was more effective in treating youth with depression, anxiety, and conduct disorder than training in and the use of standard manualized treatments. If replicated, these findings suggest that the future in intervention research may lie in the development of and training in broader treatment protocols that can be flexibly integrated and tailored to the specific patient. More research in this area is needed, and psychoanalytic researchers should continue to heed this call, contributing as this volume shows to the development of treatment models and to the sophisticated measurement and understanding of outcomes.

Furthermore, psychodynamic approaches are likely to continue to influence future decisions concerning the classification and treatment of psychiatric disorders only if more evidence is provided for the validity of psychodynamic views on these issues. Hence, there is an urgent need for large-scale studies concerning the nature of psychiatric disorders and their classification that make use of assessment instruments rooted in contemporary psychoanalytic approaches. Finally, the clinical utility of psychodynamic approaches compared to other models of psychopathology needs to be investigated further (Spitzer, First, Shedler, Westen, & Skodol, 2008). Both psychoanalytic organizations and large funding agencies have an important responsibility here to ensure that psychodynamic approaches are represented in future research efforts in this area.

THE NEED FOR A DYNAMIC, LIFESPAN PERSPECTIVE

Psychoanalysis has always had a strong focus on tracing the emergence of psychopathology across the lifespan (Emde, 2005; Fonagy et al., 2006; Luyten, Mayes, et al., 2012). As this volume illustrates, it shares this interest with contemporary developmental psychopathology and the neurosciences. Indeed, both developmental psychopathology and the neurosciences are increasingly concerned with processes of *multifinality* and *equifinality* (Cicchetti & Rogosch, 1996) in explaining the developmental pathways implicated in health and disease. As discussed by Luyten and colleagues in Chapter 1, equifinality implies that there are many possible pathways toward one specific developmental outcome, rather than assuming that there is a single etiological pathway for each mental disorder or developmental outcome. Multifinality, in turn, implies that the same developmental factors may result in different developmental outcomes, depending on their interaction with other factors. Recent neuroscientific views—particularly the Developmental Origins of Health and Disease (DOHaD) paradigm (Gluckman et al., 2009)—similarly assume that (early) life experiences play an important role in "programming" and "resetting" developmental trajectories, ranging from neuroendocrine systems such as the hypothalamic–pituitary–adrenal axis, the main human stress-regulating system, to the immune system, neurocircuitry, and musculoskeletal development, resulting in changes in physiology and structure. In this context, changes in gene expression through epigenetic mechanisms such as DNA methylation have received considerable attention recently (Champagne & Curley, 2009) and are of specific interest to psychoanalytic researchers (Fonagy & Luyten, in press; Luyten, Vliegen, Van Houdenhove, & Blatt, 2008). Similarly, the strong shift in contemporary psychiatric genetics from the study of the main effects of genes to the investigation of gene–environment correlations and gene–environment interactions is equally exciting for psychoanalytically oriented researchers and clinicians alike. Gene–environment correlations refer to the finding that genes may increase exposure to certain environments (and vice versa), while gene–environment interactions involve synergistic interactions between genes and environment (e.g., certain genes may increase sensitivity to stress and thus vulnerability to psychopathology) (Plomin & Davis, 2009; Rutter, 2009).

Interestingly, there is now good evidence to suggest that the genes implicated in gene–environment correlations and interactions should be thought of not so much as "vulnerability genes," but as genes that render individuals more susceptible to environmental influences, for better or for worse (Belsky & Pluess, 2013; Ellis, Boyce, Belsky, Bakermans-Kranenburg, & van IJzendoorn, 2011). These views are particularly interesting for psychoanalytic researchers, as they suggest the existence of complex interactions between genes and environment across the lifespan. Furthermore, there are indications that the frequency of these social susceptibility genes differs as a function of the degree of individualism versus collectivism within a particular culture: Cultures with higher levels of collectivism may be characterized by a higher prevalence of social susceptibility genes. This fact serves to refocus our attention on evolutionary issues, which historically have been a central focus of psychoanalysis (Luyten & Blatt, 2013; Way & Lieberman, 2010). These findings also have important implications for intervention, as they suggest that some individuals are more susceptible to environmental influences, including psychosocial interventions, than are others. This also points to possible genetically determined limitations on the effects of psychosocial interventions (Aitchison, Basu, McGuffin, & Craig, 2005).

These views once again reinforce the need for a shift away from disorder-centered strategies toward person-oriented research and treatment strategies. This shift can open up important new perspectives for both psychoanalytic researchers and clinicians, whose interest lies primarily in understanding the person and his or her developmental history rather than one particular symptom, disorder, or developmental outcome (Luyten et al., 2008). This in turn opens up possibilities to design developmentally informed specified and targeted interventions (Fonagy & Target, 2002), as, for instance, emphasized by St. John and Lieberman in Chapter 18. Specifically, they argue that there is no neat distinction between and among children with internalizing and externalizing disorders, given the high comorbidity between these disorders, which questions the clinical utility of this distinction (Blatt & Luyten, 2009; Lahey et al., 2008). They note, for instance, that

> PTSD in particular defies neat categorization as either an internalizing or an externalizing disorder. Falling under the general heading of anxiety disorders, PTSD is often considered to be an internalizing disorder, yet many of the signs exhibited by toddlers and preschoolers suffering from PTSD—such as fighting, biting, and reckless behavior—are more immediately recognizable as externalizing behaviors. (p. 5)

At the same time, the new findings and perspectives emerging from contemporary psychiatric genetics pose some challenges to reframe accounts of the strong emphasis on the (early) environment in psychoanalytic accounts. To begin with, estimates of heredity for most psychological features hover at around 40–60% (Kendler, 2013; Plomin, DeFries, Knopik, & Neiderhiser, 2013), even for behaviors that are often believed to be completely determined by environmental factors, such as parenting behaviors (Klahr & Burt, 2013) and social support (Kendler, 1997). Second, psychiatric genetics suggests that we have to rethink the influence of parental behaviors on child development, as the child's genetic makeup is what largely determines parenting behaviors (so-called evocative gene–environment correlations) (Klahr & Burt, 2013; Marceau et al., 2013), rather than direct parent-to-child effects. To give an example of such findings, a recent study in two large samples of 909 Swedish and 405 U.S. parents reported that active evocative gene–environment processes explained the association between maternal and paternal negativity and externalizing problems in their adolescent offspring (Marceau et al., 2013). No evidence was found, by contrast, for passive gene–environment correlations or direct effects of parenting on externalizing symptoms in adolescents. As noted, these findings seriously question basic psychoanalytic assumptions concerning the influence of attachment figures on development across time, although of course not all parents may be prone to such evocative effects.

The evidence for the longitudinal stability of attachment behavior is increasingly being challenged by findings that attachment stability from childhood to adulthood is modest at best (Haltigan, Roisman, & Fraley, 2013), mainly because of its interaction with many other developmental factors, including the developmental unfolding of genetic influence (Belsky & Pluess, 2013). For instance, while studies have found little or no influence of genetic factors on attachment in childhood, a recent study found that by adolescence, around 40% of differences in attachment style are genetically determined, suggesting a potential "resetting" of attachment in adolescence influenced by genetic factors (Fearon, Shmueli-Goetz, Viding, Fonagy, & Plomin, 2013). Although several studies have provided evidence for the stability of personality and attachment across the lifespan, such findings may be somewhat misleading, as this stability seems largely explained by the stability of the environment in these studies rather than the stability of these features themselves (Fraley & Roberts, 2005). Of course, it is also true that there is genetic regulation of behavior in parents and in the notion of evoked behavior from child to parent. There is also a need to understand why some parents do not respond to this evocation and others do. Nonetheless, introducing notions of heritable contributions to the impact of environmental factors on long-term outcome does raise questions about core psychoanalytic assumptions concerning the stability of internal working models of self and others. Hence, much work remains to be done to integrate these findings into a comprehensive, psychodynamically informed theory about psychological development across the lifespan that accommodates genetic influences on evoked behavior in dyads and in families and accounts for complex interactions between heritable and shared environments over time.

THE NEED FOR FURTHER INTEGRATION WITH THE NEUROSCIENCES

The above discussion brings us to the need for further integration with the neurosciences. It must be clear from this volume that it is currently hard to imagine a discussion of psychological issues without reference to neuroscientific findings. This, of course, constitutes a major difference from the early days of psychoanalysis, when neuroscience was far too static, speculative, and concerned with basic cognitive issues to be really relevant to psychoanalysis. Freud abandoned his "Project for a Scientific Psychology" (Freud, 1895/1950), an attempt to bridge the gap between his early psychoanalytic formulations and the neurosciences of his time, for precisely these reasons.

Now, findings from the different strands within neuroscience, ranging from psychiatric genetics to neurobiology, and from imaging research, can no longer be neglected. For the first time in history, affective neuroscience in particular (Panksepp, 1998) is providing increasing insight into what happens in the brain in complex, conflict-laden (interpersonal) situations. There is increasing recognition that the brain is experience-expectant and, essentially, social: that it is a highly developed organ that has, from an evolutionary perspective, developed to allow human beings to adapt to ever-changing (social) circumstances. We can no longer dismiss these views and the findings emerging from related research as irrelevant.

At the same time, in many respects, the neurosciences are still in their infancy; many studies in this field are still plagued by important methodological limitations and small sample sizes, and have not been integrated into more comprehensive theories about brain functioning. Modeling complex social interactions in ways that are amenable to functional imaging paradigms, although a step forward, also imposes constraints on what are surely multidetermined social contexts in the real world. Furthermore, important philosophical issues concerning brain–mind relationships remain to be solved (for a recent overview, see Fotopoulou, Pfaff, & Conway, 2012). But this should not lead us to (defensively) dismiss neuroscientific research, nor should we demonstrate a self-congratulatory attitude in arguing that the neurosciences have largely confirmed psychoanalytic models of the mind. In fact, we believe that contemporary neuroscience suggests a rather different and more complex model of the mind. We should instead embrace the openness the neurosciences have shown toward psychoanalytic ideas. By embracing these new developments, psychoanalytic researchers could play an important role in the development of new neuroscientific paradigms and in the application of novel techniques and methods in the study of normal and disrupted psychological development. A particular challenge for the field in this context is the study of the effects of psychodynamic therapy on the function and connectivity of specific neural circuits. Initial findings are promising (Abbass, Nowoweiski, Bernier, Tarzwell, & Beutel, 2014), but many more imaginative research efforts, necessitating close interdisciplinary collaborations, are needed.

CHALLENGES FOR THE DEVELOPMENT, EVALUATION, AND DISSEMINATION OF PSYCHOANALYTIC TREATMENTS

Demonstrating the effects of psychodynamic treatments on the brain is not the only, and perhaps not most important, challenge psychodynamic treatment approaches face. More than ever, psychoanalysis is confronted with questions about whether the various treatment approaches it continues to inspire are effective (from both a psychological and a cost perspective) and what the effective mechanisms of its treatments are (see Leichsenring, Kruse, & Rabung, Chapter 23).

These questions are not that easy to answer. First, although it is generally assumed that any treatment should be based on insights into the nature of psychopathology (Kazdin, 2007, 2011), different treatment approaches, based on often very different conceptualizations of psychopathology and employing very different interventions, have generally shown similar effects in most disorders (Lambert, 2013; Miller, Wampold, & Varhely, 2008; Wampold, Minami, Baskin, & Callen Tierney, 2002). This so-called Dodo bird verdict (Luborsky et al., 2002) is at odds with the emphasis in the psychoanalytic tradition on the specificity of psychoanalytic treatments and their effects. Extant research suggests that there are no qualitative differences in the outcome of longer-term psychoanalysis versus briefer forms of dynamic treatment and between psychodynamic treatments and other types of treatment (Grant & Sandell, 2004; Kächele, 2010).

By contrast, estimates suggest that theory-specific interventions (such as transference interpretations in psychodynamic treatments) explain only about 15% of the variance in outcome (Lambert & Barley, 2002). Common factors (e.g., providing support) (30%), expectancy and placebo effects (15%), and extratherapeutic factors (35–40%) (e.g., spontaneous remission, positive changes in patients' lives) would be responsible for the bulk of the variance in outcomes (see also Luyten et al, Chapter 1). Furthermore, there is ample evidence for therapist and patient effects on treatment outcome (Blatt, Zuroff, Hawley, & Auerbach, 2010). These factors pose considerable constraints on any effort to demonstrate the "unique" effects of psychodynamic treatments and on attempts to demonstrate a unique relationship between typical psychodynamic interventions and therapeutic outcome. Perhaps psychoanalytic researchers and clinicians must begin to accept that *all* psychosocial interventions focus on relatively similar psychological processes (Blatt et al., 2010) and neurobiological systems, either by altering top-down regulation or by changing bottom-up processes, or a combination of both (Luyten, Blatt, & Mayes, 2012).

Recently, we have formulated an even broader theory of change in the context of psychotherapy that further limits claims of "unique" effects of any specific treatment approach (Fonagy & Luyten, in press; Fonagy, Luyten, & Allison, 2013). We argue that effective treatment involves the reactivation of three social learning processes: (1) learning happening within the context of a specific form of psychotherapy, with the patient being provided with a language that helps him or her to understand and make sense of problems; (2) the effects of psychotherapy, whatever its theoretical orientation, on the development and/or recovery of the capacity for mentalizing (i.e., the ability to understand the self and others in terms of mental states such as feelings and desires); and (3) learning beyond therapy, that is, social learning from others outside the treatment setting—an evolutionary prewired process and capacity that all psychotherapies, but psychoanalytic treatments in particular, may have neglected, although it perhaps provides the most powerful arena for change.

Treatment research in general and psychodynamic treatment research in particular face a daunting task in attempting to unravel these processes. Several studies have already paved the way and have provided evidence for a relationship between (specific) psychoanalytic interventions and outcome (Baldwin, Wampold, & Imel, 2007; Hawley, Ho, Zuroff, & Blatt, 2006; Høglend et al., 2006; Safran, Muran, & Eubanks-Carter, 2011), but we now need wide-ranging and detailed studies that are powered to detect relationships between process and outcome *across* rather than *within* different treatments. More research on the identification of characteristics of effective therapists (Ackerman & Hilsenroth, 2001; Baldwin et al., 2007; Zuroff, Kelly, Leybman, Blatt, & Wampold, 2010), regardless of their theoretical orientation, is needed. Similarly, studies on the influence of relevant patient features, and their interaction with the therapeutic alliance and process in different types of intervention, promise to shed further light on the mechanisms of change in effective treatments.

These studies may also give rise to more comprehensive treatments that allow treatment tailoring, as is outlined for instance by Blatt in Chapter 7 (see also Blatt et al., 2010).

This discussion leads us to a second issue—the relationship between theory and technique. The psychodynamic tradition has undeniably been characterized by a relatively strong divide between them (Fonagy, 2003b). This is best exemplified by the huge imbalance between the major developments in psychoanalytic theory and the rather modest changes in psychoanalytic technique. At the same time, it is important to acknowledge that there are many exceptions to this rule, such as brief dynamic treatments (Malan, 1963; Sifneos, 1979), longer-term supportive-expressive therapy (Luborsky, 1984), and, more recently, work on the development of transference-focused psychotherapy (Clarkin et al., 2001) and mentalization-based treatment (Bateman & Fonagy, 2006) for borderline personality disorder. Perhaps not coincidentally, the closer relationship between theory and technique that characterizes these treatments emerged in the context of a close dialogue between clinical practice, theorizing, and systematic research. More research in this area is needed and should be particularly attentive to potential harmful and iatrogenic effects of intensive psychoanalytic treatments, such as the use in patients with borderline personality disorder of strongly insight-oriented treatments encouraging regression that far surpasses these patients' capacities, which therefore are likely to be associated with iatrogenic effects, as reflected by comparisons between follow-along and treatment studies (Fonagy & Bateman, 2006). Finally, even if the field manages to produce more convincing evidence supporting the effectiveness of psychoanalytic treatments and their purported mutative factors, there is still the problem of the dissemination of these treatments and psychoanalytic training, which we discuss next.

CHALLENGES FOR PSYCHOANALYTIC TRAINING

The issues discussed so far raise important questions concerning the training of psychoanalytic therapists. Psychoanalytic training traditionally emphasizes four issues: the study of theory, individual cases, supervision, and personal psychoanalysis. With some exceptions, the language of poetics dominates psychoanalytic training, and psychodynamic professionals have built their identity around this model. It almost naturally follows that these practitioners feel threatened by the language of schematics, particularly in combination with the growing pressures of managed care and evidence-based medicine. As a result, research often remains a foreign language at best and a "foreign body" at worst in psychoanalytic training.

Rigidity and orthodoxy have often resulted from this relatively traditional approach to training, and methods to increase therapeutic effectiveness (such as the use of role-play or taping of sessions) (Diener, Hilsenroth, & Weinberger, 2007) have often been discouraged. Research and methods associated with the systematic examination of psychodynamic treatment (such as routine outcome monitoring) are often met with fierce resistance in psychoanalytic circles (Lemma, Target, & Fonagy, 2011). However, several research groups have shown that these attitudes toward research are relatively easy to change as clinicians become more acquainted with research (Clarkin et al., 2001; Henton & Midgley, 2012; Lemma et al., 2011; Taubner, Buchheim, Rudyk, Kachele, & Bruns, 2012). Furthermore, there are clear signs that research is gaining a more prominent role in psychoanalytic training, although these efforts are often still quite limited (Emde & Fonagy, 1997; Wallerstein, 2009).

The integration of research and clinical approaches in psychoanalytic training still has a long way to go, and many psychoanalytic practitioners continue to have no or very little exposure to research and research findings. At a time when the "scientist–practitioner" model is increasingly used in training, it may be time for a more fundamental reevaluation of psychoanalytic models of clinical training (Kernberg, 2000; Luyten, Blatt, & Corveleyn, 2006). Although this many not always be an easy process, as evidenced by recent attempts to reform psychoanalytic training programs (Kernberg, 2012), it may lead to a new generation of psychoanalytic researchers and practitioners for whom the translation of research findings to clinical practice is self-evident (Kächele, Schachter, & Thomä, 2009). There are similar pressures and ongoing efforts to revise training for practitioners in a range of psychotherapeutic approaches, and the more developers of psychoanalytic training programs begin to collaborate with those working within other training perspectives, the more shared approaches to innovative pedagogy for mental health practice may emerge.

DISCUSSION AND CONCLUSIONS

Contemporary psychodynamic approaches to psychopathology are currently undergoing a clear revival. They have considerably changed in terms of their theoretical outlook, attitude to evidence, treatment approach, and stance toward other neighboring disciplines. Yet, these theories have retained their roots in the rich tradition characteristic of psychoanalytic thought—and they are not likely to lose them in the future. It is our hope that this novel brand of psychoanalysis—one that is able to retain what is valuable in what is old, and add what is valuable in what is new—could end not just our "not-so-splendid isolation" from other branches of science (Fonagy, 2003a), but also our isolation from each other within psychoanalysis.

REFERENCES

Abbass, A. A., Nowoweiski, S. J., Bernier, D., Tarzwell, R., & Beutel, M. E, (2014). Review of psychodynamic psychotherapy neuroimaging studies. *Psychotherapy and Psychosomatics, 83*(3), 142–147.

Ackerman, S. J., & Hilsenroth, M. J. (2001). A review of therapist characteristics and techniques negatively impacting the therapeutic alliance. *Psychotherapy: Theory, Research, Practice, Training, 38*, 171–185.

Aitchison, K., Basu, A., McGuffin, P., & Craig, I. (2005). Psychiatry and the "new genetics": Hunting for genes for behaviour and drug response. *British Journal of Psychiatry, 186*, 91–92.

Baldwin, S. A., Wampold, B. E., & Imel, Z. E. (2007). Untangling the alliance–outcome correlation: Exploring the relative importance of therapist and patient variability in the alliance. *Journal of Consulting and Clinical Psychology, 75*, 842–852.

Bateman, A. W., & Fonagy, P. (2006). *Mentalization based treatment for borderline personality disorder: A practical guide.* Oxford, UK: Oxford University Press.

Belsky, J., & Pluess, M. (2013). Genetic moderation of early child-care effects on social functioning across childhood: A developmental analysis. *Child Development, 84,* 1209–1225.

Blatt, S. J. (2008). *Polarities of experience: Relatedness and self definition in personality development, psychopathology, and the therapeutic process.* Washington, DC: American Psychological Association.

Blatt, S. J., & Luyten, P. (2009). A structural-developmental psychodynamic approach to psychopathology: Two polarities of experience across the life span. *Development and Psychopathology, 21,* 793–814.

Blatt, S. J., & Luyten, P. (2010). Reactivating the psychodynamic approach to classify psychopathology. In T. Millon, R. F. Krueger, & E. Simonsen (Eds.), *Contemporary directions in psychopathology: Scientific foundations of the DSM-V and ICD-11* (pp. 483–514). New York: Guilford Press.

Blatt, S. J., Zuroff, D. C., Hawley, L. L., & Auerbach, J. S. (2010). Predictors of sustained therapeutic change. *Psychotherapy Research, 20,* 37–54.

Casey, B. J., Craddock, N., Cuthbert, B. N., Hyman, S. E., Lee, F. S., & Ressler, K. J. (2013). DSM-5 and RDoC: Progress in psychiatry research? *Nature Reviews. Neuroscience, 14,* 810–814.

Caspi, A., Houts, R. M., Belsky, D. W., Goldman-Mellor, S. J., Harrington, H., Israel, S., et al. (2013). The p Factor: One general psychopathology factor in the structure of psychiatric disorders? *Clinical Psychological Science, 2,* 119–137.

Champagne, F. A., & Curley, J. P. (2009). Epigenetic mechanisms mediating the long-term effects of maternal care on development. *Neuroscience and Biobehavioral Reviews, 33,* 593–600.

Cicchetti, D., & Rogosch, F. A. (1996). Equifinality and multifinality in developmental psychopathology. *Development and Psychopathology, 8,* 597–600.

Clarkin, J. F., Foelsch, P. A., Levy, K. N., Hull, J. W., Delaney, J. C., & Kernberg, O. F. (2001). The development of a psychodynamic treatment for patients with borderline personality disorder: A preliminary study of behavioral change. *Journal of Personality Disorders, 15,* 487–495.

Costa, P. T., & McCrae, R. R. (2010). Bridging the gap with the five-factor model. *Personality Disorders, 1,* 127–130.

Cuthbert, B., & Insel, T. (2013). Toward the future of psychiatric diagnosis: The seven pillars of RDoC. *BMC Medicine, 11,* 126.

Cuthbert, B. N., & Kozak, M. J. (2013). Constructing constructs for psychopathology: The NIMH research domain criteria. *Journal of Abnormal Psychology, 122,* 928–937.

Diener, M. J., Hilsenroth, M., & Weinberger, J. (2007). Therapist affect focus and patient outcomes in psychodynamic psychotherapy: A meta-analysis. *American Journal of Psychiatry, 164,* 936–941.

Doron, G., & Moulding, R. (2009). Cognitive behavioral treatment of obsessive compulsive disorder: A broader framework. *Israel Journal of Psychiatry and Related Science, 46,* 257–263.

Eapen, V. (2012). Neurodevelopmental genes have not read the DSM criteria: Or, have they? *Frontiers in Psychiatry, 3,* 75.

Ellis, B. J., Boyce, W. T., Belsky, J., Bakermans-Kranenburg, M. J., & van IJzendoorn, M. H. (2011). Differential susceptibility to the environment: An evolutionary–neurodevelopmental theory. *Development and Psychopathology, 23,* 7–28.

Emde, R. N. (2005). A developmental orientation for contemporary psychoanalysis. In E. S. Person, A. M. Cooper, & G. O. Gabbard (Eds.), *The American Psychiatric Publishing textbook of psychoanalysis* (pp. 117–130). Washington, DC: American Psychiatric Publishing.

Emde, R. N., & Fonagy, P. (1997). An emerging culture for psychoanalytic research? Editorial. *International Journal of Psycho-Analysis, 78,* 643–651.

Fearon, P., Shmueli-Goetz, Y., Viding, E., Fonagy, P., & Plomin, R. (2013). Genetic and environmental influences on adolescent attachment. *Journal of Child Psychology and Psychiatry.*

Fonagy, P. (2003a). Genetics, developmental psychopathology and psychoanalytic theory: The case for ending our (not so) splendid isolation. *Psychoanalytic Inquiry, 23*, 218–247.

Fonagy, P. (2003b). Some complexities in the relationship of psychoanalytic theory to technique. *Psychoanalytic Quarterly, 72*, 13–47.

Fonagy, P., & Bateman, A. (2006). Progress in the treatment of borderline personality disorder. *British Journal of Psychiatry, 188*, 1–3.

Fonagy, P., & Luyten, P. (in press). A multilevel perspective on the development of borderline personality disorder. In D. Cicchetti (Ed.), *Development and psychopathology* (3rd ed.). New York: Wiley.

Fonagy, P., Luyten, P., & Allison, E. (2013). Teaching to learn from experience: Epistemic mistrust, personality, and psychotherapy. *Manuscript submitted for publication.*

Fonagy, P., & Target, M. (2002). Psychodynamic approaches to child therapy. In F. W. Kaslow & J. Magnavita (Eds.), *Comprehensive handbook of psychotherapy: Vol. I. Psychodynamic/object relations* (pp. 105–129). New York: Wiley.

Fonagy, P., & Target, M. (2007). The rooting of the mind in the body: New links between attachment theory and psychoanalytic thought. *Journal of the American Psychoanalytic Association, 55*, 411–456.

Fonagy, P., Target, M., & Gergely, G. (2006). Psychoanalytic perspectives on developmental psychopathology. In D. Cicchetti & D. J. Cohen (Eds.), *Developmental psychopathology: Vol. 1. Theory and method* (2nd ed., pp. 701–749). Hoboken, NJ: Wiley.

Fotopoulou, A., Pfaff, D., & Conway, M. A. (2012). *From the couch to the lab: Trends in psychodynamic neuroscience.* Oxford, UK: Oxford University Press.

Fraley, R. C., & Roberts, B. W. (2005). Patterns of continuity: A dynamic model for conceptualizing the stability of individual differences in psychological constructs across the life course. *Psychological Review, 112*, 60–74.

Freud, S. (1950). Project for a scientific psychology. In J. Strachey (Ed. & Trans.), *The standard edition of the complete psychological works of Sigmund Freud* (Vol. 1, pp. 281–293). London: Hogarth Press. (Original work published 1895)

Freud, S. (1959). An autobiographical study. In J. Strachey (Ed. & Trans.), *The standard edition of the complete psychological works of Sigmund Freud* (Vol. 20, pp. 7–74). London: Hogarth Press. (Original work published 1925)

Gill, M. M. (1976). Metapsychology is not psychology. In M. M. Gill & P. S. Holzman (Eds.), *Psychology versus Metapsychology: Essays in Memory of George S. Klein.* New York: International Universities Press.

Gluckman, P. D., Hanson, M. A., Bateson, P., Beedle, A. S., Law, C. M., Bhutta, Z. A., et al. (2009). Towards a new developmental synthesis: adaptive developmental plasticity and human disease. *Lancet, 373*, 1654–1657.

Grant, J., & Sandell, R. (2004). Close family or mere neighbors?: Some empirical data on the differences between psychoanalysis and psychotherapy. In P. Richardson, H. Kächele, & C. Renlund (Eds.), *Research on psychoanalytic psychotherapy with adults* (pp. 81–108). London: Karnac Books.

Haltigan, J. D., Roisman, G. I., & Fraley, R. C. (2013). The predictive significance of early caregiving experiences for symptoms of psychopathology through midadolescence: enduring or transient effects? *Development and Psychopathology, 25*, 209–221.

Hawley, L. L., Ho, M.-H. R., Zuroff, D. C., & Blatt, S. J. (2006). The relationship of perfectionism, depression, and therapeutic alliance during treatment for depression: Latent difference score analysis. *Journal of Consulting and Clinical Psychology, 74*, 930–942.

Henton, I., & Midgley, N. (2012). "A path in the woods": Child psychotherapists' participation in a large randomised controlled trial. *Counselling and Psychotherapy Research, 12*, 204–213.

Høglend, P., Amlo, S., Marble, A., Bogwald, K. P., Sorbye, O., Sjaastad, M. C., et al. (2006). Analysis of the patient–therapist relationship in dynamic psychotherapy: An experimental study of transference interpretations. *American Journal of Psychiatry, 163*, 1739–1746.

Kächele, H. (2010). Distinguishing psychoanalysis from psychotherapy. *International Journal of Psychoanalysis, 91,* 35–43.

Kächele, H., Schachter, J., & Thomä, H. (2009). *From psychoanalytic narrative to empirical single case research. Implications for psychoanalytic practice.* New York: Routledge.

Kahl, K. G., Winter, L., & Schweiger, U. (2012). The third wave of cognitive behavioural therapies: What is new and what is effective? *Current Opinion in Psychiatry, 25,* 522–528.

Kazdin, A. E. (2007). Mediators and mechanisms of change in psychotherapy research. *Annual Review of Clinical Psychology, 3,* 1–27.

Kazdin, A. E. (2011). Evidence-based treatment research: Advances, limitations, and next steps. *American Psychologist, 66,* 685–698.

Kendler, K. S. (1997). Social support: a genetic-epidemiologic analysis. *American Journal of Psychiatry, 154,* 1398–1404.

Kendler, K. S. (2013). What psychiatric genetics has taught us about the nature of psychiatric illness and what is left to learn. *Molecular Psychiatry, 18,* 1058–1066.

Kernberg, O. F. (2000). A concerned critique of psychoanalytic education. *International Journal of Psychoanalysis, 81,* 97–120.

Kernberg, O. F. (2012). Suicide prevention for psychoanalytic institutes and societies. *Journal of the American Psychoanalytic Association, 60,* 707–719.

Kernberg, O. F., & Caligor, E. (2005). A psychoanalytic theory of personality disorders. In M. F. Lenzenweger & J. F. Clarkin (Eds.), *Major theories of personality disorder* (2nd ed., pp. 114–156). New York: Guilford Press.

Klahr, A. M., & Burt, S. A. (2013). Elucidating the etiology of individual differences in parenting: A meta-analysis of behavioral genetic research. *Psychological Bulletin, 140,* 544–586.

Krueger, R. F., Skodol, A. E., Livesley, W. J., Shrout, P. E., & Huang, Y. (2007). Synthesizing dimensional and categorical approaches to personality disorders: Refining the research agenda for DSM-V Axis II. *International Journal of Methods in Psychiatric Research, 16* (Suppl. 1), S65–S73.

Lahey, B. B., Rathouz, P. J., Van Hulle, C., Urbano, R. C., Krueger, R. F., Applegate, B., et al. (2008). Testing structural models of DSM-IV symptoms of common forms of child and adolescent psychopathology. *Journal of Abnormal Child Psychology, 36,* 187–206.

Lambert, M. (2013). The efficacy and effectiveness of psychotherapy. In M. Lambert (Ed.), *Bergin and Garfield's handbook of psychotherapy and behavior change* (6th ed., pp. 169–218). Hoboken, NJ: Wiley.

Lambert, M. J., & Barley, D. E. (2002). Research summary on the therapeutic relationship and psychotherapy outcome. In J. C. Norcross (Ed.), *Psychotherapy relationships that work* (pp. 17–32). Oxford, UK: Oxford University Press.

Lemma, A., Target, M., & Fonagy, P. (2011). *Brief dynamic interpersonal therapy. A clinician's guide.* Oxford, UK: Oxford University Press.

Luborsky, L. (1984). *Principles of psychoanalytic psychotherapy: A manual for supportive-expressive (SE) treatment.* New York: Basic Books.

Luborsky, L., Rosenthal, R., Diguer, L., Andrusyna, T. P., Berman, J. S., Levitt, J. T., et al. (2002). The Dodo bird verdict is alive and well—mostly. *Clinical Psychology: Science and Practice, 9,* 2–12.

Luyten, P. (2015). Unholy questions about five central tenets of psychoanalysis that need to be empirically verified. *Psychoanalytic Inquiry, 35,* 5–23.

Luyten, P., & Blatt, S. J. (2011). Integrating theory-driven and empirically-derived models of personality development and psychopathology: A proposal for DSM-V. *Clinical Psychology Review, 31,* 52–68.

Luyten, P., & Blatt, S. J. (2013). Relatedness and self-definition in normal and disrupted personality development: Retrospect and prospect. *American Psychologist, 68,* 172–183.

Luyten, P., Blatt, S. J., & Corveleyn, J. (2006). Minding the gap between positivism and hermeneutics in psychoanalytic research. *Journal of the American Psychoanalytic Association, 54,* 571–610.

Luyten, P., Blatt, S. J., & Mayes, L. C. (2012). Process and outcome in psychoanalytic psycho-therapy research: The need for a (relatively) new paradigm. In R. A. Levy, J. S. Ablon, & H. Kächele (Eds.), *Handbook of evidence-based psychodynamic psychotherapy: Bridging the gap between science and practice* (2nd ed.). New York: Humana Press/Springer.

Luyten, P., Mayes, L. C., Target, M., & Fonagy, P. (2012). Developmental research. In G. O. Gab-bard, B. Litowitz, & P. Williams (Eds.), *Textbook of psychoanalysis* (2nd ed., pp. 423–442). Washington, DC: American Psychiatric Press.

Luyten, P., Vliegen, N., Van Houdenhove, B., & Blatt, S. J. (2008). Equifinality, multifinality, and the rediscovery of the importance of early experiences: Pathways from early adversity to psychiatric and (functional) somatic disorders. *Psychoanalytic Study of the Child, 63,* 27–60.

Malan, D. H. (1963). *A study of brief psychotherapy.* New York: Plenum Press.

Marceau, K., Horwitz, B. N., Narusyte, J., Ganiban, J. M., Spotts, E. L., Reiss, D., et al. (2013). Gene–environment correlation underlying the association between parental negativity and adolescent externalizing problems. *Child Development, 84,* 2031–2046.

McWilliams, N. (2011). *Psychoanalytic diagnosis: Understanding personality structure in the clinical process* (2nd ed.). New York: Guilford Press.

Miller, S., Wampold, B., & Varhely, K. (2008). Direct comparisons of treatment modalities for youth disorders: a meta-analysis. *Psychotherapy Research, 18,* 5–14.

Panksepp, J. (1998). *Affective neuroscience: The foundations of human and animal emotions.* Oxford, UK: Oxford University Press.

PDM Task Force. (2006). *Psychodynamic Diagnostic Manual.* Silver Spring, MD: Alliance of Psychoanalytic Organizations.

Plomin, R., & Davis, O. S. (2009). The future of genetics in psychology and psychiatry: Micro-arrays, genome-wide association, and non-coding RNA. *Journal of Child Psychology and Psychiatry, 50,* 63–71.

Plomin, R., DeFries, J. C., Knopik, V. S., & Neiderhiser, J. M. (2013). *Behavioral genetics* (6th ed.). New York: Worth.

Rapaport, D., & Gill, M. M. (1959). The points of view and assumptions of metapsychology. *International Journal of Psycho-Analysis, 40,* 153–162.

Rutter, M. (2009). Understanding and testing risk mechanisms for mental disorders. *Journal of Child Psychology and Psychiatry and Allied Disciplines, 50,* 44–52.

Safran, J. D., Muran, J. C., & Eubanks-Carter, C. (2011). Repairing alliance ruptures. *Psycho-therapy, 48,* 80–87.

Shahar, G. (2010). Poetics, pragmatics, schematics, and the psychoanalysis-research dialogue. *Psy-choanalytic Psychotherapy, 24,* 315–328.

Shedler, J., & Westen, D. (2010). The Shedler–Westen Assessment Procedure: Making personality diagnosis clinically meaningful. In J. F. Clarkin, P. Fonagy, & G. O. Gabbard (Eds.), *Psy-chodynamic psychotherapy for personality disorders. A clinical handbook* (pp. 125–161). Washington, DC: American Psychiatric Publishing.

Sifneos, P. E. (1979). *Short-term dynamic psychotherapy: Evaluation and technique.* New York: Plenum Press.

Skodol, A. E., Bender, D. S., Morley, L. C., Clark, L. A., Oldham, J. M., Alarcon, R. D., et al. (2011). Personality disorder types proposed for DSM-5. *Journal of Personality Disorders, 25,* 136–169.

Spitzer, R. L., First, M. B., Shedler, J., Westen, D., & Skodol, A. E. (2008). Clinical utility of five dimensional systems for personality diagnosis: A "consumer preference" study. *Journal of Nervous and Mental Disease, 196,* 356–374.

Target, M., & Fonagy, P. (1994). The efficacy of psychoanalysis for children: Prediction of out-come in a developmental context. *Journal of the American Academy of Child and Adolescent Psychiatry, 33,* 1134–1144.

Taubner, S., Buchheim, A., Rudyk, R., Kachele, H., & Bruns, G. (2012). How does neurobio-logical research influence psychoanalytic treatments?—Clinical observations and reflections from a study on the interface of clinical psychoanalysis and neuroscience. *American Journal of Psychoanalysis, 72,* 269–286.

Wallerstein, R. S. (2009). What kind of research in psychoanalytic science? *International Journal of Psychoanalysis, 90,* 109–133.

Wampold, B. E., Minami, T., Baskin, T. W., & Callen Tierney, S. (2002). A meta-(re)analysis of the effects of cognitive therapy versus "other therapies" for depression. *Journal of Affective Disorders, 68,* 159–165.

Watson, D., Clark, L. A., & Chmielewski, M. (2008). Structures of personality and their relevance to psychopathology II. Further articulation of a comprehensive unified trait structure. *Journal of Personality, 76,* 1485–1522.

Way, B. M., & Lieberman, M. D. (2010). Is there a genetic contribution to cultural differences?: Collectivism, individualism and genetic markers of social sensitivity. *Social Cognitive and Affective Neuroscience, 5,* 203–211.

Weisz, J. R., Chorpita, B. F., Palinkas, L. A., Schoenwald, S. K., Miranda, J., Bearman, S. K., et al. (2012). Testing standard and modular designs for psychotherapy treating depression, anxiety, and conduct problems in youth: A randomized effectiveness trial. *Archives of General Psychiatry, 69,* 274–282.

Westen, D., Shedler, J., & Bradley, R. (2006). A prototype approach to personality disorder diagnosis. *American Journal of Psychiatry, 163,* 846–856.

Wilamowska, Z. A., Thompson-Hollands, J., Fairholme, C. P., Ellard, K. K., Farchione, T. J., & Barlow, D. H. (2010). Conceptual background, development, and preliminary data from the unified protocol for transdiagnostic treatment of emotional disorders. *Depression and Anxiety, 27,* 882–890.

Zuroff, D. C., Kelly, A. C., Leybman, M. J., Blatt, S. J., & Wampold, B. E. (2010). Between-therapist and within-therapist differences in the quality of the therapeutic relationship: Effects on maladjustment and self-critical perfectionism. *Journal of Clinical Psychology, 66,* 681–697.

Author Index

Subject Index